AF479203

HUMAN BLOOD COAGULATION

HAEMOSTASIS AND THROMBOSIS

Human Blood Coagulation, Haemostasis and Thrombosis

EDITED BY

ROSEMARY BIGGS

BSc, PhD, MD, FRCP, MA

*Formerly, Director, Oxford Haemophilia Centre
and Lecturer in Haematology,
University of Oxford
Fellow of Linacre College, Oxford*

AND

C. R. RIZZA

MD, FRCPE

*Director, Oxford Haemophilia Centre,
Clinical Lecturer in Haematology
University of Oxford*

THIRD EDITION

BLACKWELL SCIENTIFIC PUBLICATIONS

OXFORD LONDON EDINBURGH

BOSTON PALO ALTO MELBOURNE

© 1972, 1976, 1984 by
Blackwell Scientific Publications
Editorial offices:
Osney Mead, Oxford, OX2 0EL
8 John Street, London, WC1N 2ES
9 Forrest Road, Edinburgh, EH1 2QH
52 Beacon Street, Boston
Massachusetts 02108, USA
706 Cowper Street, Palo Alto
  California 94301, USA
99 Barry Street, Carlton
Victoria 3053, Australia

First published 1972
Second edition 1976
Third edition 1984

Set and printed at
Alden Press, Oxford
Bound by Standard Bookbinding Co Ltd
Standard Road, London NW10

DISTRIBUTORS

USA
  Blackwell Mosby Book Distributors
  11830 Westline Industrial Drive
  St Louis, Missouri 63141
Canada
  Blackwell Mosby Book Distributors
  120 Melford Drive, Scarborough
  Ontario, M1B 2X4
Australia
  Blackwell Scientific Book Distributors
  31 Advantage Road, Highett
  Victoria 3190

British Library
Cataloguing in Publication Data

Human blood coagulation, haemostasis
  and thrombosis.—3rd ed.
  1. Blood—Coagulation, Disorders of
  I. Biggs, Rosemary   II. Rizza, C.R.
  616.1'57   RC647.C55

ISBN 0-632-00838-5

Preface to
Third Edition

Six years have passed since the publication of the second edition of *Human Blood Coagulation, Haemostasis and Thrombosis*. During that time there have been important advances in many aspects of blood coagulation and haemostasis. This has required complete re-writing of many of the chapters for this edition as well as the addition of several new chapters. As with the previous editions, the aim of the book is to review well established facts and theories on the subject and in the more clinically orientated chapters, to give advice and information which would be of value to a practising clinician. Unlike the second edition, this edition does not contain appendices giving detailed descriptions of laboratory reagents and methods. This subject would require a book to itself and indeed there are now several publications available which deal solely with this aspect of the field.

We are grateful to the contributors for their hard work in helping us to produce this book and we hope that the readers will find it stimulating, interesting and instructive.

Preface to
First Edition

Three editions of *Human Blood Coagulation and Its Disorders*, written by myself and Professor R.G.Macfarlane, appeared in 1953, 1957 and 1962 respectively. These editions represented our personal experience in research on blood coagulation and our local experience in treating patients, together with our own selection from the steadily growing literature on haemostasis and thrombosis. By 1969 the literature had expanded massively and we no longer felt capable to write from our own knowledge about the whole field. We thus decided that the time had come to replace the original book by a volume contributed to by many experts. Since Professor Macfarlane has retired, the task of editing has fallen to me.

The present volume has attempted to cover much the same subject matter as the original volume and some of the material from the last edition of *Human Blood Coagulation and Its Disorders* has been retained. Since the sections have been written by different people there is necessarily some overlap of material from one chapter to another. There is also variation in emphasis and opinion in the different chapters. There are, naturally, also differences in the way various authors have approached their subjects. Some may hold the view that it is an editor's job to eliminate these differences to produce a uniform point of view, a standard length of chapter and a limitation on the number of references quoted. I have not taken this view. All of those contributing to the book are acknowledged experts in their own subjects and, with very minor alterations, I have accepted their contributions as written. I should like to acknowledge my personal indebtedness to all of them for the considerable effort that they have made and to say that I think they have written an authoritative and most interesting book and I hope that our readers will find it as useful as I do.

The Technical Appendix contains many standard methods included in *Human Blood Coagulation and Its Disorders* and some additional methods provided by contributors to the book.

April 1972   Rosemary Biggs

Contributors

D. E. G. AUSTEN, BSc, PhD, C Chem, FRSC *Principal Scientific Officer, Oxford Haemophilia Centre, Churchill Hospital, Oxford*

TREVOR W. BARROWCLIFFE, *Division of Blood Products, National Institute for Biological Standards and Control, Holly Hill, Hampstead, London, NW3 6RB*

R. F. BAUGH, BS, MS, PhD *Director of Research and Development for Hemotec, Inc, formerly Assistant Research Biochemist, University of California, San Diego, School of Medicine, Department of Pathology M-012, La Jolla, California 92093, USA*

BRUCE BENNETT, MB,ChB, MD, MRCP, FRCP, MRCPath *Reader in Medicine, University of Aberdeen, Aberdeen Royal Infirmary, Foresterhill, Aberdeen, AB9 2ZB*

ROSEMARY BIGGS, BSc, PhD, MD, FRCP, MA *Formerly, Director, Oxford Haemophilia Centre, Churchill Hospital, Oxford; University Lecturer in Haematology, Oxford University*

G. V. R. BORN, MA, MB, CHB, DPhil, FRS *Professor of Pharmacology, King's College, University of London, Strand, London, WC2 2LS*

A. S. DOUGLAS, BSc, MD, FRCP (Lond, Ed, & Glas), FRCPath *Regius Professor of Medicine, University of Aberdeen; Honorary Consultant Physician, Aberdeen Royal Infirmary and Woodend Hospital*

M. P. ESNOUF, MA, BSc, DPhil *Department of Clinical Biochemistry, University of Oxford, Radcliffe Infirmary, Oxford*

R. M. HARDISTY, MD, FRCP, FRCPath *Professor of Haematology, Institute of Child Health, London University, Honorary Consultant in Haematology, Hospital for Sick Children, Great Ormond Street, London*

S. HEPTINSTALL, BSc, PhD *Lecturer, Department of Medicine, University Hospital, Queen's Medical Centre, Nottingham, NG7 2UH*

CECIL HOUGIE, MD *Professor of Pathology, University of California, San Diego, School of Medicine, Department of Pathology, M-012, La Jolla, California 92093, USA*

LEON W. HOYER, MD *Professor of Medicine, Head, Hematology Division, University of Connecticut Health Center, Farmington, Connecticut 06032, USA*

T. B. L. KIRKWOOD, MA, MSc, PhD Member of Scientific Staff, Computing Laboratory, National Institute for Medical Research, The Ridgeway, Mill Hill, London NW7 1AA

J. M. MATTHEWS, MB, ChB *Associate Specialist, Oxford Haemophilia Centre, Churchill Hospital, Oxford*

J. R. A. MITCHELL, MD, BSc, MA, DPhil, FRCP *Professor of Medicine, University Hospital, Queen's Medical Centre, Nottingham*

DEREK OGSTON, DSc, PhD, MD, FRCP *Professor of Medicine, Aberdeen Royal Infirmary, Foresterhill, Aberdeen AB9 2ZB*

C. R. RIZZA, MD, FRCPE *Director, Oxford Haemophilia Centre, Churchill Hospital, Oxford; Clinical Lecturer in Haematology, University of Oxford*

I. L. RHYMES, FIMLS *Chief Medical Laboratory Scientific Officer, Oxford Haemophilia Centre, Churchill Hospital, Oxford*

J. K. SMITH, BSc, PhD, FRSC *Chief Project Scientist, Blood Products Laboratory, Plasma Fractionation Laboratory, Churchill Hospital, Oxford*

T. J. SNAPE, BA, PhD *Head of Quality Control, Blood Products Laboratory, Elstree, Herts*

Contents

Chapter 1
Early Stages of Blood Coagulation and the Intrinsic Activation of Prothrombin

C. HOUGIE *and* R. F. BAUGH

Introduction

The intrinsic coagulation system may be considered to consist of those components which are involved in activating factor X to Xa via the factor VIII:factor IX:phospholipid:Ca^{2+} complex. Factor X is the focal point at which the intrinsic and extrinsic coagulation systems converge, and although over the past several years it has become increasingly evident that the concept of two separate systems for blood coagulation is no longer valid, from a diagnostic and didactic viewpoint the concept remains useful. Our understanding of *in vivo* intrinsic blood coagulation remains far from complete. Two central questions which remain unanswered are (1) how is intrinsic coagulation initiated and, (2) what is the nature and function of factor VIII, the antihaemophilic factor? Until these questions are resolved, considerable controversy will exist concerning the mechanism of intrinsic coagulation.

Intrinsic coagulation can be conveniently divided into three stages: contact activation, factor IX activation, and the formation of the factor VIII:factor IX:phospholipid:Ca^{2+} complex which activates factor X (Table 1). Most of our knowledge concerning each of these stages has been gathered from *in vitro* studies. Extrapolation of concepts developed in this manner to the *in vivo* situation may be misleading. The number of variables involved *in vivo* cannot yet be reproduced and independently analysed in a controlled manner in an *in vitro* setting. A review of the literature shows that a variety of other systems or components has been postulated to interact with intrinsic coagulation. These include platelets, vessel walls, various types of leucocytes, components of the immune, kinin, complement, and fibrinolytic systems. Rarely accounted for in coagulation studies is the fluid dynamics of the vascular system. Many of these interacting components do so with the contact phase of intrinsic coagulation; and prekallikrein, factor XII, and high molecular weight kininogen are components of both the kinin and fibrinolytic systems. The multi-faceted role of the contact factors suggests that *in vivo* the initiation of intrinsic coagulation is linked to a variety of physiologic responses which affect the coagulation process *in vivo* but are not evident in test-tube coagulation.

Another point to be considered when examining the human intrinsic clotting system is that much of our knowledge has been gathered in studies on

Table 1. Clotting factors of intrinsic coagulation.

Factor	Common name	Molecular weight	Concentration in $\simeq 1$ ml plasma
Factor XII	Hageman factor	76 000	40 μg
Prekallikrein	—	85 000–88 000	25–40 μg
High molecular weight kininogen	HMWK	120 000	80 μg
Factor XI	Plasma thromboplastin antecedent	124 000	4–7 μg
Factor IX	Christmas factor	55 000	3–4 μg
Factor VIII	Antihaemophilic factor	Unknown	0.2 μg

clotting factors derived from non-human sources. The existence of the clotting factors has usually been recognized first from clinical studies of human plasmas which did not clot adequately in standard *in vitro* clotting tests. Generally, enough information was gained from these studies to identify the clotting factor in a non-human plasma from which the factor was subsequently purified. Once the non-human clotting factor was characterized, the clotting factor was then isolated from human plasma. There are several good reasons for this approach. The identification of the factor is initially most easily accomplished by noting clinical symptoms in humans and using mixing experiments of various deficient plasmas to establish the identity of a new factor. However, obtaining enough human plasma for isolation of the factor, when none of its physical or chemical properties are known, is an expensive undertaking. The demand for human plasma in therapeutic treatments is such that large volumes of human plasma are not generally available for experimental uses, a prerequisite when developing purification procedures. Clotting factors are notoriously susceptible to proteolysis and specific proteolytic inhibitors cannot be added to human plasma intended for therapeutic use; accordingly, outdated human plasma is not generally suitable for the initial fractionation of a new clotting factor. For these reasons, it was more feasible to obtain and characterize the clotting factor from non-human sources. Once the physical and chemical properties were known, the human clotting factor could be isolated without inordinate waste being incurred in developing a purification procedure. Although there has been general agreement between the results obtained from non-human and human sources, enough differences exist to suggest that extrapolation of non-human clotting factor studies to human coagulation may be misleading. This has been evident with studies on bovine and human high molecular weight kininogen as detailed below. This approach has generally resulted in a lag period of several years between the discovery of a clotting factor in humans and its eventual characterization. The first physical and chemical data available are usually from a non-human factor and are not necessarily representative of the human factor.

Contact phase of intrinsic coagulation

With the exception perhaps of factor VIII, less is known of the contact phase of blood coagulation than any other area of clotting. The term 'contact phase' is a deceptive one because it refers to a test-tube phenomenon not easily translated into physiologic terms. When freshly collected plasma is exposed to a negatively charged surface, several clotting factors are activated, i.e. converted from the zymogen to the active protease. These factors are factor XII, prekallikrein, and factor XI. Thus simple contact with a surface leads to apparent proteolytic activity, so-called 'contact activation'. Contact activation can be demonstrated with a number of different substances such as various glasses, kaolin and ellagic acid, which are clearly not physiological. Four clotting factors are involved in the contact phase of clotting, three enzymes and one cofactor. The enzymes, factor XIIa, factor XIa and kallikrein exist in plasma as zymogens, that is, inactive precursors of the enzymes. Once activated, each is a protease with limited specificity, the protease cleaving only certain specific peptide bonds in a limited number of substrates. This is in contrast to a broad range protease which shows little substrate specificity. High molecular weight kininogen is both a substrate for kallikrein and a cofactor in the activation of factor XII, prekallikrein and factor XI. The conversion of factor XII and prekallikrein to the active proteases is believed to occur in a reciprocal cyclic manner, which is a difficult concept to grasp. Factor XIIa, in the presence of high molecular weight kininogen, activates prekallikrein to kallikrein. Conversely, kallikrein, in the presence of high molecular weight kininogen, converts XII to XIIa. Both of these activations occur via mechanisms similar to the activation of most serine class proteases, i.e. by the cleavage of the specific, limited number of peptide bonds in the zymogen which leads to the unmasking of the proteolytic activity. The principal problem is how to account for these observations by a simplified sequence of events which will explain 'contact activation'.

For several years it seemed that the answer to this dilemma might reside in the molecular structure of factor XII. It had been shown that factor XII was the component required for contact activation and it was the only zymogen capable of independent binding to a surface. With current knowledge of protein and enzyme structure it was easy to postulate that when factor XII is bound to a surface, the resulting conformational change unmasked the proteolytic site and intrinsic coagulation was initiated. The modified factor XII then activated prekallikrein to kallikrein which in turn converted factor XII to XIIa. The reciprocal activation occurring between factor XII and prekallikrein ensured the amplification of the initial response (Ratnoff and Saito 1979). The problem was to demonstrate that surface-bound factor XII had proteolytic activity which could activate either prekallikrein, factor XI or additional factor XII. This has not been easy to verify; highly purified reagents were required and results would be negated by the presence of even minute traces of either XIIa or kallikrein. In a large number of such studies the results were inconclusive, and no evidence could be found for the production of a contact-activated factor XII. This has led to the postulation of several less attractive mechanisms. There were studies indicating that factor XII underwent a conformation change when bound to a surface and that, although the bound factor XII showed no increased proteolytic activity, it was a much better substrate for kallikrein activation than was fluid phase factor XII. It has thus been suggested that (1) there exist as yet unidentified factors necessary for contact activation or, (2) a low level of proteolytic activity is present in the zymogen forms of prekallikrein and other clotting factors which can activate the bound factor XII to factor XIIa (Griffin and Beretta 1979) or, (3) low levels of proteases (possibly activated clotting factors) are always present in plasma, and the binding of factor XII to a surface makes factor XII susceptible to activation by them (Kaplan 1978).

An area which has received little attention concerns the interaction of the contact phase with platelets. Some intriguing observations have been made which suggest platelets may interact with the contact phase of coagulation but little effort has been spent on delineating these interactions. Platelets are known to interact with several coagulation factors, i.e. thrombin, factor V and factor X, and interactions have been reported involving factor VIII and IX (see Baugh and Hougie 1981). Two links occurring between platelets and clotting factors involved in contact activation have been suggested. A platelet-derived activator of factor XI has been described, suggesting a possible relationship between factor XI and platelet function (Walsh 1972). An observation made on several von Willebrand's patients suggests another relationship (Cramer *et al.* 1976). In approximately 1 in 5 of these patients, compared to approximately 1 in 15 of normal patients, the factor XII level is significantly lower than factor XII levels of normal controls. Von Willebrand's patients have a plasma protein defect resulting in diminished platelet adherence at the site of vascular lesions. Thus, in a disorder characterized by defective platelet function, there is often a lowered level of one of the contact factors. However, the link is tenuous at least and the relationship unknown.

Factor XII

Factor XII, or Hageman factor, appears to be the key enzyme of the contact phase of intrinsic blood coagulation (Colman and Wong 1977). The activated zymogen is a serine protease which is inhibited by diisopropyl fluorophosphate (DFP), an active site inhibitor of serine proteases (Kurachi and Davie 1977, Meier *et al.* 1977, Revak, Cochrane and Griffin 1977). Human factor XII circulates as a single polypeptide chain of a molecular weight of *c.* 80 000. The molecule has internal disulphide bonds which appear to be important in the activation of the molecule. A variety of plasma proteases have been shown to convert factor XII to factor XIIa, but when considering rates of activation, kallikrein appears to be the most potent. Activation can lead to two different forms of factor XII depending on whether the initial cleavage takes place inside or outside the internal disulphide loop (Fig. 1) (Revak, Cochrane and Griffin 1977, Revak *et al.* 1978). The two forms differ in both physical properties and enzymatic activities and Griffin and Beretta (1979) have suggested that the two forms be designated α-factor XIIa and β-factor XIIa, according to whether the cleavage occurs within or outside the disulphide loop. Kallikrein activates surface-bound factor XII by cleaving a peptide bond inside the disulphide loop to produce the two-chain, disulphide-linked enzyme, α-factor XIIa (mol.wt = 76 000) with a light chain with a mol.wt of 28 000 and a heavy chain of 52 000 daltons. It is this form of factor XII which is most active in converting factor XI to factor XIa. Cleavage by kallikrein can also occur just outside the disulphide loop, producing a 52 000 mol.wt proteolytically inactive fragment which contains the surface-binding sites of factor XII and the 28 000 mol.wt, β-factor XIIa. β-factor XIIa is a poor activator of factor XI, but is still capable of a significant rate of activation of prekallikrein. α-Factor

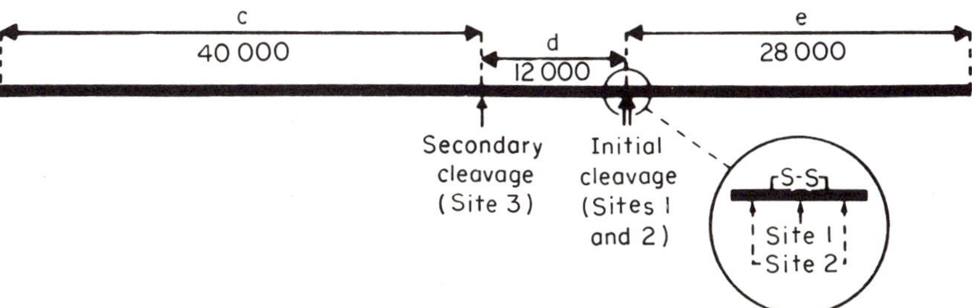

Fig. 1. Cleavage patterns for the activation of factor XII. Sites 1 and 2 involve cleavage in the vicinity of the disulphide loop. Cleavage at site 1 produces a two chain disulphide linked α factor XIIa, while cleavage at site 2 gives a single chain β factor XIIa of reduced molecular weight. Cleavage at site 3 occurs only after prolonged incubation with kallikrein. (Reprinted with permission from Revak, Cochrane and Griffin (1977) and the *Journal of Clinical Investigation*.)

XIIa is the surface-bound form of factor XIIa while β-factor XIIa has lost its surface-binding properties and is found in the fluid phase.

One question concerning factor XII is whether it is capable of autoactivation. Can either form of factor XIIa activate factor XII? Conflicting data exists concerning this point and no direct evidence has been produced which supports the autoactivation of factor XII. Using a spectrophotometric assay with a synthetic colorimetric substrate for kallikrein in a factor XII-linked assay system, Silverberg *et al.* (1980) suggested the kinetics of colour formation of the hydrolysed substrate supported the autoactivation of factor XII. The formation of XIIa was not followed and due to the extreme susceptibility of factor XII to activation by other proteases, the presence of contaminating proteases could not be totally excluded. The direct demonstration of the activation of factor XII by factor XIIa has not been achieved and serious questions remain as to whether factor XII is capable of autoactivation.

The initial event which results in the formation of XIIa still remains uncertain. As stated earlier, the most attractive hypothesis for XII activation was the conformational unmasking of the factor XII proteolytic site following binding to a negatively charged surface. The conformational change was apparent upon binding; kaolin-bound factor XII was shown to be much more susceptible to activation by a variety of proteases including factor XIa, kallikrein, plasmin, trypsin and chymotrypsin, and McMillan *et al.* (1974) had shown a conformational change did occur in factor XII structure by following the circular dichoism spectrum in the presence of activating agents. The formation of an active site following binding has not been demonstrated. The unmasking of the proteolytic site was measured by following the rate of incorporation of isotopically labelled DFP. Bound factor XII incorporated DFP at a rate the same as unbound factor XII; thus it did not appear that the active site was exposed by the conformational change (Griffin and Beretta 1979). The zymogens of many serine proteases incorporate DFP at a measurable rate varying from $1/600$ to more than $1/1000$ of the rate of the activated protease. Factor XII displayed such behaviour and it has been suggested that this limited proteolytic activity, which is also present in the zymogen prekallikrein, could be enough to explain the activation of intrinsic coagulation when factor XII is surface bound. Thus, the trigger for contact activation would be the production of a significantly better substrate, bound factor XII, rather than the unmasking of a proteolytic site.

Recently, both bovine and human factor XII prepared by the research group of Dr Earl Davie have been shown to have significantly enhanced proteolytic activity following binding to a negatively charged surface without any demonstrable cleavage of the factor XII zymogen. Kurachi *et al.* (1983) used SDS disc gel electrophoresis to follow the activation of purified factor XI by both purified factor XII and factor XII[a]. These studies indicated that not only was a negatively charged surface needed for factor XII to activate factor XI, but factor XI was also required to express the proteolytic activity in factor XII. This suggested that factor XI induced an additional conformational change and that this could be a reason why no enhanced DFP incorporation into surface bound factor XII has been measured. Other noteworthy observations from these studies were that factor XIa could activate factor XII, and high molecular weight kininogen produced a two- to five-fold enhancement in the rate of factor XI activation by factor XII, which was dependent on both the concentration and type of activating agent used. Three activating agents were investigated in these studies: dextran sulphate, kaolin, and sulphatides (glycosphingolipids containing sulphur). These observations appear to partially confirm the hypothesis of the unmasking of a proteolytic site (Fig. 2), but

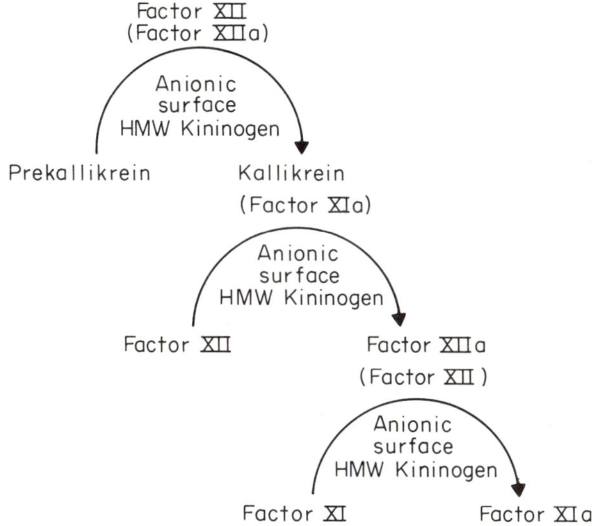

Fig. 2. A proposed mechanism for the surface activation of blood coagulation in the presence of an anionic surface (Reprinted with permission from Kurachi *et al.* (1983) and *Advances in Experimental Medicine and Biology.*)

further confirmation will be required before they can be considered on firm ground. In contrast to contact activation, enzymes (kinin-like) from cultured rabbit endothelial cell homogenates have been shown to activate rabbit factor XII in a specific manner, i.e. the enzymes do not activate prekallikrein or factor XI (Wiggins *et al.* 1980). Such an activation of factor XII would have significance *in vivo* but should have little bearing on 'contact activation' in an *in vitro* setting.

Prekallikrein

There is general agreement as to the role of prekallikrein in intrinsic blood coagulation and the function of the activated enzyme, kallikrein, is to increase the amount of factor XIIa. Prekallikrein circulates as a single-chained zymogen with a molecular weight of 85 000 or 87 000 (Mandle and Kaplan 1977, Bouma *et al.* 1980, Scott, Lui, and Colman 1979). Two forms of the zymogen, with approximately the same molecular weight, are found in plasma and both forms have been identified as prekallikreins. The plasma concentration of prekallikrein is estimated to be in the range of 25–40 μg/ml. The significant differences between the two forms of plasma prekallikrein have not been identified, but could be due to genetic differences, differences in carbohydrate content, or partial degradation. Immunologically, the forms are indistinguishable and both can be activated to form kallikrein. Kallikrein is a serine-class, limited protease and has the same molecular weight as its precursor, prekallikrein. The activation of prekallikrein by factor XIIa leads to a disulphide-linked two-chained molecule with a heavy chain of *c.* 52 000 and a light chain of 37 000 or 42 000. The variability in molecular weight seen with prekallikrein is preserved in the light chain of kallikrein. It has been reported that the active site serine of kallikrein resides in the light chain (Mandle and Kaplan 1977).

The physiological role of prekallikrein in coagulation, as with factor XII and high molecular weight kininogen, is enigmatic. The genetic absence of prekallikrein (Fletcher trait) does not lead to a haemorrhagic disorder despite the recognition of a substantial number of patients with this abnormality. Thus the data regarding the role of prekallikrein in clotting come strictly from *in vitro* analysis. Only one plasma-derived activator of prekallikrein has been described, factor XIIa. No other plasma activator has been found. Other proteases have been noted to activate prekallikrein (trypsin, urokinase) but these are not normally found in plasma. Interestingly it appears that the vascular lining may not contain proteases that activate prekallikrein, as the rabbit endothelial cell homogenate described by Wiggins *et al.* (1980) activated only factor XII. Thus, the activation of prekallikrein appears to be dependent on the activation of factor XII.

Kallikrein has several factor XII-linked functions. It is necessary for the expression of the fibrinolytic activity found in plasma (Bouma *et al.* 1980). Plasma kinin-forming activity is also dependent on the presence of kallikrein (Wuepper 1973). In both cases, kallikrein is directly involved. Kallikrein can cleave plasminogen to plasmin, and although not the most active plasminogen activator known, it is nevertheless the only plasminogen activator which has been found in plasma. The kinin-forming ability of kallikrein is the result of its ability to cleave high molecular weight kininogen (HMWK) and release the vasoactive nonapeptide, bradykinin. Bradykinin and similar kinins bring about increased vascular permeability, contraction of smooth muscle, pain and chemotactic activity in leucocytes. Each of these activities should have significant effect on the physical formation and dissolution of a blood clot and are dependent on the activation of factor XII, illustrating the coordination of several physiological processes through a single initial stimulus.

High molecular weight kininogen (HMWK)

Human plasma contains two types of kininogens which are differentiated by their molecular weights. Kininogens are substrates for kallikreins which release kinins via limited proteolysis of the kininogen. The plasma kininogens are referred to as high molecular weight kininogen (110 000–120 000) and low molecular weight kininogen (80 000) and it has been reported they share several immunological determinants (Kerbiriou, Bouma and Griffin 1980). Bradykinin, a nonapeptide, is the principal kinin released from both (Fig. 3). It is only within the last ten years that it has been realized that HMWK possessed additional physiological activity. In the clotting system, it is now recognized that HMWK is synonymous with the clotting factor which has been variously

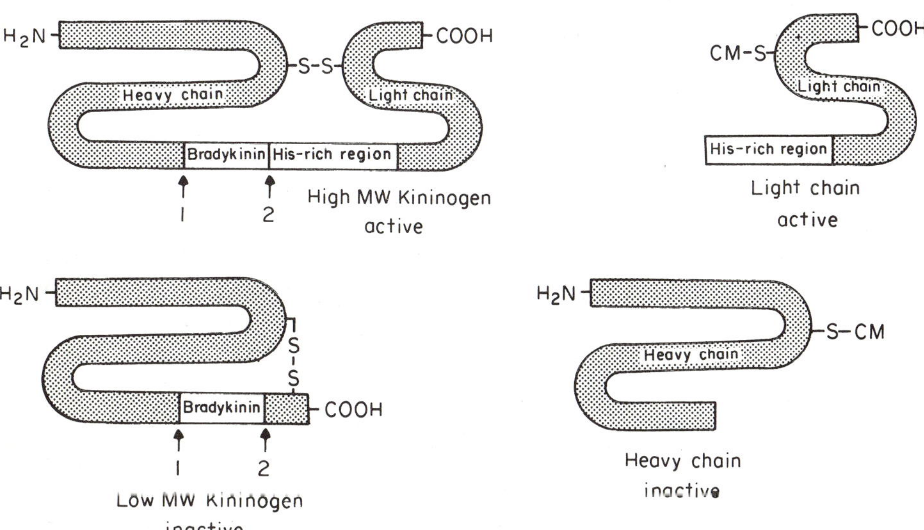

Fig. 3. Structural models for high and low molecular weight kininogens. (Reprinted with permission from Kerbiriou, Bouma and Griffin (1980) and the American Society of Biological Chemists.)

termed as contact activation cofactor, Fitzgerald factor, Williams factor, Flaujeac factor or Reid factor.

HMWK characterization is not yet complete and there appear to be some significant differences between bovine and human HMWK with respect to the action of kallikrein. Following release of the nonapeptide bradykinin, bovine HMWK (kinin-free HMWK) has little procoagulant activity (Han *et al.* 1978), while human HMWK still possesses procoagulant activity. This is attributed to the fact that bovine kallikrein releases a histidine-rich region from bovine HMWK, while human kallikrein leaves this region intact in human HMWK (Kerbiriou and Griffin 1979). This region is believed to be intimately involved in the action of HMWK in the clotting system and has led to various hypotheses concerning the function of HMWK as a procoagulant.

HMWK circulates in plasma as a single-chained polypeptide with a molecular weight of 110 000 to 120 000 daltons. Initially it was thought to circulate as a two-chained molecule, but as has been the case with several clotting factors, as purification procedures improve, it is becoming apparent that HMWK is a single-chain molecule which is easily degraded during purification. The molecule may circulate either as a dimer or complexed with either prekallikrein or factor XI (Thompson, Mandle and Kaplan 1977, Thompson, Mandle and Kaplan 1979, Kerbiriou, Bouma and Griffin 1980, Schiffman, Mannhalter and Tyner 1980). The role of HMWK in coagulation is that of a regulatory cofactor, similar to factor V and factor VIII. Kinetically HMWK accelerates the rate of conversion of factor XII to XIIa, prekallikrein to kallikrein, and factor XI to XIa. As with both factor V and factor VIII it is difficult to assess whether HMWK must first be activated before it can function as a procoagulant. There is some evidence which suggests that activation by kallikrein must occur before the procoagulant activity is expressed (Kato *et al.* 1979), but the interpretation of the experimental data supporting this conclusion is not straightforward.

The action of human kallikrein on human HMWK has been studied by a handful of investigators and, with minor variations, generally speaking the results are similar. Kerbiriou, Bouma and Griffin (1980) suggested that native HMWK, a single-chain protein of molecular weight 110 000, was cleaved to a two-chain disulphide-linked protein by an unresolved number of steps. The two-chain molecule had a molecular weight of 95 000. During this process, bradykinin was released, and in the reduced form the chains were shown to have molecular weights of 65 000 and 44 000. The light chain (44 000 mol.wt) was shown to retain the procoagulant activity. Schiffman, Mann-halter and Tyner (1980) found that HMWK initially had a molecular weight of 121 000, and proteolysis by kallikrein led to a series of intermediate products, but the final product, a two-chained kinin-free HMWK, had a molecular weight of 95 000. In this instance the chains were 65 000 and 54 000 daltons, which was significantly more than the molecular weight of the 95 000 dalton unreduced molecule. According to these investigators, the 120 000 dalton mol.wt HMWK is cleaved to a 102 000 molecular weight intermediate which has two chains of approximately the same size (65 000). This involved the removal of 19 000 mol.wt units from the protein. The second step leading to the 95 000 mol.wt HMWK involved the removal of approximately 7000 mol.wt units from one of the two 65 000 mol.wt chains, giving the final 95 000 mol.wt HMWK (a 65 000 mol.wt chain and a 54 000 mol.wt chain). The molecular weight differences noted between the chains and the intact, unreduced molecule at the intermediate and final stages of activation were assumed to arise out of artifacts of molecular weight measurements with SDS disc gel electrophoresis, a phenomenon quite common with carbohydrate-containing proteins. These studies did not elucidate at which step bradykinin was released, but it is known that a two-chain HMWK which still possesses kinin-forming activity can be isolated from kallikrein-treated HMWK. Thus, it is probable that bradykinin is not released in the conversion to the 102 000 mol.wt form. The investigators did not have any data to show that a difference existed between the two 65 000 mol.wt chains. Following the second step, however, the 54 000 mol.wt chain contained no measurable carbohydrate while the remaining 65 000 mol.wt chain still contained carbohydrate. The procoagulant activity was found in the light chain of the final product.

The function of HMWK appears to be multi-faceted. It not only provides a source of bradykinin but probably circulates complexed with almost all of the plasma factor XI and prekallikrein (approximately 90 per cent of the plasma concentration of each). Scott and Colman (1980) have suggested that HMWK may have a stabilizing effect on prekallikrein in plasma, as HMWK-deficient patients were shown to have decreased levels of prekallikrein which could be increased by administering plasma containing HMWK. The binding sites for both factor XI and prekallikrein appear to be the same, but plasma contains an excess of HMWK in comparison to both factor XI and prekallikrein, so both are nearly totally complexed. This binding site is in the light chain of cleaved HMWK. The molar ratio of binding is 1 : 1 for both factor XI and prekallikrein. It appears that a 1 : 1 molar ratio between HMWK and factor XII also exists (Kurachi *et al.* 1983). Thus, current data suggest HMWK has a surface binding region which is rich in histidine content. The region interacts with a surface near a factor XII molecule to form a complex which contains either HMWK and factor XII or HMWK and prekallikrein. The net result is to bring the reactants of the contact phase into intimate contact.

Factor XI

The recognition of factor XI (plasma thromboplastin antecedent, PTA) as a clotting component was first described by Rosenthal, Dreskin and Rosenthal (1953). In contrast to factor XII, prekallikrein and HMWK, some, although not all, patients with a deficiency of factor XI occasionally bleed excessively following surgery or injury. Factor XI is a serine protease zymogen which, when activated, has limited proteolytic activity. The observation that some factor XI-deficient patients have a bleeding problem while those deficient in factor XII, prekallikrein or HMWK do not, has suggested that factor XI may be activated via pathways independent of factor XII. It has, therefore, been suggested that platelets release a protease capable of activating factor XI following stimulation of the release reactions, but verification of this proposal has not been forthcoming (Walsh 1972). Several pathways have been described in which components of the extrinsic coagulation system can activate intrinsic system components yet none of these involve factor XI. Thus, it remains unknown why some patients with factor XI deficiency bleed, while excessive bleeding with factor XII deficiency does not occur.

Factor XI circulates at estimated concentrations of 4–7 μg/ml. Nearly all factor XI is estimated to be complexed with HMWK in plasma. The molecular weight of factor XI is 124 000 daltons and its molecular configuration is unique for a proteolytic zymogen (Fig. 4). The molecule is composed of two identical chains linked by an interchain disulphide bond (Bouma and Griffin 1977, Kurachi and Davie 1977). Each chain in the zymogen contains a potential proteolytic active site, and each chain can be activated. Factor XI has been demonstrated to be activated to factor XIa by trypsin and by factor XIIa, although it is believed that the trypsin activation has no physiological significance. The activation of factor XI involves the cleavage of each chain between an interchain disulphide loop to give factor XIa, which is composed of four chains, two light and two heavy. No evidence has been found for the presence of an activation peptide so no change in molecular weight occurs during activation. The chain molecular weights for factor XIa are 35 000 for

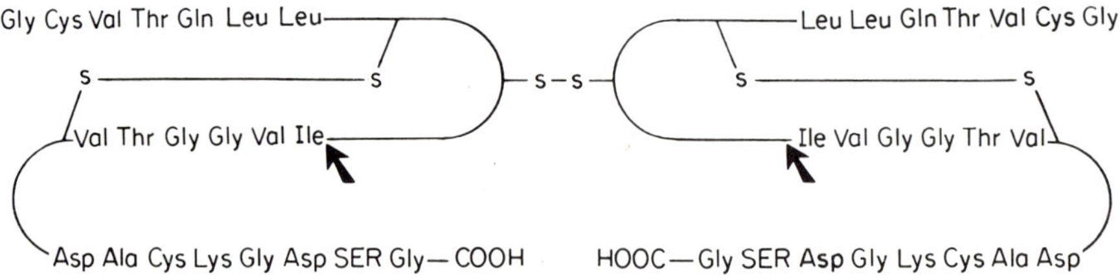

Fig. 4. Partial structure of human factor XI. The two chained zymogen structure with the connecting disulphide link is shown. The arrows indicate the cleavage points by factors XIIa. The raised letter serine indicates the two active site serines. The location and number of intrachain disulphide bonds are not known. (Reprinted with the permission of Kurachi and Davie (1977) and the American Chemical Society.)

the heavy chains and 25 000 for the light chains. The enzymatic sites reside in the light chains (Kurachi and Davie 1977).

Factor IX and factor VIII interaction

The next phase of blood coagulation involves factor IX (Christmas factor) and factor VIII. Factor IX is a vitamin K-dependent plasma glycoprotein synthesized in the liver and present in human plasma at a concentration of approximately 5 μg/ml (Østerud, Bouma and Griffin 1978). Like the other vitamin K-dependent plasma proteins, the amino-terminal region of factor IX contains 12 γ-carboxyglutamic acid residues which bind Ca^{2+} ions, these in turn linking the protein to phospholipid. The bovine molecule has been completely sequenced and has 416 amino acid residues with carbohydrate residues linked to four asparaginyl residues (Katayama *et al.* 1979). The precursor or zymogen molecule is a single chain protein with a molecular weight of approximately 56 000 daltons, while the physiologically active form (factor IXa) is a two-chain serine protease. This protease is referred to as factor IXaβ to differentiate it from the protease referred to as factor IXaα which is the result of the cleavage of factor IX by an enzyme in Russell's viper venom.

The sequence of events that occurs during the conversion of bovine factor IX to factor IXaβ by factor XIa was first determined in 1974 by the elegant studies of Fujikawa and colleagues. The first step is the cleavage of an arginine–alanine bond by factor XIa to give rise to a two-chain intermediate held together by disulphide bonds. This intermediate has no enzymatic activity. In the second step an arginine–valine bond is cleaved, giving rise to an activation peptide and the active enzyme IXaβ (Fig. 5). As a result of these reactions, the molecular weight of the precursor is reduced from 56 000 to 46 000 daltons. The cleavage of human factor IX is similar (Fig. 6) but the first cleavage can occur at either the arginine–alanine or arginine–valine bonds (Di Scipio, Kurachi and Davie 1978, Østerud, Bouma and Griffin 1978).

These molecular events were elucidated in large part using the technique of sodium dodecyl sulphate-polyacrylamide gel electrophoresis (SDS PAGE) in

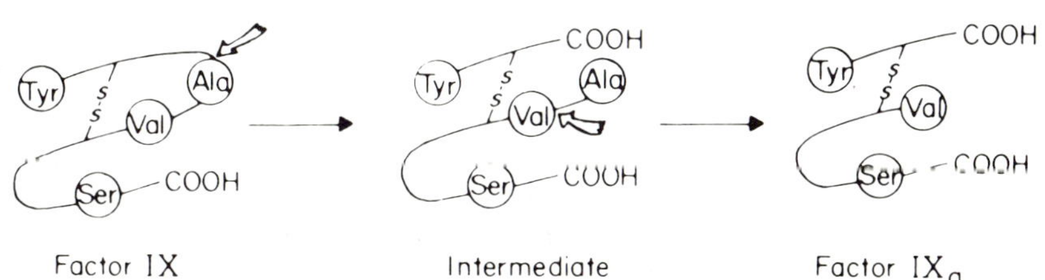

Fig. 5. Activation of bovine factor IX. (Reprinted with permission from Fujikawa *et al* (1974b) and the American Chemical Society.)

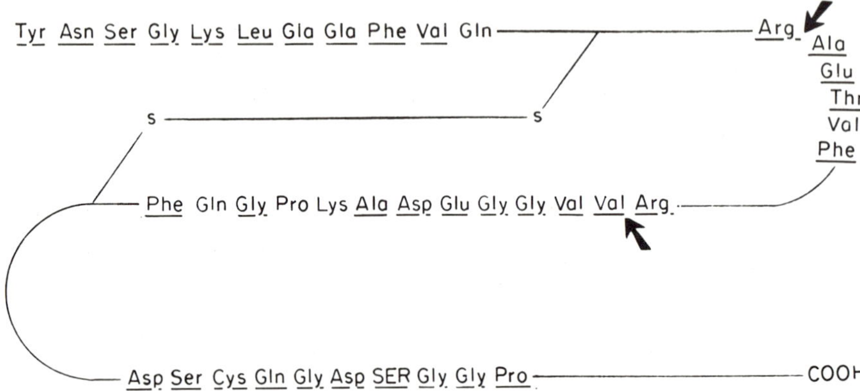

Fig. 6. Cleavage of human IX to IXᵃ. The two arrows indicate the sites of cleavage by XIᵃ. In the bovine species, the first cleavage is at the arginyl-alanine bond, while in the case of the human molecule the first cleavage may occur at either site. (Reprinted with permission from Di Scipio, Kurachi and Davie (1978) and the *Journal of Clinical Investigation.*)

which migration of proteins through a gel matrix is governed principally by size rather than charge. If a reducing agent such as β mercaptoethanol as well as SDS is included in the gel to reduce interchain disulphide bonds, the released disulphide-linked polypeptide sub-units can be visualized on the gel after staining, and their number and molecular size deduced. Since it is a single chain molecule, the factor IX zymogen gives a single band whether reduced or unreduced while factor IXa (a two-chain molecule) gives a single band in the unreduced gel and two bands following reduction (Fig. 7a,b). In both the studies of Fujikawa *et al.* (1974b) on bovine factor IX and Di Scipio *et al.* (1978) on human factor IX, the course of the reaction was followed by incubating amounts of factor XIa, too small to give a visible band on the gel, with highly purified factor IX and Ca^{2+} and analysing subsamples at intervals. During the

---

Figs 7a and b.
(a) SDS polyacrylamide gel electrophoresis of factor IX following activation with factor XIᵃ. Each gel is a 2.5 μl sample containing 12.5 μg of protein removed from the reaction mixture at the indicated time and then incubated at 37° for 4 h with 2 per cent SDS in the absence of reducing agent before electrophoresis. The gel pattern at the far right is a control sample of factor IXᵃ.
(b) SDS polyacrylamide gel electrophoresis of factor IX activation with factor XIa after reduction of the reactants. Samples and conditions identical to (a) except the protein was incubated with 2 per cent SDS and 5 per cent 2-mercaptoethanol before electrophoresis. H_{Ala} and H_{Val} refer to NH_2-terminal amino acids. (Reprinted with permission from Fujikawa *et al.* (1974b) and the American Chemical Society.)

FACTOR IX
FACTOR IX$_A$
TIME (MIN.)
0   1   2   3   5   10   15   20   30   IX$_A$ CONTROL

Fig. 7a

IX
H$_{ALA}$
H$_{VAL}$
L
TIME (MIN.)
0   1   2   3   5   10   15   20   30   IX$_A$ CONTROL

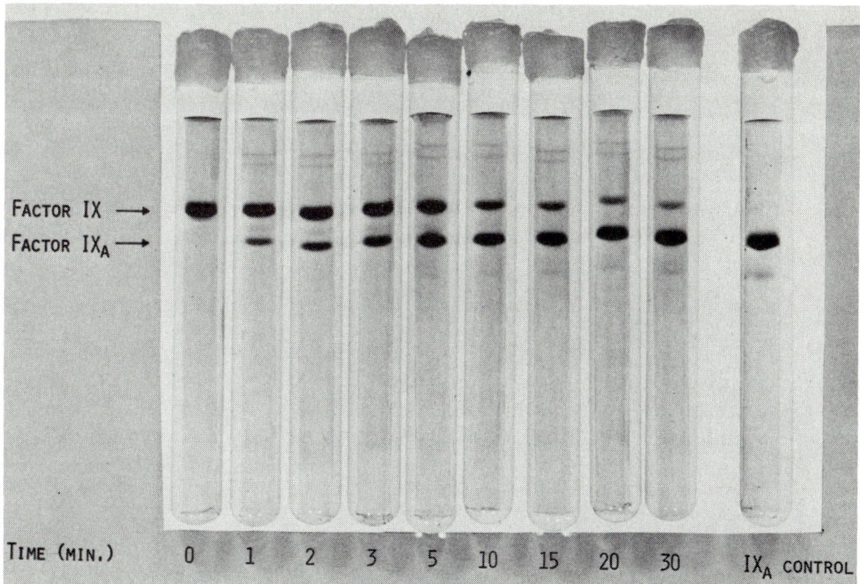

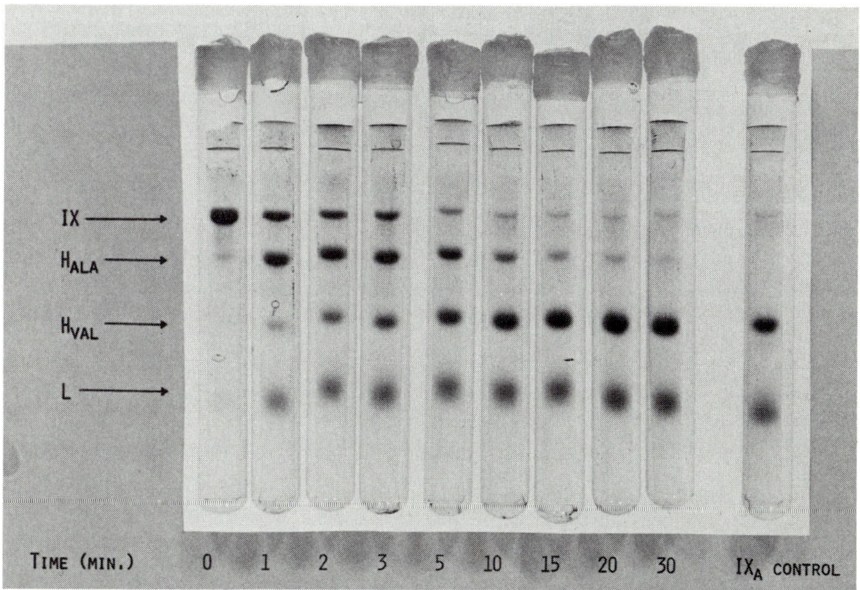

Fig. 7b

first few minutes of incubation a new, faster-moving band corresponding to factor IXa appears on the unreduced gel (Fig. 7a). This band (IXa) increases in intensity as the reaction proceeds while the original band (representing the precursor molecule) decreases in intensity and disappears on completion of the reaction (Fig. 7a). The shift in position of the band is attributable to a reduction in size of the factor IX molecule from 55 000 daltons to the 44 000 daltons with release of an 11 000 dalton polypeptide molecule (not shown on the gel). When the samples are reduced (Fig. 7b) the single band of factor IX decreases in intensity in the first few minutes with the appearance of three new bands, representing polypeptide chains. The two faster-moving proteins (labelled H_{VAL} and L) correspond to the two polypeptide chains which are found in factor IXa (Fig. 7b, last gel on the right). The protein band just ahead of factor IX (labelled H_{ALA}) appeared very rapidly and then disappeared in the next 15 to 20 minutes. These findings are best explained by the formation of a two-chain intermediate and the cleavage of the heavy chain of this intermediate to give rise to factor IXa. Factor IXa has a heavy chain smaller than that of the intermediate, but the light chain is identical in size so that only three new major bands, two heavy chains and one light chain, are observed in the reduced gels during the course of the reaction.

Confirmation of this hypothesis was obtained using preparative procedures in which relatively large amounts of purified factor IX were partially activated, the reaction stopped, the intermediates reduced, S-pyridylethylated, and then isolated by gel filtration (Fujikawa *et al.* 1974b). Two heavy chains, but only one type of light chain (16 000), were found. The smaller heavy chain corresponded to that of the factor IXa molecule and had a molecular weight of 27 300 daltons while the larger, which was derived from the intermediate, had a molecular weight of 38 800. In addition, a polypeptide (mol.wt $\simeq$ 11 000), referred to as the activation peptide, was also isolated. The light chain was found to have the same amino-terminal sequence, namely, Tyr-Asn-Ser-Gly, as the parent molecule, and therefore must have arisen from its amino-terminal end. Both the heavy chain of the intermediate and the activation peptide contained the sequence Ala-Glu-Thr-Ile-Phe, indicating that this peptide must have been split off the heavy chain of the intermediate in the second step of the reaction. It is this cleavage which gives rise to the smaller heavy chain of IXa which has as its first four residues at the amino-terminal end, Val-Val-Gly-Gly.

The first intermediate formed in the activation of human factor IX is very difficult to demonstrate, suggesting that the cleavage of the arginine–valine bond occurs at a much faster rate than that of the arginine–alanine bond (Østerud, Bouma and Griffin 1978). The critical event in the activation of both human and bovine factor IX is the cleavage of the internal arginine–valine bond. This probably permits formation of a new ion pair between the valine and the aspartic acid residue adjacent to the active serine (Di Scipio, Kurachi and Davie 1978). This would be analogous to the activation mechanism which has been established for the pancreatic serine proteases (Di Scipio, Kurachi and Davie 1978).

The activation of factor IX by the protease in Russell's viper venom occurs in a single step and involves only the cleavage of the internal arginine–valine peptide bond (Lindquist, Fujikawa and Davie 1978). No change in factor IX is observed on SDS gel electrophoresis during activation by the protease, but in the reduced gel a new major protein band with a molecular weight of approximately 28 000 daltons is found. This suggests that the precursor molecule has been split into two chains that migrate at essentially the same rate on gel electrophoresis (Lindquist *et al.* 1978).

The conversion of factor X to Xa by activated IXa in the absence of factor VIII is very slow and there is an absolute requirement for calcium ions (Suomela, Blombäck and Blombäck 1977, Hultin and Nemerson 1978, Neal and Chavin 1979). Phospholipid also appears to be essential (Schiffman, Rapaport and Chong 1960, Lundblad and Davie 1964, Brown and Hougie 1982) and the occasional finding that factor IXa can convert X to Xa in the absence of added phospholipid (Suomela, Blombäck and Blombäck 1977, Neal and Chavin 1979) may be attributable to the presence of phospholipid in one of the reagents. In a study of the phospholipid requirements for the IXa–VIII interaction, combinations of phospholipids found to be active were phosphatidic acid:phosphatidyl choline (3:2), phosphatidyl serine:phosphatidyl choline (1:1), and phosphatidyl serine:phosphatidyl ethanolamine (1:2) (Lundblad and Davie 1964). Phosphatidyl serine alone had only slight activity while phosphatidyl choline alone, phosphatidic acid alone or an equimolar mixture of phosphatidyl choline and phosphatidyl ethanolamine had relatively little effect (Lundblad and Davie 1964, Brown and Hougie 1983). Isolated human and bovine platelets were far less effective in fulfilling the phospholipid requirement than isolated phospholipid fraction (Lundblad and Davie 1964). However, washed platelets which have first been treated with thrombin, then washed, are more effective than phospholipid (Elödi, Váradi and Vörös 1981).

The conversion of factor X to factor X^a is greatly accelerated by factor VIII (antihaemophilic factor), the procoagulant protein which is deficient or abnormal in haemophilia. This factor has not yet been characterized and relatively little is known about its physico-chemical structure. In plasma it circulates as a complex with the von Willebrand's factor (see Chapter 5) and in the absence of this protein rapidly loses activity. Factor VIII can be separated from von Willebrand's factor by a variety of relatively simple procedures, such as sucrose density ultracentrifugation (Brown, Carton and Hougie 1982) or gel filtration (Owen and Wagner 1972), but such preparations have relatively little biological activity and are very unstable.

The formation of a more active species of factor IXa on incubation with factor VIII, or vice versa, has not been demonstrated. Moreover, the reaction product of factor IXa, factor VIII, phospholipid and calcium can be inactivated by the addition of either an antibody against factor VIII or an antibody against factor IX which suggests formation of a complex (Østerud and Rapaport 1970). The reaction of factor IXa with factor VIII therefore does not appear to be of the enzyme-substrate type. That factor VIII forms a complex with factor IXa, phospholipid and calcium was first suggested by experiments using a molecular sieve technique (Hougie, Denson and Biggs 1967). Bovine factor VIII (2000-fold purified) and factor IXa prepared from bovine plasma were incubated with phospholipid (PL) and calcium. When maximum coagulant activity developed, the reaction mixture was applied to a Sephadex G-200 column and eluted with buffer containing calcium. The active product which converts factor X to Xa and is referred to as 'tenase' (Váradi and Hemker 1976) was found to be totally excluded from the gel pores (being the first protein to pass through the column) and this suggested the formation of a IXa-VIII-PL-CA^{2+} complex. On the other hand, when elution was carried out by buffer alone, each reactant appeared in the position it would have been found in if chromatographed separately. Activated factor IX was also found to complex with phospholipid in the presence of calcium. But as factor VIII and phospholipid when applied alone in the presence or absence of calcium were both excluded from the gel, and appeared in the void volume fractions, these experiments were not conclusive and it was not possible to demonstrate complexing of these two reagents by this technique.

Chuang, Sargeant and Hougie (1974), using the same technique, then showed the factors could be dissociated to their pre-complex forms and recombined to once again form 'tenase'. The factor VIII and factor IXa have to be complexed to the same phospholipid micelle for maximum activity. Thus if factor VIII and factor IXa are allowed to bind phospholipid separately before they are incubated together, the 'tenase' generates more slowly than when the proteins are allowed to bind to the same phospholipid micelle (Chuang, Sargeant and Hougie 1974, Váradi and Hemker 1976).

At a calcium concentration of 30 mmol, the complex was found to display maximal activity when the concentrations of factors VIII and IXa were each 1 unit/ml (their plasma concentrations); under these conditions, 1 mol of factor IXa was found to activate 23 mol of factor X in 30 seconds (Elödi and Váradi 1979). However, others have found that a large excess of factor VIII to factor IXa is required to saturate the IXa (Brown, Baugh and Hougie 1978, Hultin and Nemerson 1978).

The formation of 'tenase' is markedly accelerated if factor VIII is activated by trace amounts of thrombin (Pitlick, Lundblad and Davie 1969, Østerud *et al.* 1971, Hultin and Nemerson 1978, Brown, Baugh and Hougie 1980, Ofosu *et al.* 1981). Thrombin-activated factor VIII forms 'tenase' at a rate 10–20 times faster than unactivated factor VIII in the presence of factor IXa, phospholipid and calcium, but the final amount of 'tenase' formed is the same (Pitlick, Lundblad and Davie 1969, Brown, Baugh and Hougie 1980). When unactivated factor VIII is used to form the complex, there is a short lag phase in which little or no activity develops and this is decreased or abolished by prior treatment of the factor VIII with thrombin (Pitlick, Lundblad and Davie 1969, Hultin and Nemerson 1978). There have been reports in which thrombin did not accelerate the reaction (Neal and Chavin 1979) but the preparations of factor VIII used in these studies may already have been fully activated by thrombin. Exposure of factor VIII to thrombin during some stage of the purification procedure is difficult to avoid and there is no physico-chemical method of detecting such activation. Thrombin increases the binding affinity of factor VIII for phospholipid so that thrombin-activated factor VIII is bound at much lower concentrations of phospholipid than unactivated factor VIII (Andersson and Brown 1981). This is probably at least in part dependent on the fact that native factor VIII binds strongly both to phospholipid and to von Willebrand's factor, and therefore more phospholipid must be added to effectively compete with von Willebrand's factor for factor VIII binding. On the other hand, thrombin-activated factor VIII does not seem to bind to von Willebrand's factor and less phospholipid is necessary for binding to occur (Andersson and Brown 1981). In this connection, it should be noted that in all the reported kinetic studies, no attempts were made to separate the von Willebrand's factor from factor VIII.

Thrombin may also have a role in modulating the formation of 'tenase'. Small amounts of thrombin with its high affinity for factor VIII (Brodén, Andersson and Sandberg 1980) convert it into a far more reactive form, the thrombin-modified factor VIII accelerates the intermediate phases of blood coagulation leading to a burst of thrombin activity and subsequent fibrin formation. As high levels of thrombin are formed, the factor VIII is subsequently destroyed, rapidly decelerating and eventually stopping fibrin formation. This series of reactions may provide an elegant biochemical control for blood coagulation (Davie, Lundblad and Hougie 1966).

The formation of the factor VIII-factor IXa-PL-Ca^{2+} complex is remarkably analogous to that of the factor V-factor Xa-PL-Ca^{2+} complex. The activities of both factors V and VIII are greatly enhanced by traces of thrombin. Neither of the two proteins appears to have an enzymatic action on any other clotting proteins, and their roles are generally considered to be regulatory ones. The biochemical structures of factor IX and X are similar with very homologous amino acid sequences, particularly in their catalytic region (Katayama *et al.* 1979) and the target of each of the complexes is a vitamin K-dependent clotting protein.

Factor X

This is a glycoprotein present in human plasma in a precursor form at a concentration of approximately 8 μg/ml (Fair, Plow and Edgington 1979). It is composed of two polypeptide chains held together by a disulphide bond(s). The bovine molecule, which has a molecular weight of 55 000 daltons, has been well characterized (Jackson and Hanahan 1968, Fujikawa, Legaz and Davie 1972, Jackson 1972) and sequenced (Enfield *et al.* 1975, Titani *et al.* 1975). The human molecule is composed of two chains and it is very similar to bovine factor IX but has a molecular weight of 59 000 daltons (Di Scipio *et al.* 1977). The amino-terminal sequence of the light chain of human factor X is identical to that of the bovine species but the heavy chain is larger and differs from that of bovine factor X in its amino-terminal sequence (Di Scipio *et al.* 1977).

The conversion of factor X to its active enzymatic form (Xa) involves the cleavage of a single specific arginyl–isoleucine peptide bond in the heavy chain of the precursor molecule (Fig. 8). This results in the formation of a glycopeptide with a molecular weight of 11 000 daltons and a protein with a molecular weight of 44 000 daltons. This protein constitutes one form of activated factor X or Xa and is referred to as factor Xα. No change is observed in the light chain during the activation reaction. In a second, slower and

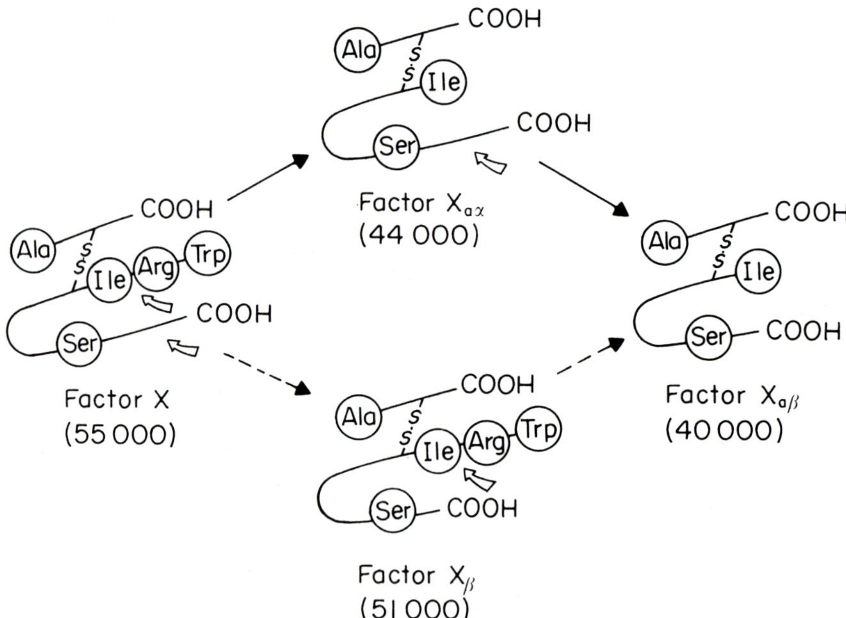

Fig. 8. Activation of bovine factor X. (Reprinted with permission from Fujikawa *et al.* (1974a) and the American Chemical Society.)

relatively unimportant step, factor Xaα is degraded by hydrolysis of a peptide bond(s) in the carboxyl-terminal region of the heavy chain; this releases another glycopeptide fragment(s), and removes the remaining carbohydrate, giving rise to factor Xaβ which has a molecular weight of 40 000 daltons (Fujikawa *et al.* 1974a). Factor X can also be converted to an inactive partially degraded protein referred to as factor Xβ (molecular weight 51 000) by an initial cleavage of the glycopeptide fragment(s) from the carboxyl-terminal region of the heavy chain (Fig. 8). The peptide bond cleaved in this reaction is the same as that involved in the conversion of factor Xaα to factor Xaβ. Factor Xβ can be converted directly to factor Xaβ by cleavage of the specific arginyl–isoleucine bond in the amino-terminal region of the heavy chain.

This mechanism of factor X to Xa conversion by the intrinsic system is the same as that induced by tissue factor and factor VII, trypsin or the protease from Russell's viper venom (Radcliffe and Barton 1973, Fujikawa *et al.* 1974a).

The subsequent events in the coagulation sequence involving the conversion of prothrombin to thrombin by the factor Xa: factor V:PL:Ca^{2+} complex are described elsewhere in detail.

REFERENCES

Andersson L.-O. & Brown J.E. (1981) Interaction of factor VIII-von Willebrand factor with phospholipid vesicles. *Biochemical Journal* **200**, 161–7.

Baugh R. & Hougie C. (1981) Structure and function in blood coagulation. In *Recent Advances in Blood Coagulation*. Poller L. (ed.). pp. 81–107. Churchill Livingstone, Edinburgh.

Bouma B. & Griffin J. (1977) Human blood coagulation factor XI. Purification, properties, and mechanism of activation by activated factor XII. *Journal of Biological Chemistry* **252**, 6432–7.

Bouma B., Miles L., Berreta G. & Griffin J. (1980) Human plasma prekallikrein. Studies of its activation by activated factor XII and of its inactivation by diisopropyl phosphofluoridate. *Biochemistry* **19**, 1151–60.

Brodén K., Andersson L.-O. & Sandberg H. (1980) Kinetics of activation of human factor VIII by thrombin. *Thrombosis Research* **19**, 299–307.

Brown J.E., Baugh R.F. & Hougie C. (1978) Substrate inhibition of the intrinsic generation of activated factor X (Stuart factor). *Thrombosis Research* **13**, 893–900.

Brown J.E., Baugh R.F. & Hougie C. (1980) The inhibition of the intrinsic generation of activated factor X by heparin and hirudin. *Thrombosis Research* **17**, 267–72.

Brown J.E., Carton C. & Hougie C. (1982) Unpublished observations.

Brown J.E. & Hougie C. (1982) Unpublished observations.

Chuang T.F., Sargeant R.B. & Hougie C. (1974) The effect of calcium ions on the properties of factor IX and its activated form. *British Journal of Haematology* **27**, 281–7.

Colman R. & Wong P. (1977) Participation of Hageman factor dependent pathways in human disease states. *Thrombosis and Haemostasis* **4**, 751–5.

Cramer A.D., Melaragno A.J., Phifer S.J. & Hougie C. (1976) Von Willebrand disease San Diego, a new variant. *Lancet* **II**, 12–14.

Davie E.W., Hougie C. & Lundblad R.L. (1969) Mechanisms of blood coagulation. In *Recent Advances in Blood Coagulation*. Poller L. (ed.). pp. 13–28. Churchill Livingstone, Edinburgh.

Di Scipio R.G., Hermodson M.A., Yates S.G. & Davie E.W. (1977) A comparison of human prothrombin, factor IX (Christmas factor), factor X (Stuart factor), and protein S. *Biochemistry* **16**, 698–706.

Di Scipio R.G., Kurachi K. & Davie E.W. (1978) Activation of human factor IX (Christmas factor). *Journal of Clinical Investigation* **61**, 1528–38.

Elödi S. & Váradi K. (1979) Optimization of conditions for the catalytic effect of the factor IXa–factor VIII complex: probable role of the complex in the amplification of blood coagulation. *Thrombosis Research* **15**, 617–29.

Elödi S., Váradi K. & Vörös E. (1981) Kinetics of formation of factor IXa–factor VIII complex on the surface of platelets. *Thrombosis Research* **21**, 695.

Enfield D.L., Ericsson L.H., Walsh K.A., Neurath H. & Titani K. (1975) Bovine factor X (Stuart factor). Primary structure of the light chain. *Proceedings of the National Academy of Sciences, USA* **72**, 16–19.

Fair D.S., Plow E.F. & Edgington T.S. (1979) Combined functional and immunochemical analysis of normal and abnormal human factor X. *Journal of Clinical Investigation* **64**, 884–94.

Fujikawa K., Coan M.H., Legaz M.E. & Davie E.W. (1974a) The mechanism of activation of bovine factor X (Stuart factor) by intrinsic and extrinsic pathways. *Biochemistry* **13**, 5290–9.

Fujikawa K., Legaz M.E. & Davie E.W. (1972) Bovine factors X_1 and S_2 (Stuart factor). Isolation and characterisation of bovine factor IX (Christmas factor). *Biochemistry* **11**, 4882–91.

Fujikawa K., Legaz M.E., Kato H. & Davie E.W. (1974b) The mechanism of activation of bovine factor IX (Christmas factor) by bovine factor XIa (activated plasma thromboplastin antecedent). *Biochemistry* **13**, 4508–16.

Griffin J. & Beretta G. (1979) Molecular mechanisms of surface-dependent activation of Hageman factor. In *Tokyo International Symposium on Kinins*. Moriya H. & Suzuki T. (eds). Plenum Press, New York.

Han Y., Kato H., Iwanaga S., Oh-ishi S. & Katori M. (1978) Primary structure of bovine high-molecular-weight kininogen. *Journal of Biochemistry* **83**, 213–21.

Hougie C., Denson K.W.E. & Biggs R. (1967) A study of the reaction product of factor VIII and factor IX by gel filtration. *Thrombosis et Diathesis Haemorrhagica* **18**, 211–22.

Hultin M.B. & Nemerson Y. (1978) Activation of factor X by factors IXa and VIII; a specific assay for factor IXa in the presence of thrombin-activated factor VIII. *Blood* **52**, 928–40.

Jackson C.M. (1972) Characterisation of two glycoprotein variants of bovine factor X and demonstration that the factor X zymogen contains two polypeptide chains. *Biochemistry* **11**, 4873–82.

Jackson C.M. & Hanahan D.J. (1968) Studies on bovine factor X. II. Characterisation of purified factor X. Observations on some alterations in zone electrophoretic and chromatographic behaviour occurring during purification. *Biochemistry* **7**, 4506–17.

Kaplan A.P. (1978) Initiation of the intrinsic coagulation and fibrinolytic pathways of man: the role of surface Hageman factor, prekallikrein, high molecular weight kininogen, and factor XI. *Progress in Hemostasis and Thrombosis* 4, 127.

Katayama K., Ericsson L.H., Enfield D.L., Walsh K.A., Neurath H., Davie E.W. & Titani K. (1979) Comparison of amino acid sequence of bovine coagulation factor IX (Christmas factor) with that of other vitamin K-dependent plasma proteins. *Proceedings of the National Academy of Sciences USA* 76, 4990–4.

Kato H., Sugo T., Ikari N., Hashimoto N., Maryuma I., Han Y., Iwanaga S. & Fujii S. (1979) Role of bovine high-molecular-weight (HMW) Kininogen in contact-mediated activation of bovine factor XII. In *Kinins II.* Suzuki T. & Moriya H. (eds). *Advances in Experimental Medicine and Biology,* 120A.

Kerbiriou D., Bouma B. & Griffin J. (1980) Immunochemical studies of human high molecular weight kininogen and of its complexes with plasma prekallikrein or kallikrein. *Journal of Biological Chemistry* 255, 3952–8.

Kerbiriou D. & Griffin J. (1979) Human high molecular weight kininogen: studies of structure–function relationships and of proteolysis of the molecule occurring during contact activation of plasma. *Journal of Biological Chemistry* 254, 12020–7.

Kurachi K. & Davie E.W. (1977) Activation of human factor XI (plasma thromboplastin antecedent) by factor XIIa (activated Hageman factor). *Biochemistry* 16, 5831–9.

Kurachi K., Ohkubo I., Heimark R., Fujikawa K. & Davie E.W. (1983) Initiation of intrinsic blood coagulation. *Advances in Experimental Medicine and Biology* 156, 39–44.

Lindquist P.A., Fujikawa K. & Davie E.W. (1978) Activation of bovine factor IX (Christmas factor) by factor XIa (activated plasma thromboplastin antecedent) and a protease from Russell's viper venom. *Journal of Biological Chemistry* 253, 1902.

Lundblad R.L. & Davie E.W. (1964) Unpublished observations cited by Davie E.W., Hougie C. and Lundblad R.L. (1969) Mechanisms of blood coagulation. In *Recent Advances in Blood Coagulation.* Poller L. (ed.). pp. 13–28. Churchill Livingstone, Edinburgh.

McMillan C., Saito H., Ratnoff O. & Walton A. (1974) The secondary structure of human Hageman factor (factor XII) and its alteration by activating agents. *Journal of Clinical Investigation* 54, 1312–22.

Mandle R. & Kaplan A. (1977) Hageman factor substrates. Human plasma prekalli-krein: mechanism of activation by Hageman factor and participation in Hageman factor-dependent fibrinolysis. *Journal of Biological Chemistry* 252, 6097–104.

Meier H., Pierce J., Colman R. & Kaplan A. (1977) Activation and function of human Hageman factor (the role of high molecular weight kininogen and prekallikrein). *Journal of Clinical Investigation* 60, 18–31.

Neal G.G. & Chavin S.I. (1979) The role of factors VIII and IX in the activation of bovine blood coagulation factor X. *Thrombosis Research* 16, 473–84.

Ofosu F., Blajchman M.A., Modi G. & Hirsh J. (1981) The factor VIII-independent activation of factor X by factors IXa and VII in plasma. *Thrombosis Research* 21, 23.

Østerud B., Bouma B.N. & Griffin J.H. (1978) Human blood coagulation factor IX, purification, peptides and mechanism of activation by activated factor IX. *Journal of Biological Chemistry* 253, 5946–51.

Østerud B. & Rapaport S.I. (1970) Synthesis of intrinsic factor X activator. Inhibition of the function of formed activator by antibodies to factor VIII and to factor IX. *Biochemistry* 9, 1854.

Østerud B., Rapaport S.I., Schiffman S. & Chong M.M.Y. (1971) Formation of intrinsic factor X-activator activity, with special reference to the role of thrombin. *British Journal of Haematology* **21**, 643.

Owen W. G. & Wagner R. H. (1972) Antihemophilic factor: separation of an active fragment following dissociation by salts or detergents. *Thrombosis et Diathesis Haemorrhagica* **27**, 502–15.

Pitlick F.A., Lundblad R.L. & Davie E.W. (1969) The role of heparin in intrinsic blood coagulation. *Journal of Biomedical Material Research* **3**, 95.

Radcliffe R.D. & Barton P.G. (1973) Comparisons of the molecular forms of activated bovine factor X. *Journal of Biological Chemistry* **248**, 6788–95.

Ratnoff O.D. & Saito H. (1979) Interactions among Hageman factor, plasma prekallikrein, high molecular weight kininogen, and plasma thromboplastin antecedent. *Proceedings of the National Academy of Sciences USA* **76**, 958.

Revak S., Cochrane C., Bouma B. & Griffin J. (1978) Surface and fluid phase activities of two forms of activated Hageman factor produced during contact activation of plasma. *Journal of Experimental Medicine* **147**, 719–29.

Revak S., Cochrane C. & Griffin J. (1977) The binding and cleavage characteristics of human Hageman factor during contact activation. A comparison of normal plasma with plasmas deficient in factor XI, prekallikrein, or high molecular weight kininogen. *Journal of Clinical Investigation* **59**, 1167–75.

Rosenthal R., Dreskin O. & Rosenthal N. (1953) New hemophilia-like disease caused by deficiency of a third plasma thromboplastin factor. *Preceedings of the Society for Experimental Biology and Medicine* **82**, 171–4.

Schiffman S., Mannhalter C. & Tyner K. (1980) Human high molecular weight kininogen. Effects of cleavage by kallikrein on protein structure and procoagulant activity. *Journal of Biological Chemistry* **255**, 6433–8.

Schiffman S., Rapaport S.I. & Chong M.M.Y. (1960) The mandatory role of lipid in the interaction of factors VIII and IX. *Proceedings of the Society for Experimental Biology and Medicine* **123**, 736.

Scott C. & Colman R. (1980) Function and immunochemistry of prekallikrein-high molecular weight kininogen complex in plasma. *Journal of Clinical Investigation* **65**, 413–21.

Scott C., Lui Y. & Colman R. (1979) Human plasma prekallikrein: a rapid high-yield method for purification. *European Journal of Biochemistry* **100**, 77–83.

Silverberg M., Dunn J., Garen L. & Kaplan A. (1980) Auto-activation of human Hageman factor; demonstration utilizing a synthetic substrate. *Journal of Biological Chemistry* **255**, 7281–6.

Suomela H., Blombäck M. & Blombäck B. (1977) The activation of factor X evaluated by using synthetic substrate. *Thrombosis Research* **10**, 267–81.

Thompson R., Mandle R. & Kaplan A. (1977) Association of factor XI and high molecular weight kininogen in human plasma. *Journal of Clinical Investigation* **60**, 1376–80.

Thompson R., Mandle R. & Kaplan A. (1979) Studies of binding of prekallikrein and factor XI to high molecular weight kininogen and its light chain. *Proceedings of the National Academy of Sciences USA* **76**, 4862–6.

Titani K., Fujikawa K., Enfield D.L., Ericsson L.H., Walsh K.A. & Neurath H. (1975) Bovine factor X_1 (Stuart factor): amino-acid sequence of heavy chain. *Proceedings of the National Academy of Sciences USA* **72**, 3082–6.

Váradi K. & Hemker H.C. (1976) Kinetics of the formation of the factor X activating enzyme of the blood coagulation system. *Thrombosis Research* **8**, 303–17.

Vennerød A.M., Ørstavik K.H., Laake K., Fagerhol M. & Ly B. (1977) Purification of human factor IX. *Thrombosis Research* **11**, 663–72.

Walsh P. (1972) The role of platelets in the contact phase of blood coagulation. *British Journal of Haematology* **22**, 237–54.

Wiggins R., Loskutoff D., Cochrane C., Griffin J. & Edgington T. (1980) Activation of rabbit Hageman factor by homogenates of cultured rabbit endothelial cells. *Journal of Clinical Investigation* **65**, 197–206.

Wuepper K. (1973) Prekallikrein deficiency in man. *Journal of Experimental Medicine* **138**, 1345–55.

Chapter 2
Thrombin–Fibrinogen Reaction and Fibrin Stabilization

M. P. ESNOUF

The explosive violence which characterizes the formation of the fibrin clot has caught the eye of investigators from many disciplines for almost a century. As our understanding of the mechanism of this reaction has increased, it has been recognized that three proteins are involved, namely fibrinogen, thrombin and factor XIII. The formation of the fibrin clot takes place in three distinct phases. The enzymic conversion of fibrinogen, by thrombin, to a soluble fibrin monomer is followed by a physical process, the spontaneous polymerization of the monomer, to give insoluble fibrin. In the last phase, which involves a second enzyme factor XIIIa, the polymer is 'stabilized' by the formation of interchain isopeptide bonds.

Fibrinogen

Fibrinogen is the most abundant clotting factor in plasma ranging in concentration from 2–5 g/l. The physico-chemical properties of the protein are characteristic of both globular and fibrous proteins. The protein has a high molecular weight, 340 000 (Caspary and Kekwick 1957), as calculated from sedimentation studies, which also suggested that it was a rod-shaped molecule. Further support for the elongated shape of the molecule came from the early electron microscope studies of Hall and Slayter (1959), who, using a shadow casting technique, obtained photographs which showed that the molecule consisted of two globular spheres (60 Å) connected by a 'thread-like' region to a central sphere (50 Å), the overall length of the molecule being 475 Å. Probably the thread connecting the spheres gave rise to the X-ray diffraction patterns characteristic of fibrous proteins seen much earlier by Astbury and his colleagues. Later electron microscope studies using negative staining techniques (Koppel 1966) did not support the rod-shaped model for fibrinogen, but, with the return of shadow casting techniques (Fowler and Erickson 1979), the work of Hall and Slayter (1959) has been vindicated and it is apparent that their model is in remarkable agreement with the more recent ideas of fibrinogen structure.

Fibrinogen is a dimer of three separate polypeptide chains α, β, and γ, which can be separated in a denaturing solvent after reduction by sulphydryl reagents. The molecular weights of the individual chains are $\alpha = 63\,000$, $\beta = 56\,000$, $\gamma = 47\,000$ (McKee, Mattock and Hill 1970). The sum of the molecular weights of these chains (166 000) confirms the dimeric nature of fibrinogen. Further fragmentation of fibrinogen can be achieved by digestion with plasmin (Marder 1971). The first degradation product (Fig. 9), fragment X (mol.wt 240 000), is formed with the loss of the exposed regions at the C-terminus of the α chains which contain a high proportion of polar residues. In the next phase, two products are formed, an asymmetric fragment Y (mol.wt 155 000) and an equivalent amount of a core fragment D (mol.wt 83 000). Fragment Y is further degraded to a second core fragment E (mol.wt 50 000) and an equimolar amount of fragment D. Fragment D corresponds to the terminal globular regions of the Hall and Slayter model, while fragment E is the central nodule.

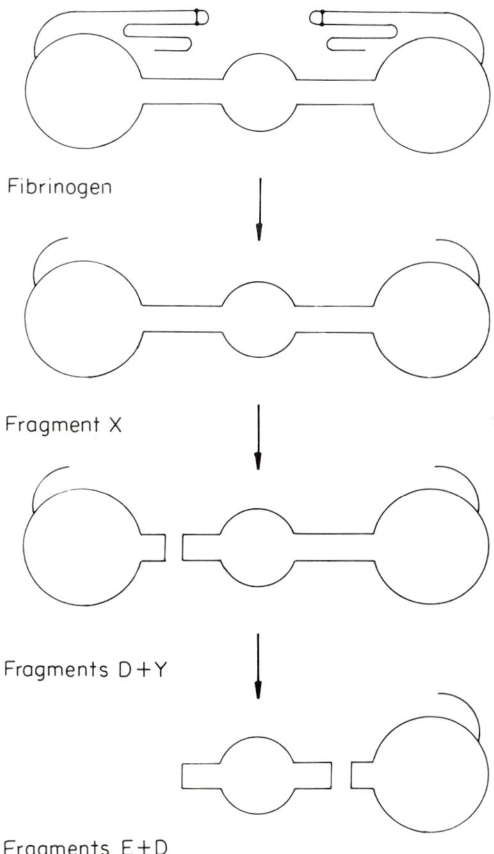

Fig. 9. A schematic illustration of the course of the degradation of fibrinogen by plasmin.

The primary structure of fibrinogen has been determined taking advantage of the selective cleavage of the molecule by plasmin, coupled with the dissociation of the cleaved polypeptide chains after reduction of the disulphide bonds. Selective cleavage of methionine residues by cyanogen bromide has been used to determine the positions of the interchain disulphide bonds. The α chain contains 610 amino acid residues (Doolittle *et al.* 1979), the β chain 461 (Watt, Takagi and Doolittle 1979) and the γ chain 411 (Henschen and Lottspeich 1977), and since fibrinogen is a dimer it therefore contains 2964 amino acids which gives a molecular weight of 329 840. In addition to amino acids, fibrinogen also contains four carbohydrate chains with a combined molecular weight of 10 000, one on each of the β and γ chains. Thus, the calculated molecular weight is in good agreement with that obtained from hydrodynamic measurements.

Fibrinogen contains 58 Cys residues, all in disulphide bonds (Henschen 1964). The position of these bonds connecting the two halves of the molecule and the three polypeptide chains is crucial to our understanding of the structure of the protein. Fibrinogen monomers are covalently linked in the N-terminal region by a disulphide bond between the two Aα chains at Cys^{28} and the two γ chains are similarly joined by a pair of bonds between Cys^{8} and Cys^{9}. This region, referred to as the N-terminal disulphide knot (Blombäck *et al.* 1976), is contained within the plasmin degradation product, fragment E. There are no interconnecting bonds between the pairs of Bβ chains in this region, instead they are linked to the Aα chains through Cys^{36} (α) to Cys^{65} (β) (Blombäck *et al.* 1976). The next group of structurally significant disulphide bonds are present in the thread joining the fragment D and E regions. These take the form of two disulphide rings connecting the α chain (Cys^{49}) to the γ chain (Cys^{19}); the γ chain (Cys^{23}) to the β chain (Cys^{76}) and the β chain (Cys^{80}) to the α chain (Cys^{49}). This interconnecting ring is repeated 111–112 residues later; between these two disulphide rings the three polypeptide chains form a supercoil (Doolittle, Goldbaum and Doolittle 1978), which must have given rise to the X-ray diffraction pattern seen earlier by Astbury and his colleagues.

The remaining bonds form intrachain disulphide loops in the β and γ chains in the fragment D region and in the α chain outside the fragment D region (Bouma, Takagi and Doolittle 1978). The recent structural work by Doolittle and his colleagues has enabled them to propose an overall shape for the fibrinogen molecule, which is in good agreement with the trinodular form, as seen in electron micrographs using the shadow casting technique (Fig. 10).

Fibrin formation

The conversion of fibrinogen to fibrin, by thrombin, involves the rapid removal of the 16 residue A peptide from the N-terminus of the Aα chain followed by the

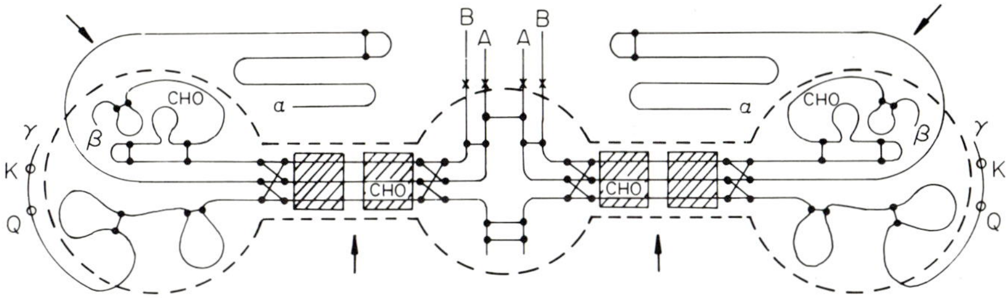

Fig. 10. A diagrammatic representation of the fibrinogen molecule (adapted from Bouma, Takagi and Doolittle 1978), showing the individual polypeptide chains set inside the dotted outline of the trinodular shape of the molecule. The disulphide bonds are shown thus (O————O). The hatched areas indicate the supercoiled region. CHO represents the carbohydrate side chains. K and Q are the Lys and Gln residues involved in the cross-linking of the γ chains. The arrows indicate the primary regions of plasmin attack. A————X and B————X represent the fibrinopeptides A and B.

slower cleavage of the 14 residue B peptide from the N-terminus of the Bβ chain, an Arg-Gly bond being cleaved in both instances. The fact that the peptides are removed sequentially suggests that following the loss of the A peptide a conformational change must take place exposing the B peptide to attack by thrombin (Blombäck *et al.* 1978).

Whereas the biochemical events prior to the polymerization of the fibrin are clear, there is still some uncertainty as to the mechanism of polymerization. In the early work, Ferry (1952) proposed that polymerization which followed the removal of the negatively charged fibrinopeptides was driven by hydrogen bond formation and dipole–dipole interactions. A more sophisticated view of the polymerization process, while embodying the charged peptide notion, is that the peptides mask specific polymerization sites. Heene and Matthias (1973) had already shown that fibrin bonded to Sepharose could bind fibrinogen, indicating that fibrinogen has sites available to interact with fibrin. Kudryk, Reuterby and Blombäck (1973) also showed that fragment D would bind to fibrin-Sepharose and in a later paper Kudryk *et al.* (1974) demonstrated that thrombin treatment of the N-terminal disulphide knot region coupled to Sepharose would also bind fibrinogen and fragment D. The conclusion to be drawn from these experiments is that the unmasked binding sites are present in the fragment D region, and that the masked sites are contained in the N-terminal region. To test this hypothesis, Laudano and Doolittle (1978, 1980) synthesized a series of peptides corresponding to the amino-terminal segments of the α and β chains which would be exposed by the removal of the A and B peptides. They showed that Gly-Pro-Arg peptides, the first three residues of the newly formed fibrin α chain, would bind to fibrin and fragment D and inhibited the polymerization of fibrin monomers, whereas peptides based on the N-terminus of the β chain, in which proline is replaced by histidine, do not inhibit the polymerization of fibrin monomers, but do bind to fibrinogen and fragment D. The consequence of this sort of interaction results in a staggered overlap of the fibrin molecules in which the terminal fragment D region of one module interacts with the central nodule (fragment E) of another. It remains to be seen whether peptides based on the β chain prevent further lateral association of the fibrin polymer.

Fibrin stabilization

One distinguishing feature of the fibrin formed in plasma is that it is not soluble in urea, whereas fibrin derived from purified fibrinogen dissolves in urea (Robbins 1944). The reason for this difference in the solubility of the fibrin is the presence, in plasma, of an additional protein, factor XIII (Lorand and Jacobsen 1958, Loewy *et al.* 1961). Human plasma factor XIII (mol.wt 320 000) is a tetramer composed of an *a* chain (mol.wt 75 000) and a *b* chain (mol.wt 85 000) in an a_2b_2 structure (Schwartz *et al.* 1973). Factor XIII circulates in plasma in an inactive form and is activated by thrombin or other proteolytic enzymes. In the first step, the *a* subunit is cleaved at an Arg-Gly bond releasing a peptide (mol.wt 4000) from the N-terminus, while the *b* subunit remains unchanged.

The cleaved protein has no biological activity unless Ca^{2+} is added (Cooke 1974, Cooke, Pestell and Holbrook 1974, Curtis *et al.* 1974). In the presence of Ca^{2+} two further changes in the structure of the protein occur. The first is the dissociation of the modified *a* subunits from the *b* subunits, and secondly an essential cysteine residue at the active centre of the catalytic subunit is unmasked.

The active enzyme catalyses the formation of two isopeptide bonds between specific glutamine and lysine residues on adjacent fibrinogen γ chains. The residues involved are Gln^{398} and Lys^{406} (Doolittle *et al.* 1972). It also follows from this that the chains are cross-linked in an antiparallel fashion. The formation of the γ-γ isopeptide bonds occurs in the first few minutes after clot formation and this is followed by a slow cross-linking of the α chains to give α polymers (McKee, Mattock and Hill 1970). The glutamyl acceptors in the α chains have now been located (Cottrell *et al.* 1979) and are Gln^{328} and Gln^{366}. At present the lysine donor residues have not been identified.

Thrombin

Thrombin is the physiological agent for the conversion of fibrinogen to fibrin and appears in blood following the activation of the clotting system. The mechanism of thrombin generation is discussed in detail in Chapter 3. Thrombin can be conveniently separated from prothrombin activation mixtures by making use of the fact that it is less negatively charged than its parent, prothrombin.

The primary sequence of bovine thrombin is shown in Chapter 3, Fig. 11, starting at residue Thr^{275} and extending to the C-terminus. The 49 residue A chain terminated by Arg^{323} has, at present, no recognized function.

In the case of human thrombin the A chain is 13 residues shorter (Lanchantin *et al.* 1975); this is the consequence of the substitution of Lys^{287} by Arg in human thrombin. The Arg-Thr bond so formed is readily cleaved by thrombin.

Thrombin has a considerable sequence homology with chymotrypsin and also similarities in secondary structure. Unfortunately, early attempts to gain information on the tertiary structure from X-ray diffraction studies have proved unsuccessful, but much can be inferred about its three-dimensional structure by comparison with chymotrypsin.

Thrombin has a considerably broader specificity than the other activated clotting factors, predominately cleaving bonds of the type Arg-X, where X is frequently a neutral or hydroxy amino acid, in a wide range of proteins including itself.

Freshly prepared α thrombin (mol.wt 39 000) will undergo autolysis to β thrombin (mol.wt 28 000), with the loss of two peptides from the A chain (prothrombin residues 275–287 and 305–323) and a peptide from the N-terminus of the B chain (residues 324–388) which contains the first disulphide loop and the carbohydrate chain. In addition, a seven residue peptide (residues 389–396) is probably removed (Kingdon, Noyes and Lundblad 1977). There is no change in the molecular weight during the further autolysis of β thrombin to γ thrombin because the polypeptide chain is cleaved within the second disulphide loop presumably at either Arg^{501} or Arg^{503}.

The progressive change from α to β and finally γ thrombin is accompanied by a change in the specific activity of the enzyme, but the extent of the change varies with the type of substrate used (Workman *et al.* 1977). There is a 200-fold drop in the V_{max} for the conversion of fibrinogen in going from α to β thrombin and a ten-fold drop in the rate of hydrolysis of synthetic nitroanilide substrates.

In contrast, with the synthetic ester substrates BAEE and TAME, β thrombin is about 1.5 times more active than α thrombin. γ Thrombin has very little coagulant activity but still has some esterolytic activity.

As it will be seen in the following chapter, thrombin, in addition to converting fibrinogen to fibrin and activating factor XIII, has other important functions in the coagulation system. It activates both factor V and VIII providing positive feedback and at the same time it forms part of a negative feedback loop by activating Protein C which is a potent inactivator of both factors V and VIII. Thrombin also has a profound effect on platelets causing them to aggregate and to bind the components of the prothrombin converting complex.

REFERENCES

Blombäck B., Hessel B., Hogg D. & Therkildsen L. (1978) A two-step fibrinogen-fibrin transition in blood coagulation. *Nature* **275**, 501–5.

Blombäck B., Hogg D.H., Gardlund B., Hessel B. & Kudryk B. (1976) Fibrinogen and fibrin formation. *Thrombosis Research* **8** (Supplement II) 329–46.

Bouma III. H., Takagi T. & Doolittle R.F. (1978) The arrangement of disulphide bonds in Fragment D from human fibrinogen. *Thrombosis Research* **13**, 557–62.

Caspary E.A. & Kekwick R.A. (1957) Some physicochemical properties of human fibrinogen. *Biochemical Journal* **67**, 41–8.

Cooke R.D. (1974) Calcium-induced dissociation of human plasma factor XIII and the appearance of catalytic activity. *Biochemical Journal* **141**, 683–91.

Cooke R.D., Pestell T.C. & Holbrook J.J. (1974) Calcium and thiol reactivity of human plasma clotting factor XIII. *Biochemical Journal* **141**, 675–82.

Cottrell B.A., Strong D.D., Watt K.W.K. & Doolittle R.F. (1979) Amino acid sequence studies on the α-chain of human fibrinogen. Exact location of the cross-linking acceptor sites. *Biochemistry* **18**, 5405–10.

Curtis C.G., Brown K.L., Credo R.B., Domanik R.A., Gray A., Stenberg P. & Lorand L. (1974) Calcium-dependent unmasking of active centre cysteine during activation of fibrin stabilising factor. *Biochemistry* **13**, 3774–80.

Doolittle R.F., Cassman K.G., Chen R., Sharp J.J. & Wooding G.L. (1972) Correlation of the mode of fibrin polymerization with the pattern of cross linking. *Annals of the New York Academy of Sciences* **202**, 114.

Doolittle R.F., Goldbaum D.M. & Doolittle L.R. (1978) Designation of sequences involved in the 'coiled coil' interdomainal connector in fibrinogen: construction of an atomic scale model. *Journal of Molecular Biology* **120**, 311–25.

Doolittle R.F., Watt K.W.K., Cottrell B.A., Strong D.D. & Riley M. (1979) The amino acid sequence of the α chain of human fibrinogen. *Nature* **280**, 464–8.

Ferry J.D. (1952) The mechanism of polymerization of fibrin. *Proceedings of the National Academy of Sciences USA* **38**, 566–9.

Fowler W.E. & Erickson H.P. (1979) Trinodular structure of fibrinogen. Conformation by both shadowing and negative stain electron microscopy. *Journal of Molecular Biology* **134**, 241–9.

Hall C.E. & Slayter H.S. (1959) The fibrinogen molecule: its size, shape and mode of polymerization. *Journal of Biophysical Biochemical Cytology* **5**, 11–15.

Heene D.L. & Matthias F.R. (1973) Adsorption of fibrinogen derivatives on insolubilised fibrinogen and fibrin. *Thrombosis Research* **2**, 137–54.

Henschen A. (1964) Number and reactivity of disulphide bonds in fibrinogen and fibrin. *Arkiv Kemi* **22**, 355–73.

Henschen A. & Lottspeich F. (1977) Sequence homology between γ chain and β chain in human fibrin. *Thrombosis Research* **11**, 869–80.

Kingdon H.S., Noyes C.M. & Lundblad R.L. (1977) Some aspects of the primary structure of bovine Alpha, Beta and Gamma thrombin. In *Chemistry and Biology of*

Thrombin. Lundblad R.L., Fenton J.W. & Mann, K.G. (eds). pp. 91–6. Ann Arbor Science Publishers, Michigan.

Koppel G. (1966) Electron microscopic investigation of the shape of fibrinogen molecules: a model for certain proteins. *Nature* **212**, 1608–9.

Kudryk B.J., Collen D., Woods K.R. & Blombäck B. (1974) Evidence for localisation of polymerization sites in fibrinogen. *Journal of Biological Chemistry* **249**, 3322–5.

Kudryk B.J., Reuterby J. & Blombäck B. (1973) Adsorption of plasmic Fragment D to thrombin modified fibrinogen-Sepharose. *Thrombosis Research* **2**, 297–303.

Lanchantin G.F., Friedmann J.A. & Hart D.W. (1975) Two forms of human thrombin, isolation and characterisation. *Journal of Biological Chemistry* **248**, 5956–66.

Laudano A.P. & Doolittle R.F. (1978) Synthetic peptide derivatives which bind to fibrinogen and prevent the polymerization of fibrin monomers. *Proceedings of the National Academy of Science USA* **75**, 3085–9.

Laudano A.P. & Doolittle R.F. (1980) Studies on synthetic peptides that bind to fibrinogen and prevent fibrin polymerization. Structural requirements, numbers of binding sites and species differences. *Biochemistry* **19**, 1013–19.

Loewy A.G., Dunathan K., Kriel R. & Wolfinger H.L. Jr. (1961) Fibrinase. I. Purification of substrate and enzyme. *Journal of Biological Chemistry* **236**, 2625.

Lorand L. & Jacobsen A. (1958) Studies of the polymerization of fibrin. The role of the globular: fibrin stabilising factor. *Journal of Biological Chemistry* **230**, 420.

McKee P.A., Mattock P. & Hill R.L. (1970) Subunit structure of human fibrinogen, soluble fibrin, and cross-linked insoluble fibrin. *Proceedings of the National Academy of Sciences USA* **66**, 738–44.

Marder V.J. (1971) Identification and purification of fibrinogen degradation products produced by plasmin considerations on the structure of fibrinogen. *Scandinavian Journal of Haematology Supplement* **13**, 21–6.

Robbins K.C. (1944) A study on the conversion of fibrinogen to fibrin. *American Journal of Physiology* **142**, 581.

Schwartz M.L., Pizzo S.V., Hill R.L. & McKee P.A. (1973) Human factor XIII from plasma and platelets. *Journal of Biological Chemistry* **248**, 1395–407.

Watt K.W.K., Takagi T. & Doolittle R.F. (1979) Amino acid sequence of the β chain of human fibrinogen. *Biochemistry* **18**, 68–76.

Workman E.F., Lawrence C.U., Kingdon H.S. & Lundblad R.L. (1977) Isolation and characterization of bovine thrombin. In *Chemistry and Biology of Thrombin*. Lundblad R.L., Fenton J.W. & Mann K.G. (eds). pp. 23–42. Ann Arbor Science Publishers, Michigan.

Chapter 3
Prothrombin and Related Proteins

M. P. ESNOUF

As a result of the pioneering work of Schmidt (1872) and Morawitz (1905), the so-called classical theory of blood coagulation evolved. In this scheme, prothrombin was considered to be a hypothetical substance which gave rise to thrombin during coagulation. Further support for this idea came from the work of Mellanby (1909, 1933) who isolated from plasma a substance which, although it had no coagulant activity, could be converted into an active coagulant resembling thrombin. These observations were extended by Eagle (1935) and Seegers (1940) who showed not only that thrombin was an enzyme, but the amount formed depended on the amount of prothrombin present. Since the original work of Seegers and his colleagues (see Seegers 1962), the techniques for the isolation of proteins have become much more sophisticated and, with benefit of hindsight, it is clear that the early preparations of prothrombin also contained not only the other vitamin K-dependent proteins (Factors IX, X, and VII) but also the more recently discovered vitamin K-dependent anticoagulant proteins. This latter group of proteins will be described in a later section in this Chapter together with a brief summary of the current ideas on the mode of action of vitamin K.

Isolation of vitamin K-dependent proteins

Prothrombin is present in plasma at a concentration of about 150 mg/l. It is a glycoprotein (mol.wt 70 000) containing about 7 per cent carbohydrate. Prothrombin has been purified from the plasma of a number of species, but for the present purpose only the procedures for human and bovine prothrombin will be considered. The methods currently in use start with the bulk absorption of the vitamin K-dependent proteins on barium citrate, followed by elution with citrate or EDTA buffers coupled with the decomposition of the barium citrate to the insoluble sulphate and precipitation of the high molecular weight proteins by the addition of ammonium sulphate (30 per cent saturation). The vitamin K-dependent proteins are recovered from the supernatant by raising the ammonium sulphate concentration to 65 per cent saturation. A preliminary separation of these proteins can then be achieved by chromatography on an anion exchanger, usually DEAE-Sephadex or DEAE-Sepharose.

The prothrombin-rich fractions obtained by this method can be used as the starting point for the preparation of all the human vitamin K-dependent proteins. In the case of the bovine proteins, factor X and Protein Z are well separated from the prothrombin peak and can be obtained substantially pure on the first chromatographic separation. The other bovine vitamin K-dependent proteins can be recovered from the prothrombin containing fractions as follows: Protein S, which is eluted on the leading edge of the prothrombin peak during DEAE-Sepharose chromatography, is recovered from the prothrombin-rich fractions after the removal of the other vitamin K-dependent proteins by passage down a blue dextran-Sepharose column (Stenflo and Jönsson 1979). Factor VII, which is eluted immediately after the fractions containing maximum prothrombin activity, can be separated by chromatography on benzamidine-Sepharose and is further purified by preparative gel electrophoresis (Kisiel and Davie 1975). If the single chain form of the protein is required, the blood should be collected in heparin, benzamidine hydrochloride and soya bean trypsin inhibitor in addition to the citrate anticoagulant. Factor IX, which is eluted in fractions which partially overlap the factor VII, can be separated by chromatography on heparin-Sepharose (Fujikawa *et al.* 1973). Protein C, which is eluted on the tail of the prothrombin-containing fractions is further purified by rechromatography on QAE-Sephadex (Stenflo 1976).

In the case of human prothrombin, the vitamin K-dependent proteins are recovered from DEAE-Sephadex in a different order (Di Scipio *et al.* 1977). Human Protein C can be isolated from the other proteins by chromatography on dextran sulphate agarose (Kisiel 1979) and preparative electrophoresis. Dextran-sulphate has been used by Pepper and Prowse (1977) to resolve human prothrombin, factor X and factor IX present in prothrombin concentrates. Human factor VII can be obtained from citrate eluates by chromatography and rechromatography on QAE-Sephadex followed by gel filtration. Factor VII is eluted in this system before the other vitamin K-dependent proteins (Broze and Majerus 1980).

Prothrombin

The past ten years have seen the rapid accumulation of detailed knowledge concerning the chemical and physical properties of prothrombin. The primary amino acid sequence and secondary structure is known (Fig. 11) (Magnusson *et al.* 1975). Prothrombin contains 582 amino acid residues and three carbohydrate chains which are attached to Asn^{77}, Asn^{101} and Asn^{376}. The individual chains have been sequenced (Mizuochi *et al.* 1979) and three different chain structures have been found which are terminated in N-acetyl sialic acid. It has also been shown that ten glutamic acid residues present in the

N-terminal region are further carboxylated on the γ-carbon by a post-translational process dependent on vitamin K (see later).

The structure of prothrombin has been subdivided into three regions defined by the primary thrombin and factor Xa cleavage points. Fragment 1 extends from the N-terminus to Arg[156] which is a thrombin cleavage point. The rest of the molecule from Ser[157] to the C-terminus is called prethrombin 1. Fragment 2 commences at Ser[157] and finishes at Arg[274] which is at the first position cleaved by factor Xa. The remainder of the molecule which is the single-chain precursor of thrombin is called prethrombin 2. Cleavage of the bond Arg[323]-Ser[324] by Xa, between the A and B chains of thrombin, gives the two-chain enzyme thrombin.

The secondary structures of Fragment 1 and 2 possess a unique triple-looped (Kringle) structure, which suggests that during the evolution of the protein, gene duplication has taken place. This idea is further supported by the fact that there is a considerable sequence homology in the two regions. In spite of these similarities, the Fragment 1 and Fragment 2 domains of prothrombin have different functions in the assembly of the prothrombin converting complex. Fragment 1 contains the high affinity and low affinity calcium binding sites (see later) which are essential for the rapid conversion of prothrombin. Fragment 2 provides the site for the interaction of prothrombin with factor V.

The B chain of thrombin contains the reactive serine (Ser[528]) and exhibits considerable sequence homology with the pancreatic proteases, but differs from them in that it contains carbohydrate attached to an asparagine residue (Asn[376]) and contains only three disulphide loops compared to four in the pancreatic enzymes. At present, the function, if any, of the A chain of thrombin remains obscure.

Recently, the biosynthesis of prothrombin has received some attention and five precursors have been identified in extracts of cultures of rat hepatoma cells supplied with tritiated leucine (Graves, Grabau and Munns 1980). These precursors with isoelectric points of 6.7, 7.2, 6.2, 5.8 and 5.5 all have apparent molecular weights close to mature prothrombin. The addition of vitamin K to these cultures reduces the level of the pI 6.7 species relative to the other intermediates, suggesting that the change in pI from 6.7 to 7.2 is associated with carboxylation. It is possible that conversion of a species with a pI 5.8 to 5.5 corresponds to the addition of sialic acid, to terminate the carbohydrate side-chains. The significance of the other intermediates is not clear. Prothrombin synthesis in cell-free systems has been achieved by MacGillivray, Chung and Davie (1980) using reticulocyte lysates and mRNA, enriched for prothrombin, obtained from bovine liver polysomes. The prothrombin obtained in this way contains a 23-residue signal peptide attached to the N-terminus. The nucleotide sequence of a cDNA clone, which

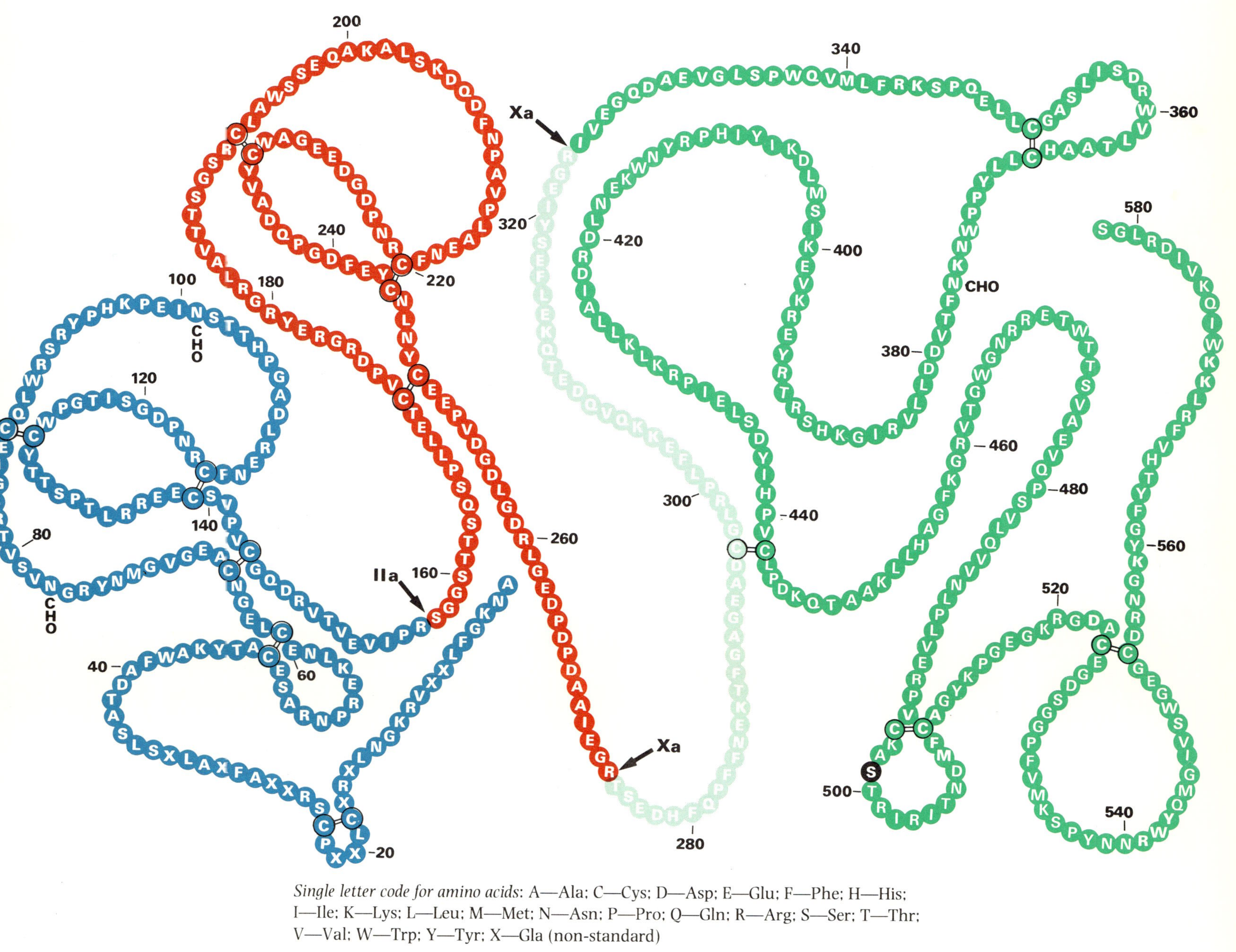

Single letter code for amino acids: A—Ala: C—Cys: D—Asp: E—Glu; F—Phe; H—His:
I—Ile; K—Lys; L—Leu; M—Met; N—Asn; P—Pro; Q—Gln; R—Arg; S—Ser; T—Thr;
V—Val; W—Trp; Y—Tyr; X—Gla (non-standard)

was obtained by reverse transcription to an enriched mRNA preparation, corresponding to prothrombin residues 433–582, confirms the amino acid sequence, except for the inversion of Asn^{506}-Asp^{507} residues (MacGillivray *et al.* 1980). An approach such as this with a cDNA clone coding for the entire prothrombin sequence will enable the exploration of the prothrombin gene. While clinically this will be of little importance, this approach will be invaluable in investigating the treatment of factor IX deficiency.

Studies on the three-dimensional structure of prothrombin have begun. Tsernoglou *et al.* (1974) have grown crystals of bovine thrombin but so far no useful information on the structure has been obtained. However, work on the structure of Fragment 1 (Aschaffenberg *et al.* 1977) has now yielded data at 0.6nm with every prospect of going to 0.3nm resolution.

The action of vitamin K

The biosynthesis of prothrombin requires vitamin K, for in the absence of vitamin K or in the presence of vitamin K antagonists, a species of prothrombin is present in plasma which has little or no biological activity. This abnormal prothrombin has an identical amino acid and carbohydrate composition with the normal protein except that the ten γ-carboxyglutamic acid residues (X in Fig. 11) are replaced by glutamic acid (Stenflo *et al.* 1974, Magnusson *et al.* 1975).

The carboxylation of these glutamic acid residues is a post-translational event and is dependent on vitamin K; unlike other biological carboxylation reactions there is no requirement for biotin or high energy phosphate. The only requirements are reduced vitamin K, molecular oxygen and carbon dioxide plus an enzyme present in rat liver microsomes (Olson and Suttie 1977). The mechanism by which the carbon dioxide is added to the γ-carbon is not clear, and has been the subject of much speculation. The carboxylation reaction is accompanied by the formation of vitamin K epoxide (Sadowski, Schnoes and Suttie 1977), but it has not been established whether carboxylation requires the formation of the epoxide. Esnouf *et al.* (1982) have found that the exposure of reduced vitamin K in 80 per cent aqueous ethanol to oxygen results in the production of vitamin K epoxide, and that during the course of this reaction two radical species of the vitamin are generated, the semiquinone and peroxyl radicals. It is suggested that the latter radical is the species of vitamin K active in carboxylation, since it should be able to withdraw a hydrogen atom from the γ-carbon of glutamic acid forming a glutamyl radical which will react directly with carbon dioxide. Attempts to find an activated carbon intermediate as opposed to the active glutamate have been unsuccessful and give further support for the mechanism based on activation of glutamic acid.

The vitamin K epoxide formed during carboxylation is recycled to the reduced form of vitamin K by the action of two enzymes, vitamin K epoxide reductase (Bell and Matschiner 1972) and vitamin K reductase (Märki and Martius 1961). In the presence of Coumarin-based drugs (oral anticoagulants) there is a selective inhibition of the vitamin K epoxide reductase (Sadowski and Suttie 1974), causing the accumulation of vitamin K epoxide at the expense of vitamin K, thereby creating a functional vitamin K deficiency. Esnouf and Prowse (1977) have shown that during oral anticoagulant therapy in humans, and in cattle receiving an equivalent dose of warfarin, about 70 per cent of the plasma prothrombin contains only seven γ-carboxyglutamic acid residues and this change was accompanied by a considerable lowering of the specific activity of the prothrombin. In the case of the abnormal bovine prothrombin, only one glutamic acid residue in each of the γ-carboxyglutamic acid pairs was carboxylated.

This seemingly minor modification of ten glutamic acid residues has a marked effect on the rate at which prothrombin is converted to thrombin by physiological activators, and is due to a failure of the abnormal prothrombin to bind calcium ions. Calcium ions have been recognized as being essential for blood coagulation for almost 100 years (Arthus and Pages 1890), but their function is only now being investigated in detail. In the case of the vitamin K-dependent proteins much of the work has been carried out with prothrombin or more particularly the Fragment 1 region, which contains a majority of the metal ion-binding sites of prothrombin. Calcium binding to Fragment 1 has been studied by a variety of techniques, and while some laboratories have reported that the metal is bound with positive cooperativity, others interpret their results as showing negative cooperativity. Jackson (1980), commenting on these disparate results, points out that the experiments carried out by different laboratories were conducted at different protein concentrations and that the observed spectral changes which were attributed to a conformational change of the protein could be accounted for, to a large extent, by self-association of the Fragment 1. However, Nelsestuen *et al.* (1980) have studied calcium binding to prothrombin, which at neutral pH did not exhibit significant self-association. They conclude that prothrombin contains ten metal binding sites, six of which are present in the Fragment 1 region and that following the addition of calcium ions there is a conformational change in the protein which cannot be attributed to self-association.

It is possible that the conformational change induced by Ca^{2+} causes the protein to bind more readily to phospholipid and interact with the other components of the prothrombinase complex.

Proteins C, S and Z

Three plasma proteins have been isolated from plasma which, like the prothrombin, depend on vitamin K for their synthesis. These proteins do not have any coagulant activity but at least one of them, Protein C, antagonizes the coagulation system. Protein C was first described by Stenflo (1976) who showed that it was a two-chain protein having a light chain (mol.wt 21 000) and heavy chain (mol.wt 42 000).

Following exposure to thrombin, trypsin or the coagulant protein from Russell's viper venom, Protein C is converted to an enzyme with the loss of an activation peptide (mol.wt 17 000) from the N-terminus of the heavy chain. This chain contains the reactive serine residue, while the vitamin K-dependent region is contained in the light chain. Activated Protein C inactivates factor V (Kisiel *et al.* 1977) and factor VIII (Vehar and Davie 1980), both these reactions being potentiated by phospholipid and calcium ions. The physiological significance of the destruction of factors V and VIII by activated Protein C was initially hard to assess, since the rate of activation of Protein C by thrombin is relatively low. However, the recent finding that there is an endothelial cell cofactor (Owen and Esmon 1981), which enhances the rate of Protein C activation some 20 000-fold, would indicate that *in vivo* Protein C is very important in regulating coagulation. This view is substantiated by the report (Marlar and Griffin 1980) of a combined factor V and factor VIII deficiency in patients which exhibit a simple autosomal recessive inheritance, which would be difficult to explain on a genetic basis. The plasmas of these patients contain normal levels of both factor V and factor VIII antigens. This apparent deficiency can be related to the absence of an inhibitor of activated Protein C which is present in normal plasma. These authors have partially purified the inhibitor and have shown that its activity is destroyed by trypsin digestion.

The action of activated Protein C on factor V is apparently stimulated (Walker 1980) by a second protein, Protein S, which like Protein C, is vitamin K-dependent and has been isolated both from human and bovine plasma as a single-chain polypeptide (mol.wt 65 000) (Kisiel 1979, Stenflo and Jönsson 1979). Incubation of Protein S with a variety of proteolytic enzymes does not yield an active enzyme. The only function for this protein which has been reported is the potentiation of factor V inactivation by Protein C. As with the other vitamin K-dependent proteins the effect of Protein S is only seen in the presence of phospholipid. A small proportion of the Protein S isolated from barium citrate eluates of bovine plasma is associated with the C_{4b} binding protein (Dahlbäck and Stenflo 1981); the functional significance of this complex is uncertain at present.

A third vitamin K-dependent protein, Protein Z, has been isolated from bovine plasma (Prowse and Esnouf 1977), and the N-terminal region has been sequenced (Petersen *et al.* 1980). The amino acid sequence of the first residues of all the plasma vitamin K-dependent proteins (Table 2) shows a high degree

Table 2. N-terminal sequence of bovine vitamin K-dependent proteins. (LC=light chain, Gla=γ-carboxy-glutamic acid.)

Protein	1 2 3 4 5 6 7 8 9 10 11 12 13 14	Reference
Prothrombin	Ala-Asn-Lys -Gly -Phe-Lue-Gla-Gla-Val -Arg-Lys -Gly-Asn-Leu-	Magnusson *et al.* (1975)
Factor X (LC)	Ala-Asn-Ser - Phe-Leu-Gla-Gla-Val -Lys -Gln -Gly-Asn-Leu-	Thøgersen *et al.* (1978)
Factor IX	Tyr-Asn-Ser -Gly -Lys -Leu-Gla-Gla-Phe-Val -Arg-Gly-Asn-Leu-	Katayama *et al.* (1979)
Factor VII	Ala-Asn- Gly -Phe-Leu- ? - ? -Leu -Leu -Pro -Gly-Ser -Leu-	Kisiel & Davie (1975)
Protein C (LC)	Ala-Asn-Ser - Phe-Leu-Gla-Gla-Leu -Arg-Pro -Gly-Asn-Val -	Stenflo (1976)
Protein S	Ala-Asn-Thr- Leu -Leu-Gla-Gla-Thr-Lys -Lys -Gly-Asn-Leu-	Stenflo & Jönsson (1979)
Protein Z	Ala-Gly -Ser -Tyr-Leu -Leu-Gla-Gla-Leu -Phe-Gla -Gly- X -Leu-	Petersen *et al.* (1980)

of homology in this region. At present the function of Protein Z is obscure. It is not activated by thrombin or by the coagulant protein from Russell's viper venom and it does not appear to act as a cofactor for the inactivation of the coagulation factors.

Conversion of prothrombin to thrombin

The conversion of prothrombin by the action of factor Xa, in the presence of factor V, phospholipid and Ca^{2+} is a complex process and is complicated by a number of parallel reactions; for clarity, they will be considered separately. First there is the cleavage of prothrombin by Xa. This is a two-step process involving the cleavage of prothrombin initially between Arg^{274} and Thr^{275} (see Fig. 11) giving Fragment 1.2 and prethrombin 2 (Esmon, Owen and Jackson 1974). This first step does not give rise to coagulant activity and in spite of the cleavage of the peptide bond, the two products associate in a non-covalent fashion. When they are electrophoresed on a polyacrylamide gel they have the same mobility as the parent prothrombin rather than migrating as separate components. This association is essential for the rapid cleavage of the second site of prothrombin at Arg^{323}-Ile^{324} between the A and B chains of thrombin, which is accompanied by the appearance of enzymic activity. The A and B chains of thrombin are joined by a disulphide bridge between Cys^{296} and Cys^{442}. This association between the two halves of the prothrombin molecule not only retains the prethrombin 2 in the prothrombin-converting complex, but also may enable the substrate to reorientate itself to facilitate the cleavage of the second peptide bond.

A complicating feature of this interaction is that the thrombin which is formed cleaves prothrombin between Arg^{156} and Ser^{157} forming Fragment 1 and prethrombin 1. Prethrombin 1 is a poor substrate for the prothrombin-converting complex since it has lost the vitamin K-dependent region and does not undergo the calcium mediated reaction. In addition, the Fragment 1 competes with the uncleaved prothrombin for the calcium mediated binding site. The net result of this is the inhibition of prothrombin conversion. In practice, in experiments where purified reagents are used, only about 30 per cent of the prothrombin is converted to thrombin. It seems that in plasma very little of the prothrombin is degraded to prethrombin 1 and Fragment 1, since at least 90 per cent of the prothrombin is converted to Fragment 1.2 (Aronson *et al.* 1977). A comprehensive review of these reactions with an extensive bibliography has been made by Suttie and Jackson (1977).

In the case of human prothrombin in which Lys^{288} is replaced by an Arg residue, there is a second thrombin cleavage point, resulting in the removal of the first 13 residues from the N-terminus of the A chain (Lanchantin,

Friedman and Hart 1975). It is unlikely that the activity of the thrombin is modified by this second cleavage.

The rate of conversion of prothrombin by factor Xa in the presence of Ca^{2+} is relatively slow. On the addition of phospholipid, the rate is stimulated *c.* 50-fold. If factor Va is added without lipid, the reaction is enhanced *c.* 350-fold. However, on adding both phospholipid and factor Va together, the rate of thrombin generation is increased *c.* 20 000-fold. The stimulation of human prothrombin activation by human protein is almost identical to that seen with bovine proteins (Jackson and Nemerson 1980). If the phospholipid is replaced by activated platelets and the clotting factor concentrations are unchanged, prothrombin conversion is increased *c.* 100 000-fold. This suggests that the assembly of the proteins on the platelet surface may be mediated by both lipid sites and by protein receptor sites. As evidence of this, Bloom *et al.* (1979) have shown that although phospholipid vesicles bind inactive factor V (k_d 7.2×10^{-8} M) more strongly than factor Va (k_d 4.4×10^{-7} M), there are approximately three times the number of binding sites for factor Va. The presence of factor Va on the lipid vesicles surface increases the affinity of factor Xa for the vesicles from k_d 2.5×10^{-6} M (without factor V) to $k_d \sim 5 \times 10^{-10}$ M and the ratio of factor Xa to factor Va on the vesicle surface is close to unity (Nesheim *et al.* 1980).

The binding of factor Va to bovine platelets, on the other hand, is considerably tighter ($k_d \sim 2 \times 10^{-10}$ M) than to phospholipid vesicles (Tracy, Nesheim and Mann 1981). Kane and Majerus (1982), comparing the results they obtained with those of Tracy, Nesheim and Mann (1981), conclude that the affinity of bovine factor Xa for bovine platelets is 10- to 20-fold less than that of human factor Xa for human platelets and that in the bovine system some of the factor Xa is bound non-productively. Bovine platelets would appear to have the same number of factor Xa and factor V binding sites, whereas in the case of human platelets there are more factor Va binding sites than factor Xa binding sites. The binding of bovine factor Va to bovine platelets is unaffected by prothrombin and factor Xa, in contrast to the human system in which both proteins stimulate the binding of factor Va to the platelets. For these reasons Kane and Majerus (1982) suggest that the bovine system may not be an appropriate model for understanding the role of human platelets in coagulation.

One further aspect of the interaction of factor Xa and factor Va on the platelet surface is the protective effect of factor Xa against the proteolysis of factor Va by Protein C_A (Dahlbäck and Stenflo 1980). In a model system using phospholipid vesicles and bovine proteins, factor Xa again protected factor Va but prothrombin added at the same concentration as factor Va had no protective effect (Nesheim *et al.* 1982). This demonstrates a clear difference in the relationship of the two factors for factor Va. The Protein C_A-mediated degradation of factor Va may be an important control mechanism *in vivo* in human plasma, because more factor Va is bound to the platelet surface than factor Xa, and is thus unprotected from the action of Protein C_A.

REFERENCES

Aronson D.L., Stevan L., Ball A.P., Franza B.R. Jr. & Finlayson J.S. (1977) Generation of the combined prothrombin activation peptide (F1:2) during the clotting of blood and plasma. *Journal of Clinical Investigation* **60**, 1410–18.

Arthus M. & Pages C. (1890) Nouvelle théorie chimique de la coagulation de sang. *Archives de Physiologie Normale et de Pathologie.* Séries 5, **2**, 739–46.

Aschaffenberg R., Blake C.C.F., Burridge J.M. & Esnouf M.P. (1977) Preliminary X-ray investigation of Fragment 1 of bovine prothrombin. *Journal of Molecular Biology* **114**, 575.

Bell R.G. & Matschiner J.R. (1972) Warfarin and the inhibition of vitamin K activity by an oxide metabolite. *Nature* **237**, 32.

Bloom J.W., Neshiem M.E. & Mann K.G. (1979) Phospholipid—binding properties of bovine factor V and factor Va. *Biochemistry* **18**, 4419–25.

Broze G.J. & Majerus P.W. (1980) Purification and properties of human coagulation factor VII. *Journal of Biological Chemistry* **255**, 1242.

Dahlbäck B. & Stenflo J. (1980) Inhibitory effect of activated Protein C in activation of prothrombin by platelet-bound factor X_a. *European Journal of Biochemistry* **107**, 331–5.

Dahlbäck B. & Stenflo J. (1981) High molecular weight complex in human plasma between vitamin K-dependent Protein S and complement C_{4b}-binding protein. *Proceedings of the National Academy of Sciences of the USA* **78**, 2512–16.

Di Scipio R.G., Hermodson M.A., Yates G.G. & Davie E.W. (1977) A comparison of human prothrombin, Factor IX (Christmas Factor), Factor X (Stuart Factor) and Protein S. *Biochemistry* **16**, 698.

Eagle H. (1935) Studies on blood coagulation. II. The formation of thrombin and fibrinogen. *Journal of General Physiology* **18**, 547.

Esmon C.T., Owen W.G. & Jackson C.M. (1974) A plausible mechanism for prothrombin activation by Factor X_a, Factor V_a, phospholipid and Ca^{++}. *Journal of Biological Chemistry* **249**, 8045–7.

Esnouf M.P., Gainey A.I., Hill H.A.O. & Thornalley P.J. (1982) The carboxylation of Preprothrombin. In *Inflammatory Diseases and Copper.* J.R.J. Sorensen (ed.). pp. 209–20. Humana Press, Clifton, New Jersey.

Esnouf M.P. & Prowse C.V. (1977) The γ carboxyglutamic acid content of human and bovine prothrombin following warfarin treatment. *Biochimica et Biophysica Acta* **490**, 471.

Fujikawa K., Thompson A.R., Legaz M.E., Meyer R.G. & Davie E.W. (1973) Isolation and characterization of bovine factor IX (Christmas Factor). *Biochemistry* **12**, 4938.

Graves C.B., Grabau C.G. & Munns T.W. (1980) Biosynthesis and processing of precursor prothrombins. In *Vitamin K Metabolism and Vitamin K-Dependent Proteins.* Suttie J.W. (ed.). p. 529. University Park Press, Baltimore.

Jackson C.M. (1980) Cooperativity of calcium binding to bovine prothrombin, prothrombin fragment 1, and Factor X. An alternative to conformational changes for explaining such behaviour. In *Vitamin K Metabolism and Vitamin K-Dependent Proteins*. Suttie J.W. (ed.). p. 16. University Park Press, Baltimore.

Jackson C.M. & Nemerson Y. (1980) Blood coagulation. *Annual Review of Biochemistry* **49**, 765–811.

Kane W.H. & Majerus P.W. (1982) The interaction of human coagulation Factor V_a with platelets. *Journal of Biological Chemistry* **257**, 3963–9.

Katayama K., Ericsson L.H., Enfield D.L., Walsh K.A., Neurath H., Davie E.W. & Titani K. (1979) Comparison of amino acid sequence of bovine coagulation Factor IX (Christmas Factor) with that of other vitamin K-dependent plasma proteins. *Proceedings of the National Academy of Sciences of the USA* **76**, 4990–4.

Kisiel W. (1979) Human plasma Protein C. *Journal of Clinical Investigation* **64**, 761.

Kisiel W., Canfield W.M., Ericsson L.H. & Davie E.W. (1977) Anticoagulant properties of bovine plasma Protein C following activation by thrombin. *Biochemistry* **16**, 5824–30.

Kisiel W. & Davie E.W. (1975) Isolation and characterisation of bovine Factor VII. *Biochemistry* **14**, 4928.

Lanchantin G.F., Friedman J.A. & Hart D.W. (1975) Two forms of human thrombin, isolation and characterisation. *Journal of Biological Chemistry* **244**, 865–75.

MacGillivray R.T.A., Chung D.W. & Davie E.W. (1980) Biosynthesis of bovine prothrombin in a cell free system. In *Vitamin K Metabolism and Vitamin K-Dependent Proteins*. Suttie J.W. (ed.). p. 546. University Park Press, Baltimore.

MacGillivray R.T.A., Friezner Degen S.J., Chandra T., Woo T.C. & Davie E.W. (1980) Cloning and analysis of a cDNA coding for bovine prothrombin. *Proceedings of the National Academy of Sciences of the USA* **77**, 5153.

Magnusson S., Petersen T.E., Sottrup-Jensen L. & Claeys H. (1975) Complete primary structure of prothrombin: isolation, structure and reactivity of ten γ carboxylated glutamic acid residues and regulation of prothrombin activation by thrombin. In *Proteases and Biological Control*. Reich E., Rifkin D.B. & Shaw E. (eds). Cold Spring Harbor Conference on Cell Proliferation **2**, 123.

Märki F. & Martius C. (1961) Vitamin K-reductasen aus rinds-und rattenleber. *Biochemische Zeitschrift* **334**, 293.

Marlar R.A. & Griffin J.H. (1980) Deficiency of Protein C inhibitor in combined Factor V/VIII deficiency disease. *Journal of Chemical Investigation* **66**, 1186–9.

Mellanby J. (1909) The coagulation of the blood. *Journal of Physiology* **38**, 28, 441.

Mellanby J. (1933) Thrombase: its preparation and properties. *Proceedings of the Royal Society (London), Series B* **113**, 93.

Mizuochi T., Yamashita K., Fujikawa K., Kisiel W. & Kobata A. (1979) The carbohydrate of bovine prothrombin. *Journal of Biological Chemistry* **254**, 6419.

Morawitz P. (1905) Die chemie der blutgerrinung. *Ergebnisse der Physiologie* **4**, 307.

Nelsestuen G.L., Resnick R.M., Wei J., Fletcher C.H. & Bloomfield V.A. (1980) Cation interactions with bovine prothrombin and prothrombin fragment 1. Stoichiometry of binding, self-association and conformational charge. In *Calcium Binding Proteins: Structure and Function*. Siegel F.G., Carafoli E., Kretsinger R.H., MacLennan D.H. & Wasserman R.H. (eds). p. 433. Elsevier North Holland, New York.

Nesheim M.E., Canfield N.M., Kisiel W. & Mann K.G. (1982) Studies of the capacity of factor Xa to protect factor Va from inactivation by activated Protein C. *Journal of Biological Chemistry* **257**, 1443–7.

Olson R.E. & Suttie J.W. (1977) Vitamin K and γ carboxyglutamate biosynthesis. *Vitamins and Hormones* **35**, 59.

Owen W.G. & Esmon C.T. (1981) Functional properties of an endothelial cell cofactor for the thrombin catalysed activation of Protein C. *Journal of Biological Chemistry* **256**, 5532–5.

Pepper D.S. & Prowse C.V. (1977) Chromatography of human prothrombin complex on dextran-sulphate agarose. *Thrombosis Research* **11**, 687.

Petersen T.E., Thøgersen H.C., Sottrup-Jensen L., Magnusson S. & Jörnvall H. (1980) Isolation and N-terminal amino acid sequence of Protein Z, a γ carboxyglutamic acid containing protein from bovine plasma. *FEBS Letters* **114**, 278–82.

Prowse C.V. & Esnouf M.P. (1977) Isolation of a new Warfarin-sensitive protein from bovine plasma. *Biochemical Society, Transactions* **5**, 255–6.

Sadowski J.A., Schnoes H.K. & Suttie J.W. (1977) Vitamin K epoxidase: Properties and relationship to prothrombin synthesis. *Biochemistry* **16**, 56.

Sadowski J.A. & Suttie J.W. (1974) Mechanism of action of coumarins. Significance of Vitamin K. *Biochemistry* **13**, 3696.

Schmidt A. (1872) Ueber die Faserstoff gerinnung. *Pflüger's Archiv für die Gesamte Physiologie des Menschen und der Tiere* **6**, 413.

Seegers W.H. (1940) Purification of prothrombin and thrombin: chemical properties of purified preparations. *Journal of Biological Chemistry* **136**, 103.

Seegers W.H. (1962) *Prothrombin.* Harvard University Press, Cambridge, M.A.

Stenflo J. (1976) A new Vitamin K-dependent protein. *Journal of Biological Chemistry* **251**, 355.

Stenflo J., Fernlund P., Eagen W. & Roepstorf P. (1974) Modifications of glutamic acid residues in prothrombin. *Proceedings of the National Academy of Sciences of the USA* **71**, 2730.

Stenflo J. & Jönsson M. (1979) Protein S, a new vitamin K-dependent protein from bovine plasma. *FEBS Letters.* **101**, 377.

Suttie J.W. & Jackson C.M. (1977) Prothrombin structure, activation and biosynthesis. *Physiological Reviews* **57**, 1–70.

Thøgersen H.C., Petersen T.E., Sottrup-Jensen L., Magnusson S. & Morris H.R. (1978) The N-terminal sequences of blood coagulation factor X and X_2 light chain. *Biochemical Journal* **175**, 613.

Tracy P.B., Nesheim M.E. & Mann K.G. (1981) Coordinate binding of Factor V_a and Factor X_a to the unstimulated platelet. *Journal of Biological Chemistry* **256**, 743–51.

Tsernoglou D., Walz D.A., McCoy L.E. & Seegers W.H. (1974) An X-ray crystallographic study of thrombin. *Journal of Biological Chemistry* **249**, 999.

Vehar G.A. & Davie E.W. (1980) Preparation and properties of bovine Factor VIII (Antihemophilic Factor). *Biochemistry* **19**, 401–10.

Walker F.J. (1980) Regulation of activated Protein C by a new protein. *Journal of Biological Chemistry* **255**, 5521–4.

Chapter 4
Extrinsic Prothrombin Activation

M. P. ESNOUF

The potent coagulant activity of tissue extracts has been known since the time of Rauschenbach (1882) and Wooldridge (1893). It was thought, on the basis of the classical theory of blood coagulation, that these extracts contained a substance which converted prothrombin to thrombin. This substance was either called 'thrombokinase' (Morawitz 1905) implying it was an enzyme, or 'thromboplastin' (Howell 1912), which is a non-committal term. The erroneous assumption, made at the time, that tissue factor acted directly on prothrombin, stimulated many attempts to isolate the active constituent from these extracts. However, with the discovery of the plasma factors V, VII and X, it can be seen in retrospect that these experiments were bound to fail, along with the assumption that tissue factor acted directly on prothrombin.

The present view of the role of tissue factor is that it forms a complex with factor VII and the complex activates factor X. Activated factor X together with factor V and phospholipid converts prothrombin to thrombin. Evidence is accumulating which shows that the tissue factor: factor VII complex is also capable of activating factor IX, thus initiating an alternative pathway for factor X activation.

Tissue factor

From the time of Howell (1912) it was thought that tissue factor was a lipoprotein complex. The first clear demonstration of this was by Chargaff, Bendich and Cohen (1944) who purified a lipoprotein complex from beef lung, which had tissue factor activity. This work was extended by Stüder (1946) who dissociated the lipid and the protein components and showed them to be inactive on their own. When the two components were recombined, activity was restored.

Williams (1964, 1966) found that microsomal preparations from human placenta, brain and bovine lung had tissue factor activity. Each of these preparations contained a lipid and protein component which was essential for activity. Hvatum and Prydz (1966) dissolved the particulate tissue factor, obtained from bovine brain, in sodium desoxycholate and on gel filtration it yielded a lipid component and a protein component with an apparent molecular weight of 50 000. When the detergent was removed the lipid and protein components reassociated yielding full coagulant activity.

The protein component of tissue factor isolated from bovine lung by Pitlick *et al.* (1971) had a considerably higher apparent molecular weight (330 000–220 000) than the brain protein. This preparation, in addition to coagulant activity, also had amino peptidase activity, although the two activities could not be separated (Nemerson and Pitlick 1971); it was concluded that the peptidase activity was coincidental to the coagulant activity, a view which was confirmed by Nemerson and Esnouf (1973) who inhibited the amino peptidase activity with *o*-phenanthroline without affecting the coagulant activity. At the same time, Bjørklid, Storm and Prydz (1973) isolated from bovine brain the protein component of tissue factor, which was a single chain polypeptide with an apparent molecular weight of 53 000. This protein had no peptidase activity in the presence or absence of phospholipid. More recently, Nemerson *et al.* (1980) have purified tissue factor from bovine brain 70 000-fold using essentially the same procedure as used by Bjørklid, Storm and Prydz (1973), but including affinity chromatography on a column of immobilized rabbit antibovine tissue factor IgG antiserum, as a final step. This protein is a single-chain polypeptide with an apparent molecular weight of 45 000.

While it is evident that tissue factor is widely distributed in the body, it remains to be answered whether its function is confined solely to the activation of the extrinsic system. In this respect, Bjørklid *et al.* (1977) conclude that the distribution of tissue factor activity in the brain does not correlate well with the vascularity of the various regions of the brain, but is more abundant in phylogenetically older structures. They suggest that tissue factor may be a constituent of primitive cells.

Factor VII

Factor VII is the plasma protein which reacts with tissue factor to form the extrinsic factor X activator. It is a vitamin K-dependent protein (see Chapter 3) which has been isolated both from bovine plasma (Kisiel and Davie 1975, Radcliffe and Nemerson 1975) and from human plasma (Broze and Majerus 1980). The protein from both species is a single-chain polypeptide and contains *c.* 13 per cent carbohydrate. The molecular weight of the bovine protein is 45 000, while that from human plasma is 48 000. Considerable precautions have to be taken to prevent proteolysis during the purification of factor VII. If protease inhibitors are not used throughout, a two-chain form of the protein will be recovered. Unlike the zymogen forms of the other coagulation factors, bovine factor VII has an unusual reactivity towards diisopropyl fluorophosphate. The human protein, on the other hand, reacts at a much slower rate with this inhibitor.

Estimates of the concentration of factor VII in plasma range from 0.1 μg to 1 μg/ml of plasma. These are based on the increase in the specific activity obtained during purification.

Factor X

Bovine factor X was the first zymogen of a serine protease found to contain two polypeptide chains linked by disulphide bonds (Fujikawa *et al.* 1972a, Jackson 1972) and is present in plasma at a concentration of 10–15 μg/ml. It has a molecular weight of 56 000 and contains 10 per cent carbohydrate. The primary amino acid sequence of both the light chain (Enfield *et al.* 1975) and the heavy chain (Titani *et al.* 1975) have been determined.

The light chain (mol.wt 16 500) is composed of 140 amino acids and contains the vitamin K-dependent region (see Chapter 3) at its N-terminus. The heavy chain (mol.wt 39 300) has 307 amino acids and, in addition to the reactive site serine (Ser^{233}), it contains two carbohydrate chains attached to Asn^{35} and Thr^{300}. The majority of the carbohydrate (*c.* 85 per cent) is attached to the Asn^{35} residue which forms part of the activation peptide Trp^1-Arg^{51} (mol.wt 11 000). This peptide is released by the physiological activators of factor X and by the coagulant protein in Russell's viper venom (Fujikawa *et al.* 1972b, Radcliffe and Barton 1973, Jesty, Spencer and Nemerson 1974). The fact that the activation peptide contains carbohydrate has been made use of by Silverberg, Nemerson and Zur (1977), who selectively tritiated the sialic acid residues and followed the activation of factor X by the release of acid soluble radioactivity. This procedure is considerably more sensitive than other procedures for measuring factor X activation. In addition, it enables one to determine the rate of factor X activation in plasma samples.

A second peptide is also cleaved from the C-terminus of the heavy chain (Gly^{291}-Leu^{307}) by autolytic digestion in the presence of Ca^{2+} and phospholipid (Jesty, Spencer and Nemerson 1974). The loss of this peptide does not influence the enzymic activity of activated factor X.

Human factor X (mol.wt 58 900) differs from bovine factor X in that the heavy chain contains an additional 15–20 residues on the amino-terminal end (Di Scipio, Hermodson and Davie 1977), a higher carbohydrate content (15 per cent) and unlike bovine factor X is only recovered as one species. Various reasons have been advanced for the difference in the chromatographic behaviour of the two species of bovine factor X. Morita and Jackson (1979) suggest that the slightly more acidic nature of X_2 can be accounted for by the sulphation of Tyr^{18}. It is possible that factor X_2 could contain more γ-carboxyglutamic acid than factor X_1 (see Chapter 3). Thøgersen *et al.* (1978)

have shown, however, that in both species there are γ-carboxyglutamate residues at 12 positions. The occupancy of γ-carboxyglutamic acid may, nevertheless, be less than 100 per cent at some positions in X_1.

A further difference between factor X_1 and X_2 is that the specific coagulant activity of factor X_{1a} is 70 per cent of that of X_{2a}, whereas the esterase activity of both forms of activated factor X is identical (Ong and Esnouf 1979).

Interaction of tissue factor, factor VII and factor X

The activation of factor X by factor VII requires tissue factor and calcium ions. During this reaction there is a considerable increase in the coagulant activity of the factor VII, which is accompanied by the conversion of the single-chain protein to a two-chain from αVIIa (Radcliffe and Nemerson 1975). A similar change in factor VII is brought about by thrombin and factor XIIa (Kisiel Fujikawa and Davie 1977). The light chain (mol.wt 18 000) contains the vitamin K-dependent region and the heavy chain (mol.wt 27 000) possesses the serine active centre. Prolonged exposure of αVIIa to factor Xa results in the loss of a small peptide from the C-terminus of the heavy chain giving βVIIa, which has no coagulant activity (Radcliffe and Nemerson 1976).

The kinetic aspects of the activation of factor X by factor αVIIa and tissue factor have been investigated by Silverberg, Nemerson and Zur (1977) using the tritiated factor X assay. They found that αVIIa, in the presence of calcium, slowly activated factor X and at plasma concentrations of factor X (0.16 μM) the addition of tissue factor enhanced the rate of factor X activation 16 000-fold. Nemerson *et al.* (1980), in a detailed kinetic analysis of this reaction, suggest that the tissue factor combines with the enzyme, enhancing its reactivity, and that the lipid component has a dual role, firstly in forming the two protein complex and secondly combining with factor X, removing it from solution. This would explain the sensitivity of tissue factor activity to the type and the amount of phospholipid added to activate the protein.

Until recently it was thought that the only substrate for the tissue factor: factor VII complex was factor X. However, Østerud and Rapaport (1977) showed that the complex will also activate factor IX. Investigating this reaction more closely and using tritiated factor IX as the substrate, Morrison-Silverberg and Jesty (1981) have shown that the activation of factor IX by the tissue factor:factor VII complex was enhanced approximately 13-fold by the presence of Xa. They propose that the formation of the tissue factor: VII:Xa occurs very rapidly, with the consequent activation of the factor VII. This activation is reversible, since, on adding an irreversible inhibitor of Xa, the complex dissociates and the factor VII activity decreases. On prolonged exposure of the factor VII to Xa, two-chain factor αVIIa is formed, which has the same activity as the complex, and the factor Xa is lost from the complex. If factor VII is exposed to factor Xa in the absence of tissue factor an abortive complex is formed.

From the above it can be seen that not only is the initial phase of the extrinsic system complex, but it may also bypass the contact phase of the intrinsic system. It is too early at this stage to say whether tissue factor-mediated factor IX activation is of importance in the human coagulation system.

Factor V

As outlined in the previous chapter, the conversion of prothrombin by Xa is considerably accelerated by the addition of a third protein, factor V. The existence of this protein was first postulated by Nolf in 1908, who called it 'thrombogen'. However, it is only comparatively recently that homogeneous preparations of the protein have been available. Factor V is a glycoprotein with a single polypeptide chain (Esmon 1979, Nesheim *et al.* 1979) and a molecular weight of 330 000. Bartlett, Latson and Hanahan (1980) have reported that bovine factor V had a molecular weight closer to 10^6 as determined from gel filtration experiments. However, these differences in the estimates of the molecular weight may be apparent rather than real, because hydrodynamic studies have revealed that the protein is highly asymmetric which would account for the anomalous behaviour of the protein on gel filtration columns. The molecular weight of the protein (330 000) calculated from sedimentation equilibrium experiments (Mann, Nesheim and Tracy 1981) confirms the value deduced from electrophoresis. Factor V isolated from human plasma has similar physical properties to the bovine protein (Dahlbäck 1980, Kane and Majerus 1981, Katzmann *et al.* 1981).

The availability of the purified protein has enabled the various groups to investigate the well-known activation of factor V caused by thrombin. From these studies it is clear that in both human and bovine factor V, the increase in coagulant activity (35–50 fold) caused by exposure to thrombin is accompanied by proteolytic cleavages of the molecule as seen by polyacrylamide gel electrophoresis of the reduced protein in the presence of SDS. Although there are some differences between the human and bovine protein in the size of the intermediate peptides produced, the activation of factor V is accompanied by the formation of a peptide with a molecular weight in the range 91 000 to 73 000. The factor V activator from Russell's viper venom also yields a fragment of the same size.

The involvement of Ca^{2+} in maintaining the structural integrity of the factor V has long been suspected and recently Hibbard and Mann (1980) have shown that factor V has two classes of Ca^{2+} binding sites, one high affinity binding site ($k_d < 10^{-8}$ M) and two low affinity sites ($k_d = 6 \times 10^{-5}$ M). The loss of factor V activity on exposure to EDTA corresponds to the removal of the Ca^{2+} ion from the high affinity site. It is likely that this site is retained in factor Va since EDTA dissociates the light chain (mol.wt 85 000) from the heavy chain (mol.wt 180 000), which can be separated by gel filtration. These chains will recombine when incubated with calcium and the coagulant activity is restored (Esmon 1979). From the above, it would appear that the activation of factor V involves the cleavage of the single-chain polypeptide (mol.wt 330 000) into a heavy chain (mol.wt 200 000–180 000) and a light chain (mol.wt 91 000–73 000) which are associated non-covalently in a domain, the integrity of which is maintained by the high affinity calcium binding site.

Purified factor Va preparations are relatively stable even in the presence of thrombin, in contrast to factor V activity in plasma after the addition of thrombin. This difference in behaviour can be ascribed to the presence of a recently described vitamin K-dependent protease, Protein C (Stenflo 1976). This protein, present in plasma, is a two-chain zymogen (see Chapter 3) and is converted to a serine protease by thrombin. Walker, Sexton and Esmon (1979) have shown that Protein C_A rapidly inactivates factor Va, but if preincubated with factor V does not alter the degree to which factor V can be activated. The inactivation of factor Va is the result of the proteolysis of both the heavy and light chains. The presence of phospholipid greatly stimulates the action of Protein C_A but is not obligatory. Factor Va is protected from the action of Protein C_A by the presence of factor Xa, but not by factor X.

The activation of Protein C by thrombin, the only known physiological activator, is a relatively slow process, so much so that it called into question the significance of this pathway in the physiological regulation of coagulation. However, recently Esmon, Owen and Esmon (1982) have isolated a protein (mol.wt 73 600) from the endothelial membrane which accelerates the activation of Protein C by thrombin some 20 000-fold. The presence of this cofactor not only establishes the importance of the Protein C in controlling coagulation but also illustrates the importance of the vessel wall as a component of the coagulation system *in vivo*.

Phospholipid

The acceleration of the factor Xa cleavage of prothrombin by factor Va is only seen in the presence of phospholipid or platelets. Historically, platelets were thought to accelerate coagulation because they released phospholipid (Platelet factor 3) during coagulation. As a result, little attention was given to the platelet membrane and much less to the chemical nature of the clotting factor receptor sites. Much of the early interest in phospholipids came from the work of Rouser and Schloredt (1958) and Wallach *et al.* (1959), who showed that ethanolamine phosphatides were most active in accelerating the coagulation of platelet-poor plasma and postulated that this group of phospholipids formed micelles of a certain critical size and that this was controlled to a great extent by the degree of unsaturation of the fatty acids esterified to the glycerol. More recent studies have shown that the phospholipid particles which are most active in binding prothrombin and factor X are mixed micelles containing phosphatidyl serine (15 per cent) and phosphatidyl choline (35 per cent) (Nelsestuen and Broderius 1977). The interaction of these proteins with the phospholipid surface is calcium dependent. The role of calcium is two-fold, firstly, inducing an obligatory conformational change in the protein (see Chapter 3), and secondly, mediating the interaction between the protein and lipid. Nelsestuen (1980) considers that prothrombin and factor X are elliptical molecules and associate with the lipid surface at one tip, the protein molecules projecting radially into the solution. The inhibitory effect of acidic phospholipid surfaces is caused by non-calcium interactions, altering the orientation of the proteins with respect to each other so that they fail to react. The most important effect of the lipid in the assembly of the prothrombin-converting complex is its interaction with factor Va, which enhances the binding of factor Xa to the complex. The importance of factor Va in the binding of factor Xa is indicated by a comparison of the affinity of factor Xa for the phospholipid surface ($k_A = 1 \times 10^6$ M^{-1}) compared with the binding of factor Xa to factor Va on the platelet surface ($k_A = 3$ to 4×10^{10} M^{-1}) (Miletich, Jackson and Majerus 1978).

The extrinsic system

The interactions described in this and the previous chapter are illustrated in Fig. 12. The only clotting factor uniquely involved in the extrinsic system is factor VII; all the other interactions are embodied in the common pathway of both the extrinsic and intrinsic system. The one departure from the classical extrinsic system is the inclusion of the activation of factor IX by the factor VII:tissue factor complex.

The physiological significance of this pathway has not yet been assessed, but the introduction of the tritiated factor assay for measuring the rates of factor IX and factor X activation in plasma should prove most informative. The use of the tritiated factor assay will also enable the biochemist to investigate in great detail the physiological significance of the interactions already found in model systems using purified factors.

The series of reactions involving the activation and inactivation of factor V are examples of positive and negative feedback control. The activation of factor V by thrombin is a clear example of positive feedback where the product of an interaction stimulates the formation of the product. Negative feedback is achieved by the inactivation of factor V in a two-step reaction initiated by thrombin. The first step involves the thrombin activation of Protein C to

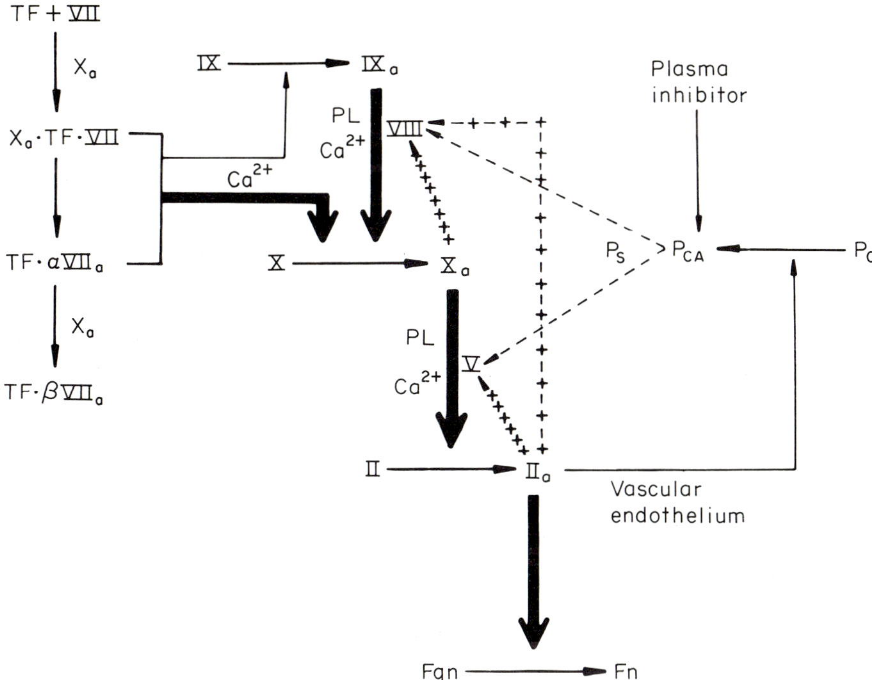

Fig. 12. The extrinsic coagulation system. Positive feedback is indicated $+ + +$ and negative feedback $- - -$. The action of thrombin on factor VIII is a combination of both activities $+ - +$.

Protein C_A, in the presence of the accelerator from the vascular endothelium. The second step is the proteolysis of factor Va, stimulated by phospholipid and an additional vitamin K-dependent protein, Protein S (Walker 1980) (see Chapter 3). Similarly, factor VIII is activated by thrombin or by Xa and inactivated by the Protein C system or by thrombin on its own.

The formation of the active complex between factor VII and Xa is a further example of positive feedback, whilst the conversion of αVIIa to βVIIa is negative feedback. In this way the coagulation system is not only able to amplify its response to the initial stimulus, but also can control the extent to which the factors are activated.

The presence of the two anticoagulant vitamin K-dependent proteins, Proteins C and S, which indirectly antagonize the coagulant vitamin K-dependent proteins, in a sense buffers the coagulation system against vitamin K deficiency or the action of oral anticoagulants. This, taken with the report that Protein C_A stimulates the release of plasminogen activator (Comp and Esmon 1980), does call for a re-examination of the effects of oral anticoagulant therapy.

REFERENCES

Bartlett S., Latson P. & Hanahan D.J. (1980) High molecular weight Factor V of bovine and human plasma. *Biochemistry* **19**, 273.

Bjørklid E., Storm E. & Prydz H. (1973) The protein component of human brain thromboplastin. *Biochemical and Biophysical Research Communications* **55**, 969.

Bjørklid E., Storm-Mathisen J., Storm E. & Prydz H. (1977) Localization of tissue thromboplastin in the human brain. *Thrombosis and Haemostasis* **37**, 91.

Broze G.J. & Majerus P.W. (1980) Purification and properties of human coagulation factor VII. *Journal of Biological Chemistry* **255**, 1242–7.

Chargaff E., Bendich A. & Cohen S.S. (1944) The thromboplastic protein; structure properties' disintegration. *Journal of Biological Chemistry* **156**, 161.

Comp P.C. & Esmon C.T. (1980) Evidence for multiple roles for activated Protein C in fibrinolysis. In *The Regulation of Coagulation*, Developments in Biochemistry, Vol. 8. Mann K.G. & Taylor F.B. (eds). p. 583. Elsevier-North Holland Pub. Co., New York.

Dahlbäck B. (1980) Human coagulation Factor V purification and thrombin catalysed activation. *Journal of Clinical Investigation* **66**, 583.

Di Scipio R.G., Hermodson M.A. & Davie E.W. (1977) Activation of human Factor X (Stuart Factor) by a protease from Russell's viper venom. *Biochemistry* **16**, 5253.

Enfield D.L., Ericsson L.H., Walsh K.A., Neurath H. & Titani K. (1975) Bovine Factor X_1 (Stuart Factor). Primary structure of the light chain. *Proceedings of the National Academy of Sciences of the USA* **72**, 16.

Esmon C.T. (1979) The subunit structure of thrombin activated Factor V. *Journal of Biological Chemistry* **254**, 964.

Esmon N.L., Owen W.G. & Esmon C.T. (1982) Isolation of a membrane-bound cofactor for thrombin catalysed activation of Protein C. *Journal of Biological Chemistry* **257**, 859–64.

Fujikawa K., Legaz M.E. & Davies E.W. (1972a) Bovine factors X_1 and X_2 (Stuart Factor) Isolation and characterization. *Biochemistry* **11**, 4882.

Fujikawa K., Legaz M.E. & Davie E.W. (1972b) Bovine factor X (Stuart Factor). Mechanism of activation by a protein from Russell's viper venom. *Biochemistry* **11**, 4892.

Hibbard L.S. & Mann K.G. (1980) The calcium binding properties of bovine Factor V. *Journal of Biological Chemistry* **255**, 638.

Howell W.H. (1912) The nature and action of the thromboplastic (zymoplastic) substance of the tissues. *American Journal of Physiology* **31**, 1.

Hvatum M. & Prydz H. (1966) Studies on tissue thromboplastin. I. Solubilization with sodium deoxycholate. *Biochimica et Biophysica Acta* **130**, 92.

Jackson C.M. (1972) Characterization of two glycoprotein variants of bovine Factor X and demonstration that the Factor X zymogen contains two polypeptide chains. *Biochemistry* **2**, 4873.

Jesty J., Spencer A.K. & Nemerson Y. (1974) The mechanism of activation of Factor X. *Journal of Biological Chemistry* **249**, 5614.

Kane W.H. & Majerus P.W. (1981) Purification and characterization of human coagulation Factor V. *Journal of Biological Chemistry* **256**, 1002.

Katzmann J.A., Nesheim M.E., Hibbard L.S. & Mann K.G. (1981) Isolation of functional human coagulation Factor V by using a hybridoma antibody. *Proceedings of the National Academy of Sciences of the USA* **78**, 162.

Kisiel W. & Davie E.W. (1975) Isolation and characterization of bovine Factor VII. *Biochemistry* **14**, 4928–34.

Kisiel W., Fujikawa K. & Davie E.W. (1977) Activation of bovine Factor VII (Proconvertin) by Factor XII_a (activated Hageman Factor). *Biochemistry* **16**, 4189.

Mann K.G., Nesheim M.E. & Tracy P.B. (1981) Molecular weight of undegraded plasma Factor V. *Biochemistry* **20**, 28.

Miletich J.P., Jackson C.M. & Majerus P.W. (1978) Properties of the Factor X_a binding site on human platelets. *Journal of Biological Chemistry* **253**, 6908.

Morawitz P. (1905) Die Chemie der Blutgerunning. *Ergebnisse der Physiologie, biologischen Chemie und experimentellen Pharmakologie* **4**, 307.

Morita T. & Jackson C.M. (1979) Bovine Factor X_1 and X_2: Activation peptide based chromatographic differences. In *Vitamin K Metabolism and Vitamin K-Dependent Proteins.* Suttie J.W. (ed.). p. 120. University Park Press, Baltimore.

Morrison-Silverberg S.A. & Jesty J. (1981) The role of activated Factor X in the control of bovine coagulation Factor VII. *Journal of Biological Chemistry* **256**, 1625.

Nelsestuen G.L. (1980) Role of calcium and phospholipid in *in vitro* thrombin generation. In *The Regulation of Coagulation*, Developments in Biochemistry, Vol. 8. Mann K.G. & Taylor F.B. (eds). p. 31. Elsevier-North Holland Pub. Co., New York.

Nelsestuen G.L. & Broderius M. (1977) Interaction of prothrombin and blood clotting Factor X with membranes. *Biochemistry* **16**, 4172.

Nemerson Y. & Esnouf M.P. (1973) Activation of a proteolytic system by a membrane lipoprotein: the mechanism of action of tissue factor. *Proceedings of the National Academy of Sciences of the USA* **70**, 310.

Nemerson Y. & Pitlick F.A. (1971) Analysis of tissue factor and peptidase activities by affinity chromatography. *Proceedings of the 2nd Meeting of the International Society on Thrombosis and Haemostasis* **42**, 1971.

Nemerson Y., Zur M., Bach R. & Gentry R. (1980) The mechanism of action of tissue factor. In *The Regulation of Coagulation*, Developments in Biochemistry, Vol. 8. Mann K.G. & Taylor F.B. (eds). p. 193. Elsevier-North Holland Pub. Co., New York.

Nesheim M.E., Myrmel K.H., Hibbard L.S. & Mann K.G. (1979) Isolation and characterization of single chain bovine Factor V. *Journal of Biological Chemistry* **254**, 508.

Nolf P. (1908) Contribution a l'étude de la coagulation du sang. Les facteurs primordiaux, leur origine. *Archives Internationales de Physiologie* **6**, 1.

Ong T.C. & Esnouf M.P. (1979) The activation of prothrombin by X_{1a} and X_{2a} and inhibition by fragment 1. *Thrombosis and Haemostasis* **42**, 325.

Østerud B. & Rapaport S.I. (1977) Activation of Factor IX by the reaction product of tissue factor and factor VII: additional pathway for initiating blood coagulation. *Proceedings of the National Academy of Sciences of the USA* **74**, 5260.

Pitlick F.A., Nemerson Y., Gottlieb A.J., Gordon R.G. & Williams W.J. (1971) Peptidase activity associated with the tissue factor of blood coagulation. *Biochemistry* **10**, 2680.

Radcliffe R.D. & Barton P.G. (1973) Comparison of the molecular forms of activated factor X. *Journal of Biological Chemistry* **249**, 6788.

Radcliffe R. & Nemerson Y. (1975) Activation and control of factor VII by activated factor X and thrombin. Isolation and characterization of a single chain form of factor VII. *Journal of Biological Chemistry* **250**, 388–95.

Radcliffe R. & Nemerson Y. (1976) Mechanism of activation of bovine Factor VII: Products of cleavage by Factor X_a. *Journal of Biological Chemistry* **251**, 4797.

Rauschenbach F. (1882) *Ueber die wechelwirkungen zwischen protoplasma und blutplasma mit einem anhang betreffend die blutplaettchen von bizzerozero.* H. Laakman, Dorpat.

Rouser G. & Schloredt D. (1958) Phospholipid structure and thromboplastic activity. *Biochemica et Biophysica Acta* **28**, 81.

Silverberg S.A., Nemerson Y. & Zur M. (1977) Kinetics of the activation of bovine coagulation Factor X by the components of the extrinsic pathway. *Journal of Biological Chemistry* **252**, 8481.

Stenflo J. (1976) A new vitamin K-dependent protein. *Journal of Biological Chemistry* **251**, 355.

Stüder A. (1946) Contribution à l'étude de la thrombokinase. In Jubilee Volume dedicated to Emile Christophe Barell. **229**, The Roche Companies, Basel.

Thøgersen H.C., Petersen T.E., Sottrup-Jensen L., Magnusson S. & Morris H.R. (1978) The N-terminal sequences of blood coagulation factor X_1 and X_2 light chains. *Biochemical Journal* **175**, 613.

Titani K., Fujikawa K., Enfield D.L., Ericsson L.H., Walsh K.A. & Neurath H. (1975) Bovine factor X_1 (Stuart Factor): Amino acid sequence of heavy chain. *Proceedings of the National Academy of Sciences of the USA* **72**, 3082.

Walker F.J. (1980) Regulation of activated Protein C by a new protein: a possible function for Protein S. *Journal of Biological Chemistry* **255**, 552.

Walker F.J., Sexton P.W. & Esmon C.T. (1979) The inhibition of blood coagulation by activated Protein C through the selective inactivation of activated Factor V. *Biochemica et Biophysica Acta* **571**, 333.

Wallach, D.F.H., Maurice P.A., Steel B.B. & Surgenor D.M. (1959) Studies on the relationship between the colloidal state and clot promoting activity of pure phosphatidyl ethanolamines. *Journal of Biological Chemistry* **234**, 2829.

Williams W.J. (1964) The activity of lung microsomes in blood coagulation. *Journal of Biological Chemistry* **239**, 933.

Williams W.J. (1966) The activity of human placenta microsomes and brain particles in blood coagulation. *Journal of Biological Chemistry* **241**, 1840–6.

Wooldridge L.C. (1893) Chemistry of the Blood. Kegan Paul, Trench, Trübner & Co., London.

Chapter 5
Factor VIII: Structure and Function

LEON W. HOYER

Although the International Committee on Thrombosis and Haemostasis clarified blood coagulation nomenclature when it introduced the general use of Roman numerals, this terminology has led to a new problem with regard to factor VIII. Unfortunately, this designation has come to have a variety of meanings that depend upon the context in which it is used and the biases of the author. The confusion is a result of the recent recognition that what had been—and to some extent still is—designated 'factor VIII' is really two quite separate proteins that circulate together as a complex in plasma.

The importance of this clarification may be more readily apparent after a brief review of the way that the term 'factor VIII' has evolved. Long before the responsible protein had been characterized, a plasma coagulant deficiency was recognized in classic haemophilia. The designation 'Factor VIII' by the International Committee (Wright 1962) was meant to be a synonym for the terms that it replaced: antihaemophilic factor, antihaemophilic globulin and platelet cofactor 1. At that time, little was known about the physical properties of the protein that was thought to have these characteristics. The detection of reduced factor VIII activity in von Willebrand's disease, in addition to defective primary haemostasis, suggested that factor VIII might have two distinct biological functions. The concept was supported by the observations that plasma transfusion corrected the two defects and that both were transmitted by a single gene in an autosomal dominant pattern. The concept of a bifunctional molecule became even more attractive when many laboratories demonstrated that a 5000-fold purified protein had both factor VIII procoagulant activity (it corrected the haemophilic plasma defect) and interacted *in vitro* with platelets in a way that was consistent with a role in primary haemostasis (Bouma *et al.* 1972). While earlier data suggested that purified antihaemophilic factor had a much higher specific activity (Michael and Tunnah 1966), most work on factor VIII was then directed towards the properties of a large protein that could be purified from cryoprecipitate without too much difficulty and which had procoagulant and platelet-related properties (Marchesi, Shulman and Gralnick 1972, Legaz *et al.* 1973, Shapiro *et al.* 1973).

                                    Chapter 5

Many concurrent studies did not support the 'bifunctional concept', however, and an alternative interpretation has gradually developed. It is now generally accepted that what had been designated plasma factor VIII is really a complex of two components that have distinct functions, biochemical and immunological properties, and genetic control. The properties of these components are summarized in Table 3 and the relationship is illustrated in Fig. 13. For the purposes of this chapter, the designation VIII:C will be used to represent the protein with antihaemophilic factor activity and VIIIR (factor VIII-related protein) will represent that molecule that has von Willebrand factor activity and is important in primary haemostasis. It is recognized that the VIII:C, VIIIR terminology is arbitrary, but it is consistent with the recent literature and the way most investigators now prefer to identify these proteins. The terms 'antihaemophilic factor' and 'von Willebrand factor' provide an equally valid terminology for the two components of the factor VIII complex.

The evidence for the distinction between the two components has been summarized in recent reviews (Koutts, Howard and Firkin 1979, Hoyer 1981) and only the most essential points will be described:

1   The two proteins can be separated when gel filtration chromatography or ultracentrifugation are carried out in buffers that have high ionic strength (1 M-NaCl or 0.24 M-CaCl$_2$) (Weiss and Kochwa 1970, Owen and Wagner 1972, Rick and Hoyer 1973).

Table 3. The components of the factor VIII complex.

VIII:C   The factor VIII procoagulant protein: the antihaemophilic factor
         Identified as:
         Factor VIII procoagulant activity (VIII:C)
             The procoagulant property of normal plasma that is measured in standard coagulation assays
         Factor VIII procoagulant antigen (VIII:CAg)
             Antigenic determinants closely associated with VIII:C
             Measured by immunoassays carried out with human antibodies

VIIIR   The factor VIII-related protein: the von Willebrand factor. A large polymeric protein that is necessary for normal platelet adhesion and bleeding time in vivo
         Identified as:
         Factor VIII-related antigen (VIIIR:Ag)
             Antigenic determinants on VIIIR that are detected by heterologous antibodies
         Ristocetin cofactor (VIIIR:RC)
             The property of normal plasma VIIIR that supports ristocetin-induced agglutination of washed normal platelets

---

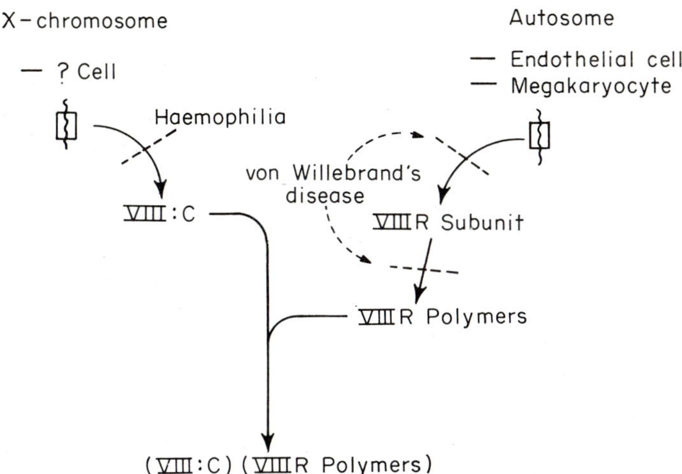

Fig. 13. The factor VIII complex in plasma. This schematic interpretation indicates the interaction of the two components, their genetic control, and the nature of the molecular defects in haemophilia and von Willebrand's disease.

2   The biological properties of the two proteins are independent. The procoagulant protein retains full VIII:C activity in the virtual absence of VIIIR (i.e. an VIII:C/VIIIR:Ag ratio over 10 000:1 (Tuddenham *et al.* 1979)) and ristocetin cofactor activity is retained when VIIIR has been separated from all detectable VIII:C protein (Olson *et al.* 1977).

3   The proteins also have unique antigenic determinants and each protein can be measured by an immunoassay that is independent of the other (Zimmerman, Ratnoff and Powell 1971, Lazarchick and Hoyer 1978).

4   The concentrations of the two proteins in plasma, as measured by both functional assays and immunoassays, can vary independently in certain conditions (Hoyer 1976, Bloom 1977).

5   The concentrations and properties of the two proteins are controlled by different genes. Non-functional VIII:C protein—or reduced concentrations of VIII:C protein—are characteristic of haemophilia, a disease transmitted by X-chromosomal inheritance. In contrast, reduced or abnormal VIIIR protein is recognized in von Willebrand's disease, a disorder in which the inheritance pattern is autosomal.

The two components of the factor VIII complex do, however, interact. Their concentrations vary together under most normal, stressful, and pathological situations, and standard purification methods separate the intact (two-component) factor VIII complex from other plasma proteins. This interaction will be considered in detail after the two components are characterized.

Factor VIII procoagulant protein: the antihaemophilic factor

Biochemical properties

Human factor VIII procoagulant protein has not yet been satisfactorily purified for standard biochemical characterization. What are often referred to as biochemical studies of antihaemophilic factor usually describe data obtained for the intact factor VIII complex. The separation of human factor VIII coagulant protein from VIIIR and other plasma proteins is very difficult, for low yield and instability magnify the effort needed to purify this trace protein.

A sufficiently large-scale effort has been possible using bovine plasma, however, and Vehar and Davie (1980) have purified VIII:C approximately 300 000-fold from large (125 litre) batches of bovine plasma. Although the yield has been very low, preliminary characterizations have been reported. The VIII:C activity elutes in Sephadex G-200 fractions that suggest a molecular weight of 250 000–300 000, but analysis by sodium dodecyl sulphate (SDS)-polyacrylamide gel electrophoresis demonstrated a triplet of protein-staining bands with molecular weights of 85 000, 88 000 and 93 000. The electrophoretic properties did not change when purified VIII:C was incubated with 2-mercaptoethanol, but it was cleaved to smaller proteins when incubated with thrombin, purified factor Xa or activated Protein C. Purified bovine VIII:C did not aggregate human platelets and antibodies to purified bovine VIII:C protein had no inhibiting effect on the platelet-aggregating activity of bovine plasma. These studies are strong evidence for the independence of the VIII:C coagulant protein from the protein responsible for platelet-aggregating activity, i.e. VIIIR.

Similar studies have not yet been possible with human factor VIII procoagulant protein. Nevertheless, a combination of functional and immunological assays have permitted a characterization of VIII:C properties in non-denaturing conditions after separation from VIIIR and most other human plasma proteins (Hoyer and Trabold 1981). Its molecular weight has been estimated to be 285 000 in these studies, a value calculated from the Sephadex G-200 elution properties (from which Stokes-radius can be estimated) and sedimentation rate (8.2 s). A similar value was obtained by Weinstein and coworkers (1981), using labelled human anti-VIII:C as a marker for the VIII:C protein in SDS-agarose/acrylamide electrophoresis.

Factor VIII procoagulant activity is relatively resistant to inactivation by reduction (Austen 1974). This property is most striking when the intact factor VIII complex is incubated with 0.05 M 2-mercaptoethanol, for there is little change in VIII:C even though ristocetin cofactor activity is completely inactivated (Counts, Paskell and Elgee 1978). Higher concentrations of reducing agents do, however, inactivate VIII:C (Blombäck *et al.* 1978). A reactive thiol group has been identified, but two studies have come to different conclusions about its proximity to the site of VIII:C function (Austen 1970, Harris, Johnson and Hodgins 1981). VIII:C functional properties are very sensitive to changes in pH and cation concentration (Weiss 1965). VIII:C is most stable between pH 6.9 and 7.2 and marked losses occur below pH 6 and above pH 8. The irreversible loss of VIII:C in EDTA and ion-exchange resin-treated plasmas demonstrates that a minimal concentration of divalent cations is required to maintain the functional conformation.

Although neither human nor bovine VIII:C has been purified in sufficient quantity for carbohydrate analysis, there is indirect evidence in both cases that the molecule contains carbohydrate residues. VIII:C separated from VIIIR is adsorbed by concanavalin A-agarose, and it can be subsequently eluted with the sugar, α-D-glucopyranoside (Tuddenham *et al.* 1979, Vehar and Davie 1980). In addition, some bacterial glucosidases and oxidases inactivate VIII:C (Austen and Bidwell 1972, Fukui *et al.* 1977).

As might be expected for a protein that has resisted purification, the plasma content of VIII:C is not known with certainty and is usually expressed by reference to standardized pools of human plasma that have been collected and stored in a way that reduces the likelihood of VIII:C activation or loss. Thus, all VIII:C (and VIII:CAg) values are arbitrary measures that indicate a relative concentration. They do not have any molecular interpretation at the present time. One can, of course, estimate the amount of protein that corresponds to a 'normal plasma level' of 1 unit/ml. From measurements of the intact human factor VIII complex and the proportion of protein that is VIII:C, the value is approximately 50 ng/unit. A similar value is obtained from the specific activity of apparently homogeneous bovine VIII:C (4500 units/mg) (Vehar and Davie 1980).

Immunological properties

Human anti-VIII:C antibodies have been recognized in some repeatedly transfused haemophilic patients and in rare individuals who form autoantibodies that inactivate VIII:C. These antibodies do not form detectable immunoprecipitates with VIII:C or with factor VIII complex, but they can detect VIII:C antigen determinants by antibody neutralization and immunoradiometric assays.

The quantitative VIII:CAg immunoassays that have been developed recently use radiolabelled human anti-VIII:C that has been purified from high titre inhibitor sera (Lazarchick and Hoyer 1978, Peake *et al.* 1979). Haemophilic and spontaneous anti-VIII:C appear to have similar properties in these assays and consistent data are obtained if one tests with a panel of antibodies (Reisner *et al.* 1980).

In general, there is excellent correlation between plasma factor VIII procoagulant activity and VIII:CAg content (Fig. 14). VIII:CAg determinants are more stable than VIII:C activity, however, and this is most striking in the case of serum in which VIII:CAg values are 60–80 per cent of those in the corresponding plasma even though there is no residual VIII:C activity (Peake *et al.* 1979). Careful studies carried out with purified VIII:C and human α-thrombin have demonstrated dose-dependent loss of VIII:CAg reactivity at low thrombin concentrations—to 60 per cent of the original value—and a qualitative change in immunoreactivity after exposure to thrombin concentrations above 0.1 unit/ml (Hoyer and Trabold 1981).

Synthesis

Despite many investigations, the site of VIII:C synthesis is not known. Both transplantation (Webster *et al.* 1971) and perfusion studies (Owen, Bowie and Fass 1979, Shaw *et al.* 1979) strongly suggest VIII:C release by the liver, but they have been limited to measurements obtained by standard coagulation assays. Firm conclusions await their confirmation by immunoassay data and by protein synthesis studies. Although the liver may have an important role in VIII:C synthesis, it must be noted that normal or increased VIII:C values are present in patients with severe hepatic disease (Bloom 1977). Thus, there is a strong suspicion that extrahepatic sources are important as well, and tissue culture studies have sought evidence for VIII:C synthesis by a ubiquitous cell type. These efforts have so far failed to detect VIII:CAg synthesis by cultured endothelial cells, monocytes, lymphocytes, or hepatocytes (Piovella *et al.* 1978, Tuddenham, Lazarchick and Hoyer 1981, and Hoyer and Forget, unpublished observations).

Function

It is generally agreed that VIII:C accelerates blood coagulation by its cofactor role in the enzymatic activation of factor X by the serine protease, factor IXa. It does so as a part of a complex that is formed with phospholipid and calcium ion, and the roles of factor IXa and VIII:C are analogous to those of factor Xa and factor Va in the prothrombin-activating complex. While factor IXa can activate factor X in the absence of the other components, this is a very slow reaction. The studies of van Dieijen and coworkers (1981) indicate that factor IXa activates (cleaves) factor X in solution with a K_m for factor X of 299 μM and a V_{max} of 2.2×10^{-3} mol factor Xa/min/mol factor IXa. While the addition of both calcium and phospholipid vesicles reduces the K_m to 0.058 μM (a value below the plasma factor X concentration of 0.2 μM). The V_{max} was unchanged by this addition and the inclusion of the intact factor VIII complex had no stimulatory effect. Thrombin-activated VIII:C increased the V_{max} by 200 000-fold, however, and rapid conversion was achieved.

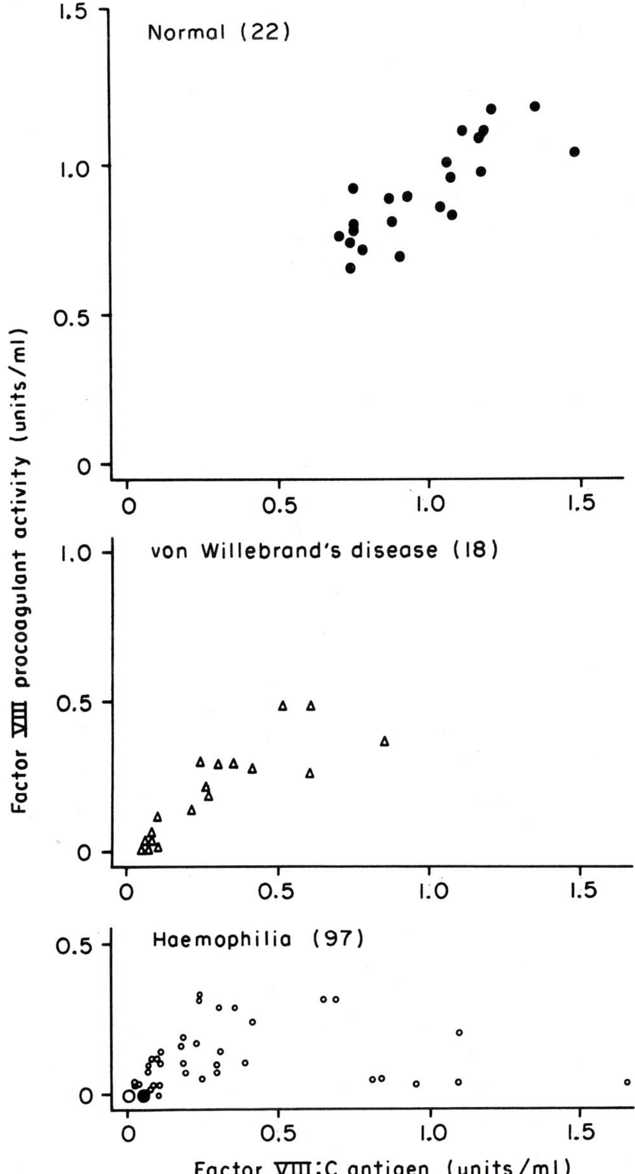

Fig. 14. The relationship of factor VIII procoagulant activity and VIII:CAg in normal individuals and in patients with haemophilia and von Willebrand's disease. In the haemophilia panel, the large open circle at the origin represents 43 plasma samples with no detectable VIII:C or VIII:CAg; the large solid circle represents 18 plasmas that had <0.01 units/ml VIII:C and 0.01–0.06 units/ml VIII:CAg.

It has been presumed that thrombin activates VIII:C by a proteolytic modification, and this effect has recently been demonstrated. Thrombin-activated human VIII:C has gel filtration, ultracentrifugation, and SDS-electrophoresis properties of a protein with a molecular weight of 116 000–120 000 daltons, a value that is significantly reduced from the 270 000–285 000 estimated for unactivated VIII:C (Hoyer and Trabold 1981, Weinstein, Chute and Deykin 1981). Factor VIII procoagulant activity is inactivated by higher concentrations of thrombin—or more prolonged exposure to the enzyme— and a further reduction in size has been identified in this case as well.

Factor VIII-related protein: the von Willebrand factor

Biochemical properties

As factor VIII-related protein (VIIIR, von Willebrand factor) comprises the bulk of the factor VIII complex, data for material that includes both components are primarily due to VIIIR properties. When purified from human, bovine or porcine plasma, factor VIII is a very large protein indeed. Initial agarose gel filtration separations suggested a molecular weight greater than 1 000 000 (Marchesi, Shulman and Gralnick 1972, Shapiro *et al.* 1973) and sedimentation equilibrium studies in 6 M guanidine indicated a value of 1.12×10^6 (Legaz *et al.* 1973). These studies and SDS-polyacrylamide gel electrophoresis analysis established that the very high molecular weight of purified factor VIII is not modified by denaturing agents (e.g. 6 M guanidine or 1 per cent SDS). Subunit structure was recognized after reduction with 2-mercaptoethanol or dithiothreitol and a single band was detected by SDS-polyacrylamide gel electrophoresis. Estimates of the molecular weight of the subunits have been between 195 000 and 240 000.

The studies carried out with highly purified factor VIII may be misleading, however, for they examine only the small fraction of VIIIR molecules (*c.* 5–10 per cent) that are recovered after purification. It is now apparent that plasma factor VIII-related protein is made up of a population of multimers that have molecular weights from *c.* 850 000 to over 12×10^6 (Hoyer and Shainoff 1980, Ruggeri and Zimmerman 1980). VIIIR heterogeneity was suspected when crossed immunoelectrophoresis demonstrated a broad arc, but discrete forms were not detected by agarose electrophoresis of purified factor VIII. The multimeric pattern only became apparent when VIIIR was examined by electrophoresis carried out in agarose, agarose/acrylamide, or dilute acrylamide gels in the presence of sodium dodecyl sulphate. The multimeric pattern has been recognized in unmodified normal human plasma (Fig. 15) as well as in purified human and porcine VIIIR, and extensive controls have been carried out to demonstrate that the size distribution is not an artifact induced by purification methods, freezing, or calcium chelation.

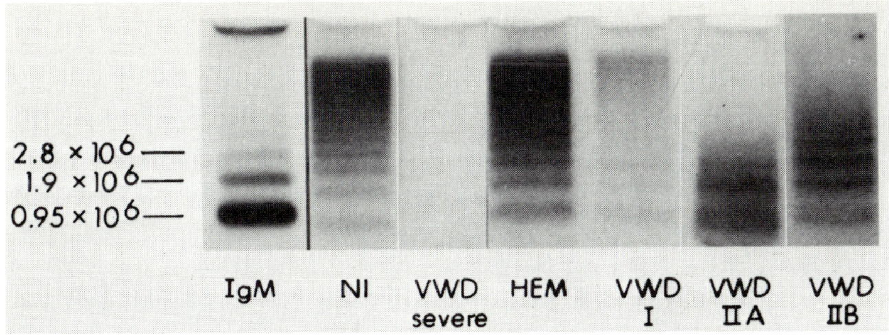

Fig. 15. The polymer pattern of human plasma VIIIR analysed by SDS-agarose electrophoresis. The migration of IgM and IgM polymers is indicated on the left and their molecular weights are noted. The VIIIR in plasma samples was identified by autoradiography after incubation with ^{125}I-labelled rabbit anti-VIIIR:Ag according to the method of Hoyer and Shainoff (1980). From the left, these plasmas are from a normal individual and patients with severe von Willebrand's disease (VIIIR:Ag < 0.01 units/ml), severe haemophilia, and Types I, IIA and IIB von Willebrand's disease.

The smallest VIIIR detected in normal human plasma has an apparent molecular weight of 850 000. This would appear to be a disulphide-bonded tetramer of the basic 200 000 molecular weight subunit. As many as eight larger bands can be detected in normal plasma and serum, and their mobilities suggest that they are composed of an integral number of tetramers. There is, in addition, a population of poorly resolved VIIIR with M_r of c. 8–12 × 10^6. Recent studies by Ruggeri and Zimmerman (1981) suggest that a somewhat more complex pattern may be detected with agarose/polyacrylamide gels and it is not yet clear how to reconcile their data with the apparent homogeneity of the reduced VIIIR subunits.

Purified human VIIIR has also been analysed by standard biochemical methods. It is a glycoprotein containing 5–6 per cent carbohydrate and an undistinguished amino acid composition (Marchesi, Shulman and Gralnick 1972, Legaz *et al.* 1973, Shapiro *et al* 1973). The blocked amino-terminal amino acid has prevented sequence analysis.

The VIIIR concentration in plasma has been determined by immunoradiometric assays in which purified VIIIR was used as the standard. The value obtained by Counts (1975) in this way, 8 μg/ml, is approximately 100 times that of VIII:C protein in human plasma.

Immunological properties

Rabbits immunized with purified human factor VIII form useful immunoprecipitating antibodies. Although these sera have variable ability to inactivate

VIII:C, they all form immunoprecipitates with VIIIR and they inactivate plasma ristocetin cofactor activity as well as other measures of VIIIR–platelet interaction (Bouma *et al.* 1972, Meyer *et al.* 1973). They are monospecific in immunoprecipitin assays if prepared with sufficiently purified factor VIII. A number of different assays have been used to detect and quantify this protein. Laurell electroimmunoassay (Zimmerman, Ratnoff and Powell 1971), immunoradiometric assays (Hoyer 1972a, Counts 1975), radioimmunoassays (Green and Reynolds 1977), ELISA assays (Bartlett *et al.* 1976), and fluorometric immunoassays (Rudzki, Tunbridge and Lloyd 1979) all give similar results.

These polyclonal rabbit antisera react with many different VIIIR antigenic determinants, and it has been estimated that over 30 IgG molecules can bind each VIIIR tetramer (Hoyer 1972b). The immunological reactivity appears to be primarily directed toward conformational antigens, since immunoreactivity is lost when the VIIIR is reduced to 200 000 molecular weight subunits. Monoclonal anti-VIIIR have recently been described by Katzmann *et al.* (1981). These non-precipitating antibodies were prepared by immunizing mice with porcine VIIIR; they had variable effects on VIIIR properties.

von Willebrand factor activity

The physiological role of factor VIII-related protein in normal platelet function has been designated 'von Willebrand factor' activity because it is deficient in patients with severe von Willebrand's disease. The prolonged bleeding time in these patients is presumed to be due to the absence of VIIIR in their plasmas and the defect is usually corrected when VIIIR-rich cryoprecipitate is infused. While the plasma defect can only be quantified by *in vitro* assays, it is always important to recognize that the bleeding time correction represents the only certain physiological measurement of this protein's function. The most generally used *in vitro* test for VIIIR function at the present time is measurement of ristocetin-induced platelet agglutination. In most instances, there is a good correlation between defective haemostasis, i.e. a prolonged bleeding time, and reduced ristocetin cofactor activity (Weiss *et al.* 1973).

The *in vitro* assessment of VIIIR function with ristocetin has become widely adopted in a rather short period of time. The initial observation was reduced or absent platelet aggregation when ristocetin was added to platelet-rich plasma (PRP) from patients with von Willebrand's disease and brisk aggregation of normal platelets (Howard and Firkin 1971). This simple measure has been adopted by many laboratories for the routine evaluation of patients with possible bleeding disorders. Unfortunately, the assessment of ristocetin-induced aggregation in patient PRP has important limitations. The major problem is its lack of sufficient sensitivity so that mild or moderate von

Willebrand's disease may be missed (Howard, Sawers and Firkin 1973). In addition, it may be falsely positive in some patients with primary platelet disorders (Weiss 1975). Ristocetin-induced aggregation is also abnormal in the platelet-rich plasma of patients with Bernard–Soulier syndrome (Howard, Hutton and Hardisty 1973). While the latter individuals have normal factor VIII levels in their plasma, their platelet membranes lack glycoprotein Ib that binds VIIIR.

Ristocetin-induced platelet aggregation can be examined in a more satisfactory way when dilutions of plasma are tested with washed normal platelets and a fixed concentration of ristocetin. These ristocetin cofactor assays can be done with freshly washed platelets or with formaldehyde-fixed platelets that remain satisfactory as test reagents for several weeks if kept in the refrigerator. The rate of ristocetin-induced aggregation is related to the amount of normal plasma factor VIII that is added and the value can be obtained from the aggregometer tracing (Weiss *et al.* 1973) or by measurement of the time required for detectable platelet agglutination (Sarji *et al.* 1974). The different methods give similar results under most conditions.

Although there is usually a good correlation of ristocetin cofactor activity *in vitro* with presumed von Willebrand factor activity *in vivo*, as judged by freedom from abnormal bleeding and by bleeding time measurements (Weiss *et al.* 1973), there are exceptions. For example, the VIIIR:RC value may become normal in von Willebrand's disease during pregnancy and in inflammatory states—or after transfusion with some factor VIII-rich concentrates—even though the bleeding time remains prolonged (Ratnoff and Saito 1974, Weiss 1974). In addition, patients with a variant form of von Willebrand's disease have long bleeding times in spite of low-normal ristocetin cofactor values and *increased* reactivity when ristocetin is added to their platelet-rich plasma (Ruggeri *et al.* 1980, Ruggeri and Zimmerman 1980). Thus, the value of ristocetin cofactor assays as measures of VIIIR function *in vitro* must not obscure the fact that they do not always reflect *in vivo* biological function. In this regard, it should also be emphasized that VIIIR:Ag and ristocetin cofactor assays measure different properties of the VIIIR protein. While immunoassays detect all VIIIR molecules with specific antigenic determinants, the protein does not always have biological activity. Moreover, artifactually increased immunoassay values are obtained for the smaller VIIIR polymers when they are compared to whole plasma standards by the Laurell electroimmunoassay method. In contrast, ristocetin cofactor measurements only identify the larger VIIIR polymers that interact with platelets (Doucet-deBruine *et al.* 1978). Thus, plasmas or plasma derivatives that lack the larger VIIIR polymers will have a very low ratio of VIIIR:RC to VIIIR:Ag and, conversely, material that is relatively enriched in large forms will have higher values for ristocetin cofactor activity than VIIIR:Ag, when compared to the whole plasma standard.

Radiolabelled purified VIIIR retains functional activity, and the ristocetin-dependent VIIIR–platelet interaction has been characterized by several investigators. The binding properties of a population of multimers are complex, however, especially when the concentration of a third component, ristocetin, affects the interaction. In general, VIIIR binding measurements correlate well with ristocetin-induced aggregation in these studies. A single class of binding sites was identified in one study (Kao, Pizzo and McKee 1979), but other investigators have identified a more complex binding pattern, both low-affinity and high-affinity sites (Morisato and Gralnick 1980). These two classes correspond to ristocetin-dependent binding of larger and smaller VIIIR polymers (Gralnick, Williams and Morisato 1981). Since physiological platelet–VIIIR interactions require the larger polymers, it is likely that the 3500 high-affinity sites mediate the essential VIII–platelet interactions.

A number of studies have suggested that VIIIR carbohydrate is important for VIIIR–platelet interactions and ristocetin-induced aggregation. While enzymatic removal of sialic acid has affected ristocetin-induced platelet aggregation in some studies (Sodetz, Pizzo and McKee 1977), other investigators have detected no reduction in VIIIR:RC reactivity after neuraminidase treatment (Gralnick 1978, DeMarco and Shapiro 1981). However, Gralnick (1978) demonstrated that oxidation or removal of the penultimate galactose abolished ristocetin-induced platelet aggregation. The oxidative inhibition was reversed by subsequent galactose reduction. VIIIR binding studies also demonstrated the effect of carbohydrate modification; this suggests that the agglutination reaction involves VIIIR binding to platelets through its carbohydrate residues.

The physiological role of VIIIR in haemostasis has been more difficult to study, since its function appears to be the stabilization of platelet–vessel wall interactions. The essential role of VIIIR in platelet adhesion has been demonstrated in a series of studies by Weiss, Baumgartner and coworkers (Weiss, Turitto and Baumgartner 1978, Baumgartner, Tschopp and Meyer 1980). They have demonstrated that VIIIR supports platelet adhesion to segments of de-endothelialized rabbit aorta when the blood-flow shear rate is high, but that VIIIR does not affect the platelet–vessel wall interaction at low shear rates. These morphometric studies have been carried out with directly sampled (native) blood as well as blood anticoagulated with citrate. In studies carried out with human renal artery segments, Sakariassen and coworkers (1979) demonstrated that VIIIR was the only plasma protein enhancing platelet adhesion to the vessel wall. Moreover, there was a good correlation between the amount of VIIIR bound and platelet adhesion when double perfusion studies were carried out in which the vessel was first perfused with VIIIR, washed, and then perfused with platelets in a medium that did not contain VIIIR. These experiments suggested that VIIIR first interacts with the subendothelium and that this is followed by platelet adhesion. The importance of VIIIR-supported platelet–platelet interactions *in vivo* is not known, but is presumed to be of less significance.

Synthesis

Immunofluorescence studies have detected human VIIIR:Ag in endothelial cells of arteries, arterioles, capillaries and veins throughout the body as well as in megakaryocytes and platelets (Bloom, Giddings and Wilks 1973, Hoyer, de los Santos and Hoyer 1973). Subsequent experiments identified both VIIIR:Ag and VIIIR:RC in the medium obtained from cultured human umbilical cord endothelial cells (Jaffe, Hoyer and Nachman 1973, 1974). Direct evidence for VIIIR synthesis by endothelial cells and megakaryocytes has also been obtained in experiments that have demonstrated the incorporation of labelled amino acids into VIIIR (Jaffe, Hoyer and Nachman 1973). The location of the endothelial cell adjacent to the blood flow has obvious advantages for the rapid release of VIIIR into the circulation and the generation of high concentrations of VIIIR near damaged vessel walls.

The interaction of VIII:C and VIIIR in the factor VIII complex

Although VIII:C and VIIIR have very distinct properties, it would be an over-simplification to suggest that they have no relationship and that they are simply two plasma proteins that happen to co-purify. Several observations indicate that they are two components of a complex that is maintained by non-covalent interactions. For example, the concentrations of the two proteins are very similar in normal plasma (Fig. 16) and in most (non-haematological) disease states. In contrast, there is no correlation between the plasma concentrations of either protein and factor V or fibrinogen (Rizza *et al.* 1975).

The interaction between the proteins remains intact when VIIIR binds to heterologous antibodies (e.g. rabbit anti- (whole) factor VIII). Thus, immuno-precipitates obtained with rabbit anti-VIIIR have coagulant activity (Bird and Rizza 1975) and anti-VIIIR coupled to agarose removes both VIII:C and VIIIR from plasma (Tuddenham *et al.* 1979). If VIII:C and VIIIR did not interact in some way, there would be no reason for VIII:C to remain with the anti-VIIIR immunoadsorbent. Unrecognized anti-VIII:C in the rabbit antisera does not effect this removal, for the VIII:C can be recovered from the beads.

A relatively high-affinity interaction between VIII:C and VIIIR can also be inferred from the effect of reducing agents. The addition of low concentrations of dithiothreitol or 2-mercaptoethanol to plasma causes a change in VIII:C properties so that it is now detected in fractions that indicate a relatively low

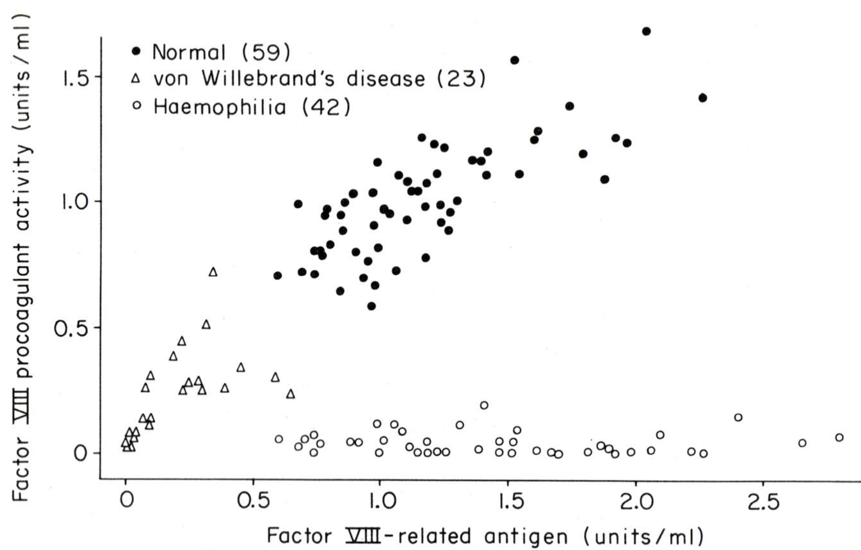

Fig. 16. The relationship of factor VIII procoagulant activity and factor VIII-related antigen in normal individuals and in patients with haemophilia and von Willebrand's disease.

molecular weight (Austen 1974, Blombäck *et al.* 1978). While a direct effect of VIII:C reduction could cause this change, this is unlikely since the high molecular weight pattern was re-established when haemophilic plasma was added. This sequence suggests that intact VIIIR in haemophilic plasma affects VIII:C properties in sucrose density gradient ultracentrifugation, agarose gel filtration, and ethanol precipitation (Blömback *et al.* 1978).

Although it is certain that VIII:C and VIIIR interact in some way, we do not know how this complex is formed other than to speculate that it is likely that electrostatic forces are important. This conclusion follows from the dissociability of the complex in high salt buffers. The biological importance of the plasma interaction is also uncertain, but VIII:C instability in the absence of VIIIR (or in plasmas that have relatively reduced VIIIR) suggests that complex formation may protect VIII:C from proteolytic inactivation (Weiss, Sussman and Hoyer 1977).

Factor VIII deficiency in haemophilia

Biochemical characterization of the plasma defect is not feasible in classical haemophilia (haemophilia A) because of the very low VIII:C concentration in even normal plasmas. Nevertheless, immunological techniques have begun to define the molecular defect as they have sought evidence for *diminished* production of normal VIII:C from the synthesis of *non-functional* VIII:C protein. Since two very different kinds of immunological analysis have been carried out, they must be clearly differentiated. The initial studies with *human* antibodies identified rare haemophilic plasmas with 'non-functional but antigenically cross-reacting AHF-like protein' detected by antibody neutralization assays (Hoyer and Breckenridge 1968, Denson *et al.* 1969). These plasmas were designated cross-reacting material positive (CRM-positive) and they are now known to have normal levels of VIII:CAg even though the VIII:C activity is very low (2–10 per cent of normal). *Rabbit* antisera to human factor VIII was subsequently employed in quantitative immunoassays of plasma samples, and normal levels of a 'factor VIII-like protein' were detected in all haemophilic plasmas by Laurell immunoprecipitin measurements (Zimmerman, Ratnoff and Powell 1971). Plasmas from patients with severe von Willebrand's disease did not form immunoprecipitates with these rabbit antisera nor did they block their VIII:C-inactivating activity. Thus, evaluations carried out with *heterologous* antisera suggested that all haemophilic plasmas have non-functional but immunologically cross-reactive material. It is now recognized that the heterologous antisera used in these studies detect VIIIR:Ag and that they do not measure VIII:C antigens. Therefore, the immunoreactivity does not demonstrate an intact factor VIII complex in haemophilia and the normal VIIIR:Ag levels are consistent with the normal bleeding time and the normal VIIIR:RC levels in haemophilia. Subsequent work has established that VIIIR purified from haemophilic plasmas is indistinguishable from normal VIIIR by standard biochemical analysis (Shapiro *et al.* 1973). Thus, VIIIR:Ag measurements differentiate haemophilia from most forms of von Willebrand's disease, but they do not provide any information about the nature of the X-chromosome defect in haemophilia.

Immunoradiometric assays for VIII:C antigenic determinant have, however, recently been described, and these assays permit both qualitative and quantitative examination of the specific defect in haemophilic plasmas. While not yet generally available, this analysis has been carried out in a number of centres and generally consistent results have been obtained.

Several different patterns can be distinguished when VIII:C and VIII:CAg levels are determined for haemophilic plasmas (Fig. 14). Most patients with severe haemophilia (VIII:C < 1 per cent of normal) have no detectable VIII:CAg. In a quarter of these plasmas there are low VIII:CAg levels, however, but these are usually 1–10 per cent of normal and it is very unusual for them to be as high as 25 per cent. There are no known clinical features that distinguish patients with no detectable VIII:CAg from those who have very low values and they appear to have the same susceptibility to inhibitor formation (McMillan *et al.* 1984).

Variable VIII:CAg levels are present in patients with mild or moderate haemophilia and a marked difference has been detected in a small subgroup of patients who have normal VIII:CAg levels even though they have very low VIII:C activity. As might be expected, these are the same plasmas as those that are CRM-positive by antibody neutralization assays (Lazarchick and Hoyer 1978).

Thus, patients with haemophilia have VIII:C deficiency transmitted by X-chromosome inheritance and they have normal VIIIR synthesis and function. Non-functional VIII:C-like molecules are synthesized by some haemophilic patients, and plasma concentrations of the immunoreactive protein are normal in rare instances. The X-chromosome mutation modifies VIII:C structure in these patients, but the nature of the structural defect has not yet been determined. The absence of detectable VIII:C in the other patients may reflect a structural defect that is so severe that antigenic reactivity is lost (as well as coagulant function) or it may indicate that VIII:C-like protein is absent from the plasma.

Most (>85 per cent) haemophilia carriers can be identified when the combination of VIII:C and VIIIR:Ag measurements is done in laboratories that have excellent quality control and sufficient expertise with reference populations of normal and obligate carrier women (Zimmerman, Ratnoff and Littell 1971, Klein *et al.* 1977). Carrier women have normal VIIIR:Ag levels; VIII:C is reduced since only half of their X-chromosomes (on average) direct normal VIII:C synthesis. The persistently abnormal VIII:C/VIIIR:Ag ratio suggests that physiological influences that affect the factor VIII complex do so in a way that modifies in a consistent manner the production, release and metabolism of the two proteins.

Factor VIII deficiency in von Willebrand's disease

Immunological and biochemical analysis has also clarified our understanding of von Willebrand's disease. In this case, the haemostatic disorder is transmitted by an autosomal locus that affects VIIIR structure and concentration. Qualitative and quantitative VIIIR defects have been identified in this disease; the reduced VIII:C levels appear to be secondary.

In its most frequent form, von Willebrand's disease is a mild or moderate bleeding disorder in which all of the components of the factor VIII complex are reduced in quantity and the bleeding time is prolonged (Table 4: Type I von Willebrand's disease). Plasma VIII:C and VIII:CAg may be slightly higher than VIIIR:Ag and VIIIR:RC, but the values are usually similar (Fig. 16). The VIIIR multimer pattern is normal on direct analysis or by crossed immunoelec-trophoresis since small quantities of all of the VIIIR polymers are present. The bleeding time may be prolonged or it may be normal. The haemostatic defect is

Table 4. Typical values in different forms of von Willebrand's disease.

	Severe	Mild–moderate		
		Type I	Type IIA	Type IIB
VIII:C (% of normal)	1	30	78	100
Bleeding time	Long	Normal–long	Long	Normal–long
VIIR:RC (% of normal)	<1	15	<10	54*
VIIIR:RAg (% of normal)	<1	18	83	80
VIIIR:Ag Crossed immunoelectrophoresis or polymer analysis	—	Normal	Abnormal	Abnormal
Genetics	Autosomal recessive	Autosomal dominant	Autosomal dominant	Autosomal dominant

* Increased ristocetin-induced agglutination in platelet-rich plasma.

often quite inconsistent in these patients, and the plasma assays and bleeding time measurements may vary from time to time (Abildgaard *et al.* 1980).

Severe von Willebrand's disease is much more easily characterized, since these patients have very low levels of both VIIIR and VIII:C, a markedly prolonged bleeding time, and a major bleeding diathesis. Family studies often demonstrate that these patients are homozygous offspring of parents with mild, or asymptomatic, von Willebrand's disease. The VIIIR:Ag and VIIIR:RC levels are usually less than 0.01 units/ml in these patients.

While most patients with severe, mild or moderate von Willebrand's disease have similar levels of the different factor VIII properties—the 'classical' pattern—other patients have normal or only slightly reduced VIII:C and VIIIR:Ag. The diagnosis of von Willebrand's disease is clarified by crossed immunoelectrophoresis in these instances (Kernoff, Gruson and Rizza 1974, Peake, Bloom and Giddings 1974). The more anodal VIIIR peak reflects an increased proportion of small VIIIR and an absence of the largest multimers (Fig. 15). The abnormal multimer distribution changes the crossed immuno-electrophoresis pattern since the electrophoretic mobility in this case is primarily an indication of size. An important consequence of the abnormal polymer distribution is impaired haemostasis, for platelet binding and a normal bleeding time appear to require the larger VIIIR forms (Doucet-deBruine *et al.* 1978, Meyer *et al.* 1980). This variant form of von Willebrand's disease in which the larger forms are missing from the plasma has been designated 'Type II' by some investigators to distinguish it from the classical 'Type I' pattern in which the polymer pattern is normal and there is a low concentration of all factor VIII components.

A further distinction has recently subdivided Type II von Willebrand's disease. Ristocetin-induced aggregation in patients with the 'Type IIB' disorder is *increased* when platelet-rich plasma is tested, and plasma VIIIR:RC levels are normal or minimally reduced (Ruggeri *et al.* 1980). In contrast, patients with more common 'Type IIA' disease have very low VIIIR:RC levels and there is no ristocetin-induced aggregation when their platelet-rich plasmas are tested. *Platelet* VIIIR:Ag is normal in Type IIB patients, however, and the basic defect in this condition may be increased platelet adsorption of large VIIIR from plasma so that the plasma is deficient in the large multimers that are essential for normal haemostasis (Ruggeri and Zimmerman 1980). The plasma VIIIR:Ag polymer pattern is also slightly different in IIA and IIB patients, for the IIA plasmas demonstrate a somewhat greater reduction in the intermediate forms (Ruggeri and Zimmerman 1980) (Fig. 15).

The importance of carbohydrate in VIIIR function has been considered in a previous section. It is, therefore, not surprising that VIIIR carbohydrate deficiency has been identified in some patients with von Willebrand's disease. The VIIIR subunits prepared from these plasmas have no detectable carbohydrate when gels are stained with PAS, and quantitative measurements of VIIIR sialic acid verify the deficiency (Gralnick and Coller 1976, Gralnick, Sultan and Coller 1977). While carbohydrate deficiency may be responsible for some instances of VIIIR dysfunction, another series of patients suggests that it is an uncommon cause of von Willebrand's disease (Zimmerman, Voss and Edgington 1979).

It is not known why VIII:C levels are low in von Willebrand's disease, for these patients have the genetic capacity to synthesize this protein. Recent studies suggest that normal VIIIR protects VIII:C from inactivation, and it is possible that the VIIIR deficiency in von Willebrand's disease leads to accelerated VIII:C inactivation *in vivo* (Weiss, Sussman and Hoyer 1977). It is also possible that plasma VIIIR levels may, in some poorly understood way, modulate VIII:C synthesis or its release into the plasma (Bloom 1979). It is likely that an understanding of the low baseline VIII:C level will clarify the mechanism of the delayed rise and prolonged survival of VIII:C (and VIII:CAg) after transfusion in von Willebrand's disease. At the present time, one can simply suggest that normal (transfused) VIIIR may stabilize VIII:C or it may influence VIII:C synthesis and release.

Summary

Normal human plasma contains a complex of two proteins that are important in haemostasis and coagulation. The factor VIII procoagulant protein (antihaemophilic factor) and the factor VIII-related protein (von Willebrand factor) are under separate genetic control, have distinct biochemical and immunological properties, and have unique and essential physiological properties. While the nature of their interaction and the details of the biochemical structures remain to be determined, the information now available permits a preliminary understanding of the molecular defects in haemophilia and von Willebrand's disease.

REFERENCES

Abildgaard C.F., Suzuki Z., Harrison J., Jefcoat K. & Zimmermann T.S. (1980) Serial studies in von Willebrand's disease: variability versus 'variants'. *Blood* **56**, 712–16.

Austen D.E.G. (1970) Thiol groups in the blood clotting action of factor VIII. *British Journal of Haematology* **19**, 477–84.

Austen D.E.G. (1974) Factor VIII of small molecular weight and its aggregation. *British Journal of Haematology* **27**, 89–100.

Austen D.E.G. & Bidwell E. (1972) Carbohydrate structure in factor VIII. *Thrombosis et Diathesis Haemorrhagica* **28**, 464–72.

Bartlett A., Dormandy K.M., Hawkey C.M., Stableforth P. & Voller A. (1976) Factor VIII-related antigen: measurement by enzyme immuno-assay. *British Medical Journal* **1**, 994–6.

Baumgartner H.R., Tschopp T.B. & Meyer D. (1980) Shear rate dependent inhibition of platelet adhesion and aggregation on collagenous surfaces by antibodies to human factor VIII/von Willebrand factor. *British Journal of Haematology* **44**, 127–39.

Bird P. & Rizza C.R. (1975) A method for detecting factor VIII clotting activity associated with factor VIII-related antigen in agarose gels. *British Journal of Haematology* **31**, 5–12.

Blombäck B., Hessel B., Savidge G., Wikstrom L. & Blombäck M. (1978) The effect of reducing agents on Factor VIII and other coagulation factors. *Thrombosis Research* **12**, 1177–94.

Bloom A.L. (1977) Physiology of factor VIII. In *Recent Advances in Blood Coagulation*. Poller L. (ed.). pp. 141–81. Churchill Livingstone, Edinburgh.

Bloom A.L. (1979) The biosynthesis of factor VIII. In *Clinics in Haematology* Vol. 8:1, pp. 53–77. Rizza C.R. (ed.). W.B. Saunders, London.

Bloom A.L., Giddings J.C. & Wilks C.J. (1973) Factor VIII on the vascular intima: Possible importance in haemostasis and thrombosis. *Nature (New Biology)* **241**, 217–19.

Bouma B.N., Wiegerinck Y., Sixma J.J., Van Mourik J.A. & Mochter I.A. (1972) Immunological characterization of purified anti-haemophilic factor A (factor VIII) which corrects abnormal platelet retention in von Willebrand's disease. *Nature (New Biology)* **236**, 104–6.

Counts R.B. (1975) Solid phase immunoradiometric assay of factor VIII protein. *British Journal of Haematology* **31**, 429–36.

Counts R.B., Paskell S.L. & Elgee S.K. (1978) Disulfide bonds and the quaternary structure of factor VIII/von Willebrand factor. *Journal of Clinical Investigation* **62**, 702–8.

De Marco L. & Shapiro S.S. (1981) Properties of human asialo-factor VIII. A ristocetin-independent platelet-aggregating agent. *Journal of Clinical Investigation* **68**, 321–8.

Denson K.W.E., Biggs R., Haddon M.E., Borrett R. & Cobb K. (1969) Two types of haemophilia (A + and A −): a study of 48 cases. *British Journal of Haematology* **17**, 163–71.

Doucet-deBruine M.H.M., Sixma J.J., Over J. & Beeser-Visser N.H. (1978) Heterogeneity of human factor VIII. II. Characterization of forms of factor VIII binding to platelets in the presence of ristocetin. *Journal of Laboratory and Clinical Medicine* **92**, 96–107.

Fukui H., Mikami S., Okuda T., Murashima N., Takase T. & Yoshioka A. (1977) Studies of von Willebrand factor: effects of different kinds of carbohydrate oxidases, SH-inhibitors and some other chemical reagents. *British Journal of Haematology* **36**, 259–70.

Gralnick H.R. (1978) Factor VIII/von Willebrand factor protein: Galactose, a cryptic determinant of von Willebrand factor activity. *Journal of Clinical Investigation* **62**, 496–9.

Gralnick H.R. & Coller B.S. (1976) Carbohydrate deficiency of the factor VIII/von Willebrand factor protein in von Willebrand's disease variants. *Science* **192**, 56–9.

Gralnick H.R., Sultan Y. & Coller B.S. (1977) von Willebrand's disease. Combined qualitative and quantitative abnormalities. *New England Journal of Medicine* **296**, 1024–30.

Gralnick H.R., Williams S.B. & Morisato D.K. (1981) Effect of the multimeric structure of the factor VIII/von Willebrand factor protein on binding to platelets. *Blood* **58**(2), 387–97.

Green D. & Reynolds N. (1977) Double-antibody radioimmunoassay for factor VIII-related antigen. *Clinical Chemistry* **23**(90), 1648–53.

Harris R.B., Johnson A.J. & Hodgins L.T. (1981) Partial purification of biologically active, low molecular weight, human antihemophilic factor free of von Willebrand factor. II. Further purification with thiol-disulfide interchange chromatography and additional evidence for disulfide bonds susceptible to limited reduction. *Biochimica et Biophysica Acta* **668**, 471–80.

Howard M.A. & Firkin B.G. (1971) Ristocetin—a new tool in the investigation of platelet aggregation. *Thrombosis et Diathesis Haemorrhagica* **26**, 363–9.

Howard M.A., Hutton R.A. & Hardisty R.M. (1973) Hereditary giant platelet syndrome: a disorder of a new aspect of platelet function. *British Medical Journal* **II**, 586–8.

Howard M.A., Sawers R.J. & Firkin B.G. (1973) Ristocetin: a means of differentiating von Willebrand's disease into two groups. *Blood* **41**, 687–90.

Hoyer L.W. (1972a) Immunologic studies of antihemophilic factor (AHF, factor VIII). IV. Radioimmunoassay of AHF antigen. *Journal of Laboratory and Clinical Medicine* **80**, 822–33.

Hoyer L.W. (1972b) Immunologic studies of antihemophilic factor (AHF, factor VIII). III. Comparative binding properties of human and rabbit anti-AHF. *Blood* **39**, 481–8.

Hoyer L.W. (1976) von Willebrand's disease. In *Progress in Hemostasis and Thrombosis*, Vol. 3. Spaet T.H. (ed.) pp. 231–87. Grune and Stratton, New York.

Hoyer L.W. (1981) The factor VIII complex: structure and function. *Blood* **58**, 1–13.

Hoyer L.W. & Breckenridge R.T. (1968) Immunologic studies of antihemophilic factor (AHF, factor VIII): Cross-reacting material in a genetic variant of hemophilia A. *Blood* **32**, 962–71.

Hoyer L.W., de los Santos R. & Hoyer J.R. (1973) Antihemophilic factor antigen. Localization in endothelial cells by immunofluorescent microscopy. *Journal of Clinical Investigation* **52**, 2737–44.

Hoyer L.W. & Shainoff J.R. (1980) Factor VIII-related protein circulates in normal human plasma as high molecular weight multimers. *Blood* **55**, 1056–9.

Hoyer L.W. & Trabold N.C. (1981) The effect of thrombin on human factor VIII. Cleavage of the factor VIII procoagulant protein during activation. *Journal of Laboratory and Clinical Medicine* **97**, 50–64.

Jaffe E.A., Hoyer L.W. & Nachman R.L. (1973) Synthesis of anti-hemophilic factor antigen by cultured human endothelial cells. *Journal of Clinical Investigation* **52**, 2757–64.

Jaffe E.A., Hoyer L.W. & Nachman R.L. (1974) Synthesis of von Willebrand factor by cultured human endothelial cells. *Proceedings of the National Academy of Sciences of the USA* **71**, 1906–9.

Kao K-J., Pizzo S.V. & McKee P. (1979) Demonstration and characterization of specific binding sites for factor VIII/von Willebrand factor on human platelets. *Journal of Clinical Investigation* **63**, 656–64.

Katzmann J.A., Mujwid D.K., Miller R.S. & Fass D.N. (1981) Monoclonal antibodies to von Willebrand's factor: Reactivity with porcine and human antigens. *Blood* **58**, 530–6.

Kernoff P.B.A., Gruson R. & Rizza C.R. (1974) A variant of factor VIII related antigen. *British Journal of Haematology* **26**, 434–40.

Klein H.G., Aledort L.M., Bouma B.N., Hoyer L.W., Zimmermann T.S. & DeMets D.L. (1977) A cooperative study for the detection of the carrier state of classic hemophilia. *New England Journal of Medicine* **296**, 959–62.

Koutts J., Howard M.A. & Firkin B.G. (1979) Factor VIII physiology and pathology in man. In *Progress in Hematology*, Vol. XI. Brown E.B. (ed.). pp. 115–45. Grune and Stratton, New York.

Lazarchick J. & Hoyer L.W. (1978) Immunoradiometric measurement of the factor VIII procoagulant antigen. *Journal of Clinical Investigation* **62**, 1048–52.

Legaz M.G., Schmer G., Counts R.B. & Davie E.W. (1973) Isolation and characterization of human factor VIII (antihemophilic factor). *Journal of Biological Chemistry* **248**, 3946–55.

McMillan C.W., Shapiro S.S., Whitehurst D.A., Hoyer L.W., Rao A.V., Lazerson J. & the Hemophilia Study Group (1984) The natural history of factor VIII inhibitors to patients with hemophilia A: A national cooperative study. II. Observations on the initial developmenmt of factor VIII inhibitors. *Blood* (in press).

Marchesi S.L., Shulman N.R. & Gralnick H.R. (1972) Studies on the purification and characterization of human factor VIII. *Journal of Clinical Investigation* **51**, 2151–61.

Meyer D., Jenkins C., Dreyfus M. & Larrieu M.-J. (1973) An experimental model for von Willebrand's disease. *Nature (London)* **243**, 293–4.

Meyer D., Obert B., Pietu G., Lavergne J.M. & Zimmermann T.S. (1980) Multimeric structure of factor VIII/von Willebrand factor in von Willebrand's disease. *Journal of Laboratory and Clinical Medicine* **95**, 590–602.

Michael S.E. & Tunnah G.W. (1966) The purification of factor VIII (anti-haemophilic globulin). Further purification and some properties of factor VIII. *British Journal of Haematology* **12**, 115–32.

Morisato D.K. & Gralnick H.R. (1980) Selective binding of the factor VIII/von Willebrand factor protein to human platelets. *Blood* **55**, 9–15.

Olson J.D., Brockway W.J., Fass D.N., Bowie E.J.W. & Mann K.G. (1977) Purification of porcine and human ristocetin-Willebrand factor. *Journal of Laboratory and Clinical Medicine* **89**, 1278–94.

Owen C.A. Jr, Bowie E.J.W. & Fass D.N. (1979) Generation of factor VIII coagulant activity by isolated, perfused neonatal pig livers and adult rat livers. *British Journal of Haematology* **43**, 307–15.

Owen W.G. & Wagner R.H. (1972) Antihemophilic factor: separation of an active fragment following dissociation by salts or detergents. *Thrombosis et Diathesis Haemorrhagica* **27**, 502–15.

Peake I.R., Bloom A.L. & Giddings J.C. (1974) Inherited variants of factor VIII-related protein in von Willebrand's disease. *New England Journal of Medicine* **291**, 113–17.

Peake I.R., Bloom A.L., Giddings J.C. & Ludlam C.A. (1979) An immunoradiometric assay for procoagulant factor VIII antigen: Results in haemophilia, von Willebrand's disease and fetal plasma and serum. *British Journal of Haematology* **42**, 269–81.

Piovella F., Giddings J.C., Peake I.R., Ricetti M., Shearn S.A.M. & Bloom A.L. (1978) Synthesis of procoagulant antihaemophilic factor *in vitro*. *Lancet* **II**, 888–9.

Ratnoff O.D. & Saito H. (1974) Bleeding in von Willebrand's disease. *New England Journal of Medicine* **290**, 1089.

Reisner H.M., Price W.A., Blatt P.M., Barrow E.S. & Graham J.B. (1980) Factor VIII coagulant antigen in hemophilic plasma: a comparison of five alloantibodies. *Blood* **56**, 615–19.

Rick M.E. & Hoyer L.W. (1973) Immunologic studies of antihemophilic factor (AHF, factor VIII). V. Immunologic properties of AHF subunits produced by salt dissociation. *Blood* **42**, 737–47.

Rizza C.R., Rhymes I.L., Austen D.E.G., Kernoff P.B.A. & Aroni S.A. (1975) Detection of carriers of haemophilia: a 'blind' study. *British Journal of Haematology* **30**, 447–56.

Rudzki A., Tunbridge L.J. & Lloyd J.V. (1979) A new simple assay for factor VIII related antigen. *Thrombosis Research* **16**, 577–86.

Ruggeri Z.M., Pareti F.I., Mannucci P.M., Ciavarella N. & Zimmerman T.S. (1980) Heightened interaction between platelets and factor VIII/von Willebrand factor in a new subtype of von Willebrand's disease. *New England Journal of Medicine* **302**, 1047–51.

Ruggeri Z.M. & Zimmerman T.S. (1980) Variant von Willebrand disease. Characterization of two subtypes by analysis of multimeric composition of factor VIII/von Willebrand factor in plasma and platelets. *Journal of Clinical Investigation* **65**, 1318–25.

Ruggeri Z.M. & Zimmerman T.S. (1981) The complex multimeric composition of factor VIII/von Willebrand factor. *Blood* **57**, 1140–3.

Sakariassen K.S., Bolhuis P.A. & Sixma J.J. (1979) Human blood platelet adhesion to artery subendothelium is mediated by factor VIII–von Willebrand factor bound to the subendothelium. *Nature* **279**, 636–8.

Sarji K.E., Stratton R.D., Wagner R.H. & Brinkhous K.M. (1974) Nature of von Willebrand factor: A new assay and a specific inhibitor. *Proceedings of the National Academy of Sciences of the USA* **71**, 2937–41.

Shapiro G.A., Andersen J.C., Pizzo S.V. & McKee P.A. (1973) The subunit structure of normal and hemophilic factor VIII. *Journal of Clinical Investigation* **52**, 2198–210.

Shaw E., Giddings J.C., Peake I.R. & Bloom A.L. (1979) Synthesis of procoagulant factor VIII, factor VIII related antigen and other coagulation factors by the isolated perfused rat liver. *British Journal of Haematology* **41**, 585–96.

Sodetz J.M., Pizzo S.V. & McKee P. (1977) Relationship of sialic acid to function and *in vivo* survival of human factor VIII/von Willebrand factor protein. *Journal of Biological Chemistry* **242**, 5538–46.

Tuddenham E.G.D., Lazarchick J. & Hoyer L.W. (1981) Synthesis and release of factor VIII by cultured human endothelial cells. *British Journal of Haematology* **47**, 617–26.

Tuddenham E.G.D., Trabold N.C., Collins J.A. & Hoyer L.W. (1979) The properties of factor VIII coagulant activity prepared by immunoadsorbent chromatography. *Journal of Laboratory and Clinical Medicine* **93**, 40–53.

van Dieijen G., Guido T., Rosing J. & Coenraad Hemker H. (1981) The role of phospholipid and factor VIIIa in the activation of bovine factor X. *Journal of Biological Chemistry* **256**, 3433–42.

Vehar G.A. & Davie E.W. (1980) Preparation and properties of bovine factor VIII (antihemophilic factor). *Biochemistry* **19**, 401–10.

Webster W.P., Zukoski C.F., Hutchin P., Reddick R.L., Mandel S.T. & Penick G.D. (1971) Plasma factor VIII synthesis and control as revealed by canine organ transplantation. *American Journal of Physiology* **220**, 1147–54.

Weinstein M., Chute L. & Deykin D. (1981) Analysis of factor VIII coagulant antigen in normal, thrombin-treated, and hemophilic plasma. *Proceedings of the National Academy of Sciences of the USA* **78**, 5137–41.

Weiss H.J. (1965) A study of the cation- and pH-dependent stability of factors V and VIII in plasma. *Thrombosis et Diathesis Haemorrhagica* **14**, 32–51.

Weiss H.J. (1974) Relation of von Willebrand factor to bleeding time. *New England Journal of Medicine* **291**, 420.

Weiss H.J. (1975) Abnormalities of factor VIII and platelet aggregation—Use of ristocetin in diagnosing in the von Willebrand syndrome. *Blood* **45**, 403–12.

Weiss H.J., Hoyer L.W., Rickles F.R., Varma A. & Rogers J. (1973) Quantitative assay of a plasma factor, deficient in von Willebrand's disease, that is necessary for platelet aggregation. Relationship to factor VIII procoagulant activity and antigen content. *Journal of Clinical Investigation* **52**, 2708–16.

Weiss H.J. & Kochwa S. (1970) Molecular forms of antihaemophilic globulin in plasma, cryoprecipitate and after thrombin activation. *British Journal of Haematology* **18**, 89–100.

Weiss H.J., Sussman I.I. & Hoyer L.W. (1977) Stabilization of factor VIII in plasma by the von Willebrand factor. *Journal of Clinical Investigation* **60**, 390–404.

Weiss H.J., Turitto V.T. & Baumgartner H.R. (1978) Effect of shear rate on platelet interaction with subendothelium in citrated and native blood. I. Shear rate-dependent decrease of adhesion in von Willebrand's disease and the Bernard–Soulier Syndrome. *Journal of Laboratory and Clinical Medicine* **92**, 750–64.

Wright I.S. (1962) The nomenclature of blood clotting factors. *Thrombosis et Diathesis Haemorrhagica* **7**, 381–2.

Zimmerman T.S., Ratnoff O.D. & Littell A.S. (1971) Detection of carriers of classic hemophilia using an immunologic assay for antihemophilic factor (factor VIII). *Journal of Clinical Investigation* **50**, 255–8.

Zimmerman T.S., Ratnoff O.D. & Powell A.E. (1971) Immunologic differentiation of classic hemophilia (factor VIII deficiency) and von Willebrand's disease, with observations on combined deficiencies of antihemophilic factor and proaccelerin (factor V) and an acquired circulating anticoagulant against antihemophilic factor. *Journal of Clinical Investigation* **50**, 244–54.

Zimmerman T.S., Voss R. & Edgington T.S. (1979) Carbohydrate of the factor VIII/von Willebrand factor in von Willebrand's disease. *Journal of Clinical Investigation* **64**, 1298–302.

Chapter 6
Naturally Occurring Inhibitors of Blood Coagulation

C. R. RIZZA

As long ago as 1905 Morawitz said 'It is probable that anticoagulants play a much more significant role in normal coagulation than was assumed in the past'. Earlier still, Schmidt (1892, cited by Morawitz 1905) stated that the presence of clot-retarding substances was probably necessary for the preservation of the fluid state of the blood.

In spite of the early realization of the importance of inhibitors of blood coagulation those substances have until recently received much less attention than the factors which promote coagulation. This is probably due partly to the difficulty of studying an inhibitor of a reaction when the reaction itself is not understood and partly to the relative infrequency of clear-cut deficiency states involving the coagulation inhibitors. The importance of the naturally occurring deficiency as a stimulus to research is clearly seen when one considers the advances in our knowledge of the blood coagulation process which have stemmed from the discovery of each new clotting factor deficiency.

The antithrombin activity of plasma is an important physiological inhibitor of the clotting process and plays an essential role in maintaining the fluidity of circulating blood. Six different activities have been described and have each been assigned a Roman numeral:

Antithrombin I refers to the removal of thrombin from the clotting system by absorption on to fibrin. This reaction is reversible and lysis of the fibrin clot brings about release of the bound thrombin apparently unaltered. The amount of thrombin recoverable from fibrin is relatively small (Seegers 1968) so that this antithrombin activity probably plays only a small role in the inhibition of thrombin.

Antithrombin II is the name given to the plasma cofactor which acts with heparin to inhibit thrombin (Howell and Holt 1918, Quick 1938). Recent work has shown that this heparin cofactor activity is closely associated with the progressive antithrombin activity (antithrombin III, AT III) of plasma and that protein fractions which contain one also contain the other. Moreover, the addition to plasma of a specific antibody to AT III brings about a loss of heparin cofactor activity as well as AT III activity and suggests very strongly that heparin cofactor activity and AT III activity are functions of the same molecule.

Antithrombin III was originally the term used to describe the plasma activity or activities which bring about progressive and irreversible inhibition of thrombin's clotting activity. It is now known that the progressive inactivation of thrombin by plasma is brought about by several substances, the most important being the material now designated as antithrombin III. In addition the α_2-macroglobulin (Lanchantin *et al.* 1966) and α_1-antitrypsin (Rimon, Shamash and Shapiro 1966, Gans and Tan 1967) components of plasma have antithrombin activity. Antithrombin III accounts for approximately 50 per cent of the progressive antithrombin activity of plasma and α_2-macroglobulin and α_1-antitrypsin each contribute about 25 per cent of the activity (Abildgaard 1967, Lane, Bird and Rizza 1975).

Antithrombin IV is a term used to describe an inhibitor activity thought to appear during clotting (Seegers, Johnson and Fell 1954).

Antithrombin V was first described by Loeliger and Hers (1957) in a patient with rheumatoid arthritis with hypergammaglobulinaemia.

Antithrombin VI refers to the antithrombin activity associated with fibrin/fibrinogen breakdown products following digestion with plasmin (Kowalski 1959, Niléhn 1967). The mode of action of the breakdown products is complex. The enzymatic action of thrombin on fibrinogen may be affected as well as the stage of fibrin polymerization depending to some extent on the molecular weight of the breakdown products.

Of the above six antithrombin activities, the activities associated with antithrombin III are the most important and most intensively studied and only those will be discussed here.

Antithrombin III (AT III)

Antithrombin III is thought to be the main inhibitor of blood coagulation and the finding of a marked tendency to thrombosis in individuals with congenital or acquired deficiency of the factor strongly supports this view. Antithrombin III acts mainly against thrombin and factor Xa but there are also important inhibitory effects on factors XIIa, XIa, IXa and possibly VIIa.

Antithrombin III is an α_2-globulin with a molecular weight of approximately 65 000 (Abildgaard 1967, Heimburger, Haupt and Schwick 1970). Analysis of the structure of AT III shows it to be a single-chain glycoprotein of 425 amino acids and four carbohydrate residues (Petersen *et al.* 1979). The activity is destroyed by ether fractionation (Kekwick and Mackay 1954), by heating to 80°C and by pH values above 9.5 and below 6. Heating to 56°C for 15 minutes results in a loss of 20–25 per cent AT III activity (Howie, Prentice and McNicol 1973, Lane, Bird and Rizza 1975). A variety of methods has been used for the separation and purification of AT III from plasma including ammonium sulphate precipitation and precipitation with alcohol. Purification methods employing the strong affinity of AT III for heparin bound to agarose are now widely used (Miller-Andersson 1974, Thaler and Schmer 1975) and yield highly purified preparations of AT III.

Interaction between thrombin and AT III

It is known that when thrombin and AT III react an irreversible complex is formed and both activities are lost. The nature of this reaction has been intensively investigated. Astrup and Darling (1942) thought the reaction was a first order reaction as did Shinowara and Buckley (1960) and Monkhouse (1970). Other workers have found a second-order reaction (Hensen and Loeliger 1963, Abildgaard 1969, Biggs *et al.* 1970, Yue, Starr and Gertler 1973). The discrepancies are most likely due to the action of other antithrombin activities in plasma as well as to the use of different test systems and different proportions of the two reactants in the test systems.

Abildgaard (1969) showed that when thrombin and purified AT III were allowed to react and then subjected to gel filtration on Sephadex G-200, protein was eluted before either thrombin or AT III alone, suggesting that a complex had formed. The position of the major peak of elution corresponded to a molecular weight of approximately 100 000 and suggested that 1 molecule of AT III had complexed with 1 molecule of thrombin. Similar results were obtained by Rosenberg and Damus (1973) using sodium dodecyl sulphate gel electrophoresis and purified thrombin and AT III. On the other hand, gel filtration studies of serum (obtained by recalcifying plasma) reveal a complex with a molecular weight of 190 000. This suggested a reaction between 2 AT III molecules and 2 thrombin molecules or between 1 AT III molecule and 4 thrombin molecules (Binder 1973). Similar results have been obtained by Pepper, Banhegyi and Cash (1977) using heparin affinity chromatography and gel filtration of serum. The reaction between thrombin and AT III is thought to involve the active serine sites in thrombin and arginine residues in AT III. Chemical modification of either of those sites prevents the reaction taking place (Rosenberg and Damus 1973). Further information concerning the reaction between thrombin and AT III has been obtained using immunological methods. Sas, Pepper and Cash (1975) have shown that when crossed immunoelectrophoresis is carried out with heparin in the first stage, different patterns of precipitation are seen depending on whether plasma or serum is electrophoresed. In the case of plasma a fast-moving component was seen along with two slower smaller components. When normal serum was electrophoresed the fast-moving component was apparently decreased in quantity but the slower-moving components became much more evident. Gel filtration studies to ascertain the nature of the precipitate peaks suggested that the slow-moving components were complexes of AT III and thrombin and possibly Xa.

There are still some features of the inactivation of thrombin by plasma which remain unexplained. For example, it is not clear why there is a discrepancy between the amount of thrombin which is neutralized when whole blood clots and the amount neutralized when it is added to plasma. It has been calculated that 1 ml of plasma contains approximately 300 units of prothrombin (Murphy and Seegers 1948) and thus has a potential for generating 300 units of thrombin. When a sample of whole blood clots very little thrombin is detectable within 10–20 minutes of clotting yet, when 300 units of thrombin are added to plasma, significant amounts of thrombin are still detectable many hours later (Klein and Seegers 1950). Clearly the addition of thrombin to plasma may in no way be comparable to the generation of thrombin in whole blood. Indeed, it may be that the early stages of blood coagulation or prothrombin conversion activate the antithrombin system in a way which the addition of thrombin fails to do.

AT III and heparin cofactor activity

As mentioned earlier there is now strong evidence that antithrombin II (heparin cofactor) activity and AT III activity are functions of the same molecule. Lyttleton (1954) drew attention to the close association between heparin cofactor and AT III and Abildgaard (1968) showed that a semi-purified preparation which contained most of the AT III activity of plasma also contained all the heparin cofactor activity. Heimburger (1967) came to the same conclusion on the basis of immunoelectrophoresis studies of AT III in the presence and absence of heparin and Rosenberg and Damus (1973) showed that a purified homogeneous preparation with progressive antithrombin activity also contained heparin cofactor activity. Furthermore, they showed that an antibody raised against the purified inhibitor precipitated equal amounts of each activity from defibrinated plasma.

The inhibitory action of AT III is greatly enhanced in the presence of heparin. In particular, the speed of inactivation of thrombin by AT III is increased when heparin is present (Quick 1938, Klein and Seegers 1950, Blombäck, Blombäck and Olsson 1963, Biggs *et al.* 1970). Heparin is thought to enhance the action of AT III by binding to the lysyl residues in the AT III molecule causing a conformational change which results in more favourable exposure of the arginine site of AT III with which the active serine site in thrombin reacts (Rosenberg and Damus 1973). There is some evidence for such a heparin-induced conformational change in AT III (Einarsson and Andersson 1977, Villaneuva and Danishefsky 1977).

Action of AT III on Xa and other activated clotting factors

In addition to inhibiting thrombin, AT III has an inhibitory effect on other activated factors in the blood. Particular attention has been paid to the effect of AT III on activated factor X (Xa) (Seegers and Marciniak 1962, Biggs *et al.* 1970, Yin, Wessler and Stoll 1971).

In 1962 Seegers and Marciniak showed that a fraction of bovine plasma containing AT III was capable of inhibiting autoprothrombin C, an activity which is now thought to correspond to factor Xa. Biggs *et al.* (1970) studied the inhibitory effect of human plasma on human factor Xa and bovine Xa and noted that in the absence of heparin the factor Xa was inhibited in much the same way as thrombin but that the presence of heparin resulted in a greatly increased inhibition of factor Xa. Indeed the heparin seemed to be more specifically related to the inactivation of factor Xa than to thrombin. Rather surprisingly they found that human plasma inhibited bovine factor Xa more effectively than it did human factor Xa. Similar observations on the different susceptibilities of human and bovine Xa have been made by Marciniak and Tsukamura (1972). Despite the apparent slowness of inactivation of human Xa by human plasma in the different *in vitro* systems very little Xa is detectable in serum within 10–20 minutes of the completion of normal blood clotting. As with inhibition of thrombin during the normal clotting process, it is possible that the early stages of coagulation may in some way enhance the inhibitory effect of AT III on factor Xa.

The fact that the thrombin AT III reaction depends upon the presence of the serine-active centre in thrombin suggests that the other serine proteases involved in blood coagulation and haemostasis may be susceptible to the action of AT III (Rosenberg and Damus 1973). This has been found to be so and the latter authors have shown that factors IXa, XIa and XIIa are inactivated by AT III and that the inhibition is greatly accelerated by heparin (Damus, Hicks and Rosenberg 1973, Harpel and Rosenberg 1976).

Assay of AT III

The inhibitory effect of AT III on blood coagulation can be assayed by measuring its antithrombin activity or its anti-Xa activity in a clotting test system. It is also possible to measure the amount of AT III antigen in plasma by immunological methods using a specific antiserum raised against AT III. Assays which measure the thrombin-inhibiting activity of AT III may be carried out by adding a relatively large amount of thrombin to the material being tested, incubating for a specified period and then determining the amount of residual thrombin by sub-sampling into fibrinogen or into a chromogenic substrate for which thrombin has a high specificity. This is the basis of the assays developed by Astrup and Darling (1942), Hallen (1962), Biggs *et al.* (1970), and Yue, Starr and Gertler (1973). A second type of assay which is a better reflection of the initial rate of reaction between thrombin and AT III has been described (Blombäck, Blombäck and Olsson 1963, Hensen and Loeliger 1963, Marciniak, Farley and DeSimone 1974). In this method relatively small amounts of thrombin are added to the material being tested for AT III activity and the incubation time is short.

Because of the ability of fibrinogen to adsorb thrombin it is usually thought desirable to defibrinate the sample before performing the test. Defibrination may be achieved by allowing the blood to clot and carrying out the test on serum, by heating the plasma (Hensen and Loeliger 1963), or by adding thrombin or the snake venom ancrod (Howie, Prentice and McNicol 1973). Defibrination with ancrod causes little loss of AT III activity from plasma whereas heating has been found to result in 25 per cent loss (Howie, Prentice and McNicol 1973). Chromogenic substrates for which thrombin has high specificity are now widely used in the second stage of the AT III assay and have resulted in new methods of assay (Blombäck *et al.* 1974, Vinazzer 1975, Blombäck 1981). Methods using those substrates would seem to have some advantages especially in laboratories with little expertise in clotting. On the other hand, problems may arise with specificity of the substrate, if it is of poor specificity or too specific so that important biological activities are not measured.

Lane, Bird and Rizza (1975) have described a method of measuring AT III activity which depends on radial diffusion of the plasma being studied in an agarose gel containing thrombin. Two advantages of this particular method are that defibrination is not required and large numbers of samples can be tested at one time.

In addition to the above assays of biological activity of AT III, it is possible to assay the AT III antigen by means of immunological methods such as the Mancini single radial immunodiffusion method (Abildgaard, Fagerhol and Egeberg 1970, Fagerhol and Abildgaard 1970, Hedner and Nilsson 1973) or by means of Laurell's electroimmunoassay (Fagerhol and Abildgaard 1970, Aberg, Nilsson and Hedner 1973, Damus and Wallace 1975). In general, there has been good correlation between the level of AT III antigen and its biological activity in plasma but Sas *et al.* (1974) have described a family in which there was a congenital deficiency of AT III biological activity associated with normal amounts of AT III antigen. Discrepancies between biological activity and immunologically detectable material have also been observed in patients treated with L-asparaginase (Conard *et al.* 1973) and in patients with repeated venous thrombosis (Nagy and Losonczy 1975). More recently Jesperson, Rasmussen and Toftgaard (1982) have reported discrepancies between functional and antigenic determination of AT III following transfusion of AT III concentrate to a patient with toxic shock syndrome and diffuse intravascular coagulation. The possibility of such discrepancies between the two methods of assay must be borne in mind when interpreting the results of immunological assays.

Assay of anti-Xa activity of AT III is carried out in a two-stage system in which a source of Xa is added to dilutions of plasma being tested and after a standard period of incubation the residual Xa is measured. This may be done by subsampling into a factor X-deficient substrate and recording the clotting time or into a chromogenic substrate and recording the change in absorbency by spectrophotometry. Clotting methods have been described by Biggs *et al.* (1970), Yue, Starr and Gertler (1973) and Marciniak and Tsukamura (1972). Assay methods using the chromogenic substrate S2222 (benzoyl-isoleucine-glutamyl-glycyl-arginine-para-nitroanilide HCl) for which factor Xa has high specificity have been described by Odegård, Lie and Abildgaard (1976).

AT III in disease

If we accept that the fluidity of the blood in the circulation depends on a fine balance between its procoagulant components and its inhibitory components, then, just as a deficiency of clot-promoting factor may result in a tendency to bleed, so we might expect a deficiency of inhibitory substances to result in a tendency to thrombose.

In 1965, Egeberg described a family with an inherited deficiency of AT III associated with recurrent episodes of venous thromboses. Seven members of the family were affected and the condition seemed to be inherited in an autosomal dominant fashion. Since Egeberg's original paper there have been several reports of inherited deficiency of AT III (von Kaulla and von Kaulla 1967, Penick 1969, van der Meer *et al.* 1973, Shapiro, Prager and Martinez 1973, Marciniak, Farley and DeSimone 1974, Sas *et al.* 1974, Gruenberg, Smallridge and Rosenberg 1975, Carvalho and Ellman 1976, Zucker, Gomperts and Marcus 1976, Odegård and Abildgaard 1977, Mackie *et al.* 1978, Matsuo *et al.* 1979, Wolf *et al.* 1979, Barbui and Rodeghiero 1981, Scully *et al.* 1981, Winter *et al.* 1982). In the majority of families so far described the level of AT III antigen where measured was reduced to the same level as the biological activity. The family described by Sas *et al.* (1974) was unusual in that normal amounts of AT III antigen were accompanied by low levels of AT III biological activity and abnormal mobility of the antigen on crossed immunoelectrophoresis (Lane 1978). The reverse was the case in the family described by Matsuo *et al.* (1979). In this family the level of biological activity was slightly higher than that of the antigen. A striking feature of many of those families is the relatively mild deficiency of AT III (40–60 per cent of average normal) which may be associated with thrombosis. Consistent with this is the finding by many workers of a narrow range of normal. If 100 per cent is taken as average normal most normal individuals fall within a range of approximately 75–140 per cent of average normal.

A reduced level of AT III has been reported in several diseases or conditions. These include venous thrombosis (von Kaulla and von Kaulla 1967, Abildgaard, Fagerhol and Egeberg 1970), disseminated intravascular clotting (Abildgaard, Fagerhol and Egeberg 1970, Damus and Wallace 1975), liver disease (Hensen and Loeliger 1963, von Kaulla and von Kaulla 1967, Abildgaard, Fagerhol and Egeberg 1970, Mannucci *et al.* 1973, Damus and Wallace 1975), septicaemia (Deutsch and Thaler 1979), following surgery (Aberg, Nilsson and Hedner 1973, Stathakis, Papayannis and Gardikas 1973), women taking oral contraceptives (Fagerhol and Abildgaard 1970, Conard, Samama and Salomon 1972). On the other hand, Hedner and Nilsson (1973) found normal or elevated levels of AT III in the majority of patients who had suffered venous thrombosis or myocardial infarction or who had undergone major surgery. Low levels, however, were found in patients suffering from cirrhosis of the liver.

The finding that levels of AT III less than 60 per cent of normal may be associated with venous thrombosis in the inherited deficiency state has prompted several groups of workers to see if the assay of AT III is of any value in identifying patients who are likely to develop venous thrombosis following surgery. So far no clear-cut answer has emerged. This is not surprising in view of the variety of tests and standards used for assaying AT III and the different types of surgical operations being studied. Even when the mean level of AT III in the patients is significantly different from that in the control group, there is usually so much overlap between the values in the two groups that the AT III assay is of little help in ascertaining whether or not a particular patient is at risk of developing venous thrombosis. It is probably wise, however, to consider patients who have AT III levels of less than 80 per cent of normal and who are undergoing major surgery, to be at risk of developing venous thrombosis. Patients with a congenital or acquired deficiency of AT III who require surgery may benefit by transfusion of AT III concentrate or fresh frozen plasma or cryoprecipitate. For long-term prophylaxis in patients with inherited deficiency of AT III and thrombotic complications, coumarin-type anticoagulants are clinically effective and should be administered on a long-term basis, possibly for the rest of the patient's life.

REFERENCES

Aberg M., Nilsson I.M. & Hedner U. (1973) Antithrombin III after operation. *Lancet* **II**, 1337.
Abildgaard U. (1967) Purification of two progressive antithrombins of human plasma. *Scandinavian Journal of Clinical and Laboratory Investigation* **19**, 190–5.
Abildgaard U. (1968) Highly purified antithrombin III with heparin cofactor activity

prepared by disc electrophoresis. *Scandinavian Journal of Clinical and Laboratory Investigation* **21**, 89–91.

Abildgaard U. (1969) Binding of thrombin to anti-thrombin III. *Scandinavian Journal of Clinical and Laboratory Investigation* **24**, 23–7.

Abildgaard U., Fagerhol M.K. & Egeberg O. (1970) Comparison of progressive antithrombin activity and concentrations of three thrombin inhibitors in human plasma. *Scandinavian Journal of Clinical and Laboratory Investigation* **26**,349–54.

Astrup T. & Darling S. (1942) Measurement and properties of antithrombin. *Acta Physiologica Scandinavica* **4**, 293–308.

Barbui T. & Rodeghiero F. (1981) Hereditary dysfunctional Antithrombin III (At-III Vincenza). *Thrombosis and Haemostasis* **45**, 97.

Biggs R., Denson K.W.E., Akman N., Borrett R. & Haddon M. (1970) Antithrombin III, antifactor Xa and heparin. *British Journal of Haematology* **19**, 283–305.

Binder R. (1973) On the complex formation of antithrombin III with thrombin. Gel filtration studies on human plasma and serum. *Thrombosis et Diathesis Haemorrhagica* **30**, 280–3.

Blombäck B., Blombäck M. & Olsson P. (1963) Studies on thrombin inactivation in normal plasma, serum and plasma fractions and its relation to heparin. *Thrombosis et Diasthesis Haemorrhagica* **9**, 368–86.

Blombäck M. (1981) Chromogenic substrates in the laboratory diagnosis of clotting disorders. In *Haemostasis and Thrombosis*. Bloom A.L. & Thomas D.P. (eds). pp. 809–23. Churchill Livingstone, Edinburgh.

Blombäck M., Blombäck B., Olsson P. & Svendsen L. (1974) The assay of antithrombin using a synthetic chromogenic substrate for thrombin. *Thrombin Research* **5**, 621–32.

Carvalho A. & Ellman L. (1976) Hereditary antithrombin III deficiency: effect of antithrombin III deficiency on platelet function. *American Journal of Medicine* **61**, 179–83.

Conard J., Durand G., Feger J. & Samama M. (1973) Acquired abnormal antithrombin III in L-asparaginase treated patients? *4th Congress, International Society on Thrombosis and Haemostasis, Vienna* (Abstracts).

Conard J., Samama M. & Salomon Y. (1972) Antithrombin III and the oestrogen content of combined oestro-progestogen contraceptives. *Lancet* II, 1148–9.

Damus P.S., Hicks M. & Rosenberg R.D. (1973) Anticoagulant action of heparin. *Nature* **246**, 355–7.

Damus P.S. & Wallace G.A. (1975) Immunological measurement of anti-thrombin III-heparin cofactor and α_2-macroglobulin in disseminated intravascular coagulation and hepatic failure coagulopathy. *Thrombosis Research* **6**, 27–38.

Deutsch E. & Thaler E. (1979) Acquired antithrombin III (AT III) deficiency in septicaemia. *Thrombosis and Haemostasis* **42**, 375.

Egeberg O. (1965) Inherited antithrombin deficiency causing thrombophilia. *Thrombosis et Diasthesis Haemorrhagica* **13**, 516–30.

Einarsson R. & Andersson L.-O. (1977) Binding of heparin to human antithrombin III as studied by measurement of tryptophan fluorescence. *Biochimica et Biophysica Acta* **490**, 104–11.

Fagerhol M.K. & Abildgaard U. (1970) Immunological studies on human antithrombin III. Influence of age, sex and use of oral contraceptives on serum concentration. *Scandinavian Journal of Haematology* **7**, 10–17.

Gans H. & Tan B.H. (1967) α_1-Antitrypsin, an inhibitor for thrombin and plasmin. *Clinica Chimica Acta* **17**, 111–17.

Gruenberg J.C., Smallridge R.C. & Rosenberg R.D. (1975) Inherited antithrombin III deficiency causing mesenteric venous infarction: a new clinical entity. *Annals of Surgery* **181**, 791–4.

Hallen A. (1962) A method for measuring antithrombin. *Thrombosis et Diathesis Haemorrhagica* **8**, 56–66.

Harpel P.C. & Rosenberg R.D. (1976) α_2-Macroglobulin and antithrombin III-heparin cofactor: modulators of hemostatic and inflammatory reactions. *Progress in Hemostasis and Thrombosis* **3**, 145–89.

Hedner U. & Nilsson I.M. (1973) Antithrombin III in a clinical material. *Thrombosis Research* **3**, 631–41.

Heimburger N. (1967) On the proteinase inhibitors of human plasma with especial reference to antithrombin. *First International Symposium on Tissue Factors in the Homeostasis of the Coagulation-Fibrinolysis System, Florence* (Abstracts).

Heimburger N., Haupt H. & Schwick H.G. (1970) Proteinase inhibitors of human plasma. In *Proceedings of the International Research Conference on Proteinase Inhibitors, Munich.* Fritz H. & Tscheche H. (eds). pp. 1–22. Walter de Gruyter, Berlin.

Hensen A. & Loeliger E.A. (1963) Antithrombin III. Its metabolism and its function in blood coagulation. *Thrombosis et Diathesis Haemorrhagica* **9**, Suppl. 1–84.

Howell W.H. & Holt E. (1918) Two new factors in blood coagulation—heparin and proantithrombin. *American Journal of Physiology* **47**, 328–41.

Howie P.W., Prentice C.R.M. & McNicol G.P. (1973) A method of antithrombin estimation using plasma defibrinated with ancrod. *British Journal of Haematology* **25**, 101–10.

Jespersen J., Rasmussen N.R. & Toftgaard C. (1982) Observations during treatment with antithrombin III concentrate of a case of tampon-related toxic shock syndrome and disseminated intravascular coagulation. Discrepancies between functional and immunologic determinations of antithrombin. *Thrombosis Research* **26**, 457–62.

Kekwick R.A. & MacKay M.E. (1954) The separation of protein fractions from human plasma with ether. *MRC Special Report, Series No. 286.* HMSO, London.

Klein P.D. & Seegers W.H. (1950) The nature of plasma antithrombin activity. *Blood* **5**, 742–52.

Kowalski E. (1959) Fibrinogen derived inhibitors of blood coagulation. *Thrombosis et Diathesis Haemorrhagica* **4**, Suppl. 211–23.

Lanchantin G.F., Plesset M.L., Freidmann J.A. & Hart D.W. (1966) Dissociation of esterolytic and clotting activities of Thrombin by trypsin-binding macroglobulin. *Proceedings of the Society for Experimental Biology and Medicine* **121**, 444–9.

Lane J.L. (1978) Some immunological investigations on antithrombin III 'Budapest'. *British Journal of Haematology* **40**, 459–70.

Lane J.L., Bird P. & Rizza C.R. (1975) A new assay for the measurement of total progressive antithrombin. *British Journal of Haematology* **30**, 103–15.

Loeliger E.A. & Hers J.F. (1957) Chronic antithrombinaemia (antithrombin V) with haemorrhagic diathesis in a case of rheumatoid arthritis with hypergammaglobulinaemia. *Thrombosis et Diathesis Haemorrhagica* **1**, 499–528.

Lyttleton J.W. (1954) The antithrombin activity of heparin. *Biochemical Journal* **58**, 15–23.

Mackie M., Bennett B., Ogston D. & Douglas A.S. (1978) Familial thrombosis: inherited deficiency of antithrombin III. *British Medical Journal* I, 136–8.

Mannucci L., Dioguardi N., Del Ninno E. & Mannucci P.M. (1973) Value of Normotest and antithrombin III in the assessment of liver function. *Scandinavian Journal of Gastroenterology* **8**, (Suppl. 19) 103–7.

Marciniak E., Farley C.H. & DeSimone P.A. (1974) Familial thrombosis due to antithrombin III deficiency. *Blood* **43**, 219–31.

Marciniak E. & Tsukamura S. (1972) Two progressive inhibitors of factor Xa in human blood. *British Journal of Haematology* **22**, 341–51.

Matsuo T., Ohki Y., Kondo S. & Matsuo O. (1979) Familial antithrombin III deficiency in a Japanese family. *Thrombosis Research* **16**, 815–23.

Miller-Andersson M., Borg H. & Andersson L.-O. (1974) Purification of antithrombin III by affinity chromatography. *Thrombosis Research* **5**, 439–52.

Monkhouse F.C. (1970) Preparation and assay of plasma antithrombin. *Methods in Enzymology* **19**, 915–24.

Morawitz P. (1905) Die Chemie der Blutgerinnung. *Ergebnisse der Physiologische biologischen Chemie und Experimental Pharmakologie* **4**, 307.

Murphy R.C. & Seegers W.H. (1948) Concentration of prothrombin and Ac-globulin in various species. *American Journal of Physiology* **154**, 134–9.

Nagy I. & Losonczy H. (1975) The significance of the chronic anticoagulant treatment in recurrent thromboemboli caused by hereditary antithrombin III deficiency. *Abstracts from Vth Congress of the International Society of Thrombosis and Haemostasis*, Paris.

Niléhn J.-E. (1967) Influence of split products of fibrinogen on results of blood coagulation tests and platelet adhesiveness. *Scandinavian Journal of Haematology* **4**, 430–40.

Odegård O.R. & Abildgaard U. (1977) Anti Xa activity in thrombophilia. Studies in a family with AT III deficiency. *Scandinavian Journal of Haematology* **18**, 86–90.

Odegård O.R., Lie M. & Abildgaard U. (1976) Antifactor Xa activity measured with amidolytic methods. *Haemostasis* **5**, 265–75.

Penick G.D. (1969) Blood states that predispose to thrombosis. In *Thrombosis*. Sherry S., Brinkhous K.M. & Genton E. (eds). National Academy of Sciences, Washington.

Pepper D.S., Banhegyi D. & Cash J.D. (1977) The different forms of AT III in serum. *Thrombosis and Haemostasis* **38**, 494–503.

Petersen T.E., Dudek-Wojciechowska G., Sottrup-Jensen L. & Magnusson S. (1979) Primary structure of anti-thrombin III (heparin co-factor). Partial homology between α_1-antitrypsin and anti-thrombin III. In *The Physiological Inhibitors of Coagulation and Fibrinolysis*. Collen D., Wiman B. & Verstraete M. (eds). pp. 43–54. Elsevier North-Holland Biomedical Press, New York.

Quick A.J. (1938) The normal antithrombin of the blood and its relation to heparin. *American Journal of Physiology* **123**, 712–19.

Rimon A., Shamash Y. & Shapiro B. (1966) The plasmin inhibitor of human plasma. IV: Its action on plasmin, trypsin, chymotrypsin and thrombin. *Journal of Biological Chemistry* **241**, 5102–7.

Rosenberg R.D. & Damus P.S. (1973) The purification and mechanism of action of human antithrombin-heparin cofactor. *Journal of Biological Chemistry* **248**, 6490–505.

Sas G., Blasko G., Banhegyi D., Jako J. & Palos L.A. (1974) Abnormal antithrombin III (antithrombin III 'Budapest') as a cause of a familial thrombophilia. *Thrombosis et Diathesis Haemorrhagica* **32**, 105–15.

Sas G., Pepper D.S. & Cash J.D. (1975) Investigations on antithrombin III in normal plasma and serum. *British Journal of Haematology* **30**, 265–72.

Schmidt A. (1892) *Zur Blutlehre.* F.C.W. Vogel, Leipzig.

Scully M.F., De Haas H., Chan P. & Kakkar V.V. (1981) Hereditary antithrombin III deficiency in an English family. *British Journal of Haematology* **47**, 235–40.

Seegers W.H. (1968) Antithrombin as proteinase inhibitor. *Annals of the New York Academy of Sciences* **146**, 593–600.

Seegers W.H., Johnson J.F. & Fell C. (1954) An antithrombin reaction related to prothrombin activation. *American Journal of Physiology* **176**, 97–103.

Seegers W.H. & Marciniak E. (1962) Inhibition of autoprothrombin C activity with plasma. *Nature* **193**, 1188–90.

Shapiro S.S., Prager D. & Martinez J. (1973) Inherited antithrombin III deficiency associated with multiple thromboembolic pneumonia. *Blood* **42**, 1001.

Shinowara G.Y. & Buckley D.J. (1960) Isolation of antithrombin globulin from human blood plasma. *Thrombosis et Diathesis Haemorrhagica* **4**, 17–30.

Stathakis N., Papayannis A.G. & Gardikas C.D. (1973) Post operative antithrombin III concentration. *Lancet* **I**, 430.

Thaler E. & Schmer G. (1975) A simple two-step isolation procedure for human and bovine antithrombin II/III (heparin cofactor): a comparison of two methods. *British Journal of Haematology* **31**, 233–43.

van der Meer J., Stoepman-van Dalen E.A. & Jansen J.M.S. (1973) Antithrombin III deficiency in a Dutch family. *Journal of Clinical Pathology* **26**, 532–8.

Villaneuva G.B. & Danishefsky I. (1977) Evidence for a heparin-induced conformational change on antithrombin III. *Biochemical and Biophysical Research Communications* **74**, 803–9.

Vinazzer H. (1975) Photometric assay of antithrombin III with a chromogenic substrate. *Haemostasis* **4**, 101–9.

von Kaulla E. & von Kaulla K.M. (1967) Antithrombin III and diseases. *American Journal of Clinical Pathology* **48**, 69–80.

Winter J.H., Fenech A., Ridley W., Bennett B., Cumming A.M., Mackie M. & Douglas A.S. (1982) Familial antithrombin III deficiency. *Quarterly Journal of Medicine* **204**, 373–95.

Wolf M., Boyer C., Lavergne J.M. & Larrieu M.J. (1979) A new variant of antithrombin III. Studies of three related cases. *Thrombosis and Haemostasis* **42**, 186.

Yin E.T., Wessler S. & Stoll P.J. (1971) Identity of plasma-activated factor X inhibitor with antithrombin III and heparin cofactor. *Journal of Biological Chemistry* **246**, 3712–19.

Yue R.H., Starr T. & Gertler M.M. (1973) Quantitative determination of total antithrombin III in plasma. *Thrombosis et Diathesis Haemorrhagica* **30**, 84–92.

Zucker M.L., Gomperts E.D. & Marcus R.G. (1976) Prophylactic and therapeutic use of anticoagulants in inherited antithrombin III deficiency. *South African Medical Journal* **50**, 1743–7.

Chapter 7
The Inheritance of Defects in
Blood Coagulation

R. BIGGS

The purpose of the present chapter is to describe as simply as possible the ways in which defects of blood coagulation are inherited and to consider the implications of the various modes of inheritance for the families of patients and for those who care for the patients themselves. To begin with, it is convenient to outline the main modes of inheritance; later, the various disease states will be classified according to their inheritance.

The inheritance of single traits

It was in the mid-nineteenth century that Gregor Mendel (1865) and later Bateson (1909) studied the inheritance of single traits in plants. Specific crosses were made and the appearance of the trait was enumerated in the first and second generations of offspring (F_1 and F_2 generations). Mendel found that if the cross was made between plants having red and white flowers then all of the first generation flowers were pink. In the second generation, arising from inbreeding plants of the F_1 generation, the plants appeared in the ratio of 1 with red flowers to 2 with pink flowers and 1 with white flowers.

Mendel realized that the observed sequence of generations could be explained if every adult plant had two characters (genes) for colour of flowers but that only one gene was transmitted to each ovum or pollen grain. Early in the twentieth century it was realized by Sutton and Boveri (1902) that the chromosomes of the cell nuclei must be the carriers of the genetic material. The reduction division (meiosis by which the double set of chromosomes is reduced to a single set) which precedes the formation of ova and pollen grains in plants and eggs and spermatozoa in animals provides exactly the mechanism envisaged by Mendel's theory of inheritance.

To return now to the red and white flowers: the mode of inheritance may be represented diagrammatically as in Fig. 17. It seems likely that each gene, for flower colour in this case, produces a single dose of pigment. When there are two genes in an individual the colour is red. One gene would produce half of the amount of pigment resulting in a pink colour and the absence of red genes would produce a white flower. Modifications of this pattern occur when one

92

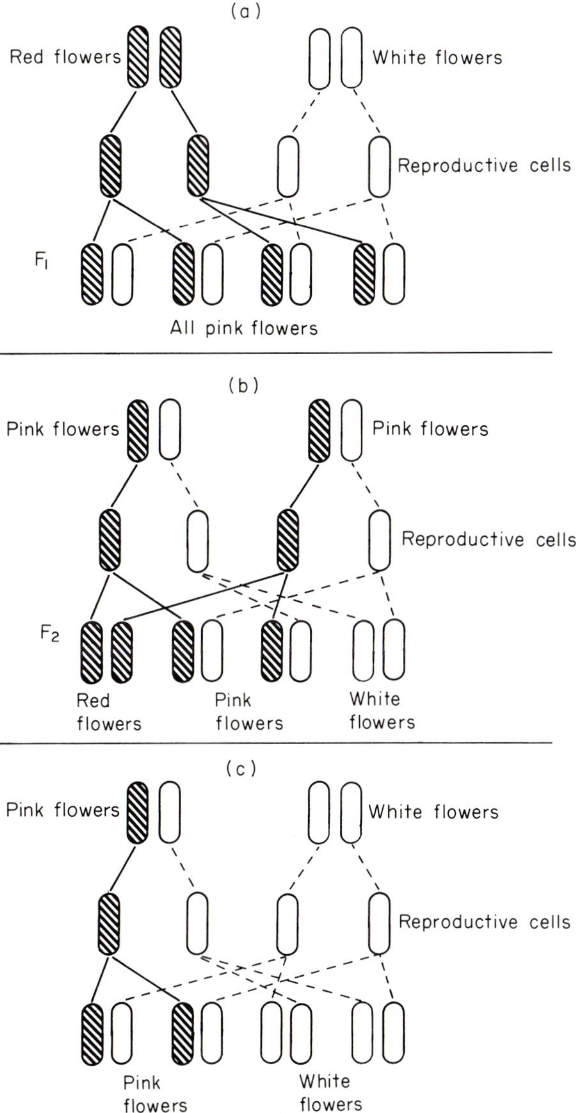

Fig. 17. The inheritance of flower colour through autosomal genes. (a) In the first generation a cross between 2 plants, one having red and the other white flowers, produces a first generation (F_1) all with pink flowers. (b) When plants with pink flowers are crossed these crosses produce a second generation (F_2) in the proportion of 1 white-flowered plant, 1 red-flowered plant and 2 pink-flowered plants. (c) In a cross between pink and white flowers the progeny appear in the proportion of 2 pink-flowered plants and 2 white-flowered plants.

gene dominates the other. Should the red gene be dominant, then those plants with only one gene controlling red colour would appear as red and be indistinguishable from those plants with two genes for red colour. It may be noted that in this sort of case the gene may still produce a single dose of colour but the human eye may be unable to distinguish between the depth of colour produced by one or two genes.

Inheritance of this kind is referred to as autosomal, and when one gene predominates then the inheritance is autosomal and dominant. The absence of colour is referred to as recessive. When a plant with one dose of colour is crossed with a white plant, half of the offspring will be pink and half white (Fig. 17c).

Sex-linked recessive inheritance

In all higher plants and animals the number of pairs of chromosomes which occur in a particular species is characteristic for that species. In man there are 48 pairs. In all species two of the chromosomes differ from the others in that they determine sex and are called sex chromosomes. In the human these sex chromosomes are called X and Y. The female has two X chromosomes and the male one X and one Y. Characteristics other than sex are carried on the X chromosomes. Thus, any gene situated on the X chromosome determines a sex-linked type of inheritance. A diagrammatic representation of sex-linked recessive inheritance is given in Fig. 18.

The practical implications of the sex-linked recessive type of inheritance of conditions such as haemophilia are as follows:

1   That all of the daughters of an affected male have one normal X chromosome and one X chromosome which carries the relevant gene. In the case of sex-linked recessive inheritance, these females (who are called carriers) are in all respects normal in appearance but have the capacity to pass the abnormality to their male offspring and through their male and female offspring to further generations.

2   All of the male offspring of an affected male are normal and cannot pass the defect to further generations.

3   In a marriage of a carrier female to a normal male, there is a 50 : 50 chance that male offspring will be affected and a 50 : 50 chance that female offspring will be carriers.

4   In the rare event of a carrier female marrying an affected male (Fig. 18c) the offspring would be in the proportion of 1 affected male to 1 normal male and 1 female haemophiliac to female carrier of haemophilia.

So far, the simple case of single gene abnormalities has been described; at a later stage more complicated situations will be considered in relation to specific disease states. The application of genetic principles to specific disease states will

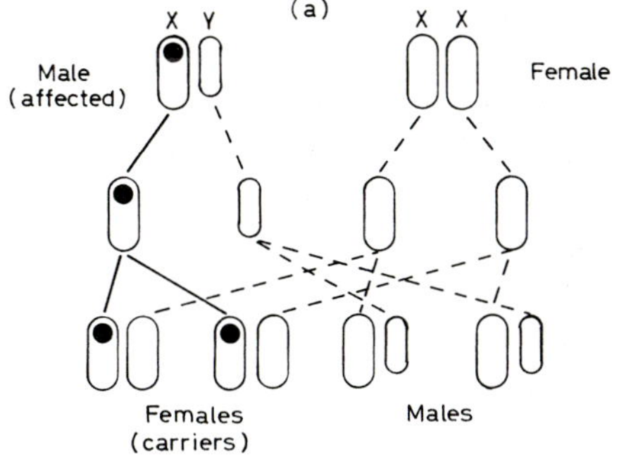

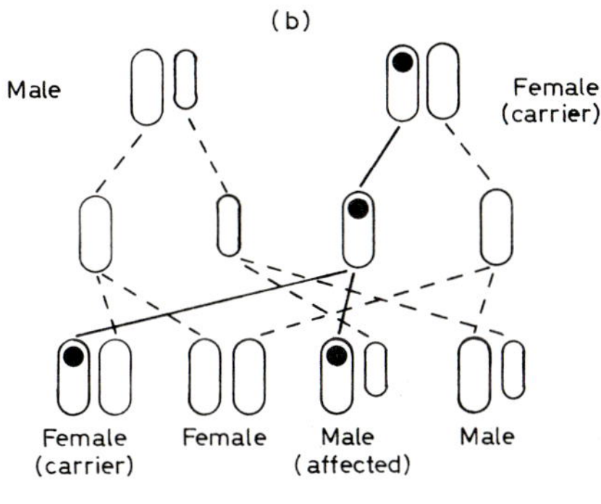

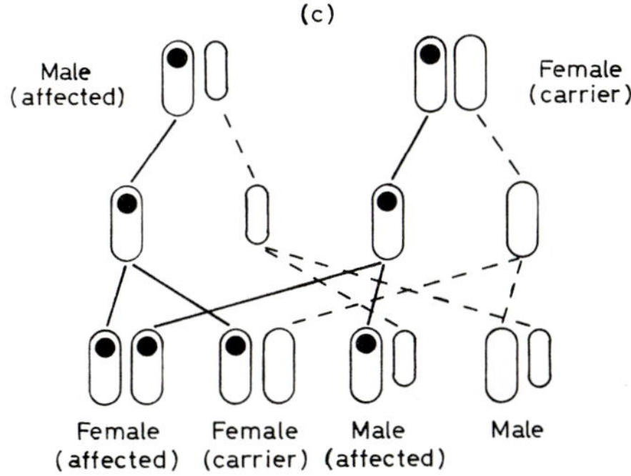

Fig. 18. Sex-linked recessive inheritance. (a) An affected male (XY) marries a normal female (XX). In this combination all of the daughters carry the defect and all of the sons are normal. (b) A carrier female marries a normal male. In this case half of the sons will be affected and half of the daughters will be carriers. (c) An affected male marries a carrier female. In this case half of the daughters will be affected with the disease and half will be carriers. Half of the sons will be normal and half will have the disease. The chromosome carrying the gene for abnormality is shown as ●.

now be discussed but first the distinction between recessive and dominant inheritance needs to be made.

What is meant by recessive or dominant?

In the example of coloured flowers, absence of colour is recessive since even a single gene for colour is expressed. If the heterozygote plants show red flower colour, indistinguishable from that of homozygous plants, then colour is dominant. In the case of disease states caused by the presence of a single abnormal gene then two sorts of criteria may be used to measure the degree of abnormality. One measure is the severity of the clinical symptoms. Historically this was the only criterion that could be used. Thus, a male patient who was crippled with haemarthroses and bled severely after injury and who inherited the defect through an apparently normal mother and had other affected male relatives would be said to have haemophilia and the inheritance would be sex-linked and recessive (since the mother had no symptoms). In the early days the laboratory tests to detect the various coagulation abnormalities had not been developed. Once such tests were available the results of tests to measure the concentration of clotting factors could be used in genetic studies. Thus in the case of factor VIII clotting activity, for example, a female with two normal X chromosomes has on average twice as much factor VIII as a carrier of haemophilia who has one normal X chromosome and one X chromosome which carries the gene for haemophilia. So it would seem that for genes which control the production of a specific substance the effect is quantitative. From the point of view of laboratory testing, factor VIII inheritance is not recessive but more like the flower colour inheritance where one gene gives pink flowers and two give red flowers. For classification it seems reasonable to give precedence to the clinical features in assessing dominance and recessiveness. The reason for this is that it is the symptoms which are of concern to the patients and to the medical services.

Even more confusing situations may arise when the laboratory tests seem relatively poorly related to the clinical manifestations of disease as may occur, for instance, with factor XI deficiency (see below). When the results of laboratory tests are not well correlated with clinical features then one may question the 'validity' of the tests. By this I mean that the test may not be related to the underlying abnormal physiology of the disease, or indeed the condition characterized by the particular test system may not qualify to be considered as a 'disease' state. These concepts will be elaborated in relation to specific conditions. A list of recognized coagulation defects and their relative frequencies is given in Table 5.

Table 5. Prevalence of the various coagulation defects.

Coagulation factor	Clinical condition	Inheritance	Prevalence per million of the population
Factor I (fibrinogen)	Afibrinogenaemia	Autosomal recessive	1.0
	Dysfibrinogenaemia	?	?
Factor II (prothrombin)	Prothrombin deficiency	? Autosomal recessive	0.1
Factor V	Factor V deficiency	Autosomal recessive	0.1
VII	Factor VII deficiency	Autosomal recessive	0.1
X	Factor X deficiency	Autosomal recessive	0.1
VIII	Haemophilia A	Sex-linked recessive	60–100
	von Willebrand's disease	Autosomal dominant	50–100
IX	Haemophilia B	Sex-linked recessive	14–18
XI	Factor XI deficiency	Autosomal	1.0
XII	Hageman defect	Autosomal	0.1
XIII	Factor XIII (fibrin stabilizing factor) deficiency	Autosomal	0.1

Laboratory tests and genetic study of coagulation defects

The development of laboratory tests has contributed to genetic study of coagulation defects. The measurement of coagulation abnormalities may be based on coagulation function tests or on immunological methods. The coagulation tests are likely to be related to the clinical features of the disease state since it is presumed that the coagulation abnormality is the cause of the observed excessive bleeding. If, however, more than one sort of coagulation test is available the results of the different tests are not always well correlated.

The immunological tests are often not well correlated with the clinical severity of excessive bleeding but give information about the nature of the defect. The defect may be due to absence of the relevant coagulation factor or to the presence of abnormal protein (molecular variant) which, though non-functional in clotting tests, may still react to immunological methods.

Conditions inherited as autosomal recessive traits

As might be expected, the conditions inherited through autosomal recessive genes are in the main those which are most rarely encountered since the abnormal genes hide in the heterozygous condition in the normal population. These are deficiencies of factors I, II, V, VII, X and in some cases of factor XI and XII. It is now proposed to consider some general features of autosomal recessive inheritance (Fig. 17).

Since the condition is recessive a pairing of an affected person and a normal person will produce all heterozygote offspring which will appear normal. A mating of two heterozygotes will result in a statistical proportion of three apparently normal offspring to one affected offspring. The combination of an affected person with a heterozygote will lead to the birth of equal numbers of affected persons and heterozygotes. These facts mean that the autosomal recessive conditions will be most commonly encountered in marriages between related persons. It is thus always worth enquiring about a possible relationship between the parents when a case of a rare autosomal recessive condition appears. It is true that a proportion of such cases results from mutation and from random mating of two heterozygotes but from the nature of the defect a rare recessive gene must be hidden in seemingly normal heterozygotes.

A brief discussion of the inheritance of each of the different coagulation defects now follows.

Afibrinogenaemia (factor I deficiency) and factor XIII deficiency

Since fibrinogen is the protein which ultimately produces the blood clot, it might be thought that fibrinogen deficiency would produce the most severe of all the haemorrhagic states caused by defective coagulation. Curiously, this is not the case. Although a proportion of patients who have complete deficiency of fibrinogen have died at fairly early ages, a number of patients survived, even without treatment, well into adult life. Complete deficiency of fibrinogen is very rare. Afibrinogenaemia occurs approximately once per million of the general population (Table 5).

The conversion of fibrinogen to fibrin takes place, as is well known, in two stages (see Chapter 2). In the first stage thrombin removes two fibrinopeptides

(A and B) from fibrinogen. The fibrin monomer resulting from this reaction then polymerizes to form fibrin strands which are then linked together under the influence of factor XIII. In addition to complete fibrinogen deficiency, a number of patients who have abnormal fibrinogen (dysfibrinogenaemia) have been described.

AFIBRINOGENAEMIA

Patients with afibrinogenaemia have no fibrinogen to be detected by either immunological or coagulation techniques. A review of cases known by 1965 is given by Kerr and a more recent record is that of Flute (1977). It was at one time thought that affected males outnumbered females (Graham 1957) but this is now not thought to be the case. Kerr (1965) noted that consanguinity had occurred in 21 of 49 marriages. The inheritance from the clinical point of view is autosomal and recessive, although those who are heterozygous for the condition usually have low levels of plasma fibrinogen. Since 10–20 per cent of the normal amount of fibrinogen is enough to promote normal haemostasis, such carriers of the condition are asymptomatic.

DYSFIBRINOGENAEMIA

Fibrinogen is a protein whose chemical structure is better understood than that of most other coagulation factors. The reactions which fibrinogen undergoes under the influence of thrombin and factor XIII are also fairly well understood (Chapter 2). In recent years a number of variants which differ from normal have been recorded. These variants may produce a retarded reaction with thrombin indicating delayed or reduced liberation of fibrinopeptides A or B or slow polymerization or both. Immunological studies usually show a normal amount of fibrinogen. The first case of dysfibrinogenaemia was recorded by Imperato and Dettori (1958). In 1973 Ménaché listed 83 cases (37 males and 46 females) in 22 families.

About 30 per cent of the patients had mildly excessive bleeding after injury but in most cases the defect was asymptomatic. The inheritance in most cases seems to be autosomal and it may be partially dominant in that heterozygotes have abnormal protein that can be detected. The distinction is academic since the condition produces no symptoms in most cases, and it is doubtful whether the majority of examples of dysfibrinogenaemia should be thought of as having a disease. It is well known that proteins are variable in normal people and there is no reason why this variability should not occur in coagulation proteins. Such variability presumably depends on the occurrence of many alternative genes (allelomorphs) at a particular chromosome site.

FACTOR XIII

Factor XIII was first described, not as a result of studying plasma from a patient, but from experimental observations on normal plasma (Laki and Lorand 1948). Laki observed that clots formed in normal plasma were insoluble in 30 per cent urea, whereas clots made in purified fibrinogen were soluble. He identified a plasma factor (factor XIII) which would render fibrinogen clots insoluble in urea. In 1960, Duckert, Jung and Schmerling discovered a patient whose plasma clots were insoluble in urea and who had a distinct haemorrhagic state. Since 1960, a number of cases have been described and the inheritance seems to be autosomal and clinically recessive though heterozygotes have low levels of factor XIII.

Prothrombin (factor II) deficiency

Prothrombin deficiency is very rare, and complete absence of prothrombin is probably incompatible with life. The cases described are all partial deficiencies and all may be cases in which the prothrombin molecule differs from normal but where some effective coagulant is formed. The early literature on 'prothrombin deficiency' was confused because prothrombin was measured by a test known as the one-stage prothrombin time. This test system is as much affected by the speed of thrombin formation as by the amount of thrombin formed. Clotting times by this method are thus greatly lengthened by deficiency of factors V, VII or X. It is impossible to distinguish these deficiencies from prothrombin deficiency in early case records.

Males and females may be affected by true prothrombin deficiency and some families have more than one affected member. The inheritance is probably autosomal and recessive.

Factor X deficiency

Factor X deficiency is rare and in several families the parents of affected persons are known to have been related (Graham, Barrow and Hougie 1957, Hougie, Barrow and Graham 1957, Bachmann 1958, Roos *et al.* 1959). Affected persons usually have levels of factor X below 5 per cent of normal but probable heterozygotes also have low levels in some families. Factor X may be measured with the one-stage prothrombin time using brain extract or Russell's viper venom as thromboplastins. Immunological methods are also available. When different methods are used different levels of factor X are recorded in some cases (Denson *et al.* 1970, Girolami *et al.* 1979). Using neutralization of antibody some patients have abnormal protein and in some no immunological protein can be detected (Denson *et al.* 1970). This suggests that there are probably a number of different molecular variants of factor X (and allelomorphic genes which control factor X production) which result in sufficient abnormality to produce symptoms. Fair and Edgington (1981) in a study of samples from 28 patients found very little difference in the level of factor X measured by different methods thus suggesting that in these cases there was little heterogeneity in the factor X.

DEFICIENCY OF FACTORS V AND VII

These two abnormalities are considered together since the two factors are both necessary for the conversion of prothrombin to thrombin using brain extract thromboplastin.

Factor V deficiency is rare, males and females are both affected and in three families the parents of affected persons were related (Brink and Kingsley 1952, Kingsley 1954, Seibert, Margolius and Ratnoff 1958). It seems likely that the condition is inherited through an autosomal recessive gene. In a family reported by Rush and Ellis (1965) unaffected heterozygotes had low factor V levels.

Factor VII deficiency is rare and is probably inherited through autosomal recessive genes. Low levels of factor VII have been found in some clinically normal persons who were relatives of affected persons (Hall *et al.* 1964). Factor VII has also been studied immunologically in affected persons and it seems that there are different molecular variants of factor VII (Hall *et al.* 1964, Girolami *et al.* 1969).

SEX-LINKED RECESSIVE INHERITANCE

Two coagulation defects are inherited through sex-linked recessive genes. These are haemophilia A and haemophilia B. The two conditions are associated with identical clinical features but abnormality of different coagulation factors (factors VIII and IX) is responsible for the defects. Seventy-five to 80 per cent of patients in this group have haemophilia A and 20–25 per cent have haemophilia B.

FACTOR VIII DEFICIENCY IN HAEMOPHILIA A

Factor VIII may be conceived as consisting of two parts, the clotting activity (VIII:C) and a carrier protein (VIIIR:Ag or factor VIII-related antigen) (see Chapter 5). In haemophilia A the clotting activity is either absent or reduced. The VIIIR:Ag is apparently normal or increased in most cases. A family tree of human sex-linked inheritance in haemophilia A is shown in Fig. 19.

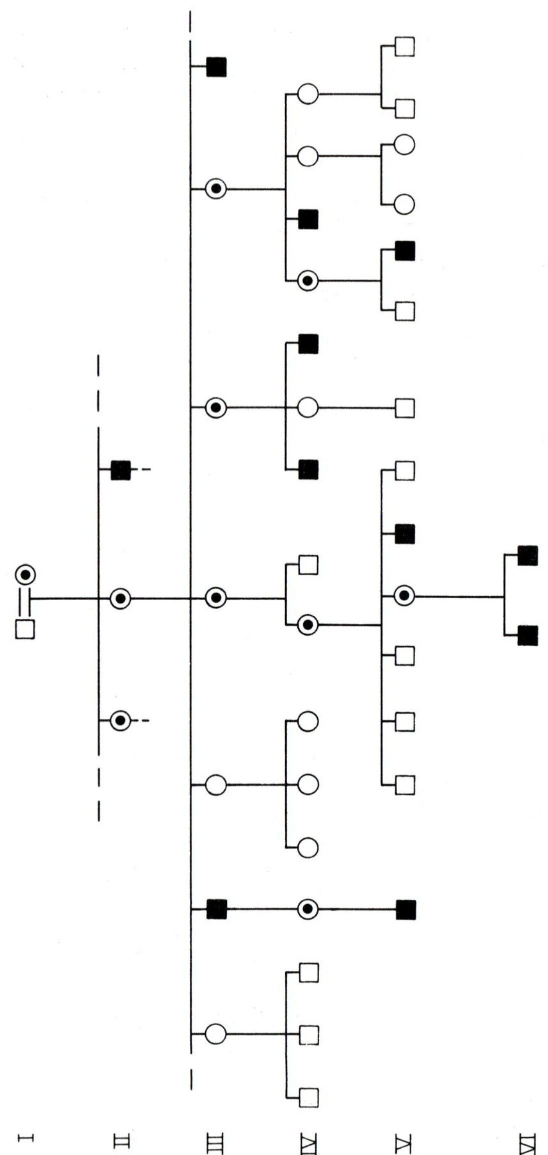

Fig. 19. Family tree of haemophilia.

As will be seen from Table 5, haemophilia A, except perhaps for von Willebrand's disease, is the most prevalent of all coagulation abnormalities. A variety of records of prevalence of haemophilia A is given in Table 6. It will be seen that the prevalence has increased considerably in recent years. This increase probably has a number of causes. The most obvious cause is better ascertainment. There has been a progressive development of specialist Haemophilia Centres in the UK and throughout the world. This development has been accompanied by increased supply of therapeutic factor VIII. These improvements have meant that most haemophilia A patients are known and treated at the Haemophilia Centres where good records are kept. In 1975, 3068 haemophilia A patients were registered in the UK and an inquiry at other hospitals revealed only 108 patients who were not also recorded by the Haemophilia Centres (Biggs and Spooner 1978).

Table 6. Prevalence of haemophilia in various populations expressed per 100 000 of the population.

Reference	Country/city	Date	Prevalence
Haldane	London, UK	1935	2.0
Andreassen	Denmark	1943	2.2
Ikkala	Finland	1960	3.7
Sjølin	Denmark	1961	3.6
Ramgren	Sweden	1962	3.35
Martin-Villar *et al.*	Spain	1971	2.3
National Hemophilia Foundation	Michigan, USA	1971	7.3
Larrain, Conte & Gonzalez	Chile	1972	3.5
National Heart and Lung Institute	USA	1972	9.0
Nilsson	Sweden	1972	5.5
Rosenberg	Brazil	1972	7–10
Sultz	New York, USA	1972	7.3
Biggs	UK	1974	6.0
Cash	Edinburgh, UK	1975	6.3
Allain	France	1976	5.3
Brackmann *et al.*	West Germany	1976	9.2
Davey	Australia	1976	5.9
Mandalaki	Greece	1976	6.25
Mannucci & Ruggeri	Italy	1976	9.8
Martin-Villar, Ortega & Magallon	Spain	1976	3.3
Masure	Belgium	1976	4.6
Nilsson	Sweden	1976	6.9
Soulier	France	1976	6.6
Rizza & Spooner	UK	1983	7.9

Another cause of increased numbers of haemophilia A patients stems from improved treatment. The patients now live longer than in the past. The average age at death in the first half of this century was 16–20 years (Andreassen 1943, Ramgren 1962). Now the average age at death is probably greater than 40 years (Biggs 1978, Rizza and Spooner 1983). Thus patients who would have died in earlier years now survive to swell the numbers. The average age of surviving patients is still below the average for normal people; it may be concluded that the increased prevalence of haemophilia A attributable to survival is not complete (Biggs 1974).

In 1935 and 1947 Haldane pointed out that any gene causing death before puberty would tend to die out unless renewed by mutation. The incidence of such a lethal disease would derive from a balance between mutation rate and early death of the affected persons. For a sex-linked gene, Haldane represented the balance as follows:

$$I = \frac{3m}{1-f}$$

Where I is the incidence at birth, f is the fitness and m is the mutation rate per generation. From the reasonably complete data of Andreassen (1943), Haldane took I to be 13.3 per 100 000 live male births or about 6.7 per 100 000 of the population, male and female.

Fitness is a measure of reproductive ability and concerns the number of children born to affected persons in comparison to those born to normal people in the same era. If one child is born to every haemophilia A patient at a particular time when two are born to normal persons then the fitness would be said to be 1 in 2 or 0.5. With the omission of one family Haldane calculated the fitness of haemophiliacs to be 0.286. The fitness is now doubtless increasing though there are as yet no figures from which to assess the extent of the increase.

A generation is taken to be 30 years. Haldane calculated the mutation rate to be 3.2 per 100 000 males per generation. This figure is similar to those of subsequent workers. Vogel (1955) estimated 2.7×10^{-5} males per generation. Ikkala (1960) gave a figure of 3.2×10^{-5} and Ramgren (1962) 2.7×10^{-5} males. Barrai *et al.* 1968 gave a much lower figure but their data about the incidence of haemophilia A was almost certainly unreliable.

Any calculations based on suppositions and Haldane's formula must be very speculative but it should perhaps be pointed out that, if Haldane's formula is correct, increased fitness will notably increase the incidence of haemophilia A. An increase from 0.286 to 0.5 or 0.8 would increase the incidence at birth from 13.3×10^{-5} to 19.2 or 48×10^{-5}. The actual figures would, of course, depend on the trend in birth rate in the general population at the time that the change in fitness occurred. It would also depend on the attitude of patients to genetic counselling at that time.

THE DETECTION OF CARRIERS OF HAEMOPHILIA A

The majority of carriers of haemophilia A are asymptomatic but on average carriers of haemophilia A are found to have half the blood concentration of factor VIII coagulant activity than is usual in normal women. The range of factor VIII:C levels in carriers is very wide, extending from less than 10 per cent of normal to 100 per cent or more. At the lower end some women in haemophilic families, who have very low factor VIII levels and suffer symptoms (Taylor and Biggs 1957), can be diagnosed as probable carriers of haemophilia A but at higher levels they are indistinguishable from normal women. The very wide range is probably due to the 'Lyonization mechanism' in females. The hypothesis that one X chromosome is inactivated in early embryonic life was put forward by Lyon (1961). According to this view the inactivation of a normal X chromosome would result in low factor VIII whereas the inactivation of the chromosome bearing the haemophilia A gene would promote a normal factor VIII level. The hypothesis has been supported by Mannucci *et al.* (1978) who found identical twins, both carriers of haemophilia A, who had dissimilar factor VIII levels (4 per cent and 36 per cent).

Only a small proportion (25–50 per cent) of carriers have sufficient low levels of factor VIII:C to allow their discrimination from normal. However, the simultaneous measurement of VIII:C and VIIIR:Ag in the same plasma sample enables one to discriminate in a proportion of cases between haemophilia A carriers and normal women. In normal women it is found that the levels of VIII:C and VIIIR:Ag are correlated. A woman with a high level of VIII:C tends also to have high VIIIR:Ag and vice versa (Fig. 20). The same applies in carriers of haemophilia but, whereas in normal women the ratio of VIII:C to VIIIR:Ag is 1, that in carriers is 0.5 (Fig. 20). It is this low ratio of VIII:C to VIIIR:Ag which makes the combined measurement of the two values so useful (Rizza *et al.* 1975, Ratnoff & Jones 1976). In fact, using both measurements 70–94 per cent of carriers of haemophilia A may be distinguishable from normal women.

THE INHERITANCE OF SPORADIC CASES OF HAEMOPHILIA A

In the case of sex-linked recessive inheritance of rarely encountered genes, it is common for there to be only one known affected person in a family. Such single cases are called sporadic cases. In some instances the condition has been passed through several generations of carrier females and maybe girls have predominated among the children in previous generations. In some instances such cases result from mutation and when this occurs the mother may be a normal woman and not a carrier of haemophilia. Using tests for VIIIR:Ag and VIII:C, Biggs and Rizza (1976) found that 39 of 41 mothers of affected single

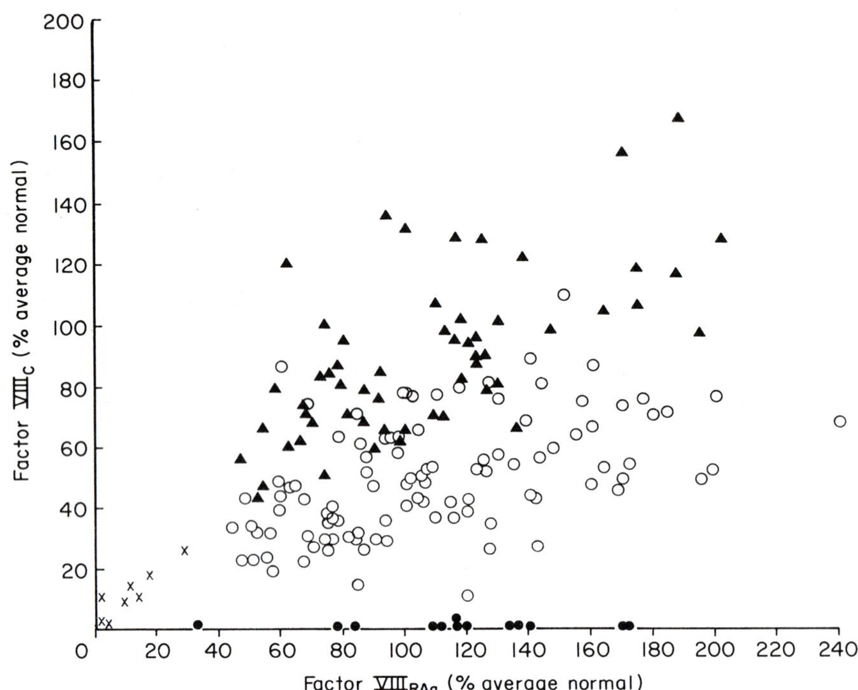

Fig. 20. The relationship between factor VIII:C and factor VIII:RAg in tests where both measurements are made on the same blood samples. X von Willebrand's disease, x haemophilia, ● normal women, ▲ proved carriers of haemophilia ○

sons were probably carriers of haemophilia. This high proportion of probable carriers suggests that the mutation rate must be substantially higher in males than in females. This idea is supported by the observations of Haldane (1947) and Graham (1979) but not by those of Barrai *et al.* (1968), Ratnoff and Jones (1976) and Ananthakrishnan and D'Souza (1979).

PROBABILITY AND GENETIC COUNSELLING IN HAEMOPHILIA A

The purpose of genetic counselling is to explain as clearly as possible to the patient (and/or members of the family) the mode of inheritance of a particular disease, in this case haemophilia A. The explanation is not always easy and understanding may be promoted by providing a booklet to which reference may be made. In addition to describing the mode of inheritance, the doctor should also make clear the steps that are now available to decrease the likelihood of an affected son being born.

Unfortunately, the whole explanation is full of the concept of probability. Certain definite and clear statements about the inheritance can be made from a study of the family tree. For example, all the daughters of a haemophilia A patient are carriers of haemophilia A and all of his sons are normal. These are the cases where no probability concept arises. For other family members there are greater or lesser *a priori* probabilities that the patient is a carrier. For example, the daughter of a known carrier has a 1 in 2 chance of being a carrier. A grand-daughter of a carrier has a 1 in 4 chance of being a carrier. Among the children of a known carrier there is a 1 in 4 chance that a haemophilic son may be born and a 1 in 4 chance of a carrier daughter.

These genetic probabilities can be modified by the results of testing for VIIIR:Ag and VIII:C (Bouma *et al.* 1975, Prentice *et al.* 1975, Elston *et al.* 1976, Graham 1977 and 1979, Klein *et al.* 1977). From prior genetic probability and the results of laboratory tests an overall probability can be calculated. It should be emphasized that an abnormal laboratory test in itself in a woman who is not known to be a member of a haemophilic family has little significance. The way that the laboratory data may be combined with *a priori* genetic information is illustrated by Graham (1979). In the case of a daughter of a known carrier the prior probability that the girl is a carrier is 1 in 2. If the laboratory results suggest that she is 10 times more likely to be a carrier than to be normal then the overall probability is 20 to 1 or 0.95. In the case of a female who is *not* a member of a haemophilic family then the prior probability that she is a carrier is likely to be less than 1 in 100 000. With this prior probability the laboratory results would need to be very convincing to give even a small probability that the woman was a carrier of haemophilia. Of course, there are women in the normal population who are not known to belong to haemophilic families but who may nevertheless be carriers (Graham 1979). The observer is, however, fairly unlikely to meet them.

Experience with haemophilic patients and their relatives suggests that a good deal of time and several interviews may be required before sex-linked inheritance is understood. The whole concept of probability is not very helpful to the patient. Bad luck is, in the human mind, something that happens to other people. A 1 in 4 chance of having a haemophilic son may not seem a great risk to a mother who wants to have children. Unfortunately, no matter how probable or improbable, the doctor is not in a position to say with certainty that a woman in a haemophilic family is *not* a carrier of haemophilia except in certain *a priori* genetic cases, for example, in the daughter of a normal male in a haemophilic family.

If a woman is a known carrier of haemophilia and wishes never to have a haemophilic child it is now possible, by selective abortion, to ensure that no affected sons are born. The sex of the child can be determined *in utero* and the presence of abnormal coagulation can be ascertained with reasonable certainty (Mibashan *et al.* 1979) and an affected male embryo can be aborted.

Factor VIII deficiency and von Willebrand's disease

As previously mentioned, factor VIII is a highly complex protein with which several activities are associated. The principal known 'related' (R) activities are discussed by Nilsson and Holmberg (1979) and are as follows:

1   VIII:C, the clotting activity.

2   VIIIR:Ag, an activity detected immunologically and measured by the Laurell (1972) technique or by immunoradiometric methods. This activity was demonstrated by Zimmerman, Ratnoff and Powell (1971).

3   VIIIR:GB, an activity associated with the adherence of platelets to glass beads.

4   VIIIR:RCF, an activity detected by the aggregation of platelets in the presence of the antibiotic ristocetin.

5   VIIIR:BT, an activity detected by a prolonged bleeding time.

von Willebrand's disease was first described in 1926 by von Willebrand from a study of a family from the Åland islands. The disease was characterized as a bleeding disorder associated with a prolonged bleeding time. The main characteristic bleeding manifestations were epistaxis, bleeding following minor injuries, such as scratches (as well as after major injuries), gastrointestinal haemorrhage and menorrhagia. The condition affected males and females equally and appeared to be inherited through an autosomal dominant gene. A typical family tree is shown in Fig. 21.

Initially the defect was thought of as an abnormality of capillary function in which capillary blood vessels failed to contract following injury. In 1953 Alexander and Goldstein showed that affected patients often (but not always) had low levels of factor VIII:C. The most severely affected patients had both long bleeding time and the lowest levels of clotting activity.

In 1971 Zimmerman, Ratnoff and Powell showed that von Willebrand's disease patients also had reduced or absent VIIIR:Ag. Sometimes VIIIR:Ag appears to be normal but a qualitatively different protein can be detected by immunoelectrophoresis (Holmberg and Nilsson 1972, Kernoff, Gruson and Rizza 1974, Rizza 1975). Absence of the VIIIR:Ag activity may also be associated with the characteristic prolonged bleeding time and by failure of the patient's plasma to agglutinate platelets in the presence of the antibiotic ristocetin (VIIIR:RCF). It seems likely that VIIIR:Ag protein plays a part in the control of bleeding by platelet plugs. Normally platelets adhere to each other and the platelet agglutinates stick to the vessel walls and through this process block small defects in the wall through which blood might otherwise seep. Failure of all the related activities may be associated with absence of, or defective, VIII:RAg.

The absent or defective VIIIR:Ag is dominantly inherited through an autosomal gene. Since absence of VIIIR:Ag is so often associated with absent

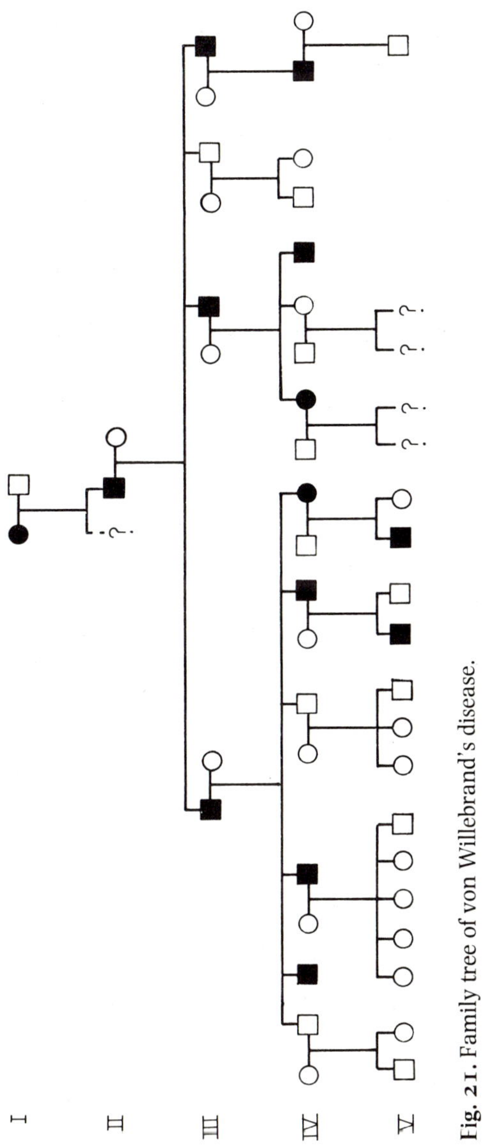

Fig. 21. Family tree of von Willebrand's disease.

VIII:C it seems that the normal factor VIII molecule must be assembled in some way from the products of at least two genes. Other complex proteins, such as blood group substances, also seem to have a similarly complicated assembly pattern. A complex structure of this sort has a strange effect on the genetic studies. For example, attempts to determine the mode of inheritance of factor VIII:C in normal people is difficult since the normal level of factor VIII:C may be associated with either a sex-linked recessive gene or with an autosomal dominant gene and the inclusion of both types in the normal variation will blur any clear pattern (Kerr *et al.* 1966).

The severity of von Willebrand's disease is very variable both from one family to another and within a particular family. The variability within a family may be due to partial dominance, the homozygous condition giving greater effect, and those who have only one abnormal gene being mildly affected. In families with wholly mild abnormality it may be that the abnormal protein (VIIIR:Ag) retains some activity.

Factor IX deficiency (haemophilia B)

Haemophilia B is inherited through a sex-linked recessive gene and has symptomatology identical with that of haemophilia A. Thus in all the early literature (prior to 1952) the two conditions were classed together as haemophilia. Haemophilia B includes mildly and severely affected patients as does haemophilia A. The degree of severity is the same in any particular family. Whereas haemophilia A patients lack factor VIII:C, haemophilia B patients lack factor IX clotting activity (IX:C). Factors VIII and IX take part in the same stage of the intrinsic clotting mechanism and this may determine the similarity of symptoms in the two diseases. Haemophilia B is less common than haemophilia A; it occurs in 5–10 males per million of the population. The mutation rate is probably $0.2–0.3 \times 10^{-5}$ live male births.

As with haemophilia A, factor IX:C has related immunological activities (IX:Ag). These related activities are not present in as high a proportion of patients as is VIIIR:Ag; as far as is known, VIIIR:Ag is present in all haemophilia A patients. Haemophilia B patients who have IX:Ag are said to be CRM+ (Cross Reacting Material positive). Among 68 kindred, Parekh Mannucci and Ruggeri (1978) found that 52 were CRM− and in 16 the affected males were CRM+. In a similar study Kasper *et al.* (1977) found that of the 71 kindred studied about one third were CRM+. Bertina and Veltkamp (1978) studied 33 patients with haemophilia B and found 14 of them to be CRM+. Kasper *et al.* (1977) and Bertina and Veltkamp (1978) used a variety of laboratory procedures and found that the patients could be divided into six (Kasper *et al.*) or seven (Bertina and Veltkamp) groups according to the results of these tests. One rather odd laboratory result is that a proportion of CRM+

cases show a long one-stage prothrombin time when ox brain is used as thromboplastin (Kidd, Denson and Biggs 1963, Hougie and Twomey 1967, Denson, Biggs and Mannucci 1968). Parekh, Mannucci and Ruggeri (1978) found five patients whose plasma gave this result. Kasper *et al.* (1977) found seven patients in this category. Bertina and Veltkamp (1978) record one case which had a grossly prolonged ox-brain prothrombin time and three others with a slightly lengthened clotting time using this test. In one case the long prothrombin time was reduced by addition of a factor IX inhibitor showing that the abnormal factor IX was responsible for the ox-brain abnormality (Bertina and Van der Linden 1982). It seems that considerable heterogeneity exists among patients who have the haemophilia B clotting defect.

Carriers of haemophilia B often have low levels of factor IX (Simpson and Biggs 1962). A study of haemophilia B carriers on a plan similar to that used for haemophilia A using IX:C and IX:Ag can of course only be carried out in those families where IX:Ag can be demonstrated. Kasper *et al.* (1977) found a good separation between carriers and normal women in those families with CRM+ affected males.

In 1983, Giannelli *et al.* studied the DNA of 5 of the 6 haemophilia B patients in the UK known to have anti-factor IX antibodies. They found gross genomic deletions in 4 of the 5 patients studied and suggested that these patients developed antibodies because they had no immunologically identifiable factor IX protein. Similar deletions were not found in 20 haemophilia B patients who had no anti-factor IX antibodies.

Using a complementary DNA (cDNA) probe derived from messenger RNA, Camerino *et al.* (1984) have found a restriction fragment length polymorphism in the region of the factor IX gene. Giannelli *et al.* (1984) using a genomic probe have determined the exact location of the polymorphism, followed its co-segregation with the abnormal factor IX gene and have demonstrated its usefulness in carrier detection.

Hopefully, similar methods will prove helpful in studying haemophilia A patients.

DEFECTS OF THE CONTACT STAGE IN COAGULATION

The initial stages of blood coagulation, as they take place in glass tubes, are complicated and tests for factors in this system often do not correlate well with clinical symptoms. A defect may be said to be 'severe' because it produces a marked abnormality *in vitro*. It may be that the mechanism detected *in vitro* has relatively little to do with normal haemostasis but is rather related to the removal of unwanted debris (such as might constitute a foreign surface) from the circulation.

Factor XI deficiency

Factor XI deficiency was described by Rosenthal, Dreskin and Rosenthal (1953). The defect causes a prolonged clotting time in glass tubes and an abnormally low consumption of prothrombin during coagulation. The majority of the known families are of Jewish origin. In (1978) Seligsohn studied 34 kindred in Israel and of these 33 had Ashkenazi Jewish ancestors. The haemorrhagic tendency is inherited through an autosomal and partially dominant gene. Leiba, Ramot and Many (1965) found that some patients with little factor XI had few symptoms whereas others who appeared to have 20–40 per cent of factor XI bled quite severely after injury. We have also noted this phenomenon. Seligsohn (1978) studied 428 healthy and haemostatically normal persons of Ashkenazi Jewish stock and found 35 with low factor XI levels. The mutation rate for this peculiarity in this particular race may be 0.03–0.057 and the frequency of homozygotes 0.1–0.3 and heterozygotes 5.5 –11 per cent of the population.

From the practical point of view it must be said that we do not know why some patients who have factor XI deficiency bleed excessively and others do not. Each kindred must be considered as an individual problem, weight being given to the clinical features as well as to the laboratory results.

Factor XII deficiency (Hageman defect)

This defect was first recorded by Ratnoff and Colopy (1955). These authors described a patient (Mr Hageman) whose blood had a very long clotting time in glass tubes but who had undergone several major operations without excessive bleeding. Thus normal haemostatic function is included in the definition of the defect. The condition is inherited through an autosomal gene and heterozygotes may have a low level of factor XII (Lucia *et al.* 1979). An immunologically related protein (XIIR:Ag) can be detected in most cases (Saito *et al.* 1979). These authors found two of 42 kindred in which no XIIR:Ag could be detected.

Two other asymptomatic contact stage deficiencies have been described (Fletcher factor by Hathaway and Alsever 1970, and Fitzgerald factor by Waldmann *et al.* 1975). These differ from factor XII deficiency in the test systems used to detect their abnormalities.

Defects of more than one coagulation factor

Occasionally a patient may lack, not one coagulation factor but two or more. Such defects are most uncommon and the most commonly described is probably a defect of both factors V and VIII (Seibert, Margolius and Ratnoff 1958, Jones *et al.* 1962). Vitamin K deficiency leads to reduction in the plasma levels of factors II, VII, IX and X. Patients who lack these four factors are known and probably these patients have a lack in some stage of the production or function of vitamin K (Biggs 1956, Newcombe *et al.* 1956).

AT III deficiency

AT III deficiency produces an excess of coagulation rather than a coagulation defect. The patients suffer from repeated episodes of intravascular clotting, the control of which may require life-long treatment with coumarin anticoagulants. The condition is inherited through an autosomal gene which may be dominant. A number of cases have now been described (e.g. Egeberg 1965, van der Meer, Stoepman-van Dalen and Jansen 1973, Marciniak, Farley and DeSimone 1974, Sas *et al.* 1974).

Conclusion

The genetics of coagulation disorders was, in the early days, mainly a question of collecting family data and recording the types of haemorrhagic manifestations characteristic of the defect. As knowledge of the mechanism of blood coagulation reactions has increased and more is known of the structure of coagulation factors, there has been a broadening of the concepts of genetic defects in blood coagulation.

Measurement of coagulation factors has led to an appreciation that the defects are probably quantitatively related to gene number. One gene for factor VIII activity, for example, seems to produce on average half the amount of factor VIII present when two such genes are included in the genotype. Half the amount of factor VIII is sufficient for normal haemostasis and thus the factor VIII gene is dominant clinically though it behaves quantitatively much like the gene for flower colour where one gene gives a pink colour and two produce red.

Knowledge of the structure of proteins has led to an appreciation of the great variety of protein structure which may retain the function of a particular coagulation activity. A good example is provided by the numerous variants of fibrinogen all of which seem to be inherited and only some of which cause any abnormality in clotting or haemostasis. It seems very likely that normal people have as great a variety of similar and normally active proteins as they have numerous tissue types. In due time maybe such proteins will be as characteristic for the individual as are finger prints. If this proves to be the case then perhaps the concept of genetic 'coagulation defects' will need to be revised. Clearly, only those abnormalities which cause clinical symptoms can be classed as defects. The symptom-free varieties will of course remain of the greatest interest in classifying the chemical attributes of molecules which retain normal activity and defining those chemical features with which defective coagulation is associated.

Another advance of great importance concerns the application of mathematical and statistical studies to the incidence of diseases in the general population and to the diagnosis of the carrier stage. Allied to these studies lie such ethical problems as the social control by the selective abortion of probable affected male embryos in haemophilia carriers and of the female embryos conceived by the wives of haemophiliacs, and birth control. The social and ethical issues raised are important since they are controversial, and those who are severely affected clinically by coagulation defects are extremely expensive to maintain in reasonable health (Biggs 1978). Vogel (1977) has emphasized the importance of keeping accurate records of the incidence of severe clinical defects. Only by keeping such records can the hypothesis about the mutation rate (in sex-linked recessive abnormalities), and its selective balance against fitness (Haldane 1935, 1947) be validated or modified. It is presumably this balance which will determine the incidence of sex-linked recessive clotting defects which, from their present relatively high incidence, are by far the most important, medically, socially and ethically.

REFERENCES

Alexander B. & Goldstein R. (1953) Dual hemostatic defect in pseudohemophilia. *Journal of Clinical Investigation* **32**, 551.

Allain J.-P. (1976) Management of haemophilia in France. *Thrombosis and Haemostasis* **35**, 553–8.

Ananthakrishnan R. & D'Souza S. (1979) Some aspects of the occurrence of new mutations in haemophilia. *Human Heredity* **29**, 90–4.

Andreassen M. (1943) *Haemofili i Danmark opera ex domo biologiae hereditairiae humanae.* Universitatis Hafniensis 6 Copenhagen.

Bachmann F. (1958) Familienunter-suchungen beim kongenitalen Stuart-Prower-Factor Mangel. *Archiv der Julius Klaus-Stiftung für Vererbungsforschung, Sozialanthropologie und Rassenhygiene* **33**, 27.

Barrai I., Cann H.M., Cavalli-Sforza L.L. & de Nicola P. (1968) The effect of parental age on rates of mutation for haemophilia and evidence for differing mutation rates for haemophilia A and B. *American Journal of Human Genetics* **20**, 175–96.

Bateson W. (1909) *Mendel's Principles of Heredity.* Cambridge University Press, Cambridge.

Bertina R.M. & Van der Linden I.K. (1982) Factor IX Deventer. Evidence for heterogeneity of hemophilia B. *Thrombosis and Haemostasis* **47**, 136–40.

Bertina R.M. & Veltkamp J.J. (1978) The abnormal factor IX of hemophilia B$^+$ variants. *Thrombosis and Haemostasis* **40**, 335–49.

Biggs R. (1956) Some observations on the blood of patients with Factor-VIII deficiency. *British Journal of Haematology* **2**, 412–20.

Biggs R. (1974) Jaundice and antibodies directed against factors VIII and IX in patients treated for haemophilia or Christmas disease in the United Kingdom. *British Journal of Haematology* **26**, 313–29.

Biggs R. (1978) *The Treatment of Haemophilia A and B and von Willebrand's Disease.* p. 92. Blackwell Scientific Publications, Oxford.

Biggs R. & Rizza C.R. (1976) The sporadic case of haemophilia A. *Lancet* **II**, 431–3.

Biggs R. & Spooner R. (1978) National survey of haemophilia and Christmas disease patients in the United Kingdom. *Lancet* **I**, 1143–4.

Bouma B.N., van der Klaauw M.M., Veltkamp J.J., Starkenburg A.E., van Tilburg N.H. &

Hermans J. (1975) Evaluation of the detection rate of hemophilia carriers. *Thrombosis Research* 7, 339–50.

Brink A.J. & Kingsley C.S. (1952) A familial disorder of blood coagulation due to deficiency of the labile factor. *Quarterly Journal of Medicine* 21, 19–31.

Camerino G., Grzeschik K.H., Jaye M., de la Salle H., Toltoshev P., Lococq J.P. & Mandel J.L. (1984) Regional localisation on the human X chromosome and polymorphism of coagulation factor IX gene (haemophilia B locus). *Proceedings of the National Academy of Sciences of the USA* (in press).

Cash J.D. (1975) Factor VIII concentrates. Transfusion and immunology. X. *Congress of the World Federation of Haemophilia*, Helsinki.

Davey M.G. (1976) 'Can a national all voluntary blood transfusion service by adequate blood component therapy cover the actual and future needs of AHF?' International Forum. *Vox Sanguinis* 31, 301–5.

Denson K.W.E., Biggs R. & Mannucci P.M. (1968) An investigation of 3 patients with Christmas disease due to an abnormal type of factor IX. *Journal of Clinical Pathology* 21, 160–5.

Denson K.W.E., Lurie A., de Cataldo F. & Mannucci P.M. (1970) The factor X defect: the recognition of abnormal forms of factor X. *British Journal of Haematology* 18, 317–27.

Duckert F., Jung E. & Schmerling D.H. (1960) A hitherto undescribed congenital haemorrhagic diathesis probably due to fibrin stabilizing factor deficiency. *Thrombosis et Diathesis Haemorrhagica* 5, 179–86.

Egeberg O. (1965) Inherited antithrombin deficiency causing thrombophilia. *Thrombosis et Diathesis Haemorrhagica* 13, 516–30.

Elston R.C., Graham J.B., Miller C.H., Reisner H.M. & Bouma B.N. (1976) Probabilistic classification of hemophilia A carriers by discriminant analysis. *Thrombosis Research* 8, 683–95.

Fair D.S. & Edgington T.S. (1981) Group analysis of abnormal factor X molecules (abstract). *Thrombosis and Haemostasis* 46, 297.

Flute P.T. (1977) Disorders of plasma fibrinogen synthesis. *British Medical Bulletin* 33, 253–9.

Giannelli F., Anson D.S., Choo K.H., Rees D.J.G., Winship P.R., Ferrari N., Rizza C.R. & Brownlee G.G. (1984) Characterisation and use of an intragenic polymorphic marker for the detection of carriers of Christmas disease (Haemophila B) *Lancet* (in press).

Giannelli F., Choo K.H., Rees D.J.G., Boyd Y., Rizza C.R. & Brownlee G.G. (1983) Gene deletions in patients with haemophilia B and anti-factor IX antibodies. *Nature* 303, 181–2.

Girolami A., Cattarozzi G., Dal Bo Zanon R., Cella G. & Toffanin F. (1979) Factor VII Padua$_2$: another factor VII abnormality with defective ox brain thromboplastin activation and a complex hereditary pattern. *Blood* 54, 46–53.

Graham J.B. (1957) Genetic problems: hemophilia and allied diseases. In *Hemophilia and Hemophilioid Diseases*. Brinkhous K.M. (ed.). p. 137. University of North Carolina Press, North Carolina.

Graham J.B. (1977) Genetic counselling in classic haemophilia A. *New England Journal of Medicine* 296, 996–8.

Graham J.B. (1979) Genotype assignment (carrier detection) in the haemophilias. In *Clinics in Haematology*. Vol. 8, pp. 115–45. Rizza C.R. (ed.). W.B. Saunders, London.

Graham J.B., Barrow E.M. & Hougie C. (1957) Stuart clotting defect II. Genetic aspects of a 'new' hemorrhagic state. *Journal of Clinical Investigation* 36, 497–503.

Haldane J.B.S. (1935) The rate of spontaneous mutation of a human gene. *Journal of Genetics* **31**, 317–26.

Haldane J.B.S. (1947) The mutation rate of the gene for haemophilia and its segregation ratios in males and females. *Annals of Eugenics* **13**, 262–71.

Hall C.A., Rapaport S.I., Ames S.B. & de Groot J.A. (1964) A clinical and family study of hereditary proconvertin (Factor VII) deficiency. *American Journal of Medicine* **37**, 172–8.

Hathaway W.E. & Alsever J. (1970) The relation of 'Fletcher factor' to factors XI and XII. *British Journal of Haematology* **18**, 161–9.

Holmberg L. & Nilsson I.M. (1972) Genetic variants of von Willebrand's disease. *British Medical Journal* **II**, 317.

Hougie C., Barrow E.M. & Graham J.B. (1957) Stuart clotting defect. I segregation of an hereditary hemorrhagic state from the heterogenous group heretofore called 'stable factor' (SPCA, proconvertin, factor VII) deficiency. *Journal of Clinical Investigation* **36**, 485–96.

Hougie C. & Twomey J.J. (1967) Haemophilia B_M: a new type of factor IX deficiency. *Lancet* **I**, 698–700.

Ikkala E. (1960) Haemophilia. A study of its laboratory clinical genetic and social aspects based on known haemophiliacs in Finland. *Scandinavian Journal of Clinical and Laboratory Investigation* **12**, Suppl. 46.

Imperato D.C. & Dettori A.G. (1958) Ipofibrinogenemia congenita con fibroastenia. *Helvetica Paediatrica Acta* **13**, 380–99.

Jones J.H., Rizza C.R., Hardisty R.M., Dormandy K.M. & MacPherson J.C. (1962) Combined deficiency of factor V and factor VIII (antihaemophilic globulin). *British Journal of Haematology* **8**, 120–8.

Kasper C.K., Østerud B., Minami J.Y., Shonick W. & Rapaport S.I. (1977) Haemophilia B: characterization of genetic variants and detection of carriers. *Blood* **50**, 351–66.

Kernoff P.B.A., Gruson R. & Rizza C.R. (1974) A variant of factor VIII related antigen. *British Journal of Haematology* **26**, 435–9.

Kerr C.B. (1965) Genetics of human blood coagulation. *Journal of Medical Genetics* **2**, 221–308.

Kerr C.B., Preston A.E., Barr A. & Biggs R. (1966) Further studies on the inheritance of factor VIII. *British Journal of Haematology* **12**, 212–33.

Kidd B., Denson K.W.E. & Biggs R. (1963) The thrombotest reagent and Christmas disease. *Lancet* **II**, 522.

Kingsley C.S. (1954) Familial factor V deficiency; the pattern of heredity. *Quarterly Journal of Medicine* **23**, 323.

Klein H.G., Aledort L.M., Bouma L.W., Hoyer L.W., Zimmerman T.S. & De Mets D.L. (1977) A cooperative study for the detection of the carrier state of classic hemophilia. *New England Journal of Medicine* **296**, 959–62.

Laki K. & Lorand L. (1948) On the solubility of fibrin clots. *Science* **108**, 280.

Larrain C., Conte G. & Gonzalez E. (1972) El problema Medico y social de la Hemofilia en Chile. *Revista Medica de Chile* **100**, 440.

Laurell C.D. (1972) Electroimmunoassay. *Scandinavian Journal of Clinical and Laboratory Investigation* **29**, Suppl. 124, 21.

Leiba H., Ramot B. & Many A. (1965) Heredity and coagulation studies in ten families with factor XI (plasma thromboplastin antecedent) deficiency. *British Journal of Haematology* **11**, 654–65.

Lucia J.F., Ercoreca L., Torres M., Giralt M. & Raichs A. (1979) Factor XII congenital deficiency. A new family study. *Thrombosis and Haemostasis* **42**, 1009–17.

Lyon M.F. (1961) Gene action in the X-chromosome of the mouse (*Mus. musculus* L.). *Nature* **190**, 372–3.

Mandalaki T. (1976) Management of haemophilia in Greece. *Thrombosis and Haemostasis* **35**, 522–30.

Mannucci P.M., Coppola R., Lombardi R., Papa M. & De Biasi R. (1978) Direct proof of extreme Lyonization as a cause of low factor VIII levels in females. *Thrombosis and Haemostasis* **39**, 544–5.

Mannucci P.M. & Ruggeri Z.M. (1976) Hemophilia care in Italy. *Thrombosis and Haemostasis* **35**, 531–6.

Marciniak E., Farley C.H. & DeSimone P.A. (1974) Familial thrombosis due to antithrombin III deficiency. *Blood* **43**, 219–31.

Martin-Villar J., Navarro J.L., Ortega F. & Yanguas J. (1971) The supply and availability of plasma concentrates in the hospitals of the Spanish social security. *Proceedings of the 1st European meeting of the World Federation of Haemophilia, Milan.*

Martin-Villar J., Ortega F. & Magallon M. (1976) Management of hemophilia in Spain. *Thrombosis and Haemostasis* **35**, 537–43.

Masure R. (1976) 'Can a national all voluntary blood transfusion service by adequate blood component therapy cover the actual and future needs of AHF?' International Forum. *Vox Sanguinis* **31**, 309–12.

Ménaché D. (1973) Abnormal fibrinogens. A review. *Thrombosis et Diathesis Haemorrhagica* **29**, 525–35.

Mendel G. (1865) Experiments in plant hybridization as translated by Bateson (1909).

Mibashan R.S., Thumpston J.K., Singer J.D., Rodeck C.H., Edwards R.J., White J.M. & Campbell S. (1979) Plasma assay of fetal factors VIII_C and IX for prenatal diagnosis of haemophilia. *Lancet* **I**, 1309–11.

National Haemophilia Foundation (1971) Michigan Chapter Quoted in NHLI Survey, Vol. 3, p. 41.

National Heart and Lung Institute (1972) *Blood Resource Study.*

Newcombe T., Matter M., Conroy L., De Marsh Q.B. & Finch C.A. (1956) Congenital hemorrhagic diathesis of the prothrombin complex. *American Journal of Medicine* **20**, 798–805.

Nilsson I.M. (1972) Personal communication.

Nilsson I.M. (1976) Management of haemophilia in Sweden. *Thrombosis and Haemostasis* **35**, 510–21.

Nilsson I.M. & Holmberg L. (1979) Von Willebrand's disease today. In *Clinics in Haematology.* Vol. 8, pp. 147–68. Rizza C.R. (ed.). W.B. Saunders, London.

Parekh V.R., Mannucci P.M. & Ruggeri Z.M. (1978) Immunological heterogeneity of haemophilia B: a multicentre study of 98 kindred. *British Journal of Haematology* **40**, 643–55.

Prentice C.R.M., Forbes C.D., Morrice S. & McLaren A.D. (1975) Calculation of predictive odds for possible carriers of haemophilia. *Thrombosis and Haemostasis* **34**, 740–7.

Ramgren O. (1962) Haemophilia in Sweden V Medical-social aspects. *Acta Medica Scandanavica* **379**, 37–60.

Ratnoff O.D. & Colopy J.E. (1955) A familial hemorrhagic trait associated with a deficiency of a clot promoting fraction of plasma. *Journal of Clinical Investigation* **34**, 602–13.

Ratnoff O.D. & Jones P.K. (1976) The detection of carriers of classic hemophilia. *American Journal of Clinical Pathology* **65**, 129–35.

Rizza C.R. (1975) Factor VIII-related antigen and von Willebrand's disease. *British*

Journal of Haematology **31**, (Suppl.), 231–45.

Rizza C.R., Rhymes I.L., Austen D.E.G., Kernoff P.B.A. & Aroni S.A. (1975) Detection of carriers of haemophilia: a 'blind' study. *British Journal of Haematology* **30**, 447–56.

Rizza C.R. & Spooner R.J.D. (1983) Treatment of haemophilia and related disorders in Britain and Northern Ireland during 1976–80: a report on behalf of the directors of haemophilia centres in the United Kingdom. *British Medical Journal* **286**, 929–33.

Roos J., van Arkel C., Verloop M.C. & Jordan F.L.J. (1959) A new family with Stuart-Prower deficiency. *Thrombosis et Diathesis Haemorrhagica* **3**, 59–76.

Rosenberg I. (1972) Hemophilia e estados ho Rio Grande do Sul. Frequencia fisiologia et hevanca. *Brazilian Journal of Medical and Biological Research* **5**, 287.

Rosenthal R.L., Dreskin O.H. & Rosenthal N. (1953) New hemophilia-like disease caused by deficiency of a third plasma thromboplastin factor. *Proceedings of the Society for Experimental Biology and Medicine* **82**, 171.

Rush B. & Ellis H. (1965) Treatment of patients with factor V deficiency. *Thrombosis et Diathesis Haemorrhagica* **14**, 74–82.

Saito H., Scott J.G., Movat H.Z. & Scialla S.J. (1979) Molecular heterogeneity of Hageman trait (factor XII deficiency). *Journal of Laboratory and Clinical Medicine* **94**, 256–65.

Sas G., Blaskó G., Bánhegyi D., Jákó J., Pálos L.A. (1974) Abnormal antithrombin III (antithrombin III 'Budapest') as a cause of a familial thrombophilia. *Thrombosis et Diathesis Haemorrhagica* **32**, 105–15.

Seibert R.J., Margolius A. & Ratnoff O.D. (1958) Observations on hemophilia, parahemophilia and coexistent hemophilia and parahemophilia. *Journal of Laboratory and Clinical Medicine* **52**, 449.

Seligsohn U. (1978) High gene frequency of factor XI (PTA) deficiency in Ashkenazi Jews. *Blood* **51**, 1223–8.

Simpson N.E. & Biggs R. (1962) The inheritance of Christmas factor. *British Journal of Haematology* **8**, 191–203.

Sjølin K. (1961) *Haemophilic Diseases in Denmark*. Blackwell Scientific Publications, Oxford.

Soulier J.P. (1976) 'Can a national all voluntary blood transfusiuon service by adequate blood component therapy cover actual and future needs of AHF?' International Forum.*Vox Sanguinis* **31**, 316–17.

Sultz H.A. (1972) *Long-term Childhood Illness*. University of Pittsburgh Press.

Taylor K. & Biggs R. (1957) A mildly affected female haemophiliac. *British Medical Journal*, **I**, 1494–6.

van der Meer J., Stoepman-van Dalen E.A. & Jansen J.M.S. (1973) Antithrombin-III deficiency in a Dutch family. *Journal of Clinical Pathology* **26**, 532–8.

Vogel F. (1955) Vergleichende Betrahtungen über die mutationsrate der geschlechts-gebunden-rezessiven Hämophilieformen in der Schweiz und in Dänemark. *Blut* **1**, 91–109.

Vogel F. (1977) A probable sex difference in some mutation rates. *American Journal of Human Genetics* **29**, 312–19.

von Willebrand E.A. (1926) Hereditär pseudohämofili. *Finska Läkaresällskapets Handlingar* **67**, 7–12.

Waldmann R., Abraham J.P., Rebuck J.W., Caldwell J., Saito H. & Ratnoff O.D. (1975) Fitzgerald factor: a hitherto unrecognized coagulation factor. *Lancet* **I**, 949–50.

Zimmerman T.S., Ratnoff O.D. & Powell A.E. (1971) Immunologic differentiation of classic hemophilia (Factor VIII deficiency) and von Willebrand's disease. *Journal of Clinical Investigation* **50**, 244–54.

Chapter 8
Clinical Features of Clotting Factor Deficiencies

C. R. RIZZA *and* J. M. MATTHEWS

Deficiencies of the blood clotting factors may be congenital or acquired. The congenital deficiencies are in general single deficiency states although there are some well-documented instances of combined clotting factor deficiencies. The acquired deficiencies of clotting factors are in general multiple and are most commonly assoiated with liver disease, vitamin K deficiency, the ingestion of coumarin-type anticoagulant drugs and defibrination secondary to intravascular clotting.

The most severe of the inherited bleeding disorders and clinically the most important is classical haemophilia (haemophilia A) which will be described first.

Haemophilia (haemophilia A)

Haemophilia is a sex-linked recessive bleeding disorder which affects males (Fig. 22). It is due to an isolated congenital deficiency of factor VIII coagulant activity.

Incidence

Haemophilia is a relatively uncommon disease; at the end of 1980 there were 4321 known haemophiliacs in the UK (Rizza and Spooner 1983). Of these, 1903 had factor VIII levels of less than 2 iu per cent and were considered to be clinically severely affected. The prevalence of the condition in the UK is therefore of the order of 8 per 100 000 of the total population or 16 per 100 000 of the male population. The prevalence of the severe form of the condition is approximately half of this. Ramgren (1962) reported that 1 in every 7000 live-born male children in Sweden is a severely affected haemophiliac. Similar figures have been reported in Finland (Ikkala 1960) and Denmark (Sjølin 1961). Estimates of the prevalence in some other countries are shown in Chapter 7 Table 6. The condition occurs throughout the world and has been seen in most racial groups. The condition is found in many breeds of dogs (Hall 1972) and has been observed in the cat (Cotter, Brenner and Dodds 1978) and the horse (Nossel, Archer and Macfarlane 1962).

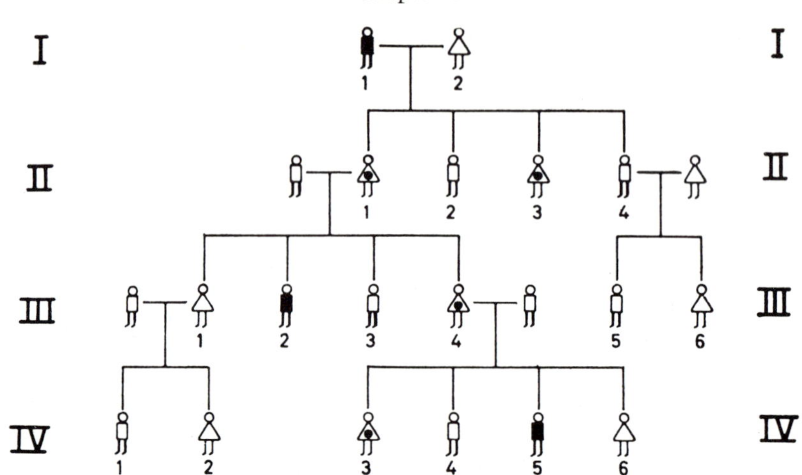

Transmission through an affected male (I,1) and carrier females (II,1 and III,4).

Fig. 22. Mode of inheritance of haemophilia and Christmas disease.

Inheritance

Haemophilia is transmitted in a sex-linked recessive manner. This mode of inheritance is shown in Fig. 22. It can be seen that if a haemophiliac marries a normal woman all their sons will be normal but all the daughters will be carriers of the condition. When a carrier marries a normal male, their sons have an equal chance of being haemophiliacs or normal and their daughters have an equal chance of being carriers or normal. In approximately 30 per cent of cases of haemophilia, there is no previous history of the condition in the family. This may be due to difficulty in obtaining a satisfactory family history or to lack of males in successive generations so that the condition may have been passed down from carrier to carrier with little opportunity to manifest itself in males. On the other hand, the appearance of haemophilia in a previously normal family may represent a mutation. In a given family, affected individuals usually show the same degree of deficiency of factor VIII so that one family may produce severely affected haemophiliacs all with undetectable levels of factor VIII in their blood; another family may have members who are less severely deficient. Some carriers of haemophilia have a reduced level of factor VIII and may bleed excessively, although not to the same extent as affected males from the same family. Bleeding in carriers may take the form of easy bruising, epistaxis, menorrhagia, post-partum haemorrhage, excessive bleeding following dental extraction and other surgical operations and following severe accidental injury.

Bleeding manifestations

The severity of the bleeding in haemophiliacs varies from patient to patient and is related to the amount of factor VIII present in the blood (Table 7). Severely affected patients with no detectable factor VIII suffer bleeding episodes, often for no known reason, into joints and muscles as well as into other sites. Immediately following injury, haemostasis may seem to be normal but recurrence of bleeding hours or even days after the initial injury is common and may then be persistent. The more mildly affected patients, with more than 2 or 3 per cent of factor VIII, still bleed after trauma but for the most part are spared the painful and crippling haemorrhages into joints and muscles experienced by the severely affected patients.

Despite a severe factor deficiency, it is unusual to see evidence of haemophilia in the newborn. Widespread bruising or cephalhaematomas are uncommon, and providing the baby is not injured or subjected to surgery, he may appear to be normal for a considerable time. Infection, premature separation of the umbilical cord or operations such as circumcision or pyloroplasty may, however, give rise to dangerous bleeding. Abnormal bruises are commonly seen for the first time from the age of three or four months when the baby becomes more active. If they occur frequently so that many bruises of different ages are present at the same time, parents may be suspected of baby

Table 7. Relationship of plasma factor VIII level to the severity of bleeding manifestations.

Plasma level of factor VIII (iu/dl)	Bleeding manifestations
>40	None
20–40	Tendency to bleed after major injury. Often not diagnosed
5–20	Bleeding after minor injury and surgery
1–5	Severe bleeding after minor injury. Occasional haemarthroses and 'spontaneous' bleeding
<1	Severe haemophilia. Spontaneous haemarthroses and muscle haemorrhages. Joint ankylosis and crippling

battering. When the child begins to stand with support his unsteadiness may result in falls which damage his lips and bruise his head or buttocks. Walking and running, kicking and jumping may produce bleeding into the joints of the ankles and knees (Fig. 23). Strain on the elbows and other joints may cause bleeding to occur there also. Not only are these haemarthroses extremely painful, but they are very damaging to the structure of joints. If not treated promptly with adequate amounts of factor VIII, restricted movement and eventual ankylosis of the joint will result. The situation is made worse by the bone changes and the disuse atrophy of muscles which result from the repeated haemarthroses and the enforced immobilization. The haemorrhages which occur into muscles can also be very painful. They restrict movement and, if tense enough, may press on nerves and blood vessels sufficiently to produce impairment of nerve function or in rare instances, gangrene. They may damage the muscle and cause fibrosis and contractures. Crippling damage to muscles and joints is the most outstanding feature of untreated severe haemophilia. Bleeding episodes occur less commonly elsewhere. The severe haemophiliac may suffer from troublesome nosebleeds, bleeding from the gums, though rarely during eruption or loss of deciduous teeth, bleeding from the kidney causing haematuria and bleeding from the alimentary tract, particularly following the ingestion of aspirin or aspirin-like drugs. Without adequate replacement therapy the severe haemophiliac becomes crippled and deprived of the social, educational, occupational and recreational aspects of a normal life.

SPECIAL FEATURES OF HAEMOPHILIC BLEEDING

Bruising

Many normal people bruise easily. Such bruises seem to affect women and children more commonly than men. The bruises tend not to spread unless a considerable degree of trauma is involved and are not lumpy unless situated in an area such as the scalp where migration of blood from the area is difficult. They are most commonly seen on the shins and thighs or sometimes on the upper arms. Haemophilic bruising may occur after some definite injury but quite often there is no known injury. Bruises are often lumpy and tend to spread. The skin over the centre of the lump is often blanched and free from discoloration. If the bruise is confined to the subcutaneous tissues, the associated lump will usually be mobile. If it originates from damaged muscle, the haematoma will be fixed to the deeper tissues and will be more painful. The amount of time for bruising to become apparent is related to the depth in the tissues of the source of bleeding. Superficial bruising is not usually a cause for concern unless it is associated with a deeper haematoma of more serious

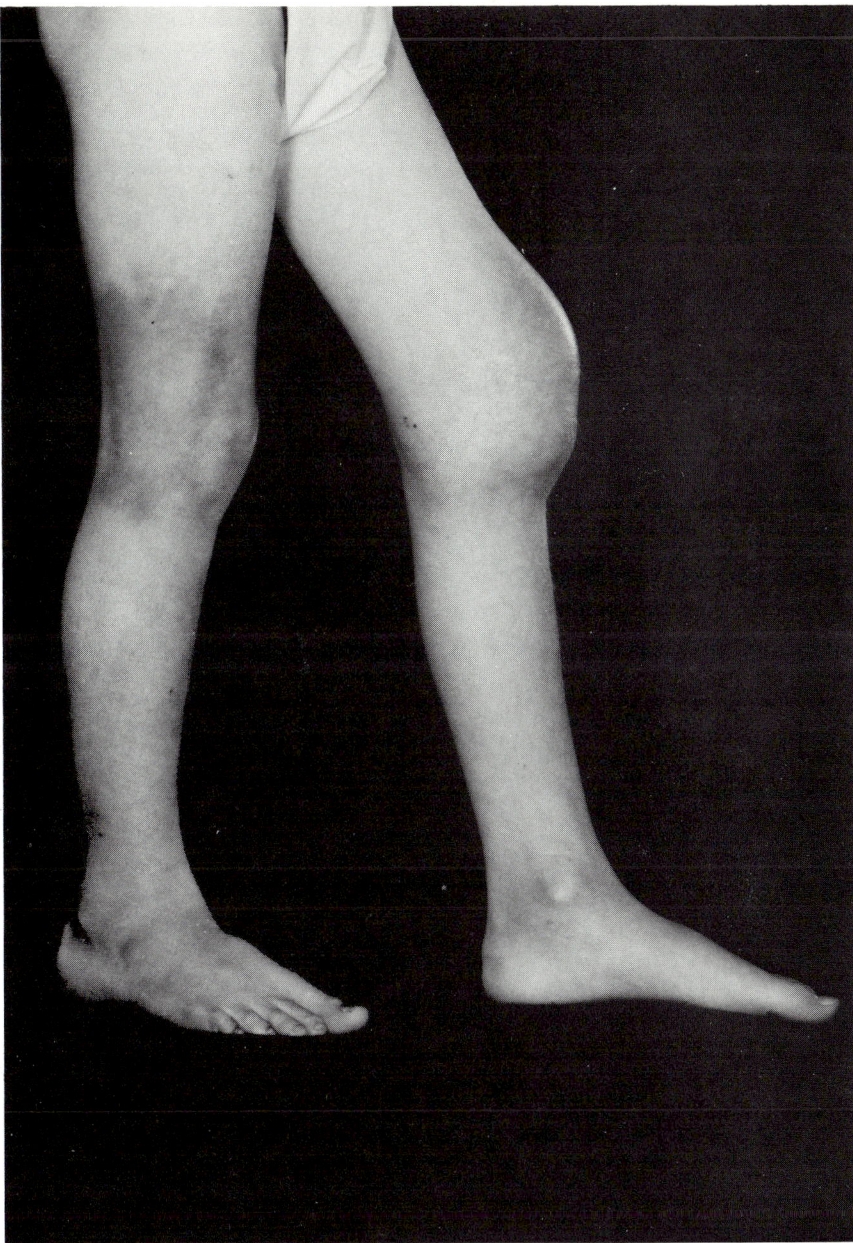

Fig. 23. Haemarthrosis of the left knee in severely affected haemophiliac (factor VIII < 1%).

significance. Superficial bruises occurring in areas such as the scalp tend to form a localized haematoma and are not infrequent in early childhood. They may be subject to repeated trauma which may induce further bleeding. Resolution, although sometimes protracted, is usually complete. Occasionally tension within the haematoma endangers the viability of the overlying skin. In such cases skin incision and evacuation of the haematoma under appropriate factor replacement is indicated. Bruises of the forehead in young haemophiliacs are sometimes followed by a black eye on one or both sides. Although one should regard any head injury of more than minor degree with seriousness, this sign is usually more dramatic than dangerous. Other superficial but sometimes uncomfortable bruises, about which advice is sometimes sought, are those which are produced by compression of skin over underlying bone, such as the linear bruise which is seen just above and along the line of the iliac crest, or the bruised perineal area from contact with a bicycle cross-bar or the type of bruise produced by nipping of the skin as produced in the anterior axillary fold by a crutch. Some of these bruises being uncomfortable and progressive require factor replacement and some may be safely left.

Wounds of skin and subcutaneous tissue

Venepuncture may be carried out safely in severe haemophiliacs providing that one does not persist in trying to enter a vein which has been damaged by previous attempts, and that when the needle is withdrawn, pressure is kept on the puncture site for several minutes continuously and the site is not rubbed thereafter. It is important when applying pressure to an antecubital vein after venepuncture to apply it with the arm fully extended so as to tense the underlying tissues and provide a firm base for pressure on the vein. Superficial scratches and needle punctures usually stop bleeding in the normal time. Cuts and lacerations may stop bleeding in a short time but recommence bleeding some time later if factor replacement is not given. Wounds which have been sutured without factor replacement may continue to bleed under the sutures with build-up of pressure, resulting in tracking of blood into surrounding tissues, distension of the wound and eventual rupture of the suture line. In the young infant superficial cuts may bleed more persistently than in the older haemophiliac and may require replacement therapy.

Haemarthroses

Severe haemophiliacs bleed more commonly into joints than elsewhere. The joints most commonly affected are knees, ankles, elbows and shoulders. In early life, as the child learns to crawl, stand, walk and run, ankle bleeds predominate. Later, as a result of changing patterns of strains, the elbow, especially the right one, becomes affected and at the same time one sees a greater incidence of knee haemarthroses. Haemarthroses of shoulders, hips, wrists and the small joints of the fingers and toes are not uncommon. The source of bleeding in a joint is thought, in most cases, to be the vessels of the synovial membrane which have been damaged by compression or nipping of the membrane between adjacent bones. The symptoms of a haemarthrosis are usually evident to the haemophiliac long before there are any signs of bleeding. To start with, he may feel a slight weakness or instability of the joint or a slightly uncomfortable or pricking sensation within it. As the amount of blood in the joint increases, it becomes more uncomfortable and its range of motion more limited. As the limited elasticity of the joint capsule is taken up pain may become agonizing. The joint is ultimately held in the position in which the volume of the joint is maximum and any attempt to change this position is extremely painful and resisted. The shoulder is held slightly abducted and internally rotated. The elbow is flexed by about 45° with the forearm slightly pronated, the hip is flexed, abducted and internally rotated, the knee is flexed by about 30–40° and the ankle is plantar-flexed. An affected joint should be immobilized in the position of maximum comfort when first treated to avoid further increase in tension and pain. Bleeding may be rapid or slow and fill the joint space in minutes or in a day or two. A severe untreated haemarthrosis is likely to take weeks if not months to resolve to a state at which weight may be borne on it. Even then, joint movement may be restricted, the associated muscles wasted and contracted, the synovial membrane and joint cartilage irrevocably damaged and there may be a resulting predisposition to further bleeds into the joint for the slightest reason. Absorption of blood from a joint depends on the volume of blood in the joint and on the state of the synovial membrane. A small volume of blood will be cleared rapidly from a joint with undamaged synovial membrane. Experimentally, a non-inflamed synovial membrane is much more capable of clearing foreign particles from a joint than is one previously inflamed and the same is true clinically. A large volume of blood produces considerable amounts of haemosiderin and other blood breakdown products and there is an associated inflammatory reaction with thickening and pigmentation of the synovial membrane. The intensity of this synovial reaction may be judged by the overlying skin temperature which may remain elevated for some four to six weeks after a single haemarthrosis and may remain warm indefinitely if the joint is subject, as is likely, to recurrent bleeds. After a severe haemarthrosis or a succession of haemarthroses, particularly in childhood, a joint may remain painlessly distended with a chronic synovitic effusion.

The pathological changes which occur in joints, the subject of small repeated bleeds, are usually slight, consisting for the most part of some synovial thickening together with superficial degenerative changes of the

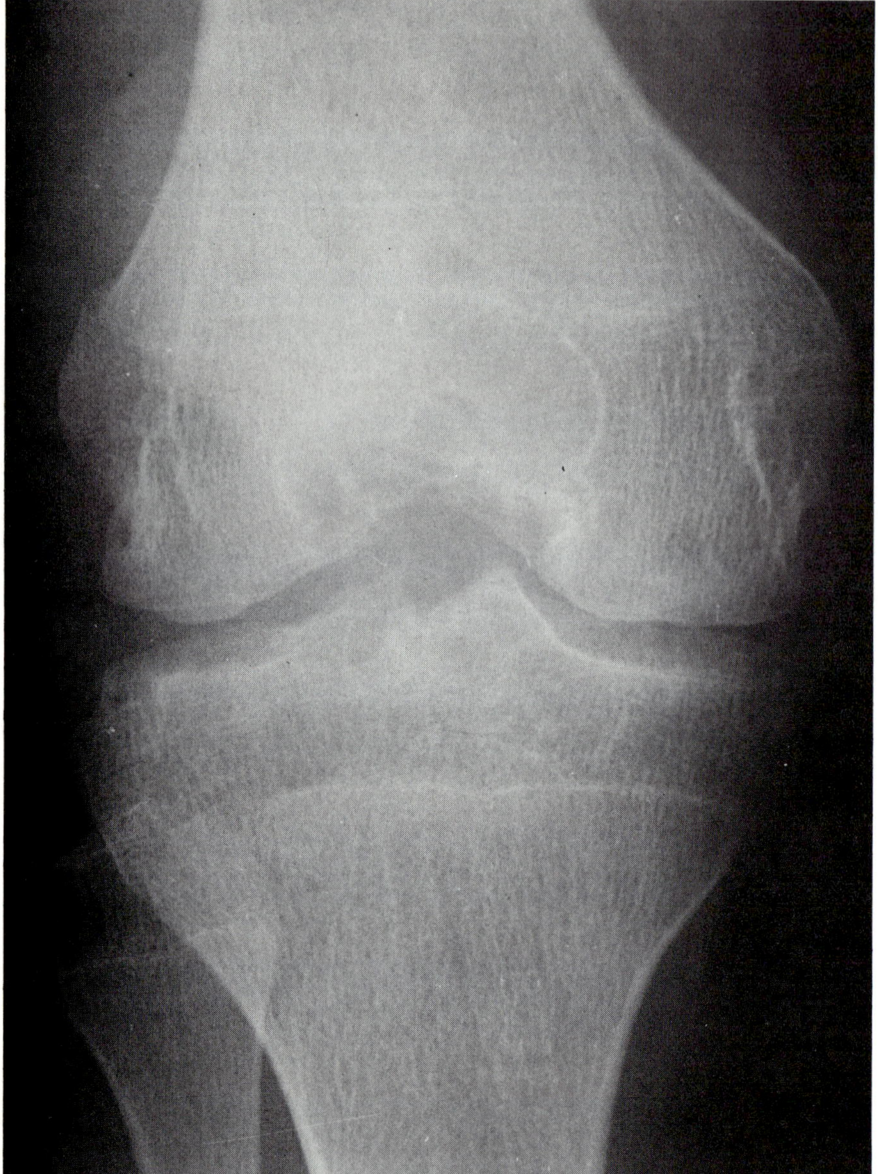

Fig. 24. Radiograph of knee showing changes of haemophilic arthropathy. Note diminution of joint space, widening if intercondylar notch, irregular joint surfaces, subchondral cysts, squaring of lower pole of patella, osteoporosis. Above, antero-posterior view. Facing page, lateral view.

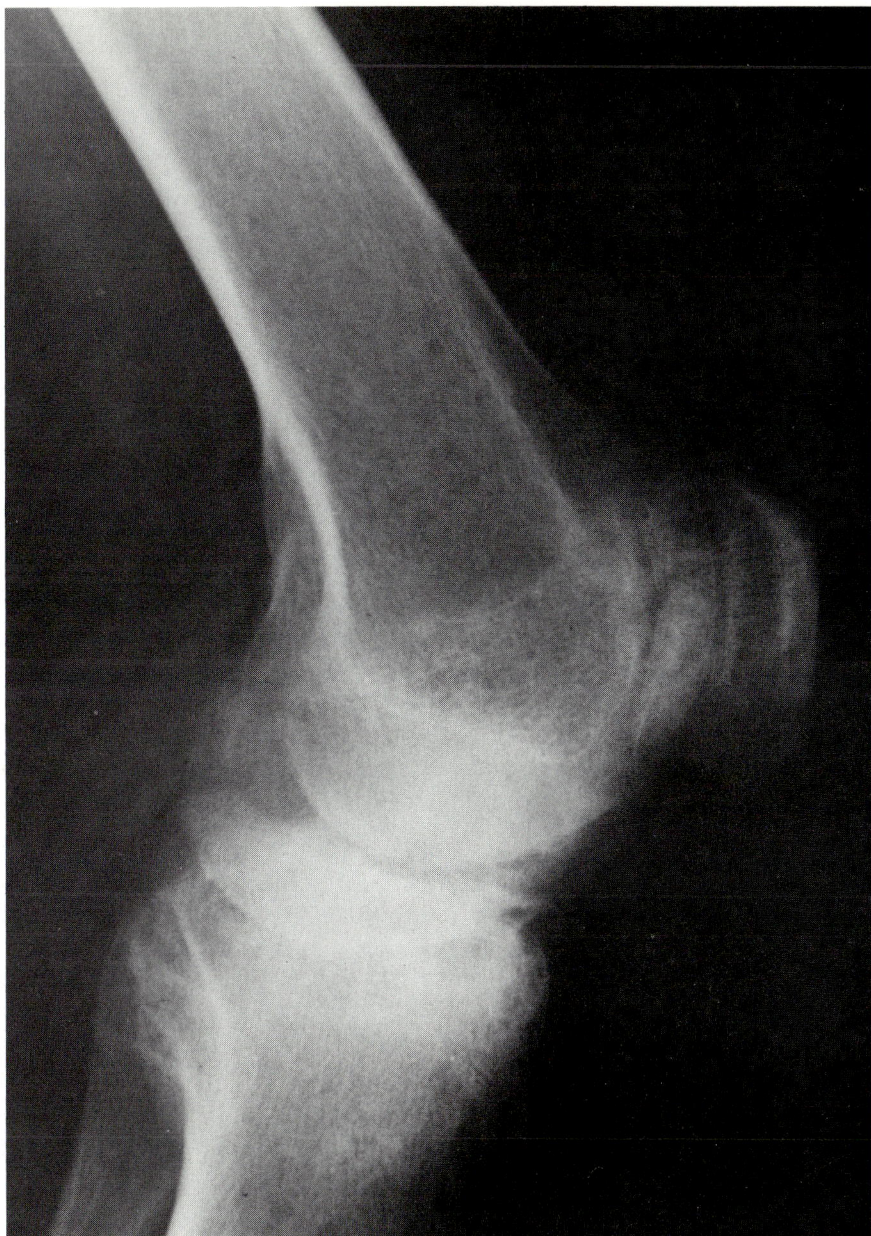

Fig. 24b.

articular cartilage. X-ray changes may be minimal. Such a joint might be expected to be the seat of some arthritic problems in later life. Severe bone and joint changes are most often related to one or more preceding severe haemarthroses with much tension and pain and prolonged disability. The capsule is distended and the synovial membrane is thickened and discoloured as a result of vascular congestion, cellular reaction and blood pigment deposition, and may show numerous vascular projections of the synovial membrane. The cartilage is often eroded exposing the cancellous bone and fragments of bone or cartilage may lie free in the joint cavity. The cartilage is usually stained with haemosiderin. X-ray examination shows irregularity of articular surface, loss of joint space and the formation of exostoses at joint margins (Fig. 24). The evidence of abnormalities of bone growth is seen in the expanded ends of long bones, and the presence of abnormal growth lines (Harris's lines). Subarticular cystic areas may be present and in the knee the intercondylar notch is often widened. Osteoporosis is sometimes marked and may predispose to fracture following slight injury. The inferior margin of the patella may be squared off.

Muscle haemorrhage

Bleeding into muscle is often spontaneous or may follow an injury such as a strain or direct blow or an intramuscular injection. Bleeding permeates the muscle fibrils within the enclosing fibrous sheath, tension increases, the function of muscle is impaired and anatomically related nerves and vessels may be endangered by pressure. If bleeding continues swelling may interfere with the skin circulation causing blistering or necrosis. When the haematoma resolves, damaged muscle tissue is repaired by a process of fibrosis with consequent contracture of the muscle. This together with the effects of any nerve damage may result in severe limb deformities. If the amount of blood is more than can be re-absorbed by the normal repair process, an intramuscular cyst may be formed and become larger over a period of time as a result of repeated bleeds into and around it. Prolonged pressure of the cyst on underlying periosteum may produce irregular thinning of the bone cortex and even lead to a pathological fracture.

The iliacus haematoma is of particular importance. It is not uncommon and its importance lies in the fact that it may cause pressure on the femoral nerve, paralyse the quadriceps muscle and render a knee which has previously been normal liable to damage. If bleeding is not controlled the tension within the iliacus sheath may increase sufficiently for the haematoma to rupture into the psoas muscle and then bleeding may occur in an unrestricted manner upwards into the retroperitoneal space and even into the chest. A chronic iliacus haematoma may also proceed to cyst formation with gross destruction of the underlying ilium.

An iliacus haematoma may develop with no history of injury. Pain is commonly first felt over the mid-inguinal point and the hip is flexed and adducted to minimize discomfort. Tingling, paraesthesiae or numbness may be felt over a small patch in front of the thigh or patella and the area of numbness may increase to affect the anterior leg from the inguinal ligament to the middle of the tibia. At the same time the quadriceps becomes weak and the patellar reflex is lost. On examination of the abdomen, a mass may be felt immediately medial to the pelvic brim at the anterior superior iliac spine extending medially to occupy the iliac fossa. The condition must be differentiated from haemarthrosis of the hip or, when involving the right side, from appendicitis. A hip haemarthrosis produces pain and tenderness in front and behind the joint. Sometimes pain may also be elicited by compressing both greater trochanters inwards thus increasing tension within the hip joint. Pain in haemarthrosis is also increased by relatively small rotatory or abduction movements of the femur. In appendicitis, pain is often initially peri-umbilical moving later towards the right iliac fossa. Guarding, rebound tenderness and right iliac fossa pain produced by pressure over the descending colon are not marked features of an iliacus haematoma and in the early stages neither are pyrexia, leucocytosis or loss of appetite, vomiting or oral fetor. Retroperitoneal haemorrhage is another important type of bleeding. Pain and tenderness are present together with guarding and rebound tenderness. Dullness to percussion may be observed and a fall in the haemoglobin usually accompanies a large haematoma. If such a haematoma originates in, or gravitates into, the pelvis it can interfere with defaecation or micturition and in the latter case catheterization may be required for a few days until treatment produces a reduction in the size of the haematoma.

Haemophilic cysts and pseudo-tumours

Haemophilic cysts are a relatively rare but much-feared complication of haemophilia (Gunning 1966, Duthie *et al.* 1973). The pathogenesis of these cysts is still not fully understood. Valderrama and Matthews (1965) have described three main types of cyst, as follows:

1   Simple cysts which are contained within the muscular fascial envelope and confined by tendinous attachments. This cyst may remain localized or may track between muscle and fascia to point internally, or externally through the skin. There is usually no involvement of bone.
2   Cysts arising in muscles with wide fibrous periosteal attachments may

start as a simple cyst but progress to cause cortical thinning and fracture of bone by interference with periosteal blood supply and by direct pressure.

3   Cysts caused by subperiosteal haemorrhage strip and raise the periosteum with resultant destruction of underlying bone as well as overlying muscle. On occasion, pseudo-tumours seem to arise from within the bone itself and may be the result of intraosseous haemorrhage.

The presence of a persistent or increasing mass in the pelvis, abdomen or limb of a haemophiliac should raise the suspicion of a haemophilic cyst. The mass is usually not tender unless there has been recent bleeding into it. The radiological appearance depends on the site and extent of the cyst and may simply show a soft tissue shadow or, in the more advanced cases, may show osteolysis, new bone formation and attempts at remodelling. Computerized axial tomography (CT) is particularly valuable for delineating the size and anatomical relations of abdominal or pelvic cysts (Fig. 25).

Gastrointestinal tract

Haematemesis and melaena occur occasionally in haemophiliacs and should be investigated in the normal manner. A local cause for the bleeding may be found but in a significant number of patients full investigation including endoscopy and sometimes even laparotomy fails to detect the cause of the

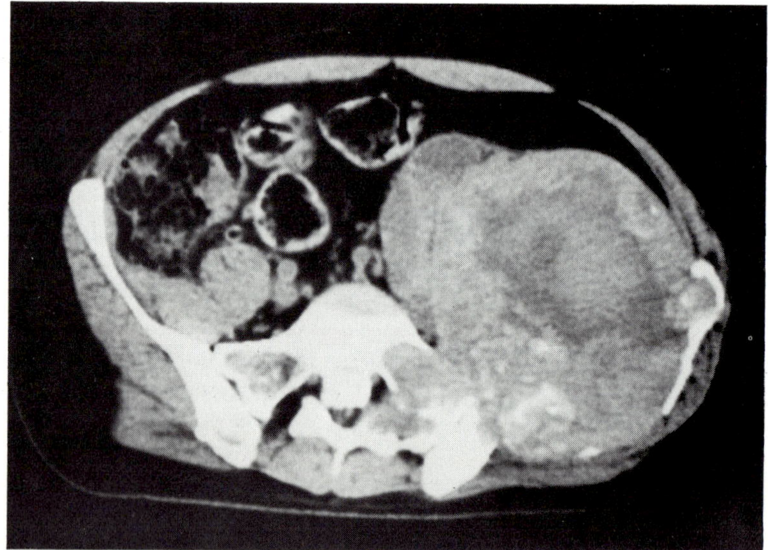

Fig. 25. CT scan of pelvis showing haemophilic cyst of left iliacus muscle. Note destruction of left ilium and invasion of sacral vertebrae.

bleeding. Haemophiliacs are especially liable to bleed from the gut following the ingestion of aspirin and other anti-inflammatory agents and this must always be enquired for when taking a history in such cases. Troublesome bleeding may occur not only from such conditions as peptic ulcer, neoplasm, ulcerative colitis or haemorrhoids but also from diverticulitis.

Kidney

Most severely affected haemophiliacs have haematuria at some time in their lives and some have it repeatedly. Most bouts of haematuria occur spontaneously without a history of injury, and radiographic examination usually fails to reveal any pathological condition. In patients with a past history of haematuria it is rarely necessary to carry out renal tract investigations unless the haematuria has become very profuse or unusually persistent. On the other hand, onset of haematuria in an older patient who has never had haematuria should be investigated as in a normal individual. Blood loss may slightly discolour the urine or it may be heavy with the passage of clots. In this case pain is common and usually one-sided. It is felt in the renal area as a dull ache increasing from time to time to an agonizingly sharp pain which is presumably due to clots entering and stretching the ureter. As a clot is passed down the ureter, pain is referred from the loin to the suprapubic area and then suddenly diminishes in intensity as the clot enters the bladder. If clots obstruct the ureter the haematuria may cease for a time but commonly recurs when the obstruction relieves itself. Some impairment of renal function may follow renal obstruction but it is unusual for function to be completely lost. Renal hypertensive disease may be an important long-term sequel (Prentice *et al.* 1971). Deformities of the renal calyx and pelvis and hydronephrosis may sometimes be seen on X-ray in patients who have suffered repeated severe episodes of haematuria (Wright, Matthews and Brock 1971). Slight haematuria seems to be innocuous and no abnormalities of renal structure or function have been attributed to it although it could be significant when considered in the context of later observation of hypertension. Haematuria is alarming to the beholder but usually involves very little blood loss. Bleeding sufficient to produce marked anaemia is uncommon. Bleeding suspected of coming from the bladder wall or from the prostatic area should be investigated in the normal way. It can be profuse enough to block urethral outflow and cause straining. Pain is referred to the tip of the penis and in such a case irrigation or even instrumental evacuation of clots may be required.

Brain

Intracranial haemorrhage is now the commonest cause of death in haemophilia (Biggs 1977). It may be extradural, subdural or intracerebral and usually follows a known injury, sometimes after a short time, sometimes a day or so later. Haemophiliacs should receive prophylactic treatment with factor VIII for 24–48 hours after a more than trivial head injury. Young children in particular should be admitted to hospital for observation for this period and not prematurely sent home. Any complaints of headache, neck stiffness, visual defects, vomiting or unusual drowsiness should be regarded with great seriousness and neurological and neurosurgical help sought without delay.

Other types of bleeding

Epistaxis usually follows some degree of trauma to the nose but when bleeding has occurred in the recent past or when the nasal mucosa is inflamed, the degree of trauma required may be minimal. Blood loss may be considerable and occasionally may be dangerous. The tendency to bleed again is increased by the rough introduction of nasal packs, by the inflammation induced by having packs in place too long, and by necrosis caused by nasal cauterization.

Bleeding from the mucous membranes of the mouth differs from skin bleeding in that the surface is moist and subject to movement of adjacent mucosal surfaces. As a consequence clots tend to be easily disturbed and washed off, and the primary haemostatic phase is often short-lived. If bleeding is slight or if treatment with factor replacement is only partially effective, a collection of blood may form under a thin film of fibrin and periodically burst into the mouth. Fibrin may be built up on a lesion little by little forming an adherent clot with the appearance of a fleshy berry-like outgrowth, greyish-red in colour. The frenulum of the upper lip is a common site of injury and haemorrhage, commonly occurring in babies who fall against the upper bar of their cot.

Bleeding into the tongue is less common but potentially dangerous and may continue until the tongue fills the mouth making it difficult to speak, swallow or even breathe. Fortunately, the resolution of such a haematoma occurs rapidly with adequate factor replacement, and temporary intubation is rarely required. The tonsil, if inflamed, is sometimes the source of bleeding from the pharynx.

Deciduous teeth usually erupt without bleeding. When dehiscence takes place it is also trouble-free unless the tooth is forcibly loosened or removed. Extraction of a single tooth in an untreated severe haemophiliac may be followed by persistent bleeding for several weeks. Extraction of fully rooted deciduous teeth in children is as serious a procedure as extraction of permanent teeth and the length of the roots of deciduous teeth in proportion to the depth of the child's jaw is in many instances greater than is the case for permanent teeth in adults. The condition of teeth and gums, particularly in older haemophiliacs who have feared dental work, may be very poor. The importance of dental hygiene must be impressed upon haemophiliacs from the earliest age.

Psychological problems in haemophilia

When haemophilia is diagnosed, usually in infancy, the parents may be shocked, angry, guilty, sad or rejecting. The father may blame the mother and take little interest in the child, leading to parental separation and much of the care and concern about the child often falls on the mother who may become depressed and even suicidal. Increasing frequency and uncertainty of occurrence of bleeds disrupts the lives of the young haemophiliac and his family but life becomes more predictable and tolerable when home treatment becomes possible and parents and child have more control over the situation.

The young haemophiliac as well as his parents adapt most easily to the social and medical problems of haemophilia if their management is knowledgeable and sympathetic and the treatment of bleeding episodes is gentle, efficient and effective. Treatment should, if possible, be carried out by the same medical and nursing staff and if this is not possible, one senior doctor should closely supervise treatment.

On occasion, children stubbornly refuse to have injections, splints or bandages and there may then be a good case for not treating certain episodes which do not present any risk, and leaving the decision for request of treatment to the child himself. The 'hyperactive child' may be a danger to himself and an increased source of anxiety to his parents and teachers. Although sedation may be useful in such circumstances there are drawbacks to such treatment.

Over-protection, particularly on the part of the mother, may lead to dependence of the child and interacting anxiety states. In adolescence particularly, the haemophiliac may react against this by pursuing forbidden dangerous activities.

Most haemophiliacs are well adapted to their disorder and get on with living their lives as best they can without major psychological disorders along the way. But some, particularly when they leave the family home, have problems and uncertainties they cannot resolve, which become evident as anxiety states or depressive illness. Still others have problems related to over-use of strong analgesic drugs to which a small number may become addicted.

The psychological problems of haemophilia may require the advice and counselling of the child psychologist, the staff of an adolescent unit or the psychiatrist and this can be arranged through the Haemophilia Centre.

Diagnosis of haemophilia

The diagnosis of severe haemophilia is usually easy and should be suspected if there is a lifelong history of prolonged and excessive bleeding following injury in a male patient with or without the relevant family history. The finding of a reduced level of factor VIII coagulant activity (VIII:C) in the blood using specific and sensitive assays together with a normal or high level of factor VIII-related antigen (VIIIR:Ag) and a normal bleeding time confirms the diagnosis. The whole blood clotting time and activated partial thromboplastin time are prolonged and the prothrombin consumption test is abnormal confirming a major defect in the intrinsic pathway of blood coagulation. The thromboplastin generation test gives abnormal results when the patient's alumina-adsorbed plasma is the source of plasma in the test system. The prothrombin time is normal.

The diagnosis of mild forms of haemophilia is occasionally difficult, especially if the factor VIII:C level is in the range 10–20 iu/dl and the patient has not been exposed to trauma sufficient to cause excessive bleeding. It is important in such patients to obtain a detailed history concerning bleeding following all forms of injury and surgery including dental extraction.

The definitive diagnosis will rest on the demonstration of a reduced level of factor VIII:C, normal level of factor VIII-related antigen and a normal bleeding time. So-called screening tests such as the activated partial thromboplastin time should be interpreted with caution. Although abnormal results will be obtained in severe haemophilia, the test may fail to detect mildly affected patients with factor VIII levels of 15–25 per cent of normal (O'Brien, North and Ingram 1981). Occasionally, there may be difficulty in distinguishing mild haemophilia from the mild variants of von Willebrand's disease. In such cases the family history may be of help in making the diagnosis but usually one must rely on further laboratory investigations such as ristocetin cofactor assay and two-dimensional immunoelectrophoresis (2DIE) of factor VIII-related antigen. In mild haemophilia, the level of ristocetin cofactor activity and the mobility of factor VIII-related antigen on 2 DIE are the same as in normal plasma whereas in the variant forms of von Willebrand's disease the level of ristocetin cofactor is often reduced and the mobility of factor VIII-related antigen increased.

It is possible to make the diagnosis of haemophilia at birth on a citrated sample of umbilical cord blood obtained by careful venepuncture and transported as soon as possible to the laboratory for assay of factor VIII:C. Factor VIII does not cross the placental barrier so that the level of the factor in a severely affected child is usually less than 1 iu/dl. Thanks to advances in the techniques of fetoscopy (Rodeck and Campbell 1978), it is now possible to diagnose haemophilia on blood samples obtained from the child *in utero* at the 16th to 20th week of pregnancy. Samples so obtained can be assayed for factor

VIII coagulant activity using modifications of conventional blood clotting assays (Mibashan *et al.* 1979) or by measuring the factor VIII coagulant antigen by means of immunoradiometric assays (Lazarchick and Hoyer 1978, Peake and Bloom 1978). The results so far obtained with these methods have been very encouraging (Firshein *et al.* 1979, Mibashan *et al.* 1979, Mibashan *et al.* 1980).

Detection of carriers

Carrier detection and genetic counselling is an important aspect of the management of the haemophilic family and requires the following:
1   Detailed information concerning the woman's pedigree, including affected and non-affected members.
2   Careful assay of factor VIII:C and factor VIII-related antigen in her blood.
    The pedigree information and the laboratory information are then combined to derive a figure for probability of carriership. In some very rare instances studies of linking between haemophilia, G6-PD deficiency and colour-blindness may be useful.

PEDIGREE INFORMATION

Haemophilia A is transmitted as an X-linked recessive condition which almost exclusively affects males. This form of inheritance results in all the sons of a haemophiliac being normal but all his daughters being obligatory carriers. There is clearly no need, from the genetic point of view, to embark on carrier studies on women who are known from their pedigree to be obligatory carriers although it is advisable to assay their factor VIII level to ensure that they are not at risk of haemorrhage during surgery. It is in the potential or possible carrier that full investigation is required. Possible carriers include (a) sisters of haemophiliacs, (b) women with a haemophilic relative, appropriately related on the maternal side of the family, and (c) mothers of single haemophiliacs with no other history of haemophilia in the family. All of the information obtained from study of the family tree must be combined with information gained from careful assay of the level of factor VIII:C and factor VIII-related antigen. Before embarking on the laboratory study it is, we believe, essential to confirm that there is indeed a bleeding disorder in the family. Ideally the affected member should be seen and investigated but failing this, well-documented evidence of haemophilia should be obtained from the laboratory which carried out the tests.

LABORATORY INFORMATION

Until the early 1970s the laboratory detection of carriers of haemophilia was based on assay of factor VIII coagulant activity. In a proportion of women with

 Chapter 8

low levels of factor VIII:C it was sometimes possible to diagnose the carrier state. But in general, the results were unsatisfactory, with the proportion of genetically proven heterozygous women detected by these assays varying from 0 per cent (Gardikas, Katsiroumbas and Kottas 1957) to 90 per cent detected (Bentley and Krivit 1960). Zimmerman, Ratnoff and Littell (1971) showed that assay of factor VIII-related antigen along with factor VIII:C greatly improved the rate of carrier detection and those two assays taken along with information from the pedigree have provided the basis for most studies of carriers. The statistical details and problems of technique have been fully discussed in an issue of the *Bulletin of the World Health Organisation* (World Health Organisation 1977). There it is recommended that each laboratory should derive its own linear discriminant based on assay of factor VIII:C and factor VIIIR:Ag in local normal women and obligatory carriers. Using this discriminant it is possible to derive a likelihood ratio which is then combined with pedigree information to derive a final probability of carrierhood. It should be remembered, however, that approximately 17 per cent of obligatory carriers may be diagnosed as normal using the above method (Barrow *et al.* 1982) and that one can never tell a woman with certainty that she is not a carrier of haemophilia. The results can be presented to her only as probabilities which she may or may not find useful.

Christmas disease (haemophilia B)

Christmas disease (factor IX deficiency) is clinically indistinguishable from classical haemophilia (factor VIII deficiency) and is characterized by prolonged bleeding which may follow injury or occur spontaneously. Like haemophilia, Christmas disease is transmitted as a sex-linked recessive disorder. The severity of bleeding is related to the level of factor IX in the blood and severe deficiency results in a severe bleeding disorder.

Incidence

The condition is less common than haemophilia and in the UK there are approximately 800 known cases, 35 per cent of which are severely affected with factor IX levels of less than 2 per cent of normal (Rizza and Spooner 1983).

As with haemophilia, it was originally thought that Christmas disease was due to the absence of the clotting factor molecule, in this case factor IX. In 1956, Fantl, Sawers and Marr observed that the plasma of one of their patients with Christmas disease was able to neutralize a factor IX antibody which had developed in another. This suggested to them that some patients with Christmas disease produced the factor IX molecule but that it was biologically inactive in blood coagulation.

Since then other workers have detected and measured factor IX antigen using a variety of techniques including inhibitor neutralizing tests (Roberts *et al.* 1968), counter immunoelectrophoresis (Yang 1978a), Laurell's electroimmunoassay (Orstavik *et al.* 1975), radioimmunoassays and immunoradiometric assays (Thompson 1977, Yang 1978b, Holmberg *et al.* 1980). On the basis of results obtained by these methods, patients with Christmas disease have been classified broadly into three groups: (a) those in whom both factor IX coagulant activity and factor IX antigen are not detected (CRM−); (b) those with normal amounts of antigen but reduced coagulant activity (CRM+); and (c) those in whom antigen and clotting activities are reduced to the same extent (CRM reduced). The CRM+ group, which accounts for 30–50 per cent of patients with Christmas disease, can be further subclassified depending on the reaction of the plasma with ox brain in the prothrombin time test; patients who show a prolonged prothrombin time in the presence of ox brain have been classified as haemophilia Bm (Hougie and Twomey 1967, Denson, Biggs and Mannucci 1968). Several variants have been described using other criteria such as the ability of the factor IX to be cleaved by XIa (Bertina and Veltkamp 1978), the binding of factor IX to Ca^{2+} (Bertina and Veltkamp 1979), or to phospholipid (Chung 1978) and electrophoretic mobility (Bertina and Veltkamp 1978) in the presence and absence of calcium ions or heparin. The severity of the bleeding symptoms does not seem to be related to the type of variant. The detection and classification of variants has been comprehensively dealt with by Bertina and van der Linden (1982). Only a very small proportion of patients with Christmas disease develop antibodies to factor IX and in the UK the figure is of the order of 1 per cent of all patients (Rizza and Spooner 1983). This incidence is considerably less than the 6–7 per cent of haemophiliacs who have antibodies to factor VIII.

Advances in our understanding of the gene defect in Christmas disease have come from the application of recombinant DNA techniques (see Chapter 7).

Diagnosis

As in the case of classical haemophilia, the diagnosis is made from the patient's clinical history, family history and specific assay of the missing blood clotting factor, in this case factor IX. In the severely affected patient, in addition to finding a low level of factor IX (<1 per cent of normal), the whole blood clotting time and activated partial thromboplastin time are prolonged and the prothrombin consumption test is abnormal. The prothrombin time (except in patients with haemophilia Bm), bleeding time and platelet count are all normal as are the levels of the other coagulation factors.

The diagnosis can be made at birth by carrying out a factor IX assay on a blood sample obtained from the umbilical cord by clean venepuncture. Although the level of factor IX in the normal neonate is considerably reduced at birth, it is usually possible to distinguish the severely affected child from the normal child.

Antenatal diagnosis of Christmas disease at the 16th–20th week of pregnancy is also now possible. Samples of blood are obtained from the child by fetoscopy and assayed for factor IX by a slight modification of the standard coagulation technique or by immunoradiometric assay of factor IX (Mibashan *et al.* 1979, Holmberg *et al.* 1980).

Bleeding in carriers of haemophilia and Christmas disease

It is not yet sufficiently known that in a proportion of female carriers of haemophilia and Christmas disease the level of factor VIII or IX may be reduced to as little as 10 or 15 per cent of normal, or sometimes even less and as a consequence the women may bleed excessively. The type of bleeding seen includes easy bruising, bleeding from cuts and scratches and epistaxis. Menorrhagia may be a problem and they may bleed heavily following accidental injuries, surgical operations and following childbirth. Such women should be managed in the same way as mild haemophiliacs so that their distressing bleeding complications may be avoided.

von Willebrand's disease

von Willebrand's disease is an inherited bleeding disorder which affects males and females and is in the majority of cases passed on in an autosomal dominant manner. In a small number of patients the condition seems to be transmitted as an autosomal recessive condition with the offspring being homozygotes and very severely affected. There is often a history of consanguinity in these families. von Willebrand's disease is one of the commonest of the inherited bleeding disorders. In Sweden, the prevalence is thought to be 10 per 100 000 of population compared with 7 per 100 000 for haemophilia (Nilsson and Holmberg 1979). The condition was first described by E.A. von Willebrand in 1926 in members of a family from Föglö in the Åland islands in the Gulf of Bothnia. The condition as described then was characterized by excessive bleeding from mucous membranes and skin following minor injuries. Bleeding into joints was rare. The platelet count was normal but the skin bleeding time was prolonged. von Willebrand believed that the disease was a form of haemophilia and called it 'pseudo-haemophilia'. The pathological defect at that time was thought to be a combined disorder of platelet function and vessel wall function. More recent work has revealed a defect in the factor VIII complex. Alexander and Goldstein (1953) reported a deficiency of factor VIII coagulant activity in two patients with all the features of von Willebrand's disease. In 1957, Nilsson *et al.* confirmed that the original family described by von Willebrand had a reduced level of factor VIII clotting activity. Nilsson *et al.* (1959) also showed that transfusion of factor VIII (fraction I–o) concentrate into patients with von Willebrand's disease resulted in a prolonged elevation of factor VIII coagulant activity in the blood accompanied by correction of the bleeding time. Moreover, the same effect was obtained even if the fraction I–o was prepared from plasma obtained from a severely affected haemophiliac. They concluded that the abnormal haemostasis in von Willebrand's disease was due to the absence of a plasma factor and that this factor was present in normal plasma and in haemophilic plasma. In addition to correcting the bleeding time, the factor stimulated synthesis or release of factor VIII coagulant activity. Several studies of von Willebrand's disease have shown decreased platelet adhesiveness *in vivo* (Borchgrevink 1960) and *in vitro* (Salzman 1963) and correction of the defect following transfusion of normal plasma, haemophilic plasma or factor VIII concentrate.

In 1971 Zimmerman, Ratnoff and Powell prepared a monospecific precipitating rabbit antibody raised against highly purified human factor VIII. Using this antibody in Laurell's electroimmunoassay, they demonstrated the presence of factor VIII-related antigen (VIIIR:Ag) in both normal and haemophilic plasma but absence or reduced levels of the antigen in the plasma of patients with von Willebrand's disease. Addition of factor VIIIR:Ag from normal plasma corrected the abnormal platelets adhesiveness in von Willebrand's disease (Bouma *et al.* 1972) and highlighted the importance of factor VIIIR:Ag for normal platelet function. Further insight into the nature of the defect in von Willebrand's disease was obtained when Howard and Firkin (1971) showed that the antibiotic ristocetin, which caused aggregation of platelets when added to normal platelet-rich plasma, failed to do so in platelet-rich plasma from patients suffering from von Willebrand's disease. Again, the defect could be corrected by the addition of normal or haemophilic plasma and was thought to be due to a quantitative or qualitative abnormality in factor VIIIR:Ag. This property of normal factor VIIIR:Ag is generally known as ristocetin cofactor (Rist Cof), factor VIII-related von Willebrand factor (VIIIR:vWF) or factor VIII-related ristocetin cofactor (VIIIR:RRCF). It is still not clear how ristocetin and ristocetin cofactor cooperate to bring about platelet aggregation but it has been suggested (Kattlove and Gomez 1975) that ristocetin probably binds to the platelet membrane and that the plasma factor causes aggregation by forming bridges between the ristocetin molecules. In contrast, the abnormality of ristocetin-induced platelet aggregation seen in Bernard–Soulier's syndrome, in which there are normal levels of ristocetin cofactor, is thought to be due to a deficiency of glycoprotein I complex on the platelet membrane and is not corrected by the addition of normal plasma. The glycoprotein I complex seems to be essential for the interaction between platelets and ristocetin cofactor and hence for platelet aggregation by ristocetin.

Variant forms of von Willebrand's disease have been described based on the level of factor VIII:C, factor VIIIR:Ag, ristocetin cofactor and the behaviour of factor VIIIR:Ag on two-dimensional immunoelectrophoresis. Several classifications have been used but one which has wide acceptance is shown in Table 8.

Type I, so-called classical von Willebrand's disease, is the commonest form of the condition and accounts for approximately 75 per cent of cases (Italian Working Group 1977, Nilsson and Holmberg 1979). There is a reduction in all activities associated with the factor VIII complex and all of the activities are reduced to the same extent. If factor VIIIR:Ag is detectable it usually has normal mobility on two-dimensional immunoelectrophoresis. The bleeding time is prolonged in the more severely affected patients. In Type II von Willebrand's disease, factor VIII:C is usually reduced as is ristocetin cofactor activity but the level of factor VIII-related antigen as measured by Laurèll's electroimmunoassay is usually normal or very slightly reduced. Immuno-radiometric assay, on the other hand, shows lower levels of factor VIIIR:Ag with characteristically non-parallel assay lines. On two-dimensional immunoelectrophoresis there is a lack of slower-moving components of factor VIIIR:Ag and an apparent increase in the faster-moving components (Fig. 26) (Kernoff, Gruson and Rizza 1974, Peake, Bloom and Giddings 1974). SDS-agarose electrophoresis shows that the larger polymeric forms which are

Table 8. Classification of von Willebrand's disease.

Type	Bleeding time	VIII:C	Ristocetin cofactor	VIIIR:Ag	Crossed immuno-electrophoresis
Type I (typical)	Normal *or* long	Usually reduced	Usually reduced	Usually reduced	Normal
Type IIa variant	Long	Reduced *or* normal	Reduced	Reduced *or* normal	Increased mobility
Type IIb variant	Long	Reduced *or* normal	Reduced *or* normal*	Reduced *or* normal	Increased mobility
Type III (Homo-zygous or double heterozygous)	Long	Greatly reduced	Greatly reduced	Absent	None visible

* When ristocetin is added to the patient's platelet-rich plasma the platelets aggregate more readily than normal.

(a)

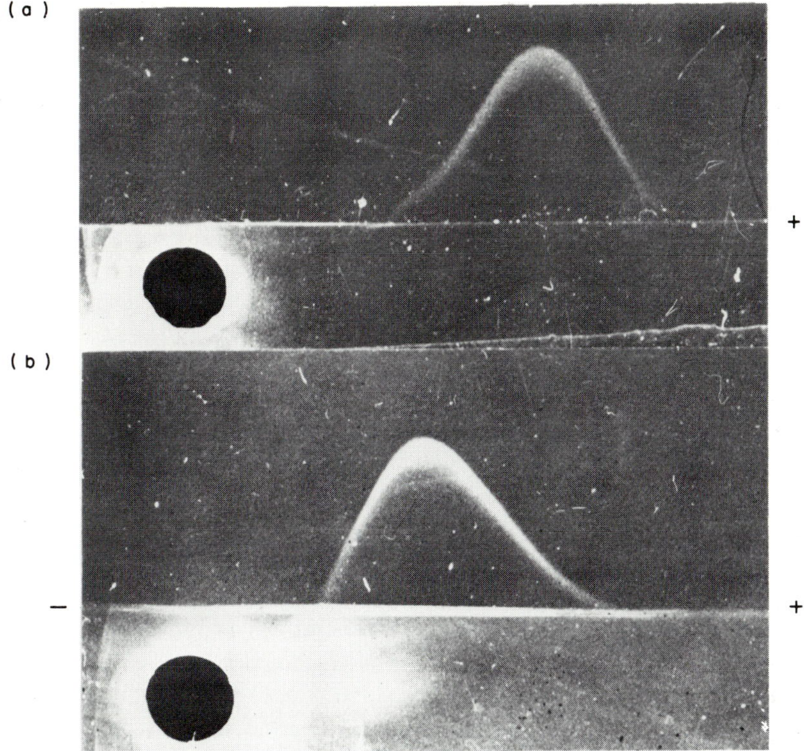

(b)

Fig. 26. Precipitation pattern obtained following two-dimensional immunoelectrophoresis of factor VIII-related antigen in (a) plasma from patient with Type II von Willebrand's disease and (b) normal plasma.

thought to be necessary for the platelet-related activities of factor VIIIR : Ag are reduced or absent. The bleeding time is usually prolonged. Recently it has been observed that some patients with Type II von Willebrand's show increased platelet aggregation compared to normal when ristocetin is added to their platelet-rich plasma (Ruggeri *et al.* 1980, Ruggeri and Zimmerman 1980). In addition, SDS-agarose electrophoresis of their plasma shows some difference between their pattern of factor VIIIR : Ag polymer distribution and that of other patients with Type II von Willebrand's. On the basis of those tests, Type II von Willebrand has been subdivided into Type IIA and Type IIB. The patients with Type IIB are those with increased platelet aggregation in the presence of ristocetin. In Type III von Willebrand's disease, there is a severe deficiency of all the activities of the factor VIII complex with severe clinical symptoms, possibly including haemarthrosis. Many of the cases of Type III von Willebrand's disease are the children of consanguineous marriages and are presumably homozygotes.

Clinical features

Patients suffering from von Willebrand's experience excessive and easy bruising and bleeding from the skin mucous membranes of the nose, gastrointestinal tract and uterus. Excessive bleeding after all forms of surgery including dental extraction is common and occurs immediately after the injury. Post-partum haemorrhage may occur 7–10 days after delivery when the level of the factor VIII complex, raised during pregnancy, has returned to its basal level.

Patients suffering from homozygous von Willebrand's are severely affected and may show a pattern of bleeding similar to that seen in haemophilia with haemarthroses and deep intramuscular haemorrhage in addition to bleeding from mucous membranes.

Diagnosis

In the majority of patients, especially those with significant symptoms, the diagnosis can be made from the patient's personal and family history and from the results of the bleeding time test and assay of the various components of the factor VIII complex. Some difficulty may be experienced in distinguishing mild von Willebrand's disease from mild haemophilia.

Typically in von Willebrand's disease the bleeding time by the Ivy method or the template method is prolonged and the levels of factor VIII:C and factor VIII-related antigen in plasma are reduced, as is the level of ristocetin cofactor. In addition, two-dimensional immunoelectrophoresis may show abnormal mobility of factor VIII-related antigen. We have found this latter test particularly useful when studying family members who have a borderline clinical history. More information concerning the multimeric pattern of factor VIII-related antigen may be obtained using SDS-agarose electrophoresis followed by fixing and reacting with affinity-purified ^{125}I-labelled antibody to factor VIII-related antigen. The multimers can then be demonstrated by autoradiography (Hoyer and Shainoff 1980, Ruggeri and Zimmerman 1980). Both clinical and laboratory manifestations of the disease may vary from member to member in the same family and from time to time in the same individual so that it may be necessary sometimes to carry out the laboratory tests on several occasions in order to confirm or refute the diagnosis.

Factor I (fibrinogen) deficiency

Disorders of plasma fibrinogen may be congenital or acquired and may arise as a quantitative defect, a qualitative defect or as a combination of these. Inherited defects of fibrinogen are extremely rare and may be due to a lack of production or diminished production of normal fibrinogen (afibrinogenaemia, hypofibrinogenaemia) or to the production in normal or reduced amounts of a structurally abnormal fibrinogen (dysfibrinogenaemia). Acquired defects, quantitative or qualitative, are seen more commonly and may be associated with a variety of pathological conditions such as disseminated intravascular coagulation, liver disease and may also appear in the neonatal period.

The inheritance of congenital afibrinogenaemia is probably autosomal with only the homozygotes being clinically affected although careful testing often shows reduced levels of fibrinogen in heterozygotes. Both sexes are affected and a large proportion of the cases described have been the offspring of consanguineous marriages. The condition was first described by Rabe and Salomon (1930). Cases have been described by Macfarlane (1938), Pinninger and Prunty (1946), Prentice (1951) and Hardisty and Pinniger (1956) and the group of disorders has recently been reviewed by Flute (1977) and Beck (1979). The condition may manifest itself at birth with prolonged bleeding from the umbilical stump. There is a tendency to bruise easily and excessively and cuts, scratches and venepunctures tend to bleed more than normal. Bleeding may occur into muscles and occasionally into joints but severe arthropathy as seen in haemophiliacs is uncommon. Bleeding may also occur from the nose or from the gastrointestinal tract. Cerebral haemorrhage has been reported and menorrhagia and post-partum haemorrhage may be troublesome in women. Persistent bleeding follows surgical operations. The patient with afibrinogenaemia has a milder bleeding disorder than does the severe haemophiliac, may lead a normal and active life and is unlikely to become crippled. The most striking laboratory findings are the infinitely prolonged whole blood clotting time, activated partial thromboplastin time and one-stage prothrombin time and the failure of the blood or plasma to clot on addition of thrombin, ancrod (Arvin) or batroxobin (Reptilase). These tests are corrected by the addition of normal plasma or fibrinogen. The levels of other clotting factors are normal. In a proportion of patients the bleeding time is prolonged. This may be due to a deficiency of platelet fibrinogen.

Inherited dysfibrinogenaemia

Qualitative disorders of fibrinogen synthesis resulting in the production of a defective protein are referred to as the 'dysfibrinogenaemias'. The first clear account of an inherited abnormal form of fibrinogen was given by Ménaché (1964) although previous workers had suggested that synthesis of an abnormal form of fibrinogen might be an inherited trait (Fanconi 1941, Ingram 1955, Imperato and Dettori 1958). Approximately 50 inherited variants have now been reported and named after the city in which they were first described (Beck 1964). Since few of the cases have been studied in detail it is not known how many of those named variants are identical.

The dysfibrinogenaemias have been classified functionally as follows:

1 Disordered fibrinopeptide release.
2 Disordered polymerization.
3 Unusual cross-linking.
4 Particular susceptibility to digestion by plasmin.

In many of the variants described, more than one of the above functional defects may be present, but in the majority of variants the main defect seems to be in the polymerization phase. Only in the case of fibrinogen Detroit has the nature of the molecular abnormality been discovered (Blombäck *et al.* 1968). Examination of the Aα chain in the region of the N-terminal disulphide knot shows that arginine has been replaced by a serine residue at position 19. For a detailed account of fibrinogen variants and their different biochemical abnormalities the reader is referred to the review by Flute (1977).

The inheritance of dysfibrinogenaemia seems to be autosomal and the sexes are affected equally. A proportion of patients bleed excessively from the mucous membranes following injury, some show abnormal wound healing and breakdown of wounds and a small number have a tendency to thrombosis. In more than half of the patients described the condition was discovered by chance during routine laboratory testing and was not associated with haemorrhagic or thrombotic manifestations. The most consistent laboratory finding is a prolonged clotting time on adding thrombin to the patient's plasma, with apparently normal or increased amounts of fibrinogen when measured by immunological or salt precipitation methods.

Factor XIII (fibrin stabilizing factor) deficiency

This uncommon disorder was first described by Duckert, Jung and Schmerling (1960) and there are now approximately 100 cases recorded in the medical literature. The prevalence in the UK is thought to be about 1 in 5 million (Lorand, Losowsky and Miloszewski 1980). Inheritance is usually autosomal recessive and there is often a history of consanguinity in the parents. In this condition, clotting by the intrinsic and extrinsic system and thrombin generation are normal but because of the absence of the fibrin stabilizing factor the clots formed *in vitro* are unstable and dissolve in the presence of reagents such as 5M urea solution or 1 per cent monochloroacetic acid. Presumably the clots formed in wounds are also unstable in the presence of the normal fibrinolytic process and this accounts for the bleeding tendency. Human factor XIII has a molecular weight of 320 000 and is composed of two types of subunit called 'a' and 'b' (Schwartz *et al.* 1973) with molecular weights of 75 000 and 85 000 respectively. In its native form, factor XIII is in the form a_2b_2. During the clotting process factor XIII is converted to the active enzyme by the action of thrombin and Ca^{2+} on the 'a' subunit which becomes enzymically active. The 'b' subunit probably plays a regulatory or protective role. The transamidase activity thus produced catalyses the formation of glutamyl-E-lysine bridges between fibrin chains, thereby rendering the fibrin clot more rigid and more resistant to lysis.

The haemorrhagic features of factor XIII deficiency can be severe and may lead to death in early life. Prolonged bleeding may occur from the umbilical stump, there is easy bruising, and muscle and joint haemorrhages have been recorded. Bleeding from mucous membranes, gastrointestinal tract and renal tract is rare. A notable feature is that 20–30 per cent of patients suffer from intracranial bleeding, often following some minor injury. Post-traumatic and post-operative bleeding characteristically occur several hours after injury and wound healing may be delayed, with abnormal scar formation (Duckert, Jung and Schmerling 1960). Repeated spontaneous abortion has been described in affected females. In view of the fact that the 'routine' tests of blood coagulation and haemostasis such as whole blood clotting time, prothrombin consumption test, prothrombin time, activated partial thromboplastin time and bleeding time are all normal in factor XIII deficiency, diagnosis of the condition requires an awareness of the possibility. A simple qualitative test for severe factor XIII deficiency can be performed by recalcifying an aliquot of the patient's plasma, allowing it to clot and then adding an equal volume of 5M urea or 1 per cent monochloroacetic acid. In the absence of factor XIII, the plasma clot will dissolve within a few hours. Assay of factor XIII activity may be carried out using the covalent incorporation of labelled synthetic amines such as fluorescent dansylcadaverine or radioactive putrescine into an added protein such as casein. Immunological assays of factor XIII are also available (Barbui *et al.* 1974, Board, Coggan and Hamer 1980).

Factor II (prothrombin) deficiency

Congenital deficiency of prothrombin is extremely rare, probably autosomal in inheritance and may affect either sex. Molecular variants causing dysprothrombinaemias have been described, as well as true hypoprothrombinaemia and account for approximately half of the families described (Owen *et al.* 1978, Bezeaud *et al.* 1979).

In hypoprothrombinaemia, the amount of prothrombin detected by clotting assay and staphylocoagulase assay is approximately the same as that found by immunoassay (Josso *et al.* 1967). In the case of dysprothrombinaemia the level of prothrombin assayed by clotting methods dependent on brain extract is reduced, whereas the amount detectable using immunological methods is normal, except in a few cases thought to be heterozygotes for both hypoprothrombinaemia and dysprothrombinaemia. The use of other pro-thrombin-converting agents such as snake venoms (*Echis carinatus, Notechis scutatus, Dispholidus typus*) or staphylocoagulase allows further classification of the dysprothrombinaemias. Shapiro and his colleagues (1969) described the first cases of dysprothrombinaemia in a large family with 11 affected members. They called this abnormal prothrombin, prothrombin Cardeza. Since then, several variant prothrombins have been described and named according to their place of origin (Josso *et al.* 1971, Girolami *et al.* 1974, Shapiro *et al.* 1974, Girolami *et al.* 1978a, Owen *et al.* 1978, Bezeaud *et al.* 1979, Rabiet *et al.* 1979). In both hypoprothrombinaemia and dysprothrombinaemia easy bruising, muscle haematomas, epistaxis and menorrhagia have been noted as well as excessive bleeding after dental extraction and other surgical operations. Haemarthroses have not been a feature of the condition (Borchgrevink *et al.* 1959, Soulier, Prou-Wartelle and Josso 1962). Diagnosis of a quantitative prothrombin deficiency is made by the use of a two-stage prothrombin assay or by tests involving Taipan or other snake venoms. The one-stage prothrombin time is insensitive to all but the most severe forms of prothrombin deficiency and may be nearly normal in moderately severe deficiencies. As mentioned above, the reduced biological activity is accompanied by a similar reduction using immunological assays. In the dysprothrombinaemias there is a deficiency of prothrombin as measured by coagulation tests using tissue extract but normal amounts of immunologically detectable prothrombin.

Factor V deficiency

Congenital factor V deficiency, which was first described by Owren in 1947, is inherited as an autosomal condition, sometimes with a family history of consanguinity. The two sexes seem to be equally affected. It is a rare condition. The nature of the molecular defect is still not clear. Using a factor V antibody which had developed in a factor V-deficient patient, Fratantoni, Hilgartner and Nachman (1972) were unable to detect antibody-neutralizing material in samples of the same patient's plasma obtained when the antibody had disappeared. From this they concluded that the genetic defect appeared to be due to lack of the protein rather than a modification of the molecule. Similar studies employing factor V antibodies which had arisen in previously normal individuals failed to detect factor V-like antigen in patients with factor V deficiency (Feinstein *et al.* 1970). We have had experience of managing factor V deficiency in two patients who bruise easily and have suffered excessive bleeding from the gums when teeth were erupting, from the nose and gastrointestinal tract and following surgical operations. One of them, a female with a factor V level of 1 per cent, has suffered at least one haemarthrosis in the knee and hip and several intramuscular haematomas involving calf and thigh, as well as menorrhagia. One of the patients has bilateral bifid renal pelves and double ureters. An association has been noted in the literature between factor V deficiency and abnormalities of renal tract, cardiovascular or skeletal systems (Seeler 1972).

In our cases haemarthroses and intramuscular haematomas have not occurred spontaneously but have always followed some injury. It would appear that a relatively low level of factor V is required in the blood to control bleeding and that this can usually be achieved by giving infusions of fresh, or fresh-frozen plasma (Borchgrevink and Owren 1961, Rush and Ellis 1965). The most characteristic laboratory finding is a prolongation of the one-stage prothrombin time and activated partial thromboplastin time which can be corrected by the addition of alumina-adsorbed normal citrated plasma. The diagnosis is confirmed by specific assays for factor V. In both of our patients the bleeding time was consistently in excess of 15 minutes, a finding also recorded by Soulier and his colleagues (1958). Occasionally the parents of severely affected patients have reduced levels of factor V of the order of 30–50 per cent of normal and are presumably heterozygotes for the condition (Rush and Ellis 1965, Seeler 1972).

Factor VII deficiency

Congenital factor VII deficiency is very rare. It was first described by Alexander *et al.* (1951). The inheritance is probably autosomal. There seems little doubt that factor VII deficiency consists of different genetic variants. Goodnight *et al.* (1971) studied four unrelated patients with hereditary factor VII deficiency employing a factor VII antibody-neutralizing technique to test for the presence of factor VII-like material. One patient had considerably more antibody-neutralizing material in his plasma than was expected from its level of factor VII clotting activity; in two patients the antibody-neutralizing material was equivalent to the factor VII activity and in the third patient there was slightly more antibody-neutralizing material compared with the clotting activity. They concluded that at least two and possibly three types of inherited factor VII deficiency existed. Similar results have been obtained by Denson, Conrad and Samama (1972), Briët *et al.* (1976) and Mazzucconi *et al.* (1977).

Girolami and his associates have studied a number of patients with mild factor VII deficiency. On the basis of antibody neutralization tests and factor VII assays carried out using tissue thromboplastin from different animals, they have defined three variants of factor VII: factor VII Verona, factor VII Padua I and factor VII Padua II (Girolami *et al.* 1977, 1978b, 1979).

The bleeding manifestations seen in factor VII deficiency are in general milder than in severe haemophilia. Some patients have lifelong bleeding problems, others have trouble in adolescence or at the onset of menstruation and yet others have little trouble throughout life. Excessive bruising, epistaxis and gastrointestinal haemorrhage occur, as well as menorrhagia in the female. Haemarthroses are said to occur less frequently than in the severe haemophiliac but we have seen two patients with several severely damaged joints as a result of recurrent haemarthroses and in one of the patients a hip replacement operation was required at the age of 27 years (see Chapter 12). Post-operative haemorrhage may occur but is not a constant finding (Ratnoff 1960, Marder and Shulman 1964). One of the patients under our care underwent tonsillectomy in childhood without transfusion therapy and did not bleed excessively, but another bled for 20 days following dental extraction.

The relationship of factor VII antigen to bleeding symptoms is not clear. Briët *et al.* (1976) noted that the presence of cross-reacting material seemed to protect against spontaneous haemorrhage but Mazzucconi *et al.* (1977) found that the clinical pictures of CRM+ and CRM− factor VII deficiency were indistinguishable.

Laboratory investigations show a prolonged one-stage prothrombin time but a normal whole blood clotting time, activated partial thromboplastin time and Russell's viper venom (Stypven) time. Specific factor VII assay, using VII-deficiency substrate plasma, confirms the diagnosis. A prolonged bleeding time has been found in a proportion of patients.

Factor X deficiency

Congenital deficiency of factor X is rare and there are only a few well-documented cases (Telfer, Denson and Wright 1956, Hougie, Barrow and Graham 1957). The inheritance is autosomal and there may be consanguinity in the parents of an affected individual. As with other clotting factors there is strong evidence for the existence of several molecular variants of the factor. Denson *et al.* (1970) studied six patients with a factor X defect. By means of antibody neutralization techniques and tests of factor X activation via the extrinsic and intrinsic system they demonstrated at least five separate abnormalities of factor X. In factor X Friuli, described by Girolami *et al.* (1970), the defect is characterized by an abnormal one-stage prothrombin time and factor X level when tissue thromboplastin is used, but normal results when Russell's viper venom is used as the activating agent. The patient's plasma contained normal amounts of cross-reacting factor X-like material which showed a line of identity with normal factor X on immunodiffusion.

Patients with factor X deficiency bleed after dental extractions and other surgery. The only patient known to us, a woman with a factor X level of 8 per cent of normal, suffered from menorrhagia and bled excessively after childbirth. Haemarthroses have been described. The half-life of transfused factor X in the circulation is approximately two to three days (Biggs and Denson 1963) and this, along with the stability of factor X in frozen plasma, makes the condition relatively easy to treat with plasma. The laboratory findings include a prolonged activated partial thromboplastin time, an abnormal thromboplastin generation test when the patient's serum is used and a long one-stage prothrombin time when either brain extract or Russell's viper venom is used. As mentioned above, in certain variants of the condition the clotting time in the presence of Russell's viper venom may be normal. The abnormal test may be corrected by the addition of normal plasma or by aged normal serum but not by alumina-adsorbed normal plasma.

Factor XI (PTA) deficiency

The condition, first described by Rosenthal, Dreskin and Rosenthal (1955) is relatively rare and those affected are usually of Ashkenazi Jewish stock (Leiba, Ramot and Many 1965, Seligsohn 1978). The condition is inherited autosomally and affects males and females. The type of bleeding seen is generally not as serious as that which is found in severe haemophilia and haemarthroses rarely occur. Bleeding usually only follows surgery or severe trauma and is rarely spontaneous. Epistaxis has been described and affected women may suffer from menorrhagia and excessive bleeding after childbirth. Surprisingly, the severity of bleeding may not be closely correlated with the degree of the deficiency state as determined by laboratory tests. The reason for this is not known. Because of this it is not easy to define the level of factor XI required for haemostasis or to control therapy by means of laboratory tests. Laboratory investigations show a normal one-stage prothrombin time, a prolonged whole blood clotting time and kaolin cephalin clotting time. The diagnosis is confirmed by specific factor XI assay employing a substrate plasma from a patient congenitally deficient in the factor. If such substrate plasma is not available the celite-eluate test of Nossel (1964) is useful for diagnostic purposes.

Factor XII (Hageman factor) deficiency

This condition, which affects the sexes equally, is transmitted as an autosomal recessive trait (Ratnoff and Colopy 1955) although in one family the condition seems dominant (Bennett *et al.* 1972). Individuals with this deficiency have a prolonged whole blood clotting time and activated partial thromboplastin time but rarely bleed excessively. Some cases in which mild bleeding has been a feature have been reported by Didisheim (1962), Nossel (1969) and Ratnoff (1977).

Fletcher and Fitzgerald factor deficiencies

Fletcher factor deficiency was first reported by Hathaway, Belhasen and Hathaway (1965) in four siblings of a consanguineous marriage. The deficiency which was not associated with bleeding symptoms was characterized by a prolonged activated partial thromboplastin time which became shorter when the period of incubation with the surface activating agent was increased. Subsequently, Wuepper (1973) showed that plasma deficient in Fletcher factor is also deficient in prekallikrein and produced strong evidence for Fletcher factor and prekallikrein being the same substance. This was confirmed by Weiss, Gallin and Kaplan (1974). The latter workers also showed that blood deficient in Fletcher factor, in addition to showing a coagulation defect, was also defective in fibrinolysis, chemotaxis and kinin generation.

Fitzgerald factor deficiency, named after the first patient described, was first reported by Waldmann and his associates (Waldmann and Abraham 1974, Waldmann *et al.* 1975). Similar cases were reported by LaCombe *et al.* (1975) and Colman *et al.* (1975) who named the defect Flaujeac and Williams deficiency respectively. Deficiency of Fitzgerald, Flaujeac and Williams factor is not associated with any haemorrhagic state and, like Fletcher factor deficiency, is characterized by a prolongation of the activated partial thromboplastin time, but in this case the abnormal clotting time is not shortened by prolonged incubation with activating agents. Fitzgerald factor has been identified as a high molecular weight kininogen.

The defect in Flaujeac and Williams trait is similar except that a wide species of kininogens seem to be deficient, low molecular weight as well as high molecular weight kininogen being affected.

Combined deficiency of factor V and factor VIII

Congenital combined deficiency of factors V and VIII is rare and was first described in two brothers by Oeri *et al.* (1954). Since then, several families have been described (Iversen and Bastrup-Madsen 1956, Jones *et al.* 1962, Seligsohn and Ramot 1969, Smit Sibinga *et al.* 1972). The condition affects males and females, is autosomal recessive in inheritance and usually results in a mild to moderate bleeding disorder. Symptoms include bruising, epistaxis, prolonged bleeding after dental extraction and other surgical procedures. Haemarthroses, menorrhagia and post-partum bleeding are infrequent. The mode of inheritance of the disorder is difficult to explain in simple terms since factor VIII:C deficiency is a sex-linked disorder and factor V deficiency is autosomal recessive. Marlar and Griffin (1980) have shown that the protease enzyme protein C which inactivates factor V and VIII acts unopposed, because of the absence of an inhibitor, in the plasma of patients with combined factor V and VIII deficiency. They suggest that the molecular basis for the combined factor V/VIII deficiency is a deficiency of protein C which has an autosomal recessive inheritance.

Alpha$_2$-antiplasmin deficiency

Koie *et al.* (1978) were the first to describe a bleeding disorder associated with α_2-antiplasmin deficiency. The bleeding manifestations were severe and included easy bruising, haemarthroses and bleeding from superficial injuries. Routine tests of blood coagulation revealed no abnormality but whole blood clot lysis time and euglobulin lysis time were markedly reduced. The patient's plasma was completely deficient in α_2-antiplasmin. More details about this family as well as other families with α_2-antiplasmin deficiency have since been reported (Aoki *et al.* 1979, Kluft, Vellenga and Brommer 1979, Miles *et al.* 1982). The condition seems to be autosomal recessive in inheritance and several members of the families described have approximately half the normal amount of α_2-antiplasmin in their plasma but do not bleed. They are presumably heterozygous for the condition. The frequency and severity of bleeding may be diminished by administration of tranexamic acid.

Acquired deficiencies of blood clotting factors

Acquired deficiencies of blood clotting factors are commoner than inherited deficiencies and usually involve more than one factor at a time unlike the inherited deficiencies which usually involve a single factor. In many instances the coagulation factor defect is only a part of some generalized disease process affecting not only those factors but also the cellular constituents of the blood, in particular platelets. The vessel wall may also be damaged and the fibrinolytic system altered. Depending on the component affected and the degree to which they are affected, the haemostatic defect may be mild or severe, with or without evidence of intravascular clotting.

Vitamin K deficiency

Vitamin K is required for the normal synthesis of factor II (prothrombin), factor VII, IX and X by the liver. It has recently been shown that all of the vitamin K-dependent clotting factors contain γ-carboxyglutamic acid and that this amino acid is responsible for the calcium binding property of these factors which is essential for full biological activity. Vitamin K is involved in the carboxylation process. In the absence of the vitamin, although the factors continue to be synthesized and can be detected immunologically, they are biologically inactive see Chapter 3.

Vitamin K is a fat-soluble substance found in the chloroplasts of many plant leaves and in some vegetable oils. Human requirements are satisfied by the average diet and in addition considerable amounts of the vitamin are synthesized by intestinal bacteria.

Vitamin K activity is associated with at least two substances which have been designated vitamin K_1 and vitamin K_2. Vitamin K_1 is phytonadione (phylloquinone) found in plants and is the only natural vitamin K available for therapy. Vitamin K_2 represents several compounds, the menaquinones. The latter substances are synthesized by bacteria, in particular Gram-positive bacteria. Vitamin K_1 and K_2 are absorbed from the intestine only if adequate amounts of bile salts are present. Following absorption, the vitamin appears to be concentrated in the liver for a short time following which there is a rapid decline. The body apparently has little storage capacity for vitamin K.

A deficiency of vitamin K and a consequent failure to synthesize factor II, VII, IX or X can result from failure of dietary intake, failure of absorption, failure of utilization or the action of drugs which are vitamin K antagonists.

Vitamin K deficiency arising from poor dietary intake is extremely rare because of the contribution made by the vitamin K synthesizing organisms in the intestine. A combination of dietary deficiency and long-term treatment with broad spectrum antibiotics which inhibit the gut organisms may result in a deficiency state.

Failure to absorb vitamin K is seen in biliary obstruction because the lipid soluble vitamin is poorly absorbed in the absence of bile salts. Inadequate absorption of vitamin K is seen also in diseases of the intestinal tract associated with malabsorption. These include sprue, regional enteritis, fibrocystic disease, ulcerative colitis and dysentery. Resection of large portions of the bowel may be followed by vitamin K deficiency and bleeding.

In hepatocellular disease such as acute hepatitis or cirrhosis of the liver the synthesis of the vitamin K-dependent factors by the hepatocyte may be impaired even in the presence of adequate amounts of vitamin K. The administration of vitamin K is usually of little value in correcting the coagulation factor deficiency unless there is also a degree of biliary obstruction as part of the disease process. Indeed the response of the coagulation factors to parenteral vitamin K has been used as a test to differentiate hepatocellular jaundice from obstructive jaundice.

Haemorrhagic disease of the newborn

Newborn infants, especially if they are premature, have a deficiency of factor II, VII, IX and X. This is due partly to poor synthesis by the immature liver and partly due to vitamin K deficiency which develops during the first few days after birth. Human milk has a low concentration of vitamin K and, in addition, the intestine of breast-fed babies seems to be deficient in organisms which synthesize vitamin K. Infants with this condition have a generalized bleeding disorder with easy bruising and bleeding from the gastrointestinal tract.

Oral anticoagulants

Certain drugs such as the coumarin anticoagulants act as antagonists of vitamin K and so interfere with the synthesis of biologically active factor II, VII, IX and X in the liver. The site of action of the drug is thought to be at the stage of post-ribosomal carboxylation of glutamic acid where vitamin K acts.

The bleeding seen in overdosage with oral anticoagulants and in other acquired deficiencies of the vitamin K-dependent clotting factors varies with the severity of the deficiency state and consists mainly of cutaneous ecchymoses, petechial haemorrhages and bleeding from the nose, gums, gastrointestinal tract and genito-urinary tract. Retroperitoneal and intracranial haemorrhages have been described as well as bleeding into muscles and joints. Gastrointestinal tract bleeding in a patient whose anticoagulant therapy is well controlled should raise the suspicion of an underlying lesion such as duodenal ulcer or a bowel neoplasm. In patients with chronic liver disease the coagulation factor deficiency may be complicated by hypersplenism and thrombocytopenia. Bleeding from associated oesophageal varices may be severe.

Bleeding during heparin therapy

Bleeding is the most important side-effect of intravenous heparin therapy and may present as superficial bruising, epistaxis, retroperitoneal bleeding, gastrointestinal or genito-urinary bleeding and wound haematomas. In a recent study of the use of intravenous heparin in the treatment of venous thrombosis 37 per cent of treated patients bled, 13 per cent of them seriously (Mant *et al.* 1977). Elderly subjects and patients with an underlying haemostatic defect seem to be at particular risk of bleeding during heparin therapy.

Low-dose heparin for the prevention of venous thrombosis during surgery seems to have a lower incidence of severe bleeding although wound haematomas may still cause problems (International Multicentre Trial 1975, Leyvraz *et al* 1983).

Acquired dysfibrinogenaemia

In 1969 von Felten, Straub and Frick reported dysfibrinogenaemia in a patient with a primary hepatoma and a coagulation defect. Study of the isolated fibrinogen revealed a defect in polymerization of fibrin. Since then, further studies in patients with severe liver disease suggest that acquired abnormalities of fibrinogen synthesis may be more common than previously thought (Soria *et al.* 1970, Lane *et al.* 1977).

In 1951 Biggs observed that the thrombin clotting time of cord blood plasma from normal neonates was delayed. Fibrinogen separated from cord blood plasma by ammonium sulphate precipitation also had a delayed clotting time compared to adult fibrinogen. This observation has been confirmed (von Felten and Straub 1969, Guillin and Ménaché 1973). The latter workers showed that fibrin monomers from fetal fibrinogen aggregated more slowly and to a lesser extent than adult monomers.

Acquired hypofibrinogenaemia

As mentioned above, reduced levels of fibrinogen may be found in conditions such as chronic liver disease and are seen in their most dramatic form in acute disseminated intravascular coagulation. This is discussed later.

Acquired isolated deficiencyy of factor X

An acquired isolated deficiency of factor X and occasionally factor IX has been observed in patients suffering from amyloid disease (Korsan-Bengsten, Hjort and Ygge 1962, Ménaché and Boivin 1962, Howell 1963, Spero *et al.* 1976, Furie, Greene and Furie 1977, McPherson *et al.* 1977, Greipp, Kyle and Bowie 1979). As a consequence of the factor X deficiency these patients may bleed into skin and muscles or from mucous membranes, spontaneously or following minor injury. The cause of the factor X deficiency is not known. Howell (1963) observed that plasma transfusions did not correct the coagulation defect in her patients and, having excluded a factor X inhibitor, suggested that amyloid deposits were selectively absorbing factor X. Support for this suggestion came from the studies of Furie, Greene and Furie (1977) who demonstrated a very rapid clearance of ^{131}I-labelled factor X from the circulation when infused into patients with amyloidosis. Further *in vitro* studies (Furie *et al.* 1981) showed that amyloid fibrils bound factor X and to a lesser extent factor IX. Laboratory tests show a prolongation of the one-stage prothrombin time, Stypven time and activated partial thromboplastin time. Specific assay for factor X reveals low levels of the factor. Factor X replacement by means of prothrombin complex concentrate has proved effective in controlling bleeding (Spero *et al.* 1976). The removal of the spleen has been followed by correction of the factor X defect (Greipp, Kyle and Bowie 1979).

Acquired isolated deficiency of factor IX

This is extremely uncommon. Handley and Lawrence (1967) reported four patients with nephrotic syndrome who had reduced levels of factor IX ranging from 5–28 per cent of normal. The levels of other clotting factors were normal. The latter authors speculated that factor IX might have been lost in the urine but failed to detect any factor IX in the patients' urine. Treatment with steroids was followed by a return to normal of the plasma factor IX level. Acquired deficiency of factor IX has also been reported in patients suffering from Gaucher's disease (Boklan and Sawitsky 1976).

Blood clotting inhibitors in systemic lupus erythematosus (SLE)

An inhibitor of blood coagulation has been found in approximately 5–10 per cent of patients with systemic lupus erythematosus (Regan, Lachner and Karpatkin 1974). The 'SLE inhibitor' or 'lupus anticoagulant' is found in a variety of other conditions including malignancy, gynaecological, urological and neurological conditions (Schleider *et al.* 1976), and occasionally in apparently normal individuals. In the study of Schleider *et al.* (1976) 50 per cent of patients wth the 'lupus anticoagulant' did not have SLE. Typically, patients show a prolongation of the activated partial thromboplastin time and the prothrombin time which is not corrected by mixing with normal plasma. Indeed, mixing with normal plasma may lead to a further prolongation of the already long clotting time. The inhibitors do not inactivate clotting factors and, providing care is taken to dilute the plasma sufficiently to prevent the inhibitor interfering with the assay system, normal levels of clotting factor are usually found. Occasionally there may be an apparent deficiency of prothrombin. The majority of inhibitors studied have been IgG immunoglobulins and are thought to act by interfering with the reaction between prothrombin activator and prothrombin. There is evidence to suggest that the inhibitor affects the phospholipid-dependent clotting reactions (Lechner 1974).

Despite abnormalities in the activated partial thromboplastin time test and prothrombin time which may be marked, most patients with SLE inhibitors do not bleed and many have undergone major surgery without excessive bleeding (Green 1972). If bleeding does take place it is probably due to concomitant thrombocytopenia. A significant number of patients with SLE inhibitors develop venous thrombosis (Lechner 1974). The administration of steroids or other immunosuppressive drugs may be followed by disappearance of the inhibitor (Gonyea, Herdman and Bridges 1968).

Diffuse intravascular coagulation (DIC)

In certain disease states procoagulant activity sufficiently powerful to trigger the blood coagulation process may enter the blood or develop in the blood and bring about disseminated intravascular clotting. As a consequence, platelets and blood coagulation factors may be consumed and the fibrin formed during the process deposited in the microcirculation, in particular in the brain, kidney, lungs and skin (McKay 1965, Regoeczi and Brain 1969, Minna, Robboy and Colman 1974). The deposition of fibrin on the vascular endothelium may be followed by an intense fibrinolytic reaction, solution of the fibrin and the appearance of fibrin breakdown products in the blood. The clinical features and laboratory findings produced by the above sequence of events may be complex and will vary with the severity of the intravascular coagulation, the sites where the fibrin microemboli lodge, the fibrinolytic reaction which follows and the nature of the underlying condition. In severe cases of DIC there is usually a depletion of platelets, factor I (fibrinogen), II, V, VIII and antithrombin III. As a result there is a breakdown in haemostasis and in many instances bleeding from wounds or venepuncture sites is the first sign of diffuse intravascular clotting. In addition, the lodging of microemboli of fibrin and platelets in small vessels may produce localized ischaemia and tissue damage with organ dysfunction. This is particularly serious when it involves kidneys, lungs or brain.

Diffuse intravascular coagulation has been observed in many disease processes. Some of those conditions are shown in Table 9.

Table 9. Clinical conditions which may be associated with disseminated intravascular clotting (DIC).

Acute variety
Shock: Haemorrhagic shock
          Anaphylactic shock
          Shock due to Gram-negative septicaemia
Burns
Obstetric causes:
          Abruptio placentae
          Amniotic fluid embolism
          Septic abortion
Intravascular haemolysis:
          Mismatched blood transfusion
          Malaria
Surgical: Operation on prostate, lungs, pancreas
          During extracorporeal circulation
Acute viral infection:
          Chickenpox
Miscellaneous:
          Snake bites
Sub-acute and chronic variety
Malignancy: Carcinomatosis, acute promyelocytic leukaemia
Retained dead fetus
Giant haemangioma (Kasabach–Merritt syndrome)

Pathogenesis

The sequence of events leading to intravascular clotting is still not well understood and will vary depending on the underlying cause. One or more of the following contributory factors may be present:

Substances such as snake venoms, tissue juice, tissue thromboplastin or other agents which can directly activate coagulation factors may gain access to the circulation. Disseminated intravascular clotting following snake bites is well known and has been extensively studied. Venoms vary in their mode of action and may act directly on fibrinogen (batroxobin, ancrod), factor X (Russell's viper venom) or on prothrombin (taipan venom) (Nahas, Denson and Macfarlane 1964).

Entrance of tissue thromboplastin into the bloodstream with activation of the clotting system has been postulated in disseminated intravascular clotting following *abruptio placentae*, operations on lungs or prostate, following injuries to the brain and in patients with carcinoma (Schneider 1952, McKay, Mansell and Hertig 1953).

Endotoxins, in particular those of Gram-negative organisms, may bring about diffuse intravascular clotting (McKay, Margaretten and Csavossy 1967). In experiments on rabbits intravenous injections of endotoxins of *E. coli* 12–24 hours after a previous injection of the endotoxin results in a severe reaction with depletion of clotting factors, circulating platelets and evidence of microemboli of platelets and fibrin in the microcirculation of the kidneys, liver, spleen and lungs. The similarity between this reaction—the generalized Shwartzman reaction—and the features of DIC in man has led to the Shwartzman reaction being used as a model for the study of DIC. The way in which the endotoxin brings about DIC is still not clearly understood but probably has several components including direct activation of factor XII, a reaction between the white cells and endotoxin to produce a powerful procoagulant and the production of widespread endothelial and tissue damage.

Certain modifying factors are probably also important for the development of the full picture: these include pregnancy (Müller-Berghaus and Schmidt-Ehry 1972), blockade of the reticulo-endothelial system (Lee, Prose and Cohen 1966), inhibition of the fibrinolytic system (Müller-Berghaus, Roka and Lasch 1973) and stimulation of the adrenergic system (Müller-Berghaus and McKay 1967, Collins *et al.* 1972).

Clinical features

DIC may present as an acute catastrophic illness as, for example, that seen following *abruptio placentae*, or may present in a more chronic form with only a mild bleeding tendency but more evidence of thrombotic complications. The latter form of DIC is seen typically in patients suffering from disseminated malignancy or in the retained dead fetus syndrome.

The commonest presenting clinical feature is bleeding from several sites including venipuncture sites, surgical wounds, the nose and gastrointestinal tract. Widespread bruising is common and intramuscular haemorrhages may be troublesome. Depending on the degree of damage of essential organs by microemboli there may be mental confusion or coma, oliguria or anuria, hypotension, cardiac arrest, hypoxia and skin necrosis.

Diagnosis

The possibility of DIC should be considered in any patient suffering from a condition which is known may be associated with DIC and who begins to bleed or has features suggestive of microembolization. Awareness of the possibility is of the utmost importance. It is essential to make the diagnosis as quickly as possible especially in the acutely ill patient. For this reason, simple tests which give quick answers are the most useful and are here dealt with first.

Thrombin time

In severe DIC the addition to plasma of a strong solution of thrombin may fail to produce a fibrin clot and this indicates gross fibrinogen depletion with or without excessive amounts of fibrin degradation products. In patients with a less severe fibrin deficiency the addition of thrombin to the plasma may result in clot formation but this takes longer than normal to come about and the clot formed is usually of poor quality and very friable. The thrombin time test is affected not only by the concentration of fibrinogen in the plasma but also by fibrinogen/fibrin breakdown products which interfere with the reaction between thrombin and fibrinogen and inhibit fibrin polymerization. Hence a prolongation of the thrombin time is, in many instances, a reflection of reduced fibrinogen level in the presence of excess amounts of fibrinogen degradation products.

One-stage prothrombin time

This simple test is sensitive to reduction in levels of fibrinogen and factors II, V, VII and X and is prolonged if there is depletion of any of these factors. Like the thrombin time it is prolonged by the presence of fibrinogen/fibrin degradation products.

Activated partial thromboplastin time (APTT)

This test of the intrinsic blood coagulation pathway is sensitive to depletion of fibrinogen and factors II, V, VIII, IX, X, XI and XII. Its main value is as a confirmatory test.

Reptilase (batroxobin) or ancrod time

These snake venoms clot plasma by acting directly on fibrinogen and usually parallel the thrombin time results. The clotting of fibrinogen by both venoms is impaired by fibrinogen degradation products but not by heparin and so may be of some value in monitoring the patient's response should he be treated with heparin.

Fibrinogen titre

This test is slightly more time-consuming than the previous tests but gives a crude estimation of the amount of fibrinogen in the plasma. The more accurate methods such as those described by Ratnoff and Menzie (1951), Ellis and Stransky (1961) or Ingram and Matchett (1960) are time-consuming and of less value in the early management of acute DIC.

Platelet count

This gives important information and is reduced in acute DIC. Normal or near normal counts may be found in chronic DIC.

Paracoagulation tests

During DIC, thrombin generated *in vivo* attacks fibrinogen, splits off fibrinopeptide A and B and thereby produces fibrin monomers. These monomers circulate in the blood as soluble complexes and can be made to precipitate by cooling the patient's serum to 4°C or by the addition of 'paracoagulants' such as protamine sulphate (protamine sulphate precipitation test) or ethanol (ethanol gelation test) (Godal *et al.* 1971, Latallo *et al.* 1971).

Although the above tests are relatively crude and sometimes difficult to reproduce they are of some value in confirming the diagnosis of DIC.

Fibrinogen/fibrin degradation products

Digestion of fibrinogen or fibrin by plasmin produces fragments of varying sizes which have been designated X, Y, D and E. These fragments still contain the antigenic sites of fibrinogen or fibrin and can be assayed using immunological techniques and appropriate antibodies (Marder and Shulman 1969). The tanned red cell, haemagglutination inhibition immunoassay (TRCHII) (Merskey, Kleiner and Johnson 1966), the staphylococcal clumping test Allington (1967) and the latex agglutination test Allington (1971) are amongst the most commonly used methods for detecting fibrin-related antigens.

Specific assays of factors V, VIII and II may show a reduced level of these factors but are time-consuming and of little value in the early management of the acute case. The same consideration applies to assays of platelet factor 4, β-thromboglobulin, fibrinopeptide A and plasminogen.

Other investigations which should be carried out because of the general information they provide include estimation of haemoglobin level, white cell count and examination of a blood film. Blood cultures should be carried out where the clinical picture suggests septicaemia.

The diagnosis of acute DIC is rarely difficult and patients with the fully developed picture will have a reduced platelet count, and fibrinogen titre, prolonged thrombin time, one-stage prothrombin time and activated partial thromboplastin time. In the case of chronic DIC diagnosis may be difficult since there may be only slight depletion of platelets and blood clotting factors. Serial estimations of platelet count, thrombin time, fibrinogen titre and FDPs may be necessary to detect the condition which may fluctuate considerably from day to day.

REFERENCES

Alexander B. & Goldstein R. (1953) Dual hemostatic defect in pseudohemophilia. *Journal of Clinical Investigation* **32**, 551.

Alexander B., Goldstein R., Landwehr G. & Cook C.D. (1951) Congenital SPCA deficiency: a new hitherto unrecognised defect with hemorrhage rectified by serum and serum fractions. *Journal of Clinical Investigation* **30**, 596–608.

Allington M.J. (1967) Fibrinogen and fibrin degradation products and the clumping of staphylococci by serum. *British Journal of Haematology* **13**, 550–67.

Allington M.J. (1971) Detection of fibrin(ogen) degradation products by a latex clumping method. *Scandinavian Journal of Haematology* Suppl. No. 13, 115–19.

Aoki N., Saito H., Kamiya T., Koie K., Sakata Y. & Kobakura M. (1979) Congenital deficiency of α_2-plasmin inhibitor associated with severe hemorrhagic tendency. *Journal of Clinical Investigation* **63**, 877–84.

Barbui T., Cartei G., Chisesi T. & Dini E. (1974) Electroimmunoassay of plasma subunits-A and -S in a case of congenital fibrin stabilizing factor deficiency. *Thrombosis et Diathesis Haemorrhagica* **32**, 124–31.

Barrow E.S., Miller C.H., Reisner H.M. & Graham J.B. (1982) Genetic counselling in haemophilia by discriminant analysis 1975–1980. *Journal of Medical Genetics* **19**, 26–34.

Barrowcliffe T.W., Kirkwood T.B.L. & Rizza C.R. (1980) Aluminium hydroxide adsorption and factor VIII clotting assays. *Lancet* **I**, 820.

Beck E.A. (1964) Abnormal fibrinogen (fibrinogen 'Baltimore') as a cause of a familial hemorrhagic disorder. *Blood* **24**, 853–4.

Beck E.A. (1979) Congenital abnormalities of fibrinogen. In Rizza C.R. (ed.). W.B. Saunders Co., London. *Clinics in Haematology.* vol. 8 pp. 169–81.

Bennett B., Ratnoff O.D., Holt J.B. & Roberts H.R. (1972) Hageman trait (factor XII deficiency): a probable second genotype inherited as an autosomal dominant characteristic. *Blood* **40,** 412–15.

Bentley H.P. Jr & Krivit W. (1960) An assay of antihemophilic globulin activity in the carrier female. *Journal of Laboratory and Clinical Medicine* **56,** 613.

Bertina, R.M. & van der Linden I.K. (1982) Detection and classification of molecular variants of factor IX. In *The Hemophilias.* Bloom A.L. (ed.). Churchill Livingstone, Edinburgh.

Bertina R.M. & Veltkamp J.J. (1978) The abnormal factor IX of haemophilia B[+] variants. *Thrombosis and Haemostasis* **40,** 335–49.

Bertina R.M. & Veltkamp J.J. (1979) A genetic variant of factor IX with decreased capacity of Ca^{++} binding. *British Journal of Haematology* **62,** 623–35.

Bezeaud A., Guillin M.-C., Olmeda F., Quintana M. & Gomez M. (1979) Prothrombin Madrid: a new familial abnormality of prothrombin. *Thrombosis Research* **16,** 47–58.

Biggs R. (1951) *Prothrombin Deficiency.* Blackwell Scientific Publications, Oxford.

Biggs R. (1977) Haemophilia treatment in the United Kingdom from 1969 to 1974. *British Journal of Haematology* **35,** 487–504.

Biggs R. & Denson K.W. (1963) The fate of prothrombin and factors VIII, IX and X transfused to patients deficient in these factors. *British Journal of Haematology* **9,** 532–47.

Blombäck M., Blombäck B., Mammen E. & Prasad A.S. (1968) Fibrinogen 'Detroit': a molecular defect in the N-terminal disulphide knot of human fibrinogen. *Nature (London)* **218,** 134–7.

Board P.G., Coggan M. & Hamer J.W. (1980) An electrophoretic and quantitative analysis of coagulation factor XIII in normal and deficient subjects. *British Journal of Haematology* **45** 633–40.

Boklan B.F. & Sawitsky W. (1976) Factor IX deficiency in Gaucher disease. *Archives of Internal Medicine* **136,** 489–92.

Borchgrevink C.F. (1960) A method for measuring platelet adhesiveness *in vivo. Acta Medica Scandinavica* **168,** 157–64.

Borchgrevink C.F., Egeberg O., Pool J.G., Skulason T., Stormorken H. & Waaler B. (1959) A study of congenital hypoprothrombinaemia. *British Journal of Haematology* **5,** 294–301.

Borchgrevink C.F. & Owren P.A. (1961) Surgery in a patient with factor V (proaccelerin) deficiency. *Acta Medica Scandinavica* **170,** 743–6.

Bouma B.N., Wiegerinck Y., Sixma J.J., van Mourik J.A. & Mochtar I.A. (1972) Immunological characterization of purified anti-haemophilic factor A (factor VIII) which corrects abnormal platelet retention in von Willebrand's disease. *Nature (New Biology),* **236,** 104–6.

Breederveld K., Giddings J.C., Ten Cate J.W. & Bloom A.L. (1975) The localization of factor V within normal human platelets and the demonstration of a platelet-factor V antigen in congenital factor V deficiency. *British Journal of Haematology* **29,** 405–12.

Briët E., Loeliger E.A., van Tilburg N.H. & Veltkamp, J.J. (1976) Molecular variant of factor VII. *Thrombosis and Haemostasis* **35,** 289–94.

Brown C.H., Kvols L.K., Hsu T.-H. & Levin J. (1972) Factor IX deficiency and bleeding in a patient with Sheehan's syndrome. *Blood* **39,** 650–7.

Chung K.S. (1978) Purification and characterization of an abnormal factor IX Alabama

(IX$_{Ala}$). *Abstract XVII, Congress of the International Society of Hematology*, Paris, p. 859.

Collins A.D., Henson E.C., Izard S.R. & Brunson I.G. (1972) Norepinephrine, endotoxin shock and the generalized Shwartzman reaction. *Archives of Pathology* **93**, 82–8.

Colman R.W., Bagdasarian A., Talamo R.C., Scott C.F., Seavey M., Guimaraes J.A., Pierce J.V., Kaplan A.P. & Weinstein L. (1975) Williams trait: human kininogen deficiency with diminished levels of plasminogen proactivator and pre kallikrein associated with abnormalities of the Hageman factor-dependent pathways. *Journal of Clinical Investigation* **56**, 1650–62.

Cotter S.M., Brenner R.M. & Dodds W.J. (1978) Hemophilia A in three unrelated cats. *Journal of the American Veterinary Association* **172**, 166–8.

Crowell E.B. (1975) Observations on a factor-V inhibitor. *British Journal of Haematology* **29**, 397–404.

Denson K.W.E., Biggs R. & Mannucci P.M. (1968) An investigation of three patients with Christmas disease due to an abnormal type of factor IX. *Journal of Clinical Pathology* **21**, 160–5.

Denson K.W.E., Conrad J. & Samama M. (1972) Genetic variants of factor VII. *Lancet* **II**, 1234 (letter).

Denson K.W.E., Lurie A., De Cataldo F. & Mannucci P.M. (1970) The factor X defect: recognition of abnormal forms of factor X. *British Journal of Haematology* **18**, 317–27.

Didisheim P. (1962) Hageman factor deficiency. *Archives of Internal Medicine* **110**, 170.

Duckert F., Jung E. & Schmerling D.H. (1960) Hitherto undescribed congenital haemorrhagic diathesis probably due to fibrin stabilizing factor deficiency. *Thrombosis et Diathesis Haemorrhagica* **5**, 179–86.

Duthie R.B., Matthews J.M., Rizza C.R. & Steel W.M. (1973) *The Management of Musculo-skeletal Problems in the Haemophilias*. Blackwell Scientific Publications, Oxford.

Ellis B.C. & Stransky A. (1961) A quick and accurate method for the determination of fibrinogen in plasma. *Journal of Laboratory and Clinical Medicine* **58**, 477–88.

Fanconi G. (1941) 'Fibrinasthenia' als Urasche einer Schiveren haemorrhagischen. Diathese bei lues congenita. *Schweizerische Medizinische Wochenschrift* **71**, 255–8.

Fantl P., Sawers R.J. & Marr A.G. (1956) Investigation of a haemorrhagic disease due to betaprothromboplastin deficiency complicated by a specific inhibitor of thromboplastin formation. *Australasian Annals of Medicine* **5**, 163–76.

Feinstein D.I., Rapaport S.I., McGhee W.G. & Patch M.J. (1970) Factor V anticoagulants: Clinical, biochemical and immunological observations. *Journal of Clinical Investigation* **49**, 1578–88.

von Felten A. & Straub P.W. (1969) Coagulation studies of cord blood with special reference to 'fetal fibrinogen'. *Thrombosis et Diathesis Haemorrhagica* **22**, 273–80.

von Felten A., Straub P.W. & Frick P.G. (1969) Dysfibrinogenemia in a patient with primary hepatoma. First observation of an acquired abnormality of fibrin monomer aggregation. *New England Journal of Medicine* **280**, 405–9.

Firshein S.I., Hoyer L.W., Lazarchick J., Forget B.G., Hobbins J.C., Clyne L.P., Pitlick F.A., Muir W.A., Merkatz I.R. & Mahoney M.J. (1979) Pre-natal diagnosis of classic hemophilia. *New England Journal of Medicine* **300**, 937–42.

Fisher S., Rikover M. & Naor S. (1966) Factor 13 deficiency with severe hemorrhagic diathesis. *Blood* **28**, 34–9.

Flute P.T. (1977) Disorders of plasma fibrinogen synthesis. *British Medical Bulletin* **33**, 253–9.

Fratantoni J.W., Hilgartner M. & Nachman R.L. (1972) Nature of the defect in congenital factor V deficiency: study in a patient with acquired circulating anticoagulant. *Blood* **39**, 751–8.

Furie B., Greene E. & Furie B.C. (1977) Syndrome of acquired factor X deficiency and systemic amyloidosis: *in vivo* studies of the metabolic fate of factor X. *New England Journal of Medicine* **297**, 81–5.

Furie B., Voo L.A., McAdam K.P.W.J. & Furie B.C. (1981) Mechanism of factor X deficiency in systemic amyloidosis. *New England Journal of Medicine* **304**, 827–30.

Gardikas C., Katsiroumbas P. & Kottas C. (1957) The antihaemophilic globulin concentration in the plasma of female carriers of haemophilia. *British Journal of Haematology* **3**, 377.

Garvey M.B. & Black J.M. (1972) The detection of fibrinogen/fibrin degradation products by means of a new antibody-coated latex particle. *Journal of Clinical Pathology* **25**, 680–2.

Giddings J.C., Shearn S.A.M. & Bloom A.L. (1975) The immunological localization of factor V in human tissue. *British Journal of Haematology* **29**, 57–65.

Girolami A., Bareggi G., Brunetti A. & Sticchi A. (1974) Prothrombin Padua: a 'new' congenital dysprothrombinemia. *Journal of Laboratory and Clinical Medicine* **84**, 654–66.

Girolami A., Cattarozzi G., Dal B.O., Zanon R., Cella G. & Toffanin F. (1979) Factor VII Padua 2: another factor VII abnormality with defective ox brain thromboplastin activation and a complex hereditary pattern. *Blood* **54**, 46–53.

Girolami A., Coccheri S., Palareti G., Poggi I., Burul A. & Cappellato G. (1978a) Prothrombin Molise: a 'new' congenital dysprothrombinemia, double heterozygosis with an abnormal prothrombin and 'true' prothrombin deficiency. *Blood* **52**, 115–25.

Girolami A., Fabris F., Dal B.O., Zanon R., Ghiotto G. & Burul A. (1978b) Factor VII Padua: a congenital coagulation disorder due to an abnormal factor VII with a peculiar activation pattern. *Journal of Laboratory and Clinical Medicine* **91**, 387–95.

Girolami A., Falezza G., Patrassi G., Stenico M. & Vettore L. (1977) Factor VII Verona coagulation disorder: double heterozygosis with an abnormal factor VII and heterozygous factor VII deficiency. *Blood* **50**, 603–10.

Girolami A., Molaro G., Lazzarin M., Scarpa R. & Brunetti A. (1970) A 'new' congenital haemorrhagic condition due to the presence of an abnormal factor X (factor X Friuli): a study of a large kindred. *British Journal of Haematology* **19**, 179–92.

Godal H.C. & Abildgaard U. (1966) Gelation of soluble fibrin in plasma by ethanol. *Scandinavian Journal of Haematology* **3**, 342–50.

Godal H.C., Abildgaard U. & Kierulf P. (1971) Ethanol gelation and fibrin monomers in plasma. *Scandinavian Journal of Haematology* (Suppl. 13), 189–91.

Gonyea L., Herdman R. & Bridges R.A. (1968) The coagulation abnormalities in systemic lupus erythematosus. *Thrombosis et Diathesis Haemorrhagica* **20**, 457–64.

Goodnight S.H., Feinstein J.I., Osterud B. & Rapaport S.I. (1971) Factor VII antibody-neutralising material in hereditary and acquired factor VII deficiency. *Blood* **38**, 1–8.

Green D. (1972) Circulatory and anticoagulants. *Medical Clinics of North America* **56**, 145–51.

Greipp P.R., Kyle R.A. & Bowie E.J.W. (1979) Factor X deficiency in primary amyloidosis: resolution after splenectomy. *New England Journal of Medicine* **301**, 1050–1.

Guillin M.-C. & Ménaché D. (1973) Fetal fibrinogen and fibrinogen Paris I: comparative fibrin monomers aggregation studies. *Thrombosis Research* **3**, 117–35.

Gunning A.J. (1966) The surgery of haemophilic cysts. In *The Treatment of Haemophilia and other Coagulation Disorders.* Biggs R. & Macfarlane R.G. (eds). pp. 262–78. Blackwell Scientific Publications, Oxford.

Hall D.E. (1972) *Blood Coagulation and Its Disorders in the Dog.* Baillière-Tindall, London.

Handley D.A. & Lawrence J.R. (1967) Factor IX deficiency in the nephrotic syndrome. *Lancet,* I, 1079–81.

Hardisty R.M. & Pinniger J.L. (1956) Congenital afibrinogenaemia: further observations on the blood coagulation mechanism. *British Journal of Haematology* 2, 139–52.

Hathaway W.E., Belhasen L.P. & Hathaway H.S. (1965) Evidence for a new plasma thromboplastin factor. I Case report, coagulation studies and physicochemical properties. *Blood* 26, 521–32.

Holmberg L., Gustavii B., Cordesius E., Kristofferson A.C., Ljung R., Löfberg L., Strömberg P. & Nilsson I.M. (1980) Pre-natal diagnosis of hemophilia B by an immunoradiometric assay of factor IX. *Blood* 56, 397–401.

Hougie C., Barrow E.M. & Graham J.B. (1957) Stuart clotting defect. I Segregation of an hereditary hemorrhagic state from the heterogeneous group heretofore called 'Stable factor' (SPCA, proconvertin, factor VII) deficiency. *Journal of Clinical Investigation* 36, 485–96.

Hougie C. & Twomey J.J. (1967) Haemophilia B_m: a new type of factor IX deficiency. *Lancet* I, 698–700.

Howard M.A. & Firkin B.G. (1971) Ristocetin—a new tool in the investigation of platelet aggregation. *Thrombosis et Diathesis Haemorrhagica* 26, 362–9.

Howell M. (1963) Acquired factor X deficiency associated with systematized amyloidosis—a report of a case. *Blood* 21, 739–44.

Hoyer L.W. & Shainoff J.R. (1980) Factor VIII-related protein circulates in normal human plasma as high molelcular weight multimers. *Blood* 55, 1056–9.

Ikkala E. (1960) Haemophilia. A study of its laboratory, clinical, genetic and social aspects based on known haemophiliacs in Finland. *Scandinavian Journal of Laboratory and Clinical Investigation* 12 (Suppl.), 46.

Imperato di C. & Dettori A.G. (1958) Ipofibrinogenemia congenita con fibrinoastenia. *Helvetica Paediatrica Acta* 13, 380–99.

Ingram, G.I.C. (1955) Variations in the reaction between thrombin and fibrinogen and their effects on the prothrombin time. *Journal of Clinical Pathology* 8, 318–23.

Ingram G.I.C. & Matchett M.O. (1960) A rapid 'side room' method for the determination of plasma fibrinogen concentration as fibrin. *Journal of Clinical Pathology* 13, 469–74.

International Multicentre Trial (1975) Prevention of fatal postoperative pulmonary embolium by low doses of heparin: an International Multicentre Trial. *Lancet* II, 45–51.

Italian Working Group (1977) Spectrum of von Willebrand's disease: a study of 100 cases. *British Journal of Haematology* 35, 101–12.

Iversen T. & Bastrup-Madsen P. (1956) Congenital familial deficiency of factor V (para haemophilia) combined with deficiency of antihaemophilic globulin. *British Journal of Haematology* 2, 265–75.

Jones J.H., Rizza C.R., Hardisty R.M., Dormandy K.M. & MacPherson J.C. (1962) Combined deficiency of factor V and factor VIII (anti haemophilic globulin). A report of three cases. *British Journal of Haematology* 8, 120–8.

Josso F., Lavergne J.M., Weilland C. & Soulier J.P. (1967) Étude immunologique de la prothrombine et de la thrombine humaine. *thrombosis et Diathesis Haemorrhagica* 18, 311–24.

Josso F., Monasterio de Sanchez J., Lavergne J.M., Ménaché D. & Soulier J.P. (1971)

Congenital abnormality of the prothrombin molecule (factor II) in four siblings: prothrombin Barcelona. *Blood* **38**, 9–16.

Kattlove H.E. & Gomez M.H. (1975) Studies on the mechanism of ristocetin-induced platelet aggregation. *Blood* **45**, 91–6.

Kernoff P.B.A., Gruson R. & Rizza C.R. (1974) A variant of factor VIII-related antigen. *British Journal of Haematology* **26**, 435–9.

Kluft C., Vellenga E. & Brommer E.J.P. (1979) Homozygous α_2-antiplasmin deficiency. *Lancet* **II**, 206.

Koie K., Kamiya T., Ogata K., Takamatsu J. & Kohakura M. (1978) α_2-Plasmin-inhibitor deficiency (Miyasato Disease). *Lancet* **II**, 1334–6.

Korsan-Bengsten K., Hjort P.F. & Ygge J. (1962) Acquired factor X deficiency in a patient with amyloidosis. *Thrombosis et Diathesis Haemorrhagica* **7**, 558–66.

Lacombe M., Varet B. & Levy J. (1975) A hitherto undescribed plasma factor acting at the contact phase of blood coagulation (Flaujeac factor): case report and coagulation studies. *Blood* **46**, 761–8.

Lane D.A., Scully M.F., Thomas D.P., Kakkar V.V., Woolf I.L. & Williams R. (1977) Acquired dysfibrinogenaemia in acute and chronic liver disease. *British Journal of Haematology* **35**, 301–8.

Latallo Z.S., Wegrzynowicz Z., Budzynski A.Z. & Kopec M. (1971) Effect of protamine sulphate on solubility of fibrinogen, its derivatives and other plasma proteins. *Scandinavian Journal of Haematology* (Suppl.) **13**, 151–62.

Lazarchick J. & Hoyer L.W. (1978) Immunoradiometric measurement of the factor VIII procoagulant antigen. *Journal of Clinical Investigation* **62**, 1048–52.

Lechner K. (1974) Acquired inhibitors in nonhemophilic patients. *Haemostasis* **3**, 65–93.

Lee L., Prose P.H. & Cohen M.H. (1966) The role of the reticuloendothelial system in diffuse, low grade intravascular coagulation. *Thrombosis et Diathesis Haemorrhagica* Suppl. No. 20, 87–95.

Leiba H., Ramot B. & Many A. (1965) Heredity and coagulation studies in ten families with factor XI (plasma thromboplastin antecedent) deficiency. *British Journal of Haematology* **II**, 654–65.

Leyvraz P.F., Richard J., Bachmann F., van Melle G., Trayvaud J.-M., Livis J.-J. & Candadjis G. (1983) Adjusted versus fixed-dose subcutaneous heparin in the prevention of deep-vein thrombosis after total hip replacement. *New England Journal of Medicine* **309**, 954–8.

Lorand L., Losowsky M.S. & Miloszewski K.J.M. (1980) Human factor XIII: Fibrin stabilising factor. *Progress in Hemostasis and Thrombosis* **5**, 245–90.

Marder V.J. (1971) Fibrinogen and fibrin degradation products. Physico-chemical and physiological considerations. *Thrombosis et Diathesis Haemorrhagica* Suppl. No. 47, 85–98.

Marder V.J. & Shulman N.R. (1964) Clinical aspects of congenital factor VII deficiency. *American Journal of Medicine* **37**, 182–94.

Marder V.J. & Shulman N.R. (1969) High molecular weight derivatives of human fibrinogen produced by plasmin. I. Physicochemical and immunological characterization. *Journal of Biological Chemistry* **244**, 2120–4.

Marlar R.A. & Griffin J.H. (1980) Deficiency of protein C inhibitor in combined factor V/VIII deficiency disease. *Journal of Clinical Investigation* **66**, 1186–9.

Mazzucconi M.G., Mandelli F., Mariani G., Briët E. & Veltkamp J.J. (1977) A CRM-positive variant of factor VII deficiency and the detection of heterozygotes with the assay of factor VII-like antigen. *British Journal of Haematology* **36**, 127–35.

Macfarlane R.G. (1938) A boy with no fibrinogen. *Lancet* **I**, 309.

McKay D.G. (1965) *Disseminated Intravascular Coagulation.* Charles C. Thomas, Springfield, Illinois.

McKay D.G., Mansell H. & Hertig A.T. (1953) Carcinoma of the body of the pancreas with fibrin thrombosis and fibrinogenopenia. *Cancer* **6**, 862–9.

McKay D.G., Margaretten W. & Csavossy I. (1967) An electromicroscope study of endotoxin shock in rhesus monkeys. *Surgery, Gynecology and Obstetrics* **125**, 825–32.

McPherson R.A., Onstad J.W., Ugoretz R.J. & Wolf P.L. (1977) Coagulopathy in amyloidosis: combined deficiency of factors IX and X. *American Journal of Haematology* **3**, 225–35.

Mant M.J., Thong K.L., Birtwhistle R.V., O'Brien B.D., hammond G.W. & Grace M.G. (1977) Haemorrhagic complications of heparin therapy. *Lancet* **I**, 1133–5.

Ménaché D. (1964) Constitutional and familial abnormal fibrinogen. *Thrombosis et Diathesis Haemorrhagica* **13**, 173–85.

Ménaché D. & Boivin P. (1962) Déficit acquis en facteur X *chez* un malade atteint d'amylose primitive: injection d'une fraction C.S.B. *Nouvelle Revue Française d'Hématologie* **2**, 868–77.

Merskey C., Kleiner G.J. & Johnson A.J. (1966) Quantitative estimation of split products of fibrinogen in human serum: Relation to diagnosis and treatment. *Blood* **28**, 1–18.

Mibashan R.S., Peake I.R., Rodeck C.H., Thumpston J.K., Furlong R.A., Gorer R., Bains O. & Bloom A.L. (1980) Dual diagnosis of prenatal haemophilia A by measurement of fetal factor VIII C and VIII C antigen (VIII C Ag). *Lancet* **II**, 994–7.

Mibashan R.S., Rodeck C.H., Thumpston J.K., Edwards R.J., Singer J.D., White J.M. & Campbell S. (1979) Plasma assay of fetal factor VIIIC and IX for pre-natal diagnosis of haemophilia. *Lancet* **II**, 1309–11.

Miles L.A., Plow E.F., Donnelly K.J., Hougie C. & Griffin J.H. (1982) A bleeding disorder due to deficiency of α_2-antiplasmin. *Blood* **59**, 1246–51.

Minna J.D., Robboy S.J. & Colman R.W. (1974) *Disseminated Intravascular Coagulation in Man.* Charles C. Thomas, Springfield, Illinois.

Müller-Berghaus G. & McKay D.g. (1967) Prevention of the generalized Shwartzman reaction in pregnant rats by alpha-adrenergic blocking agents. *Laboratory Investigation* **17**, 276–80.

Müller-Berhaus G., Roka L. & Lasch H.g. (1973) induction of glomerular microclot formation by fibrin monomer infusion. *Thrombosis et Diathesis Haemorrhagica* **29**, 375–83.

Müller-Berghaus G. & Schmidt-Ehry G.B. (1972) The role of pregnancy in the induction of the generalized Shwartzman reaction. *American Journal of Obstetrics and Gynecology* **114**, 847–9.

Nahas L., Denson K.W.E. & Macfarlane R.G. (1964) A study of the coagulant action of eight snake venoms. *Thrombosis et Diathesis Haemorrhagica* **12**, 353–67.

Nilsson I.M., Blombäck M., Jorpes E., Blombäck B. & Johansson S.A. (1957) von Willebrand's disease and its correction with human fraction I-o. *Acta medica Scandinavica* **159**, 179–88.

Nilsson I.M. & Holmberg L. (1979) von Willebrand's disease today. in *Clinics in Haematology.* Vol. 8:1. pp 147–68. Rizza C.R. (ed.). W.B. Saunders Co., London.

Nossel H.L. (1964) *The Contact Phase of Blood Coagulation.* Blackwell Scientific Publication, Oxford.

Nossel H.L., Archer R.K. & Macfarlane R.G. (1962) Equine haemophilia: report of a case and its response to multiple infusions of heterospecific AHG. *British Journal of Haematology* **8**, 335–42.

Nossel H.L., Niemetz J., Mibashan R.S. & Schulze W.g. (1966) The measurement of factor XI (plasma thromboplastin antecedent). Diagnosis and therapy of the congenital deficiency state. *British Journal of Haematology* **12**, 133.

O'Brien P.F., North W.R.S. & Ingram G.I.C. (1981) The diagnosis of mild haemophilia by the Partial Thromboplastin Time Test. WFH/ICTH Study of the Manchester Method. *Thrombosis and Haemostasis* **45**, 162–8.

O'Brien P.F., North W.R.S. & Ingram G.I.C. (1981) The diagnosis of mild haemophilia by the Partial Thromboplastin Time Test. WRH/ICTH Study of the Manchester Method. *Thrombosis and Haemostasis* **45**, 162–8.

Oeri J., Matter M., Isenschmid H., Hauser F. & Koller F. (1954) Angeborener Mangel an Faktor V (parahaemophilie) verbunden mit echter haemophilie A bei zwei brudern. *Bibliotheca Paediatrica* **58**, 575–88.

Ørstavik K.H., Østerud B., Prydz H. & Berg K. (1975) Electroimmunoassay of factor IX in hemophilia b. *thrombosis Research* **7**, 373–82.

Owen C.A., Henriksen R.A., McDuffie F.C. & Mann K.G. (1978) Prothrombin Quick: a newly identified dysprothrombinemia. *Mayo Clinic Proceedings* **53**, 29–33.

Owren P.A. (1947) The coagulation of blood, investigations on a new clothing factor. *Acta Medica Scandinavica* (Suppl. 194).

Peake I.R. & Bloom A.L. (1978) Immunoradiometric assay of procoagulant factor VIII antigen in plasma and serum and its reduction in haemophilia. *Lancet* **II**, 473–5.

Peake I.R., Bloom A.L. & Giddings J.L. (1974) Inherited variants of factor VIII related protein in von Willebrand's disease. *New England Journal of Medicine* **291**, 113–17.

Pinniger J.L. & Prunty F.T.G. (1946) Some observations on the blood clotting mechanism. The rôle of fibrinogen and platelets, with reference to a case of congenital afibrinogenaemia. *British Journal of Experimental Pathology* **27**, 200–10.

Prentice A.I.D. (1951) A case of congenital afibrinogenaemia. *Lancet* **I**, 211–13.

Prentice C.R.M., Lindsay R.M., Barr R.D., Forbes C.D., Kennedy A.D., McNicol g.P. & Douglas A.S. (1971) Renal complications in haemophilia and Christmas disease. *quarterly Journal of Medicine* **40**, 47–61.

Quick A.J. & Hussey C.V. (1962) Hereditary hypoprothrombinaemias. *Lancet* **I**, 173.

Rabe F. & Salomon E. (1920) Über Faserstoffmangel im Blute bein einem Falle von Hämophile. *Deautches Archiv für Klinische Medizin* **132**, 240–4.

Rabiet M.-J., Elion J., Labie D. & Josso F. (1979) Prothrombin Metz: Purification and characterization of a variant of human prothrombin. *Thrombosis and Haemostasis* **42**, 57.

Ramgren O. (1962) A clinical and medicosocial study of haemophilia in Sweden. *Acta Medica Scandinavica* **171** (Suppl. 379), 111–90.

Ratnoff O.D. (1960) *Bleeding Syndromes. A Clinical Manual.* Charles C. Thomas, Springfield, Illinois.

Ratnoff O.D. (1977) The surface-mediated initiation of blood coagulation and related phenomena. In *Haemostasis: Biochemistry, Physiology and Pathology.* Ogston D. & Bennett B. (eds). John Wiley & Sons, London.

Ratnoff O.D. & Colopy J.H. (1955) A familial hemorrhagic trait associated with a deficiency of clot promoting fraction of plasma. *Journal of Clinical Investigation* **34**, 602–13.

Ratnoff O.D. & Menzie C. (1951) A new method for the determination of fibrinogen in small samples of plasma. *Journal of Laboratory and Clinical Medicine* **37**, 316–20.

Regan M.G., Lachner J. & Karpatkin S. (1974) Platelet function and coagulation profile in lupus erythematosus: Studies in 50 patients. *Annals of Internal Medicine* **81**, 462–8.

Regoeczi E. & Brain M.C. (1969) Organ distribution of fibrin in disseminated intravascular coagulation. *British Journal of Haematology* **17**, 73–81.

Reid H.A., Chan K.E. & Thean P.C. (1963) Prolonged coagulation defect in Malayan viper bite. *Lancet* **I**, 617–21.

Rizza C.R. & Spooner R.J.D. (1983) Treatment of haemophilia and related disorders in

Britain and Northern Ireland during 1976–80: report on behalf of the directors of haemophilia centres in the United Kingdom. *British Medical Journal* **286**, 929–33.

Roberts H.R., Grizzle J.E., McLester W.D. & Penick G.D. (1968) Genetic variants of hemophilia B: detection by means of a specific inhibitor. *Journal of Clinical Investigation* **47**, 360–5.

Rodeck C.H. & Campbell S. (1978) Sampling of pure fetal blood by fetoscopy in second trimester of pregnancy. *British Medical Journal* **II**, 728–30.

Rosenthal R.L., Dreskin O.H. & Rosenthal N. (1955) Plasma thromboplastin antecedent (PTA) deficiency: clinical, coagulation, therapeutic and hereditary aspects of a new hemophilia-like disease. *Blood* **10**, 120.

Rosner F. (1969) Hemophilia in the Talmud and Rabbinic writings. *Annals of Internal Medicine* **70**, 833–7.

Ruggeri Z.M., Pareti F.I., Mannucci P.M., Ciavarella N. & Zimmerman T. (1980) Heightened interaction between platelets and factor VIII/von Willebrand factor in a new subtype of von Willebrand's disease. *New England Journal of Medicine* **302**, 1047–51.

Ruggeri Z.M. & Zimmerman T.S. (1980) Variant von Willebrand's disease: Characterization of two sub-types by analysis of multimeric compositions of factor VIII/von Willebrand factor in plasma and platelets. *Journal of Clinical Investigation* **65**, 1318–25.

Rush B. & Ellis H. (1965) Treatment of patients with factor-V deficiency. *Thrombosis et Diathesis Haemorrhagica* **14**, 74–82.

Salzman E.W. (1963) Measurement of platelet adhesiveness. A simple *in vitro* technique demonstrating an abnormality in von Willebrand's disease. *Journal of Laboratory and Clinical Medicine* **62**, 724–35.

Schleider M.A., Nachman R.L., Jaffe E.A. & Coleman M. (1976) A clinical study of the lupus anticoagulant. *Blood* **48**, 499–509.

Schneider C.L. (1947) The active principle of placental toxin: Thromboplastin: its inactivator in blood: Anti-thromboplastin. *American Journal of Physiology* **149**, 123–9.

Schneider C.L. (1952) Rupture of the basal (Decidual) plate in abruptio placentae: a pathway of auto extraction from the decidua into the maternal circulation. *American Journal of Obstetrics and Gynecology* **63**, 1078–90.

Schwartz M.L., Pizzo S.V., Hill R.L. & McKee P.A. (1973) Human factor XIII from plasma and platelets. *Journal of Biological Chemistry* **248**, 1395–407.

Seeler R.A. (1972) Parahemophilia. Factor V deficiency. *Medical Clinics of North America* **56**, 119–25.

Seligsohn U. (1978) High gene frequency of factor XI (PTA) deficiency in Ashkenazi Jews. *Blood* **51**, 1223–8.

Seligsohn U. & Ramot B. (1969) Combined factor-V and factor-VIII deficiency: Report of four cases. *British Journal of Haematology* **16**, 475–86.

Shapiro S.S., Maldonado M., Fradera J. & McCord S. (1974) Prothrombin San Juan: a complex new dysprothrombinemia. *Journal of Clinical Investigation* **53**, 73a.

Shapiro S.S., Martinez J. & Holburn R.R. (1969) Congenital dysprothrombinemia: an inherited structural disorder of human prothrombin. *Journal of Clinical Investigation* **48**, 2251.

Sjølin K.-E. (1961) *Haemophilic Diseases in Denmark. A Classification of the Clotting Defects in 78 Haemophilic Families.* Blackwell Scientific Publication, Oxford.

Smit Sibinga C.Th., Gökemeyer J.D.M., Ten Kate L.P. & Bos-Van Zwol F. (1972) Combined deficiency of factor V and factor VIII: Report of a family and genetic analysis. *British Journal of Haematology* **23**, 467–81.

Soria J., Soria C., Samama M., Coupier J., Girard M.L., Bousser J. & Bilski-Pasquier G.

(1970) Dysfibrinogénémies acquises dans les atteintes hépatiques sévères. *Coagulation* **3**, 37–44.

Soulier J.-P. & Prou-Wartelle O. (1966) Étude comparative des taux de cofacteur de la staphylocoagulase (CRF) et des taux de facteur II (prothrombine) dans diverses conditions. *Nouvelle Revue Française d'Hématologie* **6**, 623–36.

Soulier J.-P., Prou-Wartelle O. & Josso F. (1962) Demivie de la prothrombine vraie (facteur II). *Nouvelle Revue Française d'Hématologie* **2**, 673.

Soulier J.-P., Prou-Wartelle O., Weilland C. & Ménaché D. (1958) Déficit cogénital en proaccelérine (factor V):quelques données nouvelles. *Thrombosis et Diathesis Haemorrhagica* **2**, 250–68.

Spero J.A., Lewis J.H., Hasiba U. & Ellis L.D. (1976) Treatment of amyloidosis associated with factor X deficiency. *Thrombosis and Haemostasis* **35**, 377–81.

Svanberg L., Hedner U. & Astedt B. (1974) Value of determination of F.D.P. during pregnancy by immunochemical and latex agglutination inhibition methods. *Acta Obstetrica et Gynaecologica Scandinavica* **53**, 81–3.

Telfer T.P., Denson K.W. & Wright D.R. (1956) A 'new' coagulation defect. *British Journal of Haematology* **2**, 308–16.

Thompson A.R. (1977) Factor IX antigen by radioimmunoassay. Abnormal factor IX protein in patients on Warfarin therapy and with hemophilia B. *Journal of Clinical Investigation* **59**, 900–10.

Valderrama J.A.F. & Matthews J.M. (1965) The haemophilic pseudotumour or haemophilic subperiosteal haematoma. *Journal of Bone and Joint Surgery* **47-B**, 256–65.

Waldmann R. & Abraham J.P. (1974) Fitzgerald factor: A heretofore unrecognized coagulation factor. (Abstract.) *Blood* **44**, 934.

Waldmann R., Abraham J.P., Rebuck J.W., Caldwell J., Saito H. & Ratnoff O.D. (1975) Fitzgerald factor: A hitherto unrecognized coagulation factor. *Lancet*, I 949–50.

Weiss A.S., Gallin J.I. & Kaplan A. (1974) Fletcher factor deficiency, a diminished rate of Hageman factor activation caused by absence of pre-kallikrein with abnormalities of coagulation, fibrinolysis, chemotactic activity and kinin generation. *Journal of Clinical Investigation* **53**, 622–33.

Willebrand von E.A. (1926) Hereditäre pseudohemofili. *Finska Läkaresällskapets Handlingar* **67**, 7–12.

World Health Organisation (1977) Methods for the detection of haemophilia carriers: A memorandum. *Bulletin of the World Health Organisation* **55**, 675–702.

Wright F.W., Matthews J.M. & Brock L.G. (1971) Complications of haemophilic disorders affecting the renal tract. *Radiology* **98**, 471–6.

Wuepper K.D. (1973) Prekallikrein deficiency in man. *Journal of Experimental medicine* **138**, 1345–55.

Yang H.C. (1978a) Immunological studies of factor IX (Christmas factor) I. Counter immunoelectrophoresis method for factor IX antigen. *Thrombosis Research* **13**, 97–109.

Yang H.C. (1978b) Immunological studies of factor IX (Christmas factor) II. Immunoradiometric assay of factor IX antigen. *British Journal of Haematology* **39**, 215–24.

Zimmerman T.S., Ratnoff O.D. & Littell A.S. (1971) Detection of carriers of classic hemophilia using an immunologic assay for antihemophilic factor (factor VIII). *Journal of Clinical Investigation* **50**, 255–8.

Zimmerman T.S., Ratnoff O.D. & Powell A.E. (1971) Immunologic differentiation of classic hemophilia (factor VIII deficiency) and von Willebrand's disease, with observations on combined deficiencies of antihemophilic factor and proaccelerin (factor V) and on an acquired circulating anticoagulant against antihemophilic factor. *Journal of Clinical Investigation* **50**, 244–54.

Chapter 9
Laboratory Diagnosis of Blood
Coagulation Disorders

D. E. G. AUSTEN *and* I. L. RHYMES

The objective of this chapter is to describe the preliminary tests and the assays which are normally used in laboratory assessment of deficiencies in blood coagulation factors. Little comment is made on platelet or fibrinolysis defects because these are considered in other chapters of this book. Practical details of most of the individual assays are to be found in *A Laboratory Manual of Blood Coagulation* by D.E.G. Austen and I.L. Rhymes (1975).

Tests in general

In investigating blood coagulation defects, the principles of investigation are basically very simple. Most tests consist of mixing reagents with blood plasma, followed by a measurement of clotting time. Colorimetric end points to such methods are a possible alternative where an enzyme such as thrombin is produced in the reaction and where that enzyme causes a colour change in a substrate. In particular, useful assays of this type are available for thrombin, antithrombin and kallikrein. Immunoassays are also available for several clotting factors but these can record the presence of the factor molecules even if they are inactive in coagulation. Hence they complement clotting tests rather than replace them.

Since the recording of clotting times is so central to this subject, the advisability of automation must be considered. Individual decisions will be governed by the experience of the operators involved and the amount of practice they can expect. At present, the overall conclusion seems to be that an automated technique can measure clotting times as precisely, or more so, than can the most experienced operator using manual methods. However, automated methods are often slower when using complex test systems and may lead to sample deterioration due to delays between measurements. At the present time automation is more useful for the tests with few manipulations and of short duration, such as one-stage prothrombin times or assays of factors V, VII or X. It is much less useful for assays of the intrinsic system and difficult to use for two-stage assays of factors VIII or IX.

Preliminary tests on the patient

Before laboratory tests are performed, the first step is to take a detailed clinical history of bleeding in the patient and his family. This should be carried out by an experienced clinician and its importance cannot be overemphasized since there are occasions when clotting tests fail to adequately explain a significant bleeding history.

Two tests are made directly upon the patient. One is the bleeding time test which records the time taken for a standard skin puncture to stop bleeding and the other is the tourniquet test which examines capillary fragility by recording the number of petechiae which arise, following a period in which a sphygmomanometer cuff is applied to the upper arm, at a pressure which restricts venous flow. The bleeding time test is abnormal in platelet defects, von Willebrand's disease, afibrinogenaemia and possibly in some cases of factor V or VII deficiency. It may also be abnormal in telangiectasia if an abnormal vessel is punctured. The tourniquet test is abnormal in platelet defects and in cases of capillary fragility such as scurvy.

Preliminary tests of coagulation

Under this heading are considered all tests other than quantitative assays for specific clotting factors and inhibitors. Although non-quantitative and in most cases not specific for any one clotting factor, the correct use of a battery of these tests may often allow a qualitative diagnosis to be made. The main problem with these tests is that most lack sensitivity so that even a complete set of normal results cannot rule out a significant bleeding disorder.

Whole Blood Clotting Time (WBCT)

This simplest test of clotting is one of the few performed on blood as collected (i.e. without added anticoagulant). Insensitive to all except moderately severe deficiencies and then mainly to factors included in the earlier stages of coagulation (XII, XI, IX, VIII) this test is also much affected by experimental variables (quality of venepuncture, test-tube sizes, volumes tested, etc.) which must be rigorously controlled if useful results are to be obtained. Except as a preliminary to the Prothrombin Consumption Test, the WBCT is probably of little more than historical interest.

Prothrombin Consumption Index Test (PCI)

Conversion of prothrombin to thrombin is a time-consuming reaction normally completed within about ten minutes. However, where any defect or deficiency exists at an earlier stage of the clotting process, this conversion can be retarded to the extent that a significant amount of prothrombin is still present in serum an hour or more after coagulation is apparently complete.

The Prothrombin Consumption Test compares the amount of prothrombin present in plasma with that present in serum 60 minutes after whole blood has clotted in a glass tube. The test therefore is conveniently performed following the WBCT. No attempt is made to assay the prothrombin quantitatively. Plasma and serum are both tested by adding brain extract and calcium chloride, the thrombin generated being detected by subsampling into fibrinogen solution. The prothrombin consumption index (PCI) is obtained by expressing the shortest clotting time obtained when testing plasma as a percentage of that obtained when testing serum.

This test is insensitive and much influenced by the technical variables affecting the preceding WBCT. A high (abnormal) PCI can result either from a long fibrinogen clotting time in the plasma stage of the test or a short fibrinogen clotting time when testing the serum. In the former case an abnormality in the extrinsic pathway is likely; in the latter the abnormality is probably to be found in the intrinsic pathway. The prothrombin consumption test is of most use in detecting platelet defects and it is here that its main value probably lies.

The temptation to discard this insensitive and often inconvenient test should be resisted as there are a small number of patients with significant bleeding problems in whom the only consistently abnormal laboratory result is the PCI (due to a short clotting time in the serum phase of the test). The exact nature of the abnormality of the clotting mechanism in these cases as yet eludes explanation.

Recalcification Time, Partial Thromboplastin Time (PTT)

These two tests, both now little used for routine purposes, are of interest as stages in the development of the activated partial thromboplastin time. The recalcification time simply measures the clotting time of anticoagulated plasma on recalcification. Although influenced by all factors of the intrinsic pathway it is insensitive and, because platelet content and surface contact are not controlled, reproducibility is poor.

In the partial thromboplastin time reproducibility is improved by always using platelet-poor plasma and adding a constant quantity of a platelet substitute, e.g. cephalin. The APTT (see below) completes this line of development by standardizing the surface contact through the addition of an activator such as kaolin. It should be noted that most of the so-called PTT kits and reagents which are commercially available are, in fact, designed and provided with instructions for the performance of APTT.

Activated Partial Thromboplastin Time (APTT) (Proctor and Rapaport 1961)

This is a useful general test of clotting function being sensitive in some degree to all known clotting factors except factors VII and XIII. To platelet-poor plasma is added a contact phase activator such as kaolin, celite or ellagic acid and a platelet substitute such as cephalin or inosithin.

The clotting process is initiated by surface activation during a period of incubation after which the addition of calcium chloride allows the clotting reactions to proceed to completion. There are many variants of this basic test in use by different workers whose personal preferences are reflected in the choice of individual reagents (the 'kaolin cephalin clotting time' is still probably the most used version of the test) and in the order in which reagents are added (the platelet substitute may be added before or after the incubation period). Perhaps the greatest discrepancy between different variations of the method lies in the incubation (activation) period chosen. With most reagents a period of at least ten minutes is required to achieve maximum activation and there are those who feel that the test should be performed under these conditions. However, activation periods as short as two minutes in no way impair the sensitivity of the test although actual clotting times are a little longer—indeed, with shorter activation periods significantly greater sensitivity may be achieved to those factors involved in the activation phase of clotting.

It might well be claimed that the main problem with this test is the undue faith put in it by many laboratory and clinical workers. Although one of the more sensitive of the preliminary tests of clotting function, the APTT is in no way a screening test in the usual sense. Even with the most sensitive of reagent systems—and there is great variation between different reagents and even between different makes and batches of the same reagent—normal results can sometimes be obtained even when clotting factors are reduced to levels at which significant bleeding problems can occur (O'Brien, North and Ingram 1981). For example, it is not unknown for a patient with a factor VIII level below 10 per cent to have an APTT within the normal range.

Some workers enhance the sensitivity of this test by working with diluted plasma samples but great care is needed in selecting the degree of dilution and the diluents to be used.

One-stage Prothrombin Time (Quick)

This is a test of the extrinsic pathway and involves adding a tissue thromboplastin to plasma and then recalcifying the mixture. Together with the APTT the prothrombin time forms the basis of the 'clotting screen' in many laboratories but shares with that test the problem of lack of sensitivity. The test is influenced by all the clotting factors in the extrinsic pathway but sensitivity to deficiencies of prothrombin and fibrinogen is particularly limited.

Thrombin Time

This is a simple test in which fibrinogen in the test sample is converted to fibrin by the addition of thrombin. Prolongation of clotting times will be obtained in cases of deficiency or functional defect of fibrinogen, all factors higher in the clotting cascade having no influence on the results. Inhibitors of the thrombin–fibrinogen reaction, e.g. fibrin degradation products, will also prolong the thrombin time.

Thromboplastin Generation Test (Biggs and Douglas 1953b)

Although of considerable historical interest, the practical importance of the TGT in the routine laboratory has diminished with the increasing availability of specific assays for most of the clotting factors. Serum and adsorbed plasma from the patient and the normal control are tested in various combinations (see table below) for their efficiency in the generation of 'intrinsic thrombo-plastin' (the complex formed by activated factor X (Xa), factor V and phospholipid). The serum will normally contain factors IX, X, XI and XII while the adsorbed plasma will normally contain factors V, VIII, XI and XII (also fibrinogen). As neither serum nor adsorbed plasma contains prothrombin the clotting reactions in a mixture of the two will stop with the production of the 'thromboplastin' complex. The thromboplastin generation in the plasma/ serum mixture (cephalin is also added to provide the phospholipid element) is detected by subsampling into normal plasma when the clotting time will reflect the amount of 'thromboplastin' in the plasma/serum mixture. A clotting factor deficiency will lead to reduced or delayed 'thromboplastin' generation which will be indicated by prolonged clotting times in the second stage of the test.

Mixtures tested			*Clotting factors suspect*
Serum	*Adsorbed plasma*		*if test result abnormal*
1	Normal	Normal	—
2	Normal	Patient	V or VIII
3	Patient	Normal	IX or X
4	Patient	Patient	XI or XII if mixtures (2) and (3) are normal

Thus a patient with Christmas disease would have prolonged clotting times in mixture (3) where factor IX would be missing from the patient's serum used in the test.

The thromboplastin generation test is relatively insensitive and time-consuming, but used in conjunction with the activated partial thromboplastin time and one-stage prothrombin time, will often identify a severe deficiency of a particular clotting factor (deficiencies of factors XI and XII cannot be differentiated). This qualitative test is the basis of the two-stage assay methods for factor VIII and IX.

If, in a test mixture containing normal plasma and normal serum, the cephalin is replaced in turn by normal and patient's platelets, an indication of the effectiveness of the platelets as a phospholipid source may be obtained.

Thrombin Generation Test (Macfarlane and Biggs 1953)

The process of thrombin generation in either freshly collected whole blood or in recalcified plasma is followed by subsampling at intervals into fibrinogen solution. Any deficiency, defect or inhibitor activity in the intrinsic clotting cascade will be reflected in reduced or delayed thrombin generation. This test, which can be technically difficult, is of use mainly for research purposes or, occasionally, in the investigation of obscure coagulation defects which are not explained by simpler tests.

Mixing Tests

Mixing tests may be performed when a significant prolongation is found in a patient's plasma when tested by a simple technique such as the APTT or prothrombin time. Details vary with different workers but an equal-parts mixture of patient and normal is generally satisfactory. Correction of the abnormality will be shown by the clotting time of the mixture being near to that of the normal while failure to correct will result in a clotting time for the mixture near to that of the patient. For effective use of mixing tests, adequate difference between the clotting times for patient and normal is essential, e.g. mixing tests are best not attempted when the difference by the APTT is less than about 15–20 seconds.

Inhibitors

Mixing tests to demonstrate the presence of inhibitory states are generally reliable. However, antibodies to factor VIII which are time-consuming in their reaction may be missed if insufficient time is allowed for the reaction to take place.

Deficiencies

Mixing tests to identify a specific factor deficiency are best performed by using a panel of plasmas each totally deficient in a different clotting factor but otherwise normal. Mixtures of such plasmas with the patient's plasma will give a corrected result in all cases except when the two plasmas mixed are deficient in the same clotting factor. When suitable deficient plasmas are not available to perform this test, mixing of the patient's plasma with, in turn, adsorbed normal plasma and aged serum may give some indication of the likely deficiency in the patient (adsorbed plasma contains factors I, V, VIII, XI and XII, aged serum contains factors VII, IX, X, XI and XII). Great care must be taken to ensure that the serum used is truly aged. Traces of thrombin or Xa activity can give false corrections and hence lead to completely wrong diagnoses. Haemophilia is not infrequently diagnosed as Christmas disease as a result of this particular error.

Laboratory tests in anticoagulant therapy

Anticoagulant therapy with coumarin- or indanedione-type drugs results in reduced levels of factors II, VII, IX and X in the patient's plasma. Laboratory control of such therapy by means of specific assays is impracticable and generally unnecessary, and many simple tests have been used and modified for this purpose. The simplest test so used has always been the one-stage prothrombin time but its lack of sensitivity and its variability with different brain thromboplastin preparations has, in the past, created problems in interpretation of results and particularly in relating results obtained in different laboratories. Procedures such as the Prothrombin and Proconvertin Test, Thrombotest and Two-Seven-Ten Test have all been designed to overcome some of the drawbacks of the simple prothrombin time and all have been used with some success.

The introduction of standardized brain thromboplastins (Poller 1964, 1967) has again established the one-stage prothrombin time as the most commonly used test and has made possible consistent results both within and between laboratories. A number of reference thromboplastins are available, differing in the animal species from which the brain was obtained and in details of preparation and storage of the reagent. These have, in most cases, been standardized against the primary World Health Organisation International Reference Thromboplastin which is a human brain extract with added factor V prepared by the National Institute for Biological Standards and Control, London, and coded 67/40. The properties of a number of these reference thromboplastins together with a selection of commercially available working reagents have been compared by extensive international study (Ingram *et al.* 1979, Loeliger and van Halam Visser 1979).

Prothrombin time results used in the control of anticoagulant therapy are commonly reported as ratios, i.e. the clotting time obtained for the patient's sample divided by that obtained for the normal control. By testing a series of normal and abnormal plasmas using two different thromboplastins it is a simple matter to establish the relationship between the ratios obtained using the two different reagents. In this way any working preparation may be standardized against one of the reference thromboplastins (Denson 1971).

In Great Britain, the Manchester Comparative Reagent (MCR) (Poller 1967), a carefully standardized human brain preparation with activity similar to 67/40, is available as a routine working reagent with results being expressed as British Ratios (BR) while batches of a similar but freeze-dried material which have been subjected to more extensive standardization are distributed as the British Comparative Thromboplastin (BCT) (Hills and Ingram 1973). BCT is available as a reference material against which home-made or commercial working reagents may be calibrated as described above. Prothrombin ratios may then be adjusted to match those obtained by using BCT and such adjusted ratios are often referred to as British Corrected Ratios. As supplies of 67/40 are almost exhausted it is proposed that a batch of BCT (BCT/120) should be established as the Second WHO International Reference Thromboplastin. The recently introduced International Normalized Ratio (INR) is the ratio which would have been obtained if the WHO International Reference Thromboplastin had been used to perform the test. In practice BR and INR are identical over most of the normal and therapeutic range. British Ratios and International Normalized Ratios cannot be interpreted in terms of the levels of any specific clotting factors. Conventional therapeutic ranges are established by experience and are 2.0–4.0 for BR or 2.0–3.95 for INR.

Heparin therapy may be monitored by the use of the activated partial thromboplastin time (other simple tests have been similarly used). Heparin levels may be assayed by a technique based on the anti-factor Xa assay (Denson and Bonnar 1973) which has more recently been simplified by the use of synthetic chromogenic substrates for factor Xa.

One-stage assays of clotting factors

Clotting factors are most commonly assayed by one-stage techniques, so called because the clotting reaction, from initiation to fibrin formation, takes place as a continuous process in a single reaction mixture (cf. two-stage methods). The level of the clotting factor under investigation is made rate-determining in the reaction by ensuring that it is present only at low concentrations, whereas all other factors and reagents are present in a constant excess. The clotting factors required, other than that being assayed, are provided at normal levels in a substrate plasma which is deficient in the factor under test. For most clinical purposes it is important that the substrate plasma is totally deficient in the factor being assayed, although a trace level may be tolerable if the test sample levels are all normal or high.

Standard and test samples are tested as a series of dilutions, and the results are obtained by comparison of standard and test either graphically or by calculation as discussed later. The choice of dilutions is a matter of personal preference but a simple three dilution series, 1/10, 1/30 and 1/100, for both standard and test samples is convenient in practice while allowing adequate accuracy and validity checking. In no case should a dilution of less than 1/10 be used—where low level samples are to be assayed the range of dilutions used for the standard should be changed (e.g. 1/100, 1/300, 1/1000) in order to provide the required overlap of clotting times.

In theory it should be possible to assay all clotting factors using tests based on either the one-stage prothrombin time or the activated thromboplastin time. In practice this is not possible since in the case of factors II and X suitable substrate plasmas are virtually unobtainable. In the case of some of the other factors, where clinical deficiency states are very rare, artificial deficient substrates may be prepared, but the natural material from a severely affected patient is always preferable. The various assay methods used are outlined below.

Assays based on the one-stage prothrombin time

This method is used for the assay of factors V and VII. Substrate plasma, a dilution of standard or test sample and saline brain extract are warmed together in a clotting tube. Calcium chloride solution is added and the clotting time recorded.

Assays based on the activated partial thromboplastin time

This method is used for factors VIII, IX, XI and XII. Substrate plasma, a dilution of standard or test sample and a platelet substitute are warmed together in a clotting tube. Activator is added and the mixture incubated for 3–10 minutes (depending on the characteristics of the reagents used). Calcium chloride solution is then added and the clotting time recorded.

The choice of platelet substitute and activator is a matter of personal preference although it is important to select reagents which give an assay with adequate slope.

Assays using snake venoms

Factor II may be assayed using the venom of either the Australian taipan snake which activates factor II without the need of any other clotting factors

(Denson, Borrett and Biggs 1971) or the tiger snake which requires the presence of factor V.

Substrate plasma, a dilution of standard or test sample and cephalin are warmed together in a clotting tube (if tiger snake venom is being used adequate factor V must be ensured either in the substrate plasma or as an extra reagent). A venom/calcium chloride mixture is added and the clotting time is recorded. Alternatively, factor II may also be assayed by a two-stage method which is described later.

Factor X is assayed using the venom of Russell's viper which activates factor X directly thus bypassing clotting factors working earlier in the cascade (Denson 1961a).

Substrate plasma and a dilution of standard or test sample are warmed together in a clotting tube. A mixture of venom and cephalin is added and after 30 seconds the mixture is recalcified and the clotting time recorded.

Assay of factors VIII and IX

Factors VIII and IX can be assayed satisfactorily using a one-stage assay and previous comments about such assays apply equally well here. As with other factors in the intrinsic reaction chain, reagents for the one-stage assay of factors VIII and IX are those of the activated partial thromboplastin time plus a substrate plasma which is completely deficient in the factor to be assayed. However, in the case of factors VIII (Biggs, Eveling and Richards 1955) and IX (Sen *et al.* 1967) an alternative technique is available called the two-stage assay. The basic procedure in two-stage assays (which are based on the thromboplastin generation test) is to incubate a mixture which is lacking in prothrombin and contains the diluted test sample. In this way a complex including activated factor X develops and rises to a concentration which is a function of the amount of the factor in question, contained by the test sample. The chain of clotting reactions is then allowed to continue by subsampling into a reagent (usually normal plasma) containing prothrombin and fibrinogen. A modified version of the two-stage factor VIII assay in which the subsampling stage has been eliminated has been described (Denson 1967). Measurement of resultant clotting time becomes a function of the activated factor X which is present, and hence of the factor VIII or IX which was originally present. Measurement of factor VIII differs from that for factor IX in the constitution of the prothrombin-free mixture which is incubated. For factor VIII assay this contains phospholipid, an activated normal serum sample (to provide factor X and activated factor IX), factor V and the diluted test sample which has previously been adsorbed, using aluminium hydroxide. With factor IX assay, the mixture consists of phospholipid, a source of activated factor XI, serum from a factor IX deficient patient, factors VIII and V, and the diluted test sample. The test sample in this case is converted to serum before dilution to remove prothrombin. One advantage of the factor VIII assay carried out in this way is immediately apparent: there is no requirement for factor VIII deficient plasma. Less of an advantage exists with factor IX measurement because of the need for deficient serum but requirements for blood with very low factor IX levels are somewhat less stringent when making this serum.

The choice as to which assay is best for a given laboratory is governed by several factors. In the case of factor VIII, the two-stage assay has been shown to be more precise and it therefore should be the assay of choice for those laboratories able to maintain and monitor the reagents that are necessary. For a small laboratory carrying out infrequent assays this can be a daunting task and in such instances the one-stage assay is a more practicable alternative. The modified versions of the two-stage assay, some of which are available in kit form, are easily performed in any laboratory but may give unsatisfactory results, and in some cases be quite unusable, at the low factor VIII levels which are important in clinical practice. With the assay of factor IX the one-stage method is an even more useful alternative (and is used by the majority of laboratories) because reagents for the two-stage factor IX assay entail more time and expertise in their preparation and monitoring. Nevertheless the two-stage method is excellent if these reagents are available.

At this stage, further distinction between the two types of assay should not be made since it is still the subject of discussion and research. This arises because one-stage and two-stage assays can give different results depending upon the exact methods used. Except in rare cases such differences are less than 20 per cent. Discrepancies which are found almost always occur when a plasma is being compared to a factor concentrate (Barrowcliffe and Kirkwood 1980). When concentrate is compared with concentrate or plasma compared with plasma, the different assay methods will generally agree. It is for this reason that there is at present much discussion concerning the best material for use as standards in these assays. The existing International Standards for both factors are concentrates but an International Reference Plasma for factor VIII is available.

If results are required in terms of 'percent average normal' then a pool of twenty normal human plasmas is usually sufficient for the assay of factor IX. However, a pool of 60 is necessary if the equivalent material for factor VIII assay is required (see section on standards for assay) and in addition the plasmas must be fresh since factor VIII is relatively unstable. Such a requirement is for the most part impracticable and it is for this reason that standardization of the factor VIII assay was usually unsatisfactory before the advent of the International Standard (Bangham and Brozović 1974).

Amongst factor IX deficient patients there are clearly distinguishable variants (Meyer, Bidwell and Larrieu 1972, Suomela 1975). There has been no evidence to suggest that treatment should be different for these variants and assay of factor IX clotting activity is still the method of monitoring therapy. In order to distinguish the variants, factor IX antigen is determined by immunoelectrophoresis and, in addition, a one-stage prothrombin time is performed using bovine brain as thromboplastin (Denson, Biggs and Mannucci 1968). Plasmas from some patients give prolonged clotting times in the latter test and some show the presence of factor IX antigen. In this way the patients can be separated into several categories of variant. It seems quite likely that an analogous heterogeneity exists in factor VIII deficiency but it has not yet been worked out so clearly (Meyer *et al.* 1972).

Assay of factor VIII-related antigen, factor VIII clotting antigen and ristocetin cofactor

Relationship of the substances

Factor VIII-related antigen (factor VIIIR:Ag), factor VIII clotting antigen (factor VIII:CAg) and ristocetin cofactor are all closely related to factor VIII coagulant activity (factor VIII:C) but the degree of their association is still a matter for discussion. It is now generally agreed that factor VIIIR:Ag and ristocetin cofactor can be separated from factor VIII:CAg and factor VIII:C, without significant loss of any of their activities. Furthermore, it is generally accepted that factor VIII:CAg represents an antigenic determinant on the actual molecule which possesses the factor VIII:C (i.e. coagulant) activity but that factor VIII:CAg does not represent the actual active site of clotting itself.

Table 10. Occurrence of factor VIII-related substances.

	Factor VIII clotting activity	Factor VIII clotting antigen	Ristocetin cofactor	Factor VIII-related antigen
Normal plasma	Yes	Yes	Yes	Yes
Normal serum	No	Yes	Yes	Yes
Severe haemophilic plasma	No	No	Yes	Yes
Severe haemophilic serum	No	No	Yes	Yes
Severe von Willebrand's plasma	No	No	No	No
Severe von Willebrand's serum	No	No	No	No

Hence factor VIII:CAg can be detected when coagulant activity has been destroyed. It is not clear as yet whether factor VIIIR:Ag and ristocetin cofactor represent different functions of the same molecule or not. However, there is little evidence as yet to suggest that the two can be separated by physical techniques.

Occurrence of the substances

Factor VIIIR:Ag and ristocetin cofactor are present in the blood of haemophiliacs as well as normal subjects, while being absent or reduced in the blood of patients with von Willebrand's disease. This is summarized in Table 10. Measuring the levels of these two substances, together with the coagulant activity, will therefore present a differential diagnosis between haemophilia and von Willebrand's disease. Furthermore, the levels in the blood vary in a similar manner to coagulant activity when a person is subjected to stress, fear or exercise. As a result, the ratio of factor VIII R:Ag to factor VIII:C is largely unaffected by such conditions and is used in preference to a simple factor VIII:C determination in the detection of female carriers of haemophilia.

Factor VIII:CAg is present in normal plasma or serum and absent or reduced in the plasma or serum of haemophiliacs or patients with von Willebrand's disease. Factor VIII:C, of course, does not survive the clotting process and hence is absent in normal serum. This is again summarized in Table 10. It follows that measurement of factor VIII:CAg can be used to determine a function of inactivated factor VIII:C, for example when a sample has become clotted or partly so. A particular example of this is seen in the measurement of factor VIII in a fetus, *in utero*, when the blood samples obtained are sometimes partly clotted. Some modern research also claims that a ratio of factor VIII:CAg to factor VIII:C has special value in carrier detection but it would be premature to draw conclusions on this.

Stability of the substances

Factor VIII:C is a relatively labile activity and assays are carried out on fresh plasma samples which have been efficiently collected.

Factor VIIIR:Ag and factor VIII:CAg are essentially stable entities and can be assayed in fresh or previously frozen samples. In principle their assays can be conducted on serum samples but this is less satisfactory because small variations in levels can occur during clotting. Ristocetin cofactor is essentially stable but variations in level have been recorded with long-term storage of samples.

Factor VIIIR:Ag assay

Assay of factor VIIIR:Ag is based, as its name implies, upon an immunological test using a specific antibody. Most usual is the Laurell immunoelectrophoretic technique (Zimmerman, Ratnoff and Howell 1971, Laurell 1972, Zimmerman *et al.* 1975) where a specific heterologous antibody is included in an agarose gel while the sample introduced into a small hole, punched in the gel, is made to traverse the gel under the influence of an electric field. Antigen driven into the antibody-containing gel leads to formation of an antigen–antibody complex which immediately redissolves in the further antigen which is being driven forward. Eventually, however, the antigen sample is depleted and the antibody–antigen complex is left as a rocket-shaped precipitate whose height is a function of the quantity of antigen originally present. In normal practice these precipitates are not dense enough to be instantly visible and they are revealed by a protein staining technique. Coomassie blue is popular but a speedier alternative is 2 per cent tannic acid. The assay is normally conducted overnight in a barbitone buffer of pH 8.6. It is best to make measurements of three dilutions of each test and standard sample and to evaluate the assay result by a graphical or calculator technique as described for the assay of factor VIII coagulant activity. This immunoelectrophoretic assay is simple and elegant and is accurate for samples containing at least 5 per cent factor VIIIR:Ag.

Alternatively, several radioactive tests are available based upon the usual principles of radioimmunoassay. Two methods are popular. In one of these (the IRMA technique), the antibody is adsorbed on to the inner surface of a plastic tube, reacted with the test sample (the antigen) and then the sandwich is completed by a further reaction with a radio-labelled antibody (Peake and Bloom 1977). The amount of labelled antibody, which becomes attached, is proportional to the amount of antigen present in the test sample. Once again, samples and standards are assayed at different dilutions in performance of the assay.

An alternative method involves making a Fab fragment of the antibody and labelling it with radioactivity (Hoyer 1972). This material is reacted with the diluted test sample and, after reaction, the antigen–antibody complex is precipitated with ammonium sulphate. Since the factor VIII complex is much larger than an antibody fragment, differential precipitation is possible and unreacted labelled antibody is separated from that combined with factor VIIIR:Ag. The radioactivity present in the complex is a measure of antigen present in the test sample. ELISA (enzyme-linked immunosorbent assay) procedures of VIIIR:Ag assay are also available (Bartlett *et al.* 1976) although they are less popular. Measurement here is based upon the colorimetric detection of an enzyme coupled to the antibody. Radioactive and colorimetric assays of factor VIII-related antigen are more time-consuming and involved than the simple Laurell technique but are more sensitive, allowing accurate measurement below the 5 per cent level. They can be used in the detection of some variants of von Willebrand's disease when 'non-parallel lines' are sometimes found (indicating that the assay does not function correctly with these samples, and quantification is inadvisable).

Two-dimensional electrophoretic methods will also indicate the von Willebrand's variants because factor VIIIR:Ag in such patients usually migrates faster in an electric field than normal antigen. The usual technique is to carry out the electrophoresis first in a gel containing no antibody and then to cut out the relevant strip of gel and reset it in a gel which does contain antibody (Ganrot 1972). Electrophoresis is then continued in a direction at right angles to the initial migration. Peaks of precipitated antibody–antigen complex are obtained which, after staining, reveal the extent to which the factor VIIIR:Ag had migrated in the first dimension.

Assay of ristocetin cofactor

Assay of ristocetin cofactor is based on the premise that normal platelets will be aggregated by ristocetin if the cofactor is present, but will not aggregate in its absence. (Ristocetin is an antibiotic no longer used because of side-effects.) It is necessary to use the correct ristocetin level in order to obtain this differential effect and avoid non-specific aggregation. Two assays of ristocetin cofactor are available. In one, the test sample is mixed with fixed platelets and ristocetin in an aggregometer which measures light absorption, or scattering, by the sample. Aggregation is plotted automatically as a function of time (Weiss *et al.* 1973). Plots are compared with those of normal samples to obtain a quantitative result. The other test is to mix the reagents and allow them to react and then allow aggregated platelets to settle (Evans and Austen 1977). Unaggregated platelets are counted in a particle counter, and the percentage aggregation is compared with results using normal samples.

Assay of factor VIII:CAg

The assays of factor VIII:CAg are based on similar principles to those of factor VIIIR:Ag. However, the Laurell technique is not applicable in this case because no suitable antibody to factor VIII:CAg has been found which can build up a visible antigen–antibody precipitate. Radioactive methods are almost exclusively used and these are entirely analogous to the IRMA assays for factor VIIIR:Ag except that an antibody to factor VIII:CAg is employed (Lazarchick and Hoyer 1978, Peake and Bloom 1978, Peake *et al.* 1979). At present, the antibodies which have proved most useful are those of high titre, which have developed in a haemophiliac in response to therapy or which have occurred spontaneously in a previously normal human subject. In principle, antibodies raised in animals could be used but none sufficiently specific are available at present.

The alternative method of assay is to employ an antibody neutralization technique in which a set amount of antibody is reacted with the sample and the amount of antibody which remains is determined. This can be a very difficult assay when conventional tube techniques are employed. However, it can be carried out alternatively by a gel diffusion method (McLellan *et al.* 1981) and this could represent a simple alternative to the radioactive methods.

Standards for assay

International reference materials are available for factor VIII clotting activity, the factor-VIII related antigen, ristocetin cofactor and factor VIII clotting antigen. For some of the British factor VIII standards the content of the factor VIII-related substances is known but the accuracy of calibration is possibly less than that for factor VIII clotting activity. Plasma pools can be used as standards for these substances but it is advisable to have 60 or more individual normal plasmas to make such a pool. This is necessary because of the very wide variation in level of the substances between different normal subjects. The pool may be frozen at $-40°C$ for use since the factor VIII-related substances are essentially stable but long-term storage is inadvisable for ristocetin cofactor standards. Of course, the use of frozen pool standards does not apply to the coagulant activity, factor VIII:C, which is a labile substance.

Assay of factor II (prothrombin)

As outlined in the section on one-stage assays, the most convenient methods of measuring factor II (prothrombin) involve snake venoms which activate factor II in the presence of phospholipid. Tiger snake venom requires the presence of factor V but taipan venom does not. There is little to choose between these two methods. Some workers claim that with the tiger snake assay, results can be calculated using logarithmic graph paper but this is not our experience. Logarithmic paper seldom gives straight lines for these assay calculations except over very short dilution ranges and normally the best method is to plot clotting times against the reciprocal of the sample concentration, using reciprocal graph paper.

If therapeutic concentrates are being assayed for factor II using snake venom methods, these materials must be initially diluted in normal plasma which has been twice absorbed with alumina. Without this protein environment, the reaction appears to be altered and clotting times changed.

An alternative assay for factor II is the so-called two-stage prothrombin time (Biggs and Douglas 1953a), in which citrated plasma is clotted by recalcification in the presence of tissue extract and the mixture subsampled at intervals into fibrinogen to measure the thrombin present. In this way, a plot of thrombin generation with time can be drawn. The area under this curve, which is a measurement of total thrombin generation and proportional to the original prothrombin level, can be compared to that of a normal sample. The advantage of the method is that it measures thrombin generation in the patient's own plasma, in the presence of his own antithrombin. The test is, however, time-consuming and can give unreliable results when testing plasma samples which have been frozen.

Assay of fibrinogen

The simplest test of fibrinogen deficiency is the thrombin time test in which thrombin solution is added to the sample and the clotting time recorded. Prolonged times indicate either a low fibrinogen level or an abnormal form of fibrinogen or else the presence of an inhibitory substance. One inhibitor which could be present is that associated with fibrin degradation products and the possibility of these affecting the result can be excluded by performing a specific immunological assay for the degradation products. Another possible inhibitory substance could be heparin either as a result of the patient being on heparin therapy or because the blood sample was incorrectly collected into heparin. The effect of heparin can be excluded by repeating the clotting test using Reptilase (a commercial preparation of *Bothrops atrox* venom) in place of thrombin because this reagent is unaffected by heparin. A comparison of the results using Reptilase (Funk *et al.* 1971) and thrombin can also sometimes help to distinguish an abnormal fibrinogen from fibrinogen deficiency.

The simple thrombin time test can be converted to a semi-quantitative test by adding thrombin to serial dilutions of test plasma and finding the extent to which the sample can be diluted while still obtaining an observable clot. This is called a fibrinogen titre and results are expressed simply as the relevant dilution for the test plasma along with the equivalent dilution for normal plasma. A popular quantitative technique (Clauss 1957) involves clotting dilutions of the test and standard samples with excess thrombin and calculating the results by a parallel line plot of clotting times as for other one-stage assays.

Quantitative biochemical measurement of fibrinogen is also possible. The method is to clot the sample, wash the resultant fibrin and measure the amount of protein it contains. Usually this involves dissolving the clot and measuring the protein in solution by a conventional protein analysis such as the biuret method (Varley 1969).

Assay of factor XIII

The function of factor XIII is to stabilize fibrin formed by the action of thrombin on fibrinogen. This is achieved by the introduction of chemical cross-links in a transglutaminase reaction. Assays can therefore be based upon clot-stabilizing ability which are the most unambiguous assays or upon a measurement of transglutaminase activity.

Since factor XIII is effective even in low concentration (around 2 per cent) in human plasma, a simple qualitative test of clot stabilization is very often applied. The plasma is clotted and the resultant clot suspended in a solution of urea or acetic acid. If the clot dissolves when left overnight at 37°C then the factor XIII content of the plasma is abnormally low. Control samples consist of a normal plasma and a known abnormal one, treated identically. It is easy to convert this test into a semi-quantitative assay by serially diluting the test plasma in one which is deficient in factor XIII and performing the test on these diluted samples. Usually this modification is avoided unless absolutely necessary because the deficient plasma is rare.

Quantitative assays are possible using the transglutaminase assay (Lorand, Urayama and de Kiewret 1969) but results are not always identical to those of the clot stability assay. Positive results can be obtained in materials, for example lysed red cells, where there is no evidence of activity associated with clot stabilization. The principle of the enzymic assay is that the factor XIII is made to cross-link a labelled amine with a protein such as casein so that the amount of label which the protein acquires is a measure of the level of factor XIII. This simulates the physiological action of factor XIII in which the factor is believed to link lysine and glutamine groups in fibrinogen; the labelled amine mimics the lysyl group while casein provides the glutamine groups. The labelled amine used can be radioactive such as ^{14}C-putrescine or fluorescent such as dansylcadaverine. Sometimes, the casein is used in a chemically substituted form where the lysine groups are blocked to obviate competition with the amine.

Factor XIII can also be assayed by immunological tests such as immuno-electrophoresis but, as with all such tests, this only registers that immunological determinants are intact on the molecules and does not prove that the factor is functionally active.

An important precaution when testing for factor XIII is to ensure that the patient has not been given replacement therapy or blood transfusions for some weeks. Because the half-life of the factor is relatively long and because 2 per cent of the average normal level is adequate for clot stability, the effects of treatment persist over a long period. Use of a strictly quantitative assay will remove this restriction to some degree.

Assay of antithrombin III and anti-Xa

Antithrombin III, which is present in normal plasma, is responsible for the progressive and irreversible inactivation of thrombin, the reaction being enhanced by the presence of heparin. Many methods are available for the measurement of antithrombin III none of which is entirely satisfactory for routine use in a clinical laboratory.

Clotting methods

Tube technique (Biggs *et al.* 1970)

Dilutions of test and standard (a pool of 30 normals) plasmas are mixed with excess thrombin and the mixtures incubated for one hour. Residual thrombin, which is measured by subsampling into fibrinogen solution, is inversely proportional to the amount of antithrombin III in the original incubation mixture. In order to remove other coagulation factors all plasmas must be heated and adsorbed before testing.

Plate radial diffusion technique (Lane, Bird and Rizza 1975)

Agarose containing thrombin is poured to form a thin gel of uniform thickness on a glass plate. Wells are punched in the gel and dilutions of test and standard plasmas placed in the wells. The plate is left overnight at room temperature after which a second agarose gel, this time containing fibrinogen, is superimposed by pouring the molten agarose mixture over the first gel. After incubation at 37°C thrombin diffusing from the first gel will have clotted the fibrinogen in the second. Clear zones (of unclotted fibrinogen) in the second gel will represent areas in which antithrombin III diffusing from the wells in the first gel has inactivated the thrombin. The diameters of these clear zones will be proportional to the antithrombin III levels in the samples introduced into the relevant wells.

Immunological method

This is the conventional Laurell method in which agarose containing antibody to antithrombin III is poured to form a rectangular gel of uniform thickness. Dilutions of test and standard samples are placed in wells punched along one side of the plate. After electrophoresis, staining is used to demonstrate the precipitation peaks. Peak height is proportional to antithrombin III level.

Chromogenic method (Ødegård and Abildgaard 1978)

Thrombin is added to the plasma sample diluted in a buffered solution which contains heparin to prevent coagulation and accelerate the reaction between thrombin and antithrombin III. After a short incubation period polybrene is added to neutralize the heparin, and residual thrombin is detected by its action in releasing *p*-nitroaniline from a synthetic substrate. Light absorption by this *p*-nitroaniline is measured spectrophotometrically and the antithrombin level obtained from a standard curve produced in the same experiment.

Each of these four methods has its disadvantages. The tube clotting method is technically tedious if more than a few samples are to be tested and the preliminary heating of the plasmas, even if well controlled, may lead to some loss of antithrombin III activity. The gel diffusion method is simple and straightforward but the overnight reaction means that the technique is not applicable where urgent answers are required. The chromogenic method is simple and precise but it can be expensive unless considerable numbers of samples are being tested. Immunological methods measure the concentration of antithrombin molecules even if they are biologically inactive and hence levels measured by these techniques can be considerably in excess of the true biological activity.

Anti-Xa (Biggs *et al.* 1970)

Assay methods for anti-Xa activity are similar to those for antithrombin III. In both tube and gel clotting methods factor Xa replaces thrombin in the first stage of the tests while in the second stage fibrinogen is replaced by a mixture of cephalin and factor X-deficient plasma. In the immunological method an antibody to anti-Xa is incorporated in the gel, while in the chromogenic method the synthetic substrate used is specific for Xa.

<h3 align="center">Assay of antibodies and inhibitors</h3>

Factor VIII antibodies

Antibodies to factor VIII clotting activity arise in about 6 per cent of haemophilic patients usually as a response to treatment with materials containing factor VIII. They may also develop in individuals with otherwise normal coagulation systems but who suffer from such conditions as rheumatoid arthritis, penicillin allergy, collagen disorders, etc.

Various methods are available for detection and measurement of these antibodies, ranging from simple qualitative mixing tests to complex assay procedures. All depend on the incubation of factor VIII with the patient's plasma and on detecting the loss of factor VIII activity compared to that in a control mixture known not to contain antibodies.

Antibodies to factor VIII clotting activity are unusual in that the reaction with factor VIII is progressive with time, weak antibodies sometimes requiring several hours for the reaction to reach completion. An important consequence of this is that any test method should allow sufficient time for the neutralization of a measurable amount of factor VIII. If sufficient time is not allowed then, particularly in the case of antibodies of low potency, the loss of factor VIII activity may not be distinguishable in view of the inherent errors of the tests or assays being used.

Mixing tests

These usually utilize the activated partial thromboplastin time test and consist of mixing the patient's plasma with normal plasma. If the APTT of the mixture is corrected to near the normal figure then a potent antibody is unlikely to be present. As the only time available for the reaction between antibody and factor VIII is little more than the activation time allowed in the test—often only two minutes—antibodies of low potency may well destroy insufficient factor VIII to significantly lengthen the APTT. Longer activation times for the mixtures will improve sensitivity but weak antibodies can still easily be missed. Further improvement in sensitivity may be achieved by incubation of the mixture of the patient's plasma and normal plasma for up to an hour before performing the APTT but in such tests the provision of relevant controls can create difficulties.

Mixing tests as outlined here are non-specific and are sensitive to all antibodies and inhibitors acting in the intrinsic pathway. Confirmation that an antibody is directed against factor VIII (or any other clotting factor) can only be obtained by performing a full specific assay as described below.

Clotting assays of factor viii antibodies

There are three procedures in common use for the measurement of antibodies to factor VIII. Advantages have been claimed for each method but all depend equally on the initial preparation of mixtures in which a source of factor VIII is added to patient's and control's plasma followed, after an incubation period, by factor VIII assays. Therefore, any suggestion that one method is simpler to perform than another would seem to be fallacious.

In the technique of Biggs and Bidwell (1959), often known as the Old Oxford method, factor VIII concentrate is added to the patient's plasma and control plasma so that the factor VIII level is about average normal. After incubation for one hour factor VIII assays are performed and, taking the control as 100 per cent, the amount of factor VIII remaining in the test sample is calculated. A residual factor VIII level of 25 per cent (i.e. 75 per cent destruction) represents one unit of antibody and useful results can be obtained up to about four units of antibody. At higher antibody levels it is necessary to dilute the patient's plasma in order to obtain accurately measurable levels of residual factor VIII and it is at this stage that major problems may arise. While many samples will still give satisfactory results, antibodies of a complex nature (Biggs *et al.* 1972a,b) will often give answers which reflect the experimental conditions rather than the true antibody level. A wide range of test plasma dilutions may be found to give very little difference in residual factor VIII with the result that, when antibody potencies as measured are multiplied by the dilution factor, the final answer will depend very largely on the dilution used. A second disadvantage of this technique is that results are influenced by the starting level of factor VIII. If for any reason the starting level of factor VIII is lower than that recommended then an exaggeratedly high antibody potency will be recorded. The reverse is true if factor VIII starting levels are higher than normal.

In the technique of Rizza and Biggs (1973) the unit is defined as that amount of antibody which will neutralize 0.5 units of factor VIII. The experiment is so designed that antibody is measured in a situation of antigen excess. Factor VIII concentrate is added to dilutions of patient's plasma and to a control plasma (haemophilic plasma containing no antibody) so that the factor VIII level in the mixtures is about 100 iu/per cent (1 iu/ml). Mixtures are incubated for four hours to allow completion of the reaction, then test mixtures are assayed against the control. That dilution which would give 50 per cent residual factor VIII is obtained by graph from the experimental results, some of which should lie on each side of the 50 per cent residual point. In addition, the factor VIII level in the control sample is determined by assay against a suitable standard. Antibody units are calculated by multiplying the titre giving 50 per cent residual factor VIII (adjusted to allow for additional dilution of test samples by the addition of factor VIII) by the factor VIII level in the control sample (in units per ml). Compared to the Biggs and Bidwell technique results are much less affected by the experimental conditions used as these are all taken into account in the final calculation. Furthermore, as the antibody unit is directly related to the amount of factor VIII destroyed, this New Oxford unit should have more relevance to the possibility of neutralizing the antibody in a patient by dosage with factor VIII. Both of the Oxford methods are equally well applicable to the assay of antibodies directed against factor VIII from animal sources, the appropriate concentrate being substituted in the initial preparation of the incubation mixtures.

In the Bethesda technique (Kasper *et al.* 1975) normal plasma (the source of factor VIII) is added in equal parts to the test sample and control sample and an incubation time of two hours is used. One unit of antibody is defined as the amount which will destroy 50 per cent of the initial factor VIII. This method suffers, although to a lesser extent, from both of the main disadvantages of the Biggs and Bidwell method.

Gel diffusion assay of factor VIII antibodies

In this technique (Bird 1975, Rainsford and Hall 1976) an agarose gel of uniform thickness is prepared with factor VIII incorporated in the gel. Wells are punched in the gel and into these are placed the plasma samples, in a series of dilutions. After incubation a second gel layer is poured on top of the first gel. This second gel layer contains haemophilic plasma which, after a further incubation period, is recalcified by immersing in calcium chloride solution. In the first stage, antibody diffusing from the plasma in the wells into the gel will neutralize factor VIII, the area of neutralization corresponding to the amount of antibody in the well. In the second stage these areas of neutralized factor VIII will be demonstrated by delayed clotting which is seen as a clear zone in the superimposed gel. The area of neutralization of factor VIII is plotted against sample dilution and results for test samples compared graphically against those for a standard (parallel-line plot as described later for factor assays). The standard used is an antibody-containing plasma which has been accurately assayed by one of the clotting methods previously described.

This technique is simple, relatively sensitive and convenient when large numbers of samples are to be tested, but discrepancies may be introduced if the test and standard antibodies are not of similar characteristics.

Accuracy and comparability of methods

As no antibody assay technique can be more accurate than the factor VIII assay used in its performance, it is not surprising that the reproducibility of results by any of these methods can be disappointing. Agreement within a laboratory, by any method, is usually acceptable but when comparison is made of results obtained by different laboratories testing the same sample, then very large discrepancies may be found (Austen *et al.* 1982). This discrepancy may be so large as to make any comparison of results between different laboratories meaningless, even when the same techniques are being used.

There is no consistent relationship between the units derived by the three methods described above (Austen *et al.* 1982). In general, lowest figures are obtained by the Old Oxford and highest by the Bethesda techniques. However, variations between the characteristics of different antibodies and discrepancies between laboratories makes any more precise definition of the relationships between the different units impossible.

Antibodies to factor IX

Antibodies to factor IX develop in a very small proportion of Christmas disease patients as a result of treatment with factor IX-containing materials. Unlike antibodies to factor VIII, those to factor IX may be considered as instantaneous in their action. The methods of testing for antibodies to factor IX are similar in principle to those for antibodies to factor VIII except that no incubation period is required for the antigen–antibody reaction to take place. No unit of measurement has been established and antibody potency is described by the proportion of added factor IX destroyed at any particular dilution of the test plasma.

Other antibodies and inhibitors

Antibodies to factors other than VIII and IX have been described and tests for these are similar to those used in the investigation of antibodies to factor IX.

There are also a number of other inhibitory effects which, by blocking reactions rather than destroying clotting factors, may be effective at any stage of the clotting cascade. Tests for such inhibitors are based on mixing tests using normal and patient's plasma in test systems such as the APTT. Quantitative methods are not available but an estimate of inhibitor potency can be obtained by testing the patient's plasma in dilution. Inhibitors of the type associated with DLE are characterized by their stability on heating at 56°C.

Assay of kinin deficiencies

These deficiencies have previously been known by various names such as the Fletcher (Wuepper 1973), Flaujeac (Lacombe, Varet and Levy 1975), Fitzgerald (Saito *et al.* 1975) and Williams (Colman *et al.* 1975) traits. It is now established that the last three of these are synonymous and represent a deficiency of high molecular weight kininogen while Fletcher factor deficiency is really a lack of prekallikrein.

One-stage assays can be devised for these factors in an analogous manner to that described for factors XI and XII but the factor-deficient plasma samples, necessary as reagents, are rare. Subjects with a deficiency in these kinins usually do not experience abnormal bleeding which, in itself, removes some priority from the analysis. The activated partial thromboplastin time is prolonged when the kinin factors are reduced, providing a short incubation time such as two minutes is employed. By increasing incubation time to 10 minutes, the prolongation of clotting time is largely (often completely) corrected. A prolonged clotting time after two minutes activation combined with a near-normal clotting time after 10 minutes activation is a good indication of a kinin deficiency.

Passavoy factor deficiency (Hougie, McPherson and Aronson 1975) has also been found to prolong clotting times in the activated partial thromboplastin test but these are not corrected by prolonged incubation and it is thought unlikely that Passavoy factor is a kinin.

Controls and standards

Any test of clotting function, however precise or reproducible, is of little value unless interpreted in the light of satisfactory controls and standards. In most cases the aim is to relate patients' results to normality. However, in coagulation studies normality itself is an elusive concept. Controls and standards are often a compromise between what is desirable and what is practicable.

In this chapter controls are taken to be materials against which patient samples are compared in a non-quantitative way. All materials against which clotting factor levels are quantitatively assayed are referred to as standards, although this term is strictly only applied to primary standards (e.g. International Standards) and other materials, perhaps less precisely calibrated, are strictly reference preparations.

Controls for preliminary tests

The ideal control for preliminary non-quantitative tests of clotting should perform two functions. Firstly, it should serve to monitor the test system itself and secondly it should indicate how a patient's results compare with normality.

The consistent performance of the test system is easily controlled by the regular testing of a normal plasma or pool of normals which has been stored in aliquots either dried or frozen below $-30°C$. This will provide reproducible day-to-day results and will quickly show any variation in the activity of the reagents. It will, however, be of no direct help in interpreting patients' results for which purpose a knowledge of the normal range is required. This range can be very large (e.g. up to 15 seconds for APTT) and can only be established by the frequent testing of single fresh normal samples taken from a large panel of donors. Over a period of time the limits of the normal range will become well defined.

Assay standards

Choice of a suitable standard for the assay of individual clotting factors will be influenced mainly by the stability and normal range of the factor concerned.

In many cases the ideal might be a pool of fresh normal plasmas but the number needed in such a pool, even when the normal range of the factor in question is relatively narrow, makes this impracticable. A small fresh pool, which should never include less than five normals, may often be used when a lower standard of accuracy is acceptable, and for factor VII in particular, which has unreliable storage characteristics in any form, this option may be as good as any.

For those factors which are stable on freezing and thawing a pool of normal plasmas stored in aliquots below $-30°C$ is satisfactory, the number of individual normals required in such a pool depending on the normal range of the factor concerned. An excellent standard for all factors except factor VII is a normal or pool of normals freeze-dried in aliquots and calibrated, after drying, against either a large number of fresh normal plasmas or a primary standard. For factors V and VIII which are particularly unstable, this dried plasma standard is the only type suitable for accurate work. Recommended standards for the different factor assays are given in Table 11. The subject of standards is discussed in greater detail in Chapter 20.

Units of measurement

With the introduction of International Standards and reference materials, clotting factor assays are increasingly being reported in international units (iu) rather than in terms of average normal (AN). The first International Standards available were for factor VIII (Bangham and Brozovich 1974) and factor IX (Brozovic, Kirkwood and Robinson 1976) and in each case problems have arisen in relating iu to AN. It was intended that iu/dl and %AN should be numerically identical but this is often not the case. Depending on assay methods used and the definition of AN in any particular laboratory the discrepancy can be significant—up to 20 per cent in the case of factor VIII and considerably more in the case of factor IX. International units have also been defined for factors VIIIR:Ag, VIII:CAg and VIIIR:RCoF and also for antithrombin III but significant discrepancies between iu and locally defined AN will be much less likely in these cases.

Clotting factor levels are traditionally reported in units/ml, one unit being the activity present in 1 ml of average fresh normal plasma, i.e. units/ml $\times$ 100 = %AN. With the introduction of international units the use of the word unit on its own can obviously cause confusion. Since units/ml (as originally defined) and iu/ml can be numerically different, it is important that the type of unit referred to should always be made absolutely clear.

Other materials as standards

Emphasis has here been placed on the use of human plasma as the basis of standards for clotting factor assays and this is generally considered to be the

Table 11. Standards for factor assays.

Factors	Working standard not requiring calibration	Working standard requiring calibration	Standard for calibration purposes
II, X, XI, XII, XIII, anti-Xa	Frozen pool of 30 normal plasmas	Freeze-dried plasma	Pool of 30 normal plasma
I	Frozen pool of 30 normal plasmas	Freeze-dried plasma	Pool of 30 normal plasmas
V	None[1]	Freeze-dried plasma	Fresh pool of 30 normal plasmas
VII	Frozen pool of 30 normal plasmas	Frozen plasma	Pool of 30 normal plasmas
VIII:C in plasma	None	Freeze-dried plasma	International Reference Plasma[2] or British Standard[4]
VIII:C in concentrate	British Working Standard[3]	Freeze-dried concentrate	International Standard
VIIIR:Ag, VIII:CAg, VIIIR:RCoF	Frozen pool of 60 normal plasmas	Freeze-dried plasma	International Reference Plasma or British Standard
IX	Frozen pool of 30 normal plasmas	Freeze-dried plasma	International or British Standard
Antithrombin III	Frozen pool of 30 normal plasmas	Freeze-dried plasma	International Reference Plasma or British Standard

[1] No standard is given here because a fresh pool of many plasmas is unrealistic as a working standard. However, in practice, it can sometimes be necessary to pool a small number of fresh plasmas and accept the consequent reduction in accuracy.

[2] International Standard for Blood Coagulation Factor VIII, Human; International Reference Preparation of Factor VIII-Related Activities in Plasma; International Standard for Blood Coagulation Factor IX, Human, and International Reference Preparation of Antithrombin III, Plasma, Human, are in limited supply and may not be available to routine laboratories.

[3] British Working Standard for Blood Coagulation Factor VIII Concentrate, Human, is a concentrate mainly used by fractionation centres and similar laboratories.

[4] British Reference Preparation for Blood Coagulation Factor VIII, Human is also calibrated for the other factor VIII activities, factor IX and antithrombin III. It is available to laboratories in the UK. Some other countries have equivalent materials available.

best material for use in the assay of patient's plasma samples. However, many other materials are available for this purpose, concentrates and animal preparations being those commonly encountered. Both should be treated with caution. Concentrates and plasmas may not be consistently comparable with one another when different assay methods are used, e.g. the one-stage and two-stage methods of factor VIII assay. Materials prepared from animal sources can significantly alter the characteristics of some assay methods leading to invalid results when the material under test is of human origin.

Calculation of assay results

Clotting factor assays are based on the principle of using test systems in which all clotting factors required for the reaction are present in constant excess, the exception being the factor under test which is present in low and variable concentrations. The factor being assayed thus becomes rate-determining in the reaction and any differences in the rate of reaction, recorded as clotting times, will be due only to variations in concentration of the factor being assayed.

Traditionally, results of clotting factor assays have been obtained by graphical means in which some function of concentration (dilution) is plotted against some function of clotting time. This is done for both standard and test samples and the result is derived from comparison of the two lines so obtained. More recently, with the ready availability of computers and calculators, there has been a trend towards purely mathematical calculation of results. These methods, although based on the same principles as graphical techniques, have the advantage of removing subjectivity in the selection of best lines through a series of experimentally obtained points.

Results by graphing

All assays depend on obtaining a series of experimental points which, for each sample tested, can be plotted as a straight line. In most cases this is achieved by plotting both concentration (dilution) and clotting times on a logarithmic scale, when lines obtained for a series of samples should all be parallel to one another. Some workers find that certain one-stage assays, particularly those for factors VIII and IX, give better straight lines if clotting times are plotted on a linear scale when, with concentrations remaining on a log scale, parallel lines are again obtained. However, some types of assays will not give straight lines if plotted by these methods and in these cases other relationships must be used.

In one-stage assays of prothrombin using taipan snake venom log/log or log/linear plots will only occasionally give straight lines and then only over a very limited range of concentrations. In this assay best results are obtained by plotting concentrations on a reciprocal scale and clotting times on a linear scale. The straight lines obtained for a series of samples will not now be parallel, but will meet at a point representing an infinite concentration of prothrombin. One advantage sometimes claimed for the use of tiger snake venom in this test is that a log/log plot is more easily achieved. This is not always the case and reciprocal/linear plots are still required on many occasions.

Assays of the inhibitors antithrombin III and anti-Xa are plotted with concentrations on a linear scale and clotting times on a log scale. All lines meet at a point representing zero level of the inhibitory factor.

In all the methods of plotting outlined above concentrations are conventionally on the horizontal axis and this design will be assumed in the following paragraph.

Having drawn satisfactory lines (see later) for standard and test samples, assay results are obtained by applying the principle that a line of constant clotting time, i.e. any horizontal line, must represent constant concentration of the factor being assayed. The horizontal axis is first recalibrated so that the point at which such a line intersects the test sample line represents 100 per cent of the clotting factor. The point at which the constant clotting time line intersects the standard line may then be read off directly on the recalibrated horizontal axis to give the factor concentration in the test sample as a percentage of the standard. (If the standard does not represent 100 per cent of the factor in question then the appropriate arithmetic adjustment must be applied.) If the graph paper used has printed calibrations on the concentration axis as is usual with log or reciprocal paper, reading of results is simplified by selecting as the line of constant clotting time that which will intersect the test sample line at a printed 100 per cent point, by which means the test sample result can be read off directly from the printed scale. It should be noted that when several test samples are calculated against the same standard line then it is usual to select a different line of constant clotting time for each test sample. It may also be necessary to recalibrate the concentration axis for each or any individual sample calculated against the same standard.

Results by mathematical calculation

Calculation methods that are described here apply to those assays where standard and test samples have a parallel line relationship. They may be used with any simple pocket calculator which has facilities for logs and a single level of parenthesis. Where programming facilities are available the calculation can usually be accommodated in less than 300 programme steps—well within the capacity of many pocket or desk calculators—with the consequent improvement in speed and convenience of calculation.

The formula given here is applicable to any assay where concentration and clotting times are both on a log scale (simple modifications will accommodate clotting times on a linear scale). Standard and test samples must both be tested in the same number of dilutions with the same dilution range ratio, although actual dilutions for the two samples need not be the same.

Test sample potency as a percentage of the standard is given by the following:

$$100 \times \left(\text{antilog} \left\{ \left[\frac{\log S_1 + \log S_2 \ldots + \log S_x - \log T_1 - \log T_2 \ldots - \log T_x}{\log S_x + \log T_x - \log S_1 - \log T_1} \right] \times \left[\frac{2}{\text{Number of dilutions}} \times \frac{\log \text{of}}{\text{dilution range ratio}} \right] \right\} \right)$$

where:

1   S_1 is the clotting time for the first dilution and S_x the clotting time for the last dilution of the standard. T_1–T_x are similar for the test sample. (Note that the top line of the first bracket includes all dilutions of test and standard samples.)

2   The number of dilutions is that for each separate sample.

3   The dilution range ratio is the ratio between the first and last dilutions, e.g. dilutions used 1/16, 1/32, 1/64, 1/128 then dilution range $= \frac{128}{16} = 8$.

More complicated equations are available for cases involving different assay designs (Kirkwood and Snape 1980).

If standard and test samples are tested at different initial dilutions the appropriate correction must be applied. Likewise, if the standard does not represent 100 per cent of the factor being assayed either a correction must be applied to the final answer, or the figure 100 in the above formula may be replaced by the actual factor level of the standard.

Validity of assays

Many of the errors inherent in assays of this type may be recognized by applying tests of validity to the experimental results. Thus, errors due to poor technique, unsatisfactory reagents, etc. will be immediately noted.

Slope

This represents the rate of change of clotting time with change of concentration. If the slope is poor then a small change in clotting time will represent a large change in factor concentration, hence small errors in technique will have a disproportionate effect on the error of the final result. The slope, in this sense, is not necessarily indicated by the appearance of the plot on graph paper where alteration of the scales of the axes may give a false impression of improvement.

At least a 50 per cent increase in clotting times with a 10-fold increase in dilution is desirable, pro rata for other dilution ranges.

Straightness

No individual point should be off the line drawn by more than 5 per cent of the clotting time involved. Lines drawn through more scatter than this must be of doubtful value.

Parallelism

Where assays are based on a parallel line relationship, strictly parallel lines must be drawn. If significant adjustment of either line is required then doubt is cast on the validity of the assay.

Overlap

All lines used are portions of sigmoid curves. In order to ensure that standard and test samples are tested on the same part of the curve, dilution ranges should be adjusted so that clotting times for the two samples overlap for at least half of their dilution ranges.

Blank

The blank time should be sufficiently long that when clotting time is plotted against factor concentration a straight line can be drawn down to at most 0.1 per cent of the factor under test. Failure to achieve this will be due to unsatisfactory reagents (most likely a substrate plasma which is not zero per cent in the appropriate factor) and will lead to an assay which is insensitive and inaccurate at low factor levels.

Standards

Any assay is, of course, valueless unless the standard against which samples are compared is satisfactory in every way.

Identification of a clotting factor deficiency

In the laboratory investigation of a patient with a suspected coagulation defect it is very difficult to define a series of tests and assays which can be justified logically. In view of the lack of sensitivity of even the best preliminary or general tests of the coagulation system it is impossible, on the basis of these tests alone, to exclude a coagulation abnormality. The only sure way of excluding a clotting factor deficiency is by performing specific assays of all individual clotting factors. In practice it is seldom possible, on grounds of time and expense, to perform all assays on all patients. Indeed, the extreme rarity of most factor deficiencies would make the routine assay of all factors of questionable justification.

A very satisfactory compromise may be achieved by the routine application of a mixture of general tests and specific assays, a selection which has proved very successful being PCI, APTT, PT, qualitative test for factor XIII, VIII assay and IX assay. It must never be forgotten that the most important part of the investigation of any patient should take place before any laboratory tests are commenced. This is the evaluation of a clinical and family history of the patient, by a clinician experienced in problems of haemostasis. A positive history of bleeding cannot be negated by any number of laboratory tests—failure to explain the problem probably only underlines the limitations of test systems. In any case, where a positive bleeding history is not explained by the battery of tests suggested above, one must proceed to all other tests and assays available in order to make a diagnosis. Even the application of every general test and assays for every known clotting factor will sometimes fail to demonstrate the abnormality. Assuming the problem does not lie with platelets or tissue abnormality such instances serve only to remind one of the very limited state of knowledge which exists on the coagulation mechanisms.

REFERENCES

Austen D.E.G., Lechner K., Rizza C. & Rhymes I.L. (1982) A comparison of the Bethesda and New Oxford methods of factor VIII antibody assay. *Thrombosis and Haemostasis* **47**, 72–5.

Austen D.E.G. & Rhymes I.L. (1975) *A Laboratory Manual of Blood Coagulation.* Blackwell Scientific Publications, Oxford.

Bangham D.R. & Brozović M. (1974) Factor VIII international units and reference materials. *Thrombosis et Diathesis Haemorrhagica* **31**, 3–11.

Barrowcliffe T.W. & Kirkwood T.B.L. (1980) Standardisation of Factor VIII. Calibration of British standards for Factor VIII clotting activity. *British Journal of Haematology* **46**, 471–81.

Bartlett A., Dormandy K.M., Hawkey C.M., Stableforth P. & Voller A. (1976) Factor-VIII-related antigen: measurement by enzyme immunoassay. *British Medical Journal* **I**, 994–6.

Biggs R., Austen D.E.G., Denson K.W.E., Borrett R. & Rizza C.R. (1972a) The mode of action of antibodies which destroy factor VIII. II. Antibodies which give complex concentration graphs. *British Journal of Haematology* **23**, 137–55.

Biggs R., Austen D.E.G., Denson K.W.E., Rizza C.R. & Borrett R. (1972b) The mode of action of antibodies which destroy factor VIII. I. Antibodies which have second-order concentration graphs. *British Journal of Haematology* **23**, 125–35.

Biggs R. & Bidwell E. (1959) A method for the study of antihaemophilic globulin inhibitor with reference to six cases. *British Journal of Haematology* **5**, 379–95.

Biggs R., Denson K.W.E., Akman N., Borrett R. & Haddon M. (1970) Antithrombin III, antifactor Xa and heparin. *British Journal of Haematology* **19**, 283–305.

Biggs R. & Douglas A.S. (1953a) The measurement of prothrombin in plasma. *Journal of Clinical Pathology* **6**, 15–22.

Biggs R. & Douglas A.S. (1953b) The thromboplastin generation test. *Journal of Clinical Pathology* **6**, 23–9.

Bird P. (1975) Coagulation in agarose gels and its application to the detection and measurement of factor VIII antibodies. *British Journal of Haematology* **29**, 329–40.

Brozović M., Kirkwood T.B.L. & Robertson I. (1976) Study of a proposed international standard for blood coagulation factor IX. *Thrombosis and Haemostasis* **35**, 222–36.

Clauss A. (1957) Gerrinnungs-physiologische schnell method zur bestimmung des fibrinogens. *Acta Haematologica* **17**, 237–46.

Colman R.W., Bagdasarian A., Talamo R., Seavey M., Scott C.R. & Kaplan A. (1975) Williams' Trait: combined deficiency of plasma plasminogen proactivation, kininogen and a new procoagulant factor. *Federation Proceedings* **34**, 859.

Denson K.W.E. (1961a) The specific assay of Prower-Stuart factor and factor VII. *Acta Haemotologica* **25**, 105–20.

Denson K.W.E. (1967) The simplified two-stage assay for factor VIII using a combined reagent. Transactions of the International Committee on Haemostasis and Thrombosis. Chapel Hill, North Carolina, USA, December 1966. *Thrombosis et Diathesis Haemorrhagica* (Suppl.) **26**, 419–21.

Denson K.W.E. (1971) International and national standardisation of control of anticoagulant therapy in patients receiving coumarin and indanedione drugs with calibrated thromboplastin preparations. *Journal of Clinical Pathology* **24**, 460–3.

Denson K.W.E., Biggs R. & Mannucci P.M. (1968) An investigation of three patients with Christmas disease due to an abnormal type of factor IX. *Journal of Clinical Pathology* **21**, 160–5.

Denson K.W.E. & Bonnar J. (1973) The measurement of heparin. A method based on the potentiation of anti-factor Xa. *Thrombosis et Diathesis Haemorrhagica* **30**, 471–9.

Denson K.W.E., Borrett R. & Biggs R. (1971) The specific assay of prothrombin using the Taipan snake venom. *British Journal of Haematology* **21**, 219–26.

Evans R.J. & Austen D.E.G. (1977) Assay of ristocetin cofactor using fixed platelets and a platelet counting technique. *British Journal of Haematology* **37**, 289–94.

Funk C., Gmür J., Herold R. & Straub P.W. (1971) Reptilase-R—A new reagent in blood coagulation. *British Journal of Haematology* **21**, 43–52.

Ganrot P.O. (1972) Crossed immunoelectrophoresis. *Scandinavian Journal of Clinical and Laboratory Investigation* **29** (Suppl. 124), 39–47.

Hills A.M. & Ingram G.I.C. (1973) Monitoring successive batches of British Comparative Thromboplastin. *British Journal of Haematology* **25**, 445–51.

Hougie C., McPherson R.A. & Aronson L. (1975) Passavoy factor: A hitherto unrecognised factor necessary for haemostasis. *Lancet* **II**, 290–1.

Hoyer L.W. (1972) Immunologic studies of antihaemophilic factor (AHF, factor VIII). IV. Radioimmunoassay of A.H.F. antigen. *Journal of Laboratory and Clinical Medicine* **80**, 822–33.

Ingram G.I.C., Schmidt R.M., Eiler R.J., Loeliger E.A., Miale J.B. & Hills A.M. (1979)

Prothrombin time standardisation: Report of the expert panel on oral anticoagulant control. *Thrombosis and Haemostasis* **42**, 1073–114.

Kasper C.K., Aledort L.M., Counts R.B., Edson J.R., Fratantoni J., Green D., Hampton J.W., Hilgartner M.W., Lazerson J., Levine P.H., McMillan C.W., Pool J.G., Shapiro S.S., Sulman N.R. & van Eys J. (1975) A more uniform measurement of factor VIII inhibitors. *Thrombosis et Diathesis Haemorrhagica* **34**, 869–72.

Kirkwood T.B.L. & Snape T.J. (1980) Biometric principles of clotting and clot lysis assays. *Clinical and Laboratory Haematology* **2**, 155–67.

Lacombe M.-J., Varet B. & Levy J.-P. (1975) A hitherto undescribed plasma factor acting at the contact phase of blood coagulation (Flaujeac factor): Case report and coagulation studies. *Blood* **46**, 761–8.

Lane J.L., Bird P. & Rizza C.R. (1975) A new assay for the measurement of total progressive antithrombin. *British Journal of Haematology* **30**, 103–15.

Laurell C.-B. (1972) Electroimmuno Assay. *Scandinavian Journal of Clinical and Laboratory Investigation* **29** (Suppl. 124), 21–37.

Lazarchick J. & Hoyer L.W. (1978) Immunoradiometric measurement of the factor VIII procoagulant antigen. *Journal of Clinical Investigation* **62**, 1048–52.

Loeliger E.A. & van Halam Visser L.P. (1979) Biological properties of the thromboplastins and plasmas included in the ICTH/ICSH collaborative study on prothrombin times. *Thrombosis and Haemostasis* **42**, 1115–27.

Lorand L., Urayama T. & de Kiewret J. (1969) Diagnostic and genetic studies on fibrin stabilizing factor with a new assay based on amine incorporation. *Journal of Clinical Investigation* **48**, 1054–64.

Macfarlane R.G. & Biggs R. (1953) A thrombin generation test. *Journal of Clinical Pathology* **6**, 3–8.

McLellan D.S., Devlin J.D., Groom P. & Aronstam A. (1981) A radial immunodiffusion method for the assay of factor VIII:C antigen (VIII:CAg) in plasma. *British Journal of Haematology* **47**, 295–305.

Meyer D., Bidwell E. & Larrieu M.J. (1972) Cross-reacting material in genetic variants of haemophilia B. *Journal of Clinical Pathology* **25**, 433–6.

Meyer D., Lavergne J.-M., Larrieu M.-J. & Josso F. (1972) Cross-reacting material in congenital factor VIII deficiency. *Thrombosis Research* **1**, 183–95.

O'Brien P.F., North W.R.S. & Ingram G.I.C. (1981) The diagnosis of mild haemophilia by the partial thromboplastin time test. WFH/ICTH study of the Manchester method. *Thrombosis and Haemostasis* **45**, 162–8.

Ødegård O.R. & Abildgaard U. (1978) Antithrombin III: Critical review of assay methods. Significance of variation in health and disease. *Haemostasis* **7**, 127.

Peake I.R. & Bloom A.L. (1977) The use of an immunoradiometric assay for factor VIII related antigen in the study of atypical von Willebrand's disease. *Thrombosis Research* **10**, 27–32.

Peake I.R. & Bloom A.L. (1978) An immunoradiometric assay of procoagulant factor VIII antigen in plasma and serum and its reduction in haemophilia. *Lancet* **I**, 473–5.

Peake I.R., Bloom A.L., Giddings J.C. & Ludlam C.A. (1979) An immunoradiometric assay for procoagulant factor VIII antigen: Results in haemophilia, von Willebrand's disease and fetal plasma and serum. *British Journal of Haematology* **42**, 269–81.

Poller L. (1964) The standardisation of anticoagulant treatment. *British Medical Journal* **II**, 565–6.

Poller L. (1967) A national standard for anticoagulant therapy. The Manchester Comparative Reagent. *Lancet* I, 491–3.

Proctor R.R. & Rapaport S.I. (1961) A partial thromboplastin time with kaolin. A simple screening test for first stage plasma clotting factor deficiencies. *American Journal of Clinical Pathology* **36**, 212–19.

Rainsford S.G. & Hall A. (1976) Detection and measurement of factor VIII antibodies in an agarose gel: a modified method. *British Journal of Haematology* **33**, 309.

Rizza C.R. & Biggs R. (1973) The treatment of patients who have factor-VIII antibodies. *British Journal of Haematology* **24**, 65–82.

Saito J., Ratnoff O.D., Waldmann R. & Abraham J.P. (1975) Fitzgerald trait. *Journal of Clinical Investigation* **55**, 1082–9.

Sen N.N., Sen R., Denson K.W.E. & Biggs R. (1967) A modified method for the assay of factor IX. *Thrombosis and Diathesis Haemorrhagica* **18**, 241–51.

Suomela H. (1975) Multiple forms of human factor IX in chromatography and isoelectric focussing. *Thrombosis Research* **7**, 101–12.

Varley H. (1967) *Practical Clinical Biochemistry*, p. 236. Heinemann Medical Books, London.

Weiss H.J., Hoyer L.W., Rickles F.R., Varma A. & Rogers J. (1973) Quantitative assay of a plasma factor deficient in von Willebrand's disease that is necessary for platelet aggregation. *Journal of Clinical Investigation* **52**, 2708–16.

Wuepper K.D. (1973) Prekallikrein deficiency in man. *Journal of Experimental Medicine* **138**, 1345–55.

Zimmerman T.S., Hoyer L.W., Dickson L. & Edgington T.S. (1975) Determination of the von Willebrand's disease antigen (factor VIII-related antigen) in plasma by quantitative immunoelectrophoresis. *Journal of Laboratory and Clinical Medicine* **86**, 152–9.

Zimmerman T.S., Ratnoff O.D. & Howell A.E. (1971) Immunologic differentiation of classic hemophilia (Factor VIII deficiency) and von Willebrand's disease. *Journal of Clinical Investigation* **50**, 245–54.

Chapter 10
Antibodies to Factor VIII Clotting Activity (VIII:C)

R. BIGGS

Antibodies directed against VIII:C arise in two classes of patients; one is that of the severely affected haemophilia A patient for whom VIII:C is presumably a foreign protein and antigenic. The second class of patients consists of a miscellaneous group of previously normal people, mainly elderly, some of whom have evidence of autoimmune disease. The antibody may also occur in pregnant women after delivery. In a review of non-haemophilic patients who developed antibodies, Lechner (1974) lists 87 such cases of which 21 followed pregnancy and 66 were of unspecified aetiology. In 1981, Green and Lechner extended this list. It is proposed first to consider the antibodies of haemophilia A patients since these are the most numerous and raise most of the difficult problems in treatment.

Anti-VIII:C antibodies in haemophilia A

Biggs (1974), Biggs and Spooner (1977) and Rizza and Spooner (1983) record that about 6 per cent of haemophilia A patients have anti-VIII:C antibodies. A similar figure is noted by Brinkhous, Roberts and Weiss (1972) and Sultan and Maisonneuve (1977). In an interesting paper, Mayer *et al.* (1969) report a much higher incidence of anti-VIII:C antibodies (about 40 per cent). This high incidence is probably due to the fact that Mayer and his colleagues made a systematic study of the blood ten days after factor VIII infusions in all patients who failed to have the expected post-infusion rise in blood factor VIII levels. Many of these antibodies were transient. A study continued over 12 years in Oxford (started by Biggs 1974) from 1969 to 1981 has not shown any tendency for the proportion of patients having antibodies to increase and this is despite increase in the amount and frequency of treatment. On the other hand, Ikkala and Simonen (1971) report an incidence of 12 per cent of antibody cases in Finland and they attribute this high incidence to increased treatment.

In considering anti-VIII:C antibodies, the following topics will be discussed:

1 What sort of protein is factor VIII?
2 What sort of protein is the anti-VIII:C antibody?

3   How do VIII:C and antibody react together and how can anti-VIII:C antibody be measured?

4   Do haemophilia A patients have an abnormal protein which replaces factor VIII?

5   Why is transfused VIII:C antigenic for some haemophilia A patients, and is the tendency to form antibodies genetically controlled?

6   Do haemophilia A patients make antibodies to sites on the factor VIII molecule other than VIII:C?

7   What is the natural history of anti-VIII:C antibodies in haemophilia A patients?

8   How can haemophilia A patients who have anti-VIII:C antibodies best be treated?

What sort of protein is factor VIII?

Factor VIII is known to be a highly complex protein of high molecular weight (Austen 1978, 1979). The VIII:C component of factor VIII is essential for normal coagulation; it probably acts as a cofactor in the middle of the chain of intrinsic clotting reactions preceding the activation of factor X and of thrombin formation.

The VIII:C activity is associated with other activities, the principal ones being factor VIII-related antigen and the ristocetin cofactor (VIIIR:Ag and VIIIR:WF (RCF)). There are two less well-defined activities which may well be associated with the same chemical substance; the activity which affects the bleeding time (VIIIR:VW (BT)) and that which affects the adhesion of platelets to glass beads (VIIIR:VW (GB)). These factors are discussed in detail by Nilsson and Holmberg (1979). The properties of the various activities are listed in Table 12.

VIIIR:Ag can be detected and measured immunologically by the Laurell (1966) method using an antibody to human factor VIII raised in rabbits. This activity (VIIIR:Ag) is reduced or absent in the blood of von Willebrand's disease patients but normal or raised in amount in haemophilia A patients (Bennett, Ratnoff and Levin 1972). The protein has properties which distinguish it sharply from VIII:C. It is stable on storage, present in serum and in haemophilic blood. The ristocetin and bleeding time activities may be associated with this substance. It is probable that VIII:C is an antigenically distinct group attached to the factor VIIIR:Ag. All of these activities are referred to as 'factor-VIII-related'. Factor VIII-related antigen can be detected by immunofluorescence on the surfaces of endothelial cells and platelets. Rarely, antibodies directed against factor VIII-related activities may occur in von Willebrand's disease patients following infusion of these patients with preparations containing factor VIII.

Table 12. The properties of factor VIII:C and its related activities.

| | Activity | | | | |
	VIII:C	VIII:CAg	VIIIR:Ag	VIIIR:WF (RCF)	VIIIR:WF (BT & GB)
Presence in normal plasma	+	+	+	+	+
Presence in normal serum	−	+	+	+	+
Presence in haemophilic plasma	−	−	+	+	+
Presence in von Willebrand plasma	±	±	±	±	±
Presence in stored normal plasma	±	+	+	+	+
Presence in endothelial cells	−	?+	+	+	+
Presence on platelet granules	−	?	+	+	+

VIII:C is usually measured through its clotting activity though an immunological activity (VIII:C antigen, VIII:CAg) associated with the clotting activity can also be measured in the way described below. The absolute amount of factor VIII in normal plasma is not known and it is probably very small since purification procedures which produce activities of factor VIII of 1000 iu/mg of protein are still impure in terms of their content of other known plasma constituents such as fibrinogen. The activity of VIII:C is expressed in u/ml in terms of an International Standard which attempts to approximate 1 unit to the activity contained in 1 ml of 'average' normal plasma (Bangham *et al.* 1971).

The whole factor VIII molecule (comprising all its activities) consists of a number of subunits which may be separated following treatment of the protein with solutions of different ionic strength and gel filtration. Using ultra-centrifuge techniques it can be shown that the diffusion coefficient decreases with ionic strength. A molecule with a molecular weight of several millions composed of subunits might well be expected to have at least one VIII:C antigenic site on every subunit. A list of possible subunit sizes for parts of factor VIII is given in Table 13. The present chapter concerns only those antibodies which are directed to VIII:C and, as will be discussed below, it seems that, contrary to expectation, the factor VIII molecule does not have numerous VIII:C antigenic sites despite its complex subunit structure.

What sort of protein is the anti-VIII:C antibody?

In recent years the purification of anti-VIII:C antibodies has been improved. Using column chromatography and isoelectric focussing (Hultin *et al.* 1977) it has been found that the main constituents of most anti-VIII:C antibodies are IgG proteins. Of 45 cases studied by Shapiro (1978) 43 were IgG, one was IgA and one was IgM. The light chains were kappa in 28 cases and lambda in 4 cases and mixed in 11 cases. Hultin *et al.* (1977) record similar results. The heavy chain components were IgG3 and IgG4 in all cases studied.

Normal IgG is made up of molecules with both kappa and lambda light chains. There are usually in normal people about 65 per cent of molecules with kappa light chains and 35 per cent of lambda light chains. The restriction of the anti-VIII:C antibodies to one light chain type in any particular patient may suggest that relatively few classes of antibody-producing cells are responsible for antibody production. Other reports of the molecular constitution of the anti-VIII:C antibodies are given by Shapiro (1967), Strauss and Merler (1967), Feinstein, Rapaport and Chong (1969), Lavergne, Meyer and Reisner (1976), Lee, Tucker and Allain (1979) and Kavanagh, Wood and Davidson 1981.

Table 13. The subunit sizes of factor VIII:C from Austen (1978).

Subunit size	Reagent used	Reference
Comparable to albumin	0.4–1.65 M-NaCl	Thelin & Wagner 1961
Comparable to fibrinogen	1.0 M-NaCl	Weiss & Kochwa 1970
100 000–150 000	Succinic anhydride/Mn^{2+}	Barrow & Graham 1972
25 000–100 000	0.25 M-CaCl$_2$	Owen & Wagner 1972
169 000–194 000	1.0 M-NaCl	Weiss, Phillips & Rosner 1972
100 000	0.25 M-CaCl$_2$	Griggs *et al.* 1973
Between fibrinogen and albumin	1 M-NaCl	Rick & Hoyer 1973
230 000	1.3 M-NaCl$_2$ to 3 × 10^{-4}M-dithiothreitol	Austen 1974
690 000	Sodium periodate	Kaelin 1975

Papain digestion of antibody separates the protein molecule into three parts: two are univalent 'Fab' fragments both of which can unite with antigenic sites and the third consists mainly of heavy chain parts (Fc fragments) which do not unite with antigen directly (Strauss and Merler 1967, Roitt 1980). Pepsin digestion separates the antibody molecule into two parts, one of which is a divalent 'Fab' part which unites with antigen and the second, the Fc fragment which does not unite with antigens (Fig. 27). The main kinetic difference usually found between papain-digested antibody and whole antibody or pepsin-digested antibody is that whereas the pepsin-digested antibody and whole antibody can form precipitates when mixed with antigen, the univalent (papain-digested) antibody does not form precipitates. Since the undigested anti-VIII:C antibody does not form a visible precipitate with VIII:C

(a) Papain digestion of antibody

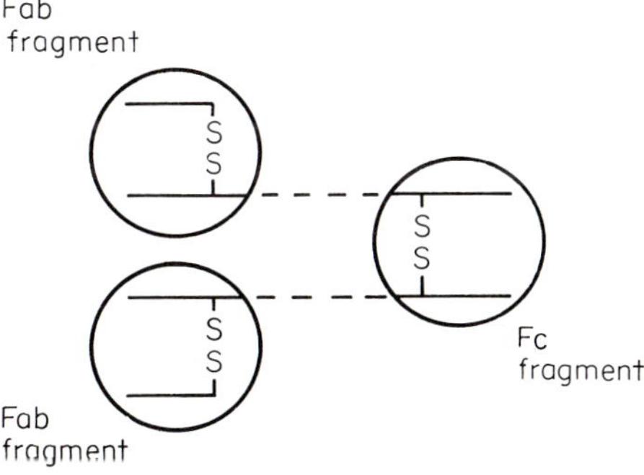

(b) Pepsin digestion of antibody

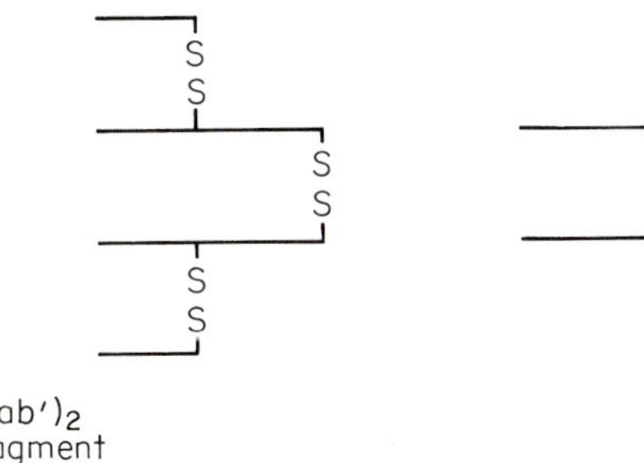

Fig. 27. The effects of papain digestion (a) and pepsin digestion (b) on the structure of antibodies.

the action of the digested anti-VIII:C antibody does not differ from that of the whole antibody in this respect.

How do VIII:C and anti-VIII:C antibody react together and how can anti-VIII:C antibody be measured?

Biggs and Bidwell (1959) studied the disappearance of factor VIII activity in mixtures of VIII:C and anti-VIII:C antibody. It was found that the destruction of factor VIII:C followed a regular pattern. When VIII:C and anti-VIII:C were incubated together the amount of residual VIII:C was proportional to the time of incubation of the mixture (Fig. 28a). The experiment was performed by incubating VIII:C and anti-VIII:C, removing samples at intervals and measuring the amount of residual factor VIII:C. The graph illustrating this type of experiment is called a time course graph (Fig. 28). When antibody was

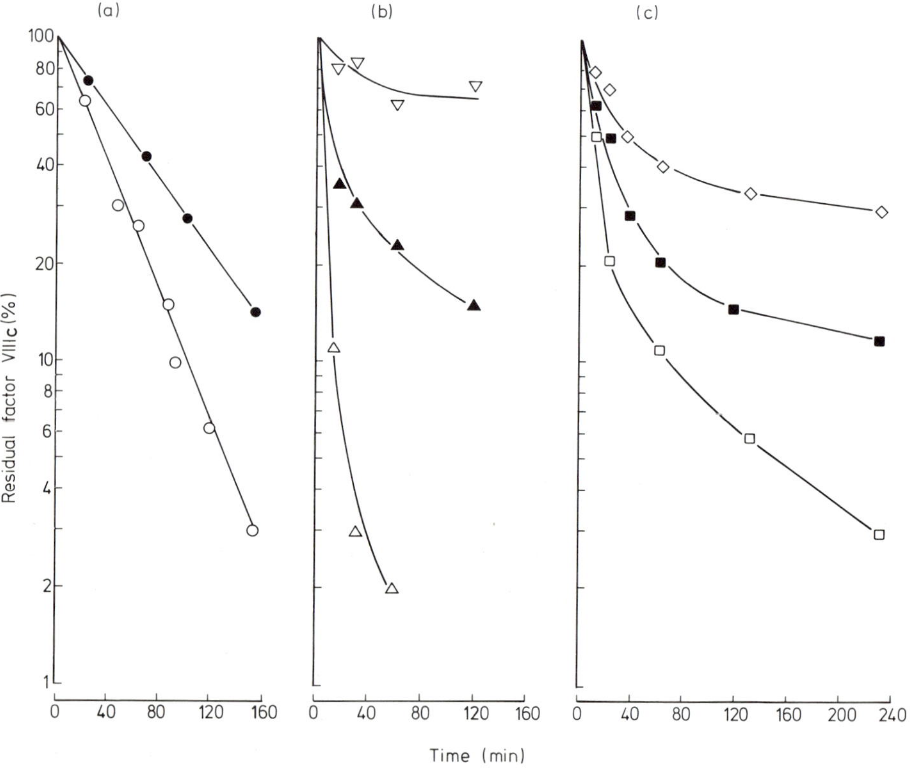

Fig. 28. Time course graphs for the destruction of VIII:C by three anti-VIII:C antibodies using two dilutions of antibody (a) and three dilutions each of antibodies (b) and (c).

present in excess the proportion of the initial factor VIII left after a given time was independent of the initial factor VIII:C concentration. In other experiments different antibody concentrations were incubated with factor VIII:C for a constant time and it was found that the amount of VIII:C destroyed was proportional to the initial antibody concentration. These and other experiments suggested that the interaction of VIII:C and anti-VIII:C (Ab) was of the type:

$$\text{VIII:C} + \text{Ab} \underset{k_2}{\overset{k_1}{\rightleftharpoons}} \text{VIII:CAb}$$

If Ab were present in excess and its concentration did not decrease appreciably during the reaction then the reaction could be written:

$$K = \frac{1}{t\text{Ab}} \log \frac{100}{\text{VIIIR}}$$

where t is the time of incubation and VIIIR is the residual VIII:C activity after time t. Under these conditions, if t is constant then the log of VIIIR will theoretically be inversely related to Ab concentration when mixtures containing varying amounts of Ab are tested, and the measurement of antibody should be independent of factor VIII concentration. This relationship (Fig. 29) was used by Biggs and Bidwell (1959) as the basis for measuring antibody activity. They defined 1 unit of antibody as that amount of antibody which would destroy 75 per cent of the initial VIII:C activity in 1 hour. It should be noted that the results in other centres could never give the same number of 'units' for a particular mixture as those in Oxford if exactly the same definition of the unit was not used. Despite this limitation the method did, for a time, provide useful local assays often reasonably consistent within one centre. Biggs and Bidwell (1959) used one particular sample of anti-VIII:C antibody in most of their experiments and they used bovine or porcine factor VIII as a source of VIII:C. As more samples of antibody were tested by this method, and as human factor VIII became more available and was used as substrate for measuring antibody, serious discrepancies from expectations based on the ideas of Biggs and Bidwell were found (Fig. 28b,c, Fig. 30). Firstly, it was found that in the time course experiments a period of rapid factor VIII destruction was often followed by a period of much slower disappearance. In part this pattern could be attributed to the fact that in most test systems antibody was usually not in excess as was assumed by Biggs and Bidwell (1959). In many cases the reaction pattern was probably due to the presence in the patient's plasma, tested for antibody, of different antibodies acting on different parts of the VIII:C site and acting at different rates and in some instances only partially destroying the factor VIII:C activity, leaving a complex of VIII:CAb with residual VIII:C activity (Biggs *et al.* 1972a,b). The altered pattern of results

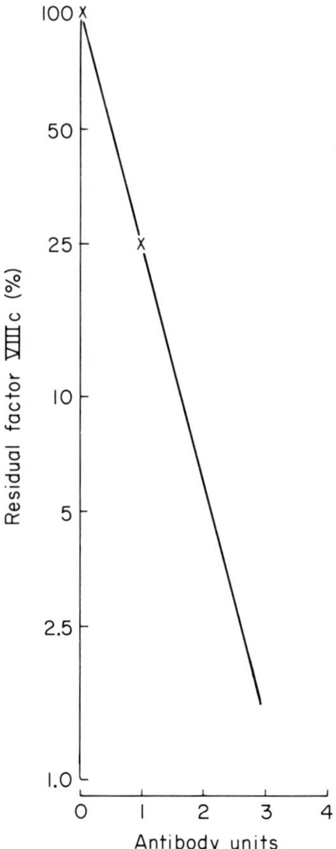

Fig. 29. Calibration graph relating logarithm of residual factor VIII to anti-VIII:C antibody concentration using the method of Biggs and Bidwell (1959).

which these deviations from second order kinetics produce are illustrated in Figs 28 and 30. In Fig. 28c it will be seen that in the time course graph a rapid initial destruction of factor VIII:C (suggesting a high antibody concentration) may be followed by a fairly sharp reduction in the speed of destruction. In this phase of slow destruction the VIII:C activity (presumably in the form VIII:CAb) remains and in the patient, may be sufficient in quantity to produce haemostasis after injury. Some previously normal patients who have acquired anti-VIII:C antibodies, always have low but recordable levels of factor VIII:C in the presence of a powerful anti-VIII:C antibody which destroys factor VIII when this is added to the patient's blood (Biggs, Denson and Nossel 1964). Presumably, the VIII:C activity in their blood is all in the form VIII:CAb.

In Fig. 30 several dilutions of five antibodies have been tested after a

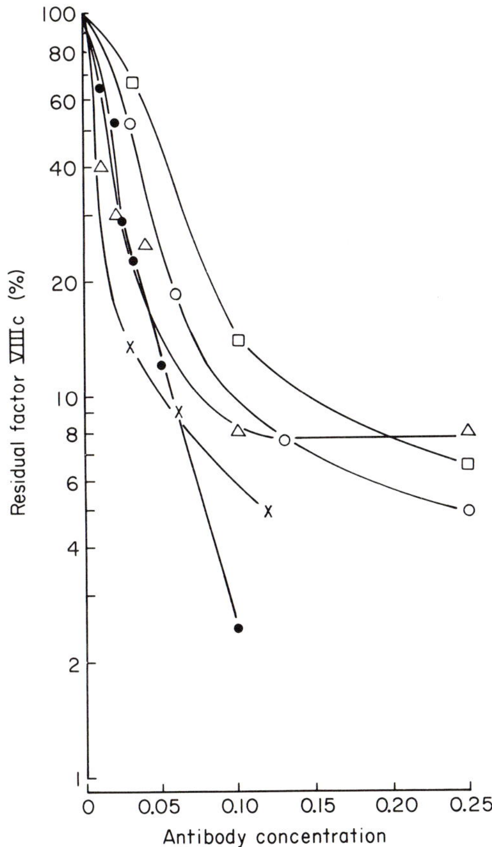

Fig. 30. Graph relating logarithm of residual factor VIII to anti-VIII:C antibody concentration for five different antibodies. In one case only (●—●) was the relationship linear as in Fig. 29.

constant incubation time and it will be seen that the logarithm of residual factor VIII:C is not linearly related to antibody concentration in four of five samples tested. Clearly, the unit of Biggs and Bidwell (1959) cannot be used to characterize this type of antibody (compare Figs 29 and 30).

From Fig. 28 (time course graphs) it will be seen that the initial fall in VIII:C concentration which occurs in mixtures of VIII:C and Ab occurs immediately after the start of incubation. Between the levels of 100 and 50 per cent of residual factor VIII:C there seems to be a reasonable linear relationship between the rate of VIII:C disappearance and antibody concentration. The immediate fall in VIII:C activity means that 1 antibody molecule is enough to neutralize 1 factor VIII:C antigenic site (Dulbecco, Vogt and Strickland 1956). Since the kinetics of VIII:C destruction seem to be most predictable in

conditions of antigen excess rather than antibody excess (as first assumed by
Biggs and Bidwell 1959), Rizza and Biggs (1973) decided to base a new unit of
antibody on a different definition. They defined the anti-VIII:C unit as that
amount of antibody which would destroy 0.5 units of VIII:C (in a mixture
initially containing 1 unit) after four hours of incubation. When antibody is
not in excess the absolute amount of factor VIII used in the test system must be
measured, since VIII:C must now be taken into account in calculating the
amount of antibody present. It will also be noted that, as before, alterations in
the definition (amount of VIII:C or time of incubation) will necessarily alter the
unit substantially.

Most antigen–antibody reactions are reversible. Biggs *et al.* 1972a were
unable to demonstrate reversibility in the reaction between VIII:C and Ab.
Allain and Frommel (1973) could recover antibody by heating antigen–antibody complexes to 37°C at pH 4.2. It may be that only those reactions with

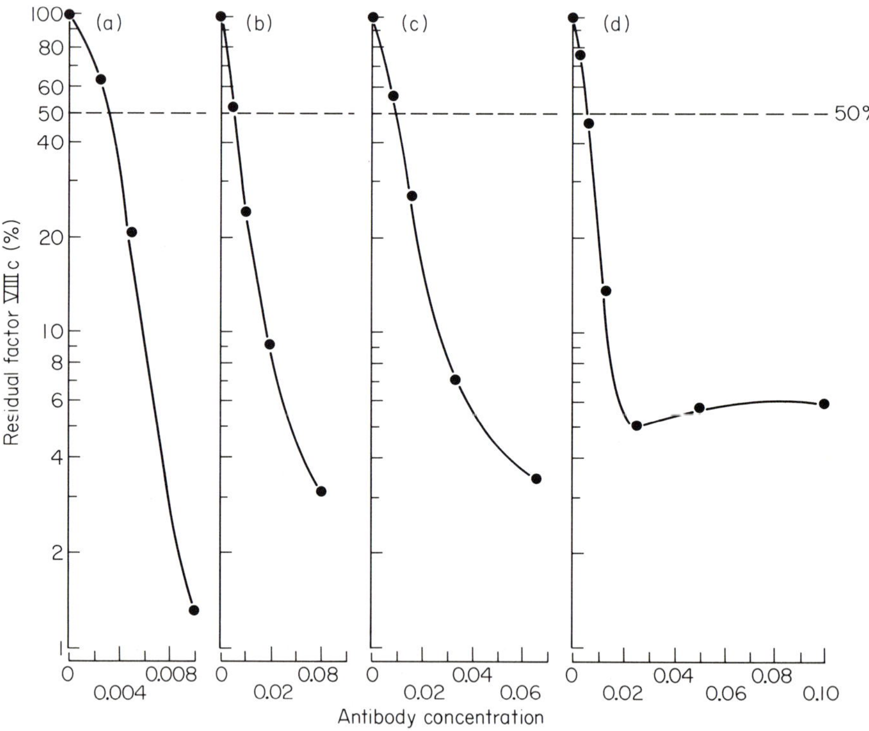

Fig. 31. Graphs illustrating the method of measuring antibody concentration for four
different antibodies (a–d) by the method of Rizza and Biggs (1973). The anti-VIII:C
antibody concentration is related to the concentration of whole plasma which is
taken to be 1.0. (See also Table 14.)

high avidity of Ab for VIII:C are demonstrated by the methods used by Biggs *et al.* (1972a,b).

In carrying out the assay of Rizza and Biggs, several dilutions of antibody are each mixed with a measured amount of factor VIII:C. The mixtures are incubated for four hours and the amounts of residual factor VIII:C are measured. The concentrations of antibody in the mixtures must be so arranged that at least one mixture gives results for residual factor VIII:C of between 20 and 60 per cent of the initial concentration (i.e. factor VIII:C is present in excess). The logarithm of residual factor VIII is plotted against antibody concentration and the amount of antibody required to produce 50 per cent destruction of the initial factor VIII is determined by interpolation. A correction is made (if necessary) for the recorded deviation of the initial factor VIII:C concentration from 1 u/ml. An example of the method is given in Fig. 31 and Table 14.

Table 14. The assay of anti-VIII:C antibody by the method of Rizza and Biggs (1973) (see also Fig. 31).

Plasma sample	Conc. Ab (whole plasma = 1)	VIII:C u/ml	Residual VIII:C %	Conc. Ab giving 50% residual VIII:C	Ab u/ml
1(a)	0.01		1.3		$\frac{2.5}{0.003}$
	0.005	2.5	21.0	0.0030	
	0.0025		63.0		= 833
2(b)	0.04		3.1		$\frac{0.46}{0.005}$
	0.02		9.1		
	0.01	0.46	23.8	0.005	= 92
	0.005		51.5		
3(c)	0.066		3.4		
	0.033		7.1		$\frac{1}{0.0085}$
	0.016	1.0	27.0	0.0085	
	0.008		56.0		= 118
	0.004		80.0		
4(d)	0.10		6.0		
	0.05		5.7		
	0.025		5.1		$\frac{1}{0.005}$
	0.0125	1.0	13.5	0.005	
	0.0062		46.0		= 200
	0.0031		76.0		

Do haemophilia A patients have an abnormal protein which replaces normal factor VIII:C?

If some haemophilia A patients lack the whole factor VIII:C antigen and some have an abnormal antigen, then it might be expected that those with no antigen might be more liable to regard the normal VIII:C antigen as foreign than those whose blood contained an abnormal antigen. For this reason a good deal of scientific effort has been expended on the attempt to divide haemophilia A patients into two groups in one of which the patients have antigen and in the other they do not. One method was to measure the amount of anti-VIII:C antibody that could be absorbed by normal and haemophilia A

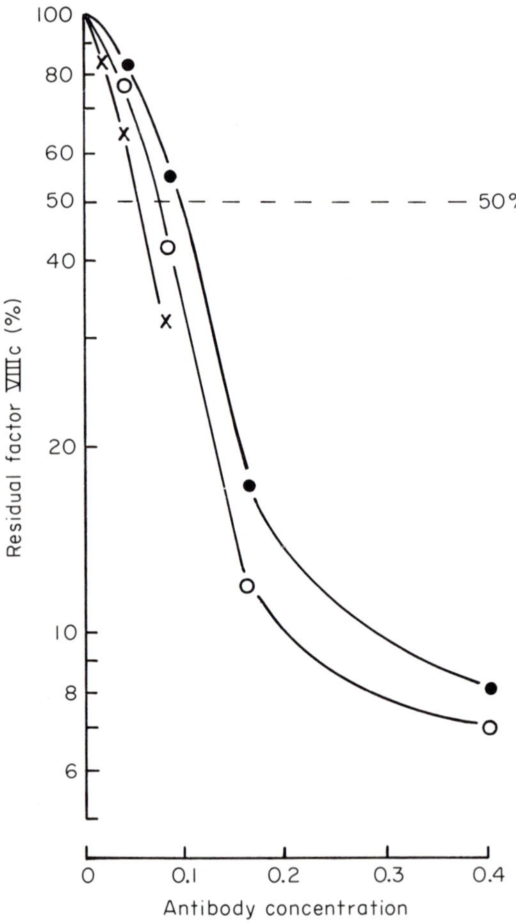

Fig. 32. Graph showing the measurement of anti-VIII:C antibody in an experiment to demonstrate absorption of anti-VIII:C antibody by VIII:C. (See also Table 15.)

patients' plasma samples. Measured amounts of antibody and VIII:C were mixed and incubated together, the amount of residual antibody after incubation measured, and the amount absorbed then obtained by subtraction. A protein similar to factor VIII:C but lacking activity might also absorb antibody. More recently, a method for measuring factor VIII:C antigen using radio-iodine labelled antibody has been described (Lazarchick and Hoyer 1978, Peake and Bloom 1978, Girma *et al.* 1981).

The method of measuring antibody by absorption is illustrated in Fig. 32 and Table 15. Factor VIII:C is incubated with a large excess of antibody. When all antibody that can attach to factor VIII:C is attached, the residual antibody is measured by dilution and addition of an excess of factor VIII:C. The practical difficulty of the method applied to factor VIII:C antibody has been discussed by Pool, Biggs and Miller (1976). The difficulty lies in the inaccuracy in measuring small differences in antibody concentration. If each antigen

Table 15. The absorption of anti-VIII:C by VIII:C (from Pool, Biggs and Miller 1976) (see also Fig. 32).

Experiment	Conc. anti-VIII:C tested	VIII:R %	Conc. anti-VIII:C giving 50% VIII:R	Anti-VIII:C u/ml
Anti-VIII:C not absorbed (control)	0.08 0.04 0.016	32 64 84	0.055	$\dfrac{1.07}{0.055} = 19.5$
Anti-VIII:C absorbed with 1.08 u/ml VIII:C	0.4 0.16 0.08 0.04	7 12 42 77	0.071	$\dfrac{1.07}{0.071} = 15.1$
Anti-VIII:C absorbed with 2.17 u/ml VIII:C	0.4 0.16 0.08 0.04	8 17 55 81	0.090	$\dfrac{1.07}{0.090} = 11.9$

In this experiment the concentration of VIII:C used to measure the antibody concentration was 1.07 u/ml. The antibody absorbed by 1 u/ml VIII:C was $19.5 - 15.1/1.08 = 4.07$ u/ml in the first experiment and $19.5 - 11.9/2.17 = 3.50$ u/ml in the second experiment. (See the first column for VIII:C concentrations used for absorption and the last column for the VIII:C concentration used to measure antibody level.)

molecule can absorb a large number of antibody molecules it follows that the difference between absorbed and unabsorbed antibody levels will be large. If, on the other hand, few antibody molecules are absorbed then the difference will be small. In the case of anti-VIII:C antibody each normal antigen molecule seems able to absorb 2–4 antibody molecules (Pool, Biggs and Miller 1976). The method is successfully applied to virus particles where this difficulty is not encountered since each virus particle has many sites for antibody attachment (Dulbecco, Vogt and Strickland 1956).

From Fig. 32 it will be clear that small differences in antibody cannot easily be measured. An experiment using different factor VIII:C levels and rabbit anti-VIII:C is recorded in Table 16. In this experiment only three of the results are from experiments in which antibody was in excess in the absorption stage and thus the difference in antibody level before and after absorption was large enough to measure reliably.

The results of several experiments shown in Table 17 give the number of sites for antibody attachment for human factor VIII:C and naturally occurring anibody as 2–3 and the number of sites for rabbit antibody as 4.5 to 5.5 (Pool, Biggs and Miller 1976). Recorded as 'units' of antibody absorbed per unit of factor VIII:C used for absorption then 1 unit of normal human factor VIII:C will absorb 3.5–4.0 units of antibody when factor VIII:C is mixed with an

Table 16. Experiments to record the amount of antibody absorbed per unit of VIII:C. Rabbit antibody and human VIII:C were used (Kernoff 1974).

F.VIII:C u/ml in absorption	Number of observations	Residual Ab u/ml	Absorbed Ab u/ml	Ab units absorbed per unit VIII:C
0	9	20.1	0	—
0.09	7	19.3	0.08	8.8
0.36	6	17.1	3.0	8.3
0.71	4	14.6	5.5	7.7
1.42	3	10.5	9.6	6.8
2.82	3	5.5	14.6	5.2
4.26	3	2.9	17.2	4.0
5.70	3	1.5	18.6	3.3

In the first series of experiments too little F.VIII:C (0.09 u/ml) was used for accurate measurement. In the last three series of experiments the amount of F.VIII:C was too high to ensure antibody excess during absorption. For the experiments giving 8.3, 7.7 and 6.8 u antibody absorbed per unit of F.VIII:C the corresponding values for the number of antibody sites per molecule of factor VIII:C are 5.40, 4.98 and 4.36.

Table 17. Experiments to show the number of antibody sites per molecule of F.VIII:C (from Pool, Biggs and Miller 1976).

Type of antibody	Type of VIII:C	Number of observations	Ab units per unit VIII:C	Number of Ab sites per molecule of VIII:C
Human 1	Human	8	4.62	2.85
	Bovine	6	3.83	2.29
Human 2	Human	2	4.75	2.94
	Bovine	2	2.15	1.10
Rabbit	Human	6	8.30	5.40
	Human	4	7.7	4.98
	Human	3	6.8	4.36

excess of antibody. This concept is important in the treatment of patients who have anti-VIII:C antibodies.

Using the method of absorption of antibody by haemophilia A plasma, the results obtained by different workers have been variable. Some authors found that all haemophilia A plasma samples contained a protein which neutralized anti-VIII:C antibodies (Shanberge and Gore 1957, Piper and Schreier 1964); others found no such protein in any samples (Adelson *et al.* 1963, Abildgaard *et al.* 1967, Uszynski 1966) and most observers found some haemophilia A plasma samples contained protein which would neutralize anti-VIII:C antibodies (Berglund 1962, Hoyer and Breckenridge 1968, Denson *et al.* 1969, Bennett and Huehns 1970, Gralnick, Abrell and Bagley 1971). The variability is probably due to the inherent difficulty of the method which might not have been appreciated by all workers. It seems likely that, as judged by absorption, a small proportion of haemophilia A patients have an VIII:C-type antigen capable of absorbing antibody but that the majority of patients do not have an antigen which will absorb anti-VIII:C antibody. Denson *et al.* 1969 suggested the terminology haemophilia A + and haemophilia A − to denote the presence or absence of neutralizing antigen. Hoyer and Breckenridge (1968) used the terms CRM + and CRM −.

In 1978 Peake and Bloom developed a technique for measuring an VIII:C protein (VIII:CAg) using highly specific anti-VIII:C antibody. A similar method is described by Girma *et al.* (1981) and Lazarchick and Hoyer (1978). In principle, the methods of Peake and Bloom and Girma *et al.* use polystyrene tubes on the inner surface of which unlabelled human anti-VIII:C antibody has been layered. Dilutions of plasma or other preparations to be tested are placed in the tubes and the VIII:C allowed to attach to the antibody. The tubes are then washed to remove any free antigen. Highly specific radio-labelled anti-VIII:C antibody is then added. The tubes are again washed to remove free antibody and the amount of bound reactivity measured. The method of Lazarchick and Hoyer is a fluid phase method in which radio-labelled antibody is allowed to react with factor VIII and the complexed antibody separated from unbound antibody by precipitation with ammonium sulphate. The radio-activity in the washed precipitate is then measured.

It has been found that severely affected haemophilia A patients have no detectable antigen by these methods but that mildly affected patients have variable amounts of antigen. Antigen is present in normal serum and in normal cord blood. These methods have proved useful in the diagnosis of haemophilia in the unborn fetus (see Chapter 8).

Despite the efforts put into all of this work, there seems to be no useful correlation between the tendency to develop anti-VIII:C antibodies and the presence or absence of antigen protein in haemophilia A patients.

Why is transfused VIII:C antigenic for some haemophilia A patients and is the tendency to form antibodies genetically controlled?

In 1974 Biggs studied the incidence of anti-VIII:C antibodies in families with more than one haemophilia A patient. She found that the incidence of antibodies in more than one family member was no greater than that in the general population of haemophilia A patients. Similar records were made by Cohn and Nielsen (1972) and Frommel and Allain (1977). This does not mean that genetic factors are not important—indeed, it would be surprising were they not involved. There is, however, no obvious reason why immunological response should be linked to the gene whose defect causes haemophilia A. Frommel *et al.* (1981) find no correlation between histocompatibility antigens and tendency to produce anti-VIII:C antibody. It is known that response to various antigens in animals is linked to major histocompatibility genes, high response to some antigens being linked to certain genes and high response to other antigens to different histocompatibility genes.

In addition to the complexity of the recipient's response to antigenic stimulus the antigenicity of various proteins is also highly unpredictable and much affected by circumstances. For example, the purification and concentration of the antigen used will affect the response as will also the duration of antigen in the body following injection. Antigen present in low concentration is likely to induce an antibody of high affinity. Rapid disappearance of antigen reduces the risk of antibody formation. Very high concentrations of antigen injected at frequent intervals may induce tolerance rather than immunization. Aggregated protein may be more immunogenic than a non-aggregated preparation.

On application to haemophilia A patients, when judged in terms of mg/ml, it seems likely that relatively low concentrations of VIII:C are used to treat the patients. All antibodies so far tested are high-affinity antibodies. It may be that the methods used to measure antibodies will detect only those antibodies of high affinity but it is also possible that the low concentration of the administered antigen determines this affinity. Most therapeutic materials did, until recently, contain much aggregated material and aggregated preparations are more antigenic than those which are pure. It is hoped that as more material of better purity becomes available the preparations may become less rather than more immunogenic. Better supplies may also affect the incidence of anti-VIII:C antibody by inducing tolerance to immunization in some patients as a result of frequent high dosage treatment.

Do haemophilia A patients make antibodies to sites on the factor VIII molecule other than VIII:C?

The injection of crude preparations of factor VIII is likely to induce the formation of many antibodies in addition to those active against the VIII:C antigenic site. Most of these antibodies would not be detected by tests at present used. Were the antibody directed towards a site very near the site for VIII:C activity it might well interfere with the destruction of factor VIII:C activity by known potent anti-VIII:C antibodies.

In 1977 Pool and Kaelin reported a study in which plasma samples from 26 severely affected haemophilic patients who did not have anti-VIII:C antibodies were incubated with factor VIII:C. After incubation the factor VIII:C was exposed to two potent anti-VIII:C antibodies. In no case was there any difference in the destruction of VIII:C activity between control samples and samples of VIII:C previously incubated with haemophilic plasma. Thus the incubation did not seem to alter the reactivity of factor VIII:C with antibody.

The natural history of anti-factor VIII:C antibodies

Patients differ from one another in their pattern of antibody production. A patient who has once produced antibody following treatment will usually do so again if challenged with a further intravenous injection of factor VIII:C. Usually the response is delayed for a few days but 5–7 days after treatment a rapid rise in antibody titre occurs. The level of antibody then rises logarithmi cally until a maximum is reached in 10 days to 2–3 weeks. The maximum reached is variable. In some patients, the level reaches 1000 u/ml (Fig. 33a,b) or more while in others the level seldom exceeds 20 u/ml (Table 18). In those patients who have low titre antibodies, the antibody usually disappears if

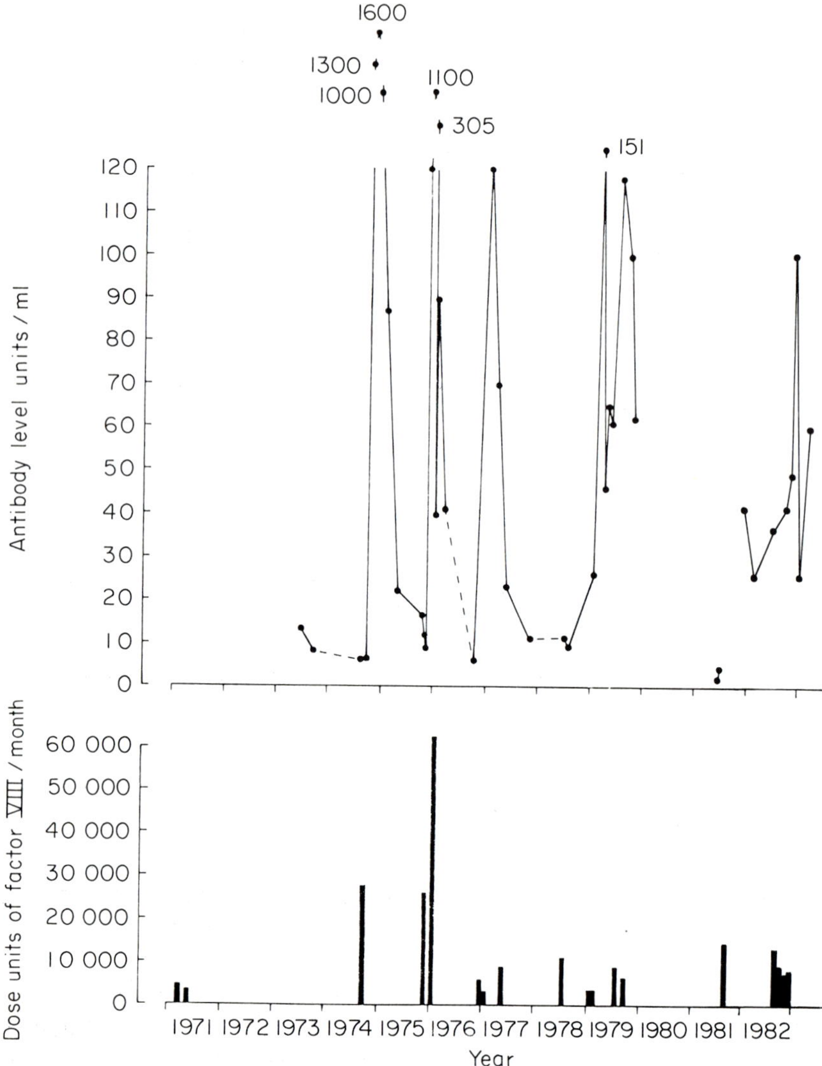

Fig. 33a. The increase and decrease in anti-VIII:C antibody concentration in a haemophilia A patient observed over periods of 11 years.

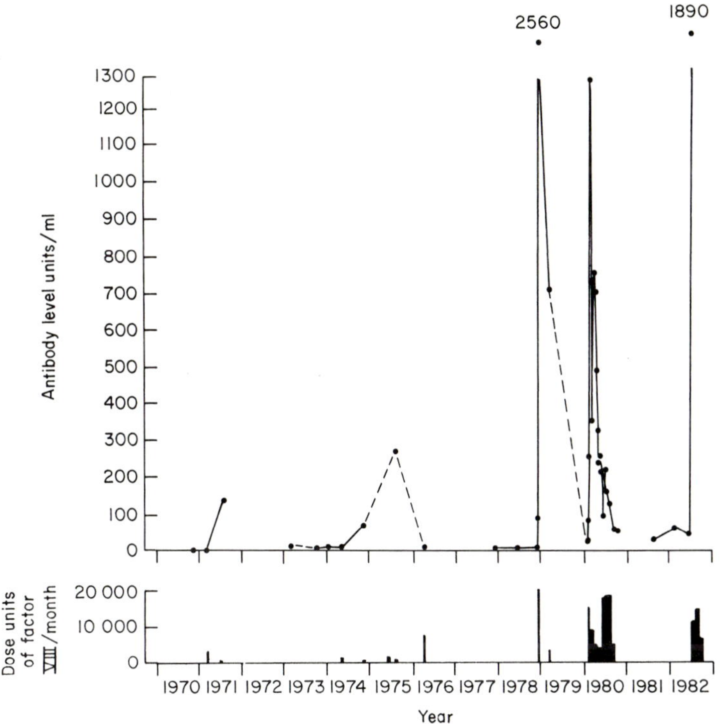

Fig. 33b. The increase and decrease in anti-VIII:C antibody in a haemophilia A patient observed over 12 years.

treatment is withheld for a period of time. The plasma of patients having high titre antibodies may have to be diluted to 1 in 1000 or even 1 in 10 000 to produce reasonably measurable levels of antibody. These high titre antibodies sometimes do not disappear completely. Having reached the maximum, they decline gradually but may remain detectable, if only at a level of a few units/ml.

The antibody levels of 30 patients having anti-VIII:C antibodies who have been treated and observed over many years are shown in Table 18. In this table the highest and lowest recorded antibody levels are listed. It will be seen that 12 patients had at some time levels above 300 u/ml: 11 had at some time levels from 22–70 u/ml and 7 had levels always below 20 u/ml.

Treatment of patients having antibodies against factor VIII:C (see also Chapter 12)

The general principles of treatment depend on rather contrary ideas: firstly, on

Table 18. The observed anti-VIII:C levels in 30 patients with haemophilia A.

Case	Lowest anti-VIII:C u/ml	Highest anti-VIII:C u/ml	Totals
1	7	1850	
2	0	485	
3	2	350	
4	10	740	
5	0	10 000	
6	4	2500	12
7	3	5560	
8	9	385	
9	9	1000	
10	0	500	
11	0	1000	
12	0	500	
13	0	33	
14	0	23	
15	0	46	
16	0	22	
17	0	68	
18	0	60	11
19	0	70	
20	3	63	
21	0	58	
22	0	58	
23	5	50	
24	1	15	
25	0	11	
26	0	1	
27	0	2	7
28	0	2	
29	0	5	
30	0	4	

preventing antibody formation by withholding treatment; secondly, on high level factor VIII:C treatment in attempt to absorb and neutralize the antibody; thirdly, on the elimination of antibody by exchange transfusion or immuno-suppressive therapy and finally on the encouragement of haemostasis despite the presence of antibody by treatment with activated prothrombin complex concentrates (which may bypass factor VIII:C) and tranexamic acid (which encourages the stability of clots).

The withholding of treatment with factor VIII:C

There is no doubt that the cessation of factor VIII replacement is always associated with a gradual fall in antibody level and that this conservative form of treatment has its place. For example, should it become necessary to perform an operation on a patient who has a low level of an anti-VIII:C antibody, then reduction in antibody titre to a manageable level prior to operation may make all the difference to the success of the operation; low titre antibodies can usually be neutralized by high dosage factor VIII:C treatment for short periods of time. An example of such a case is illustrated in Fig. 37.

Fifteen years ago it was customary to give factor VIII to antibody patients only when they had serious haemorrhagic lesions. In 1973, Rizza and Biggs noted that nearly half of the episodes of bleeding in their haemophilia A patients having anti-VIII:C antibodies were treated during the year. At the present time these patients are treated nearly as freely as patients who have no antibodies and some are on regular home therapy.

The treatment of patients using factor VIII:C

In general, patients who have anti-factor VIII:C antibodies will need at least twice the dose of factor VIII:C that would be required by a patient who lacks antibody. Three major considerations control the use of factor VIII:C for patients who have antibodies. The first concerns the amount of factor VIII required to neutralize the patient's antibody. The second is that treatment will customarily raise the antibody titre. The third consideration is the level of antibody in the patient at the time of treatment.

A useful concept in considering the effectiveness of specific treatment in these patients is 'the response to treatment'. This term is expressed as the percentage of rise in level of factor VIII:C per u/kg dose. A normal response ranges from 1.8–2.0 per cent rise u/kg.

The amount of factor VIII:C required to neutralize the circulating antibody cannot be predicted exactly. In the test-tube one unit of factor VIII:C has been found to neutralize 3–4 units of antibody, but in the circulation where antibody formation may be occurring simultaneously with neutralization by administered factor VIII one cannot count on being able to neutralize more than one unit of antibody per unit of factor VIII:C. Thus, if a patient weighing 60 kg has an antibody level of 10 u/ml he may need 25 000 units of factor VIII to neutralize his circulating anti-factor VIII antibody before a circulating level of factor VIII:C can be recorded. In practice, less factor VIII:C (which will not produce a measurable level of VIII:C) is often sufficient to produce clinical improvement. Except in cases of very dangerous bleeding or operation cases,

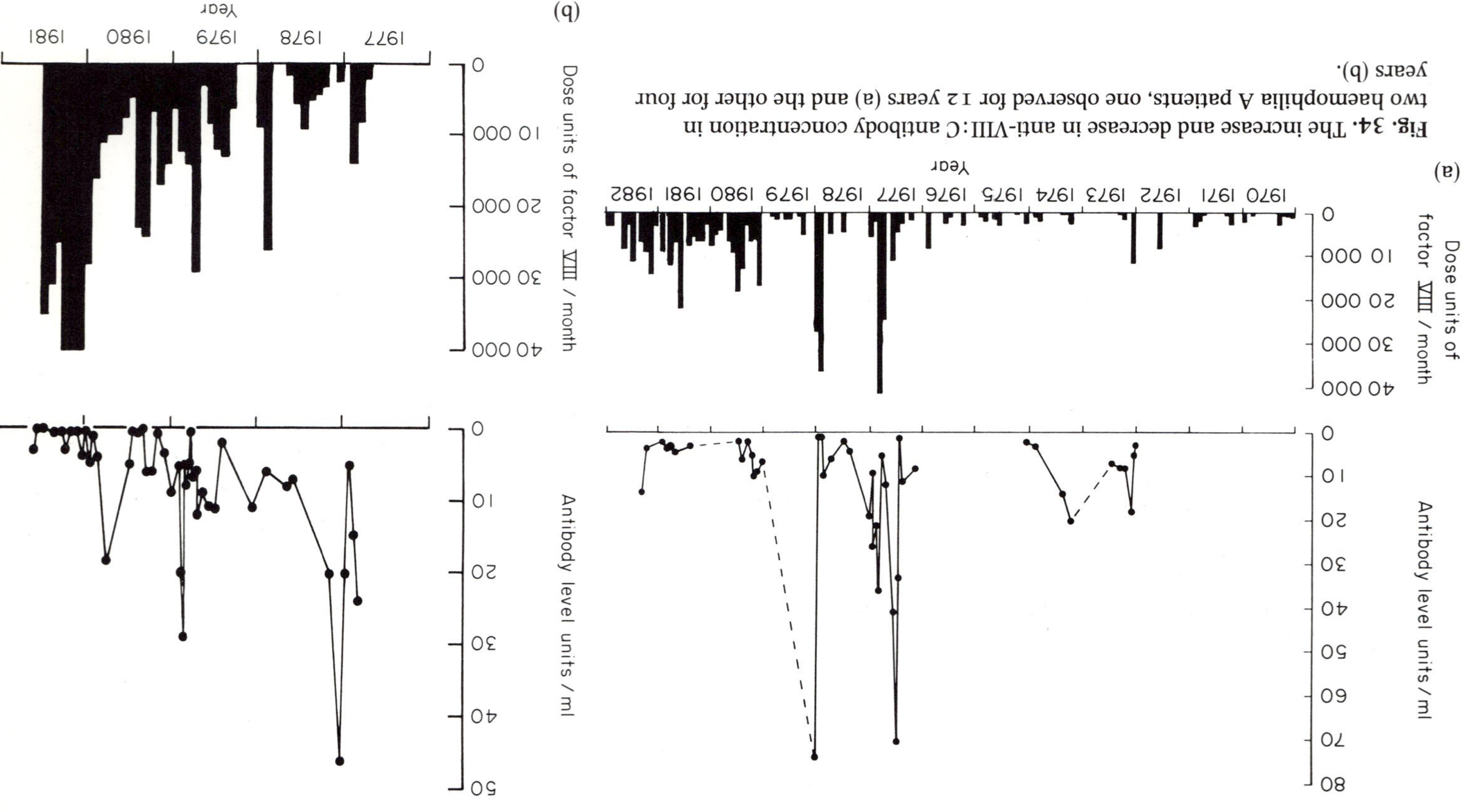

Fig. 34. The increase and decrease in anti-VIII:C antibody concentration in two haemophilia A patients, one observed for 12 years (a) and the other for four years (b).

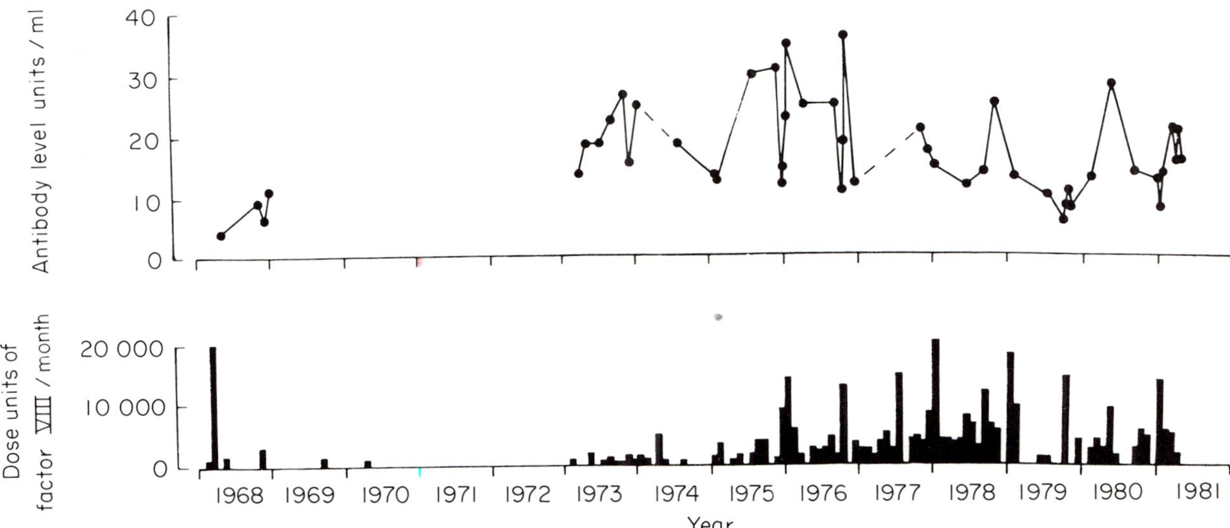

Fig. 35a. The increase and decrease in anti-VIII:C antibody concentration in haemophilia A patient, observed for 14 years.

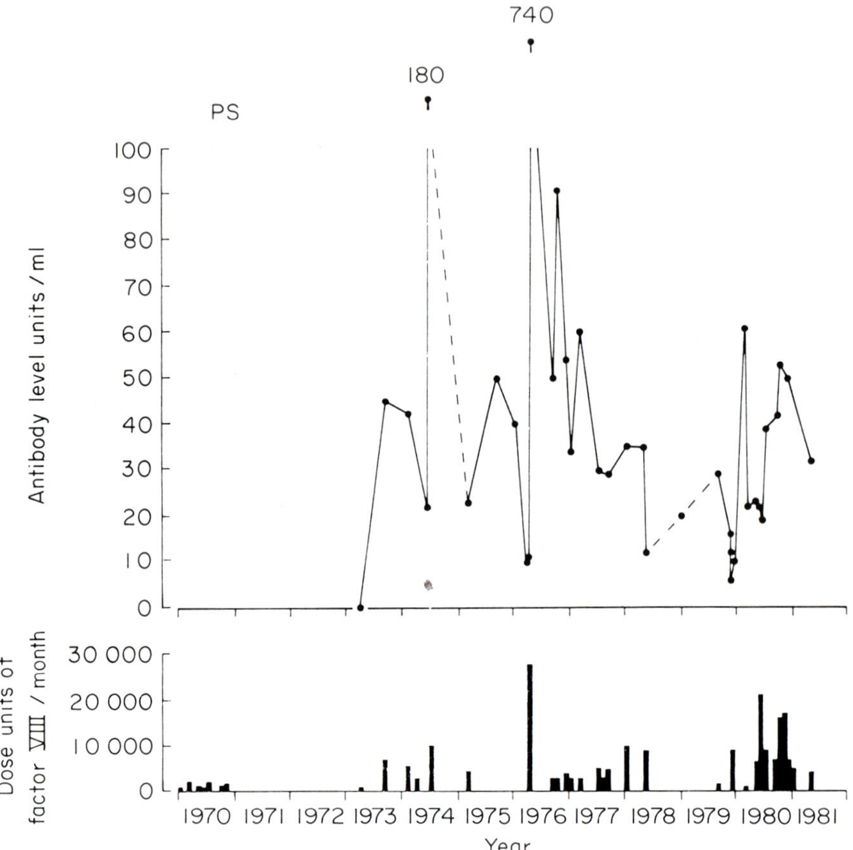

Fig. 35b. The increase and decrease in anti-VIII:C antibody concentration in a haemophilia A patient observed for 11 years.

we usually use twice the dose of factor VIII:C that would be used for patients who have no antibody. The dose for patients having antibodies is of the order of 50 u/kg.

The effect of factor VIII:C treatment on the level of antibody in patients viewed over a long time

The records of two patients appear in Fig. 33a,b. Both form high titre antibodies. One (Fig. 33a) was treated with factor VIII at infrequent intervals and an antibody response followed each large dose of factor VIII. The other patient showed the typical rise in antibody following treatment but also had one period of relatively frequent treatment during which his antibody response declined (Fig. 33b). This is also apparent in the 1980 record for Fig. 33b when repeated treatment resulted in a lesser rise in antibody titre although the antibody level never fell below 50 u/ml. Two other patients (Fig. 34a,b) both had periods between 1979 and 1981 in which they had frequent treatment and in which the high antibody response characteristic of earlier periods failed to occur. Fig. 35 shows the records of two more patients. One of them (Fig. 35a) had levels of antibody between 10 and 30 u/ml from 1968–1981 despite quite frequent treatment in the later years. The second patient (Fig. 35b) had antibody levels between zero and 60 u/ml with the exception of three peaks of 180 u/ml, 740 u/ml and 91 u/ml in 1974, 1976 and 1977 and the antibody response did not seem to be affected by treatment. Fig. 36a,b shows the records of two more patients. One (Fig. 36a) had an antibody level of 70 u/ml in 1973. After the start of high level frequent treatment the antibody of this patient disappeared and has not since recurred. The second patient (Fig. 36b) had a low titre antibody which disappeared as soon as frequent treatment was started. In the cases of four other patients having low titre antibodies it seems that the antibodies have disappeared following the start of frequent high dosage treatment. The experience in Oxford has been discussed by Rizza and Matthews (1982).

The conclusion would seem to be that frequent treatment with factor VIII:C may reduce the antibody response and, in the case of low or intermediate titre antibodies, may suppress antibody formation completely. Disappearance of antibody following prophylactic treatment has also been recorded by Shapiro (1978).

The effect of antibody level on the immediate response to factor VIII:C treatment

The response to treatment by haemophilia A patients may be judged by the patient's clinical response and by the level of factor VIII:C achieved in the blood. Usually the two indicators are related; the higher the blood level of factor VIII:C the more certain the control of haemostasis. In the case of patients who have antibodies, the patient may sometimes respond clinically even when there is no detectable post-treatment blood concentration of factor VIII:C. The clinical response in these circumstances is uncertain and would not be sufficient to protect the patient during major surgery. For major surgery it is essential to achieve substantial blood concentrations of factor VIII:C.

The conditions necessary to achieve effective blood levels of factor VIII:C in antibody patients may be illustrated by reference to patients who have been treated at the Oxford Haemophilia Centre. These cases may be considered in terms of factor VIII:C levels achieved with different doses in terms of u/kg.

As previously noted, low titre antibodies may disappear when treatment is withheld. In patients whose antibody has disappeared, the response to factor

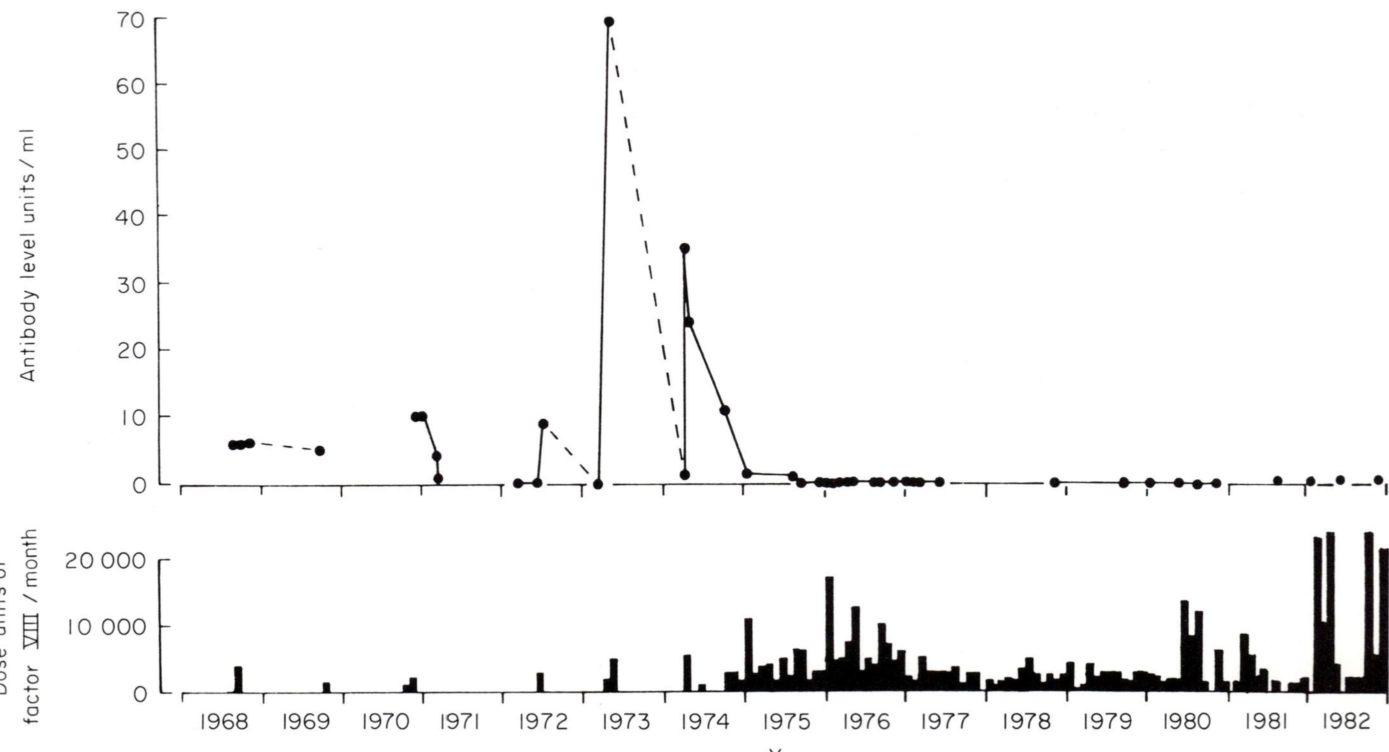

Fig. 36a. The increase and decrease in anti-VIII:C antibody in a patient observed for 14 years.

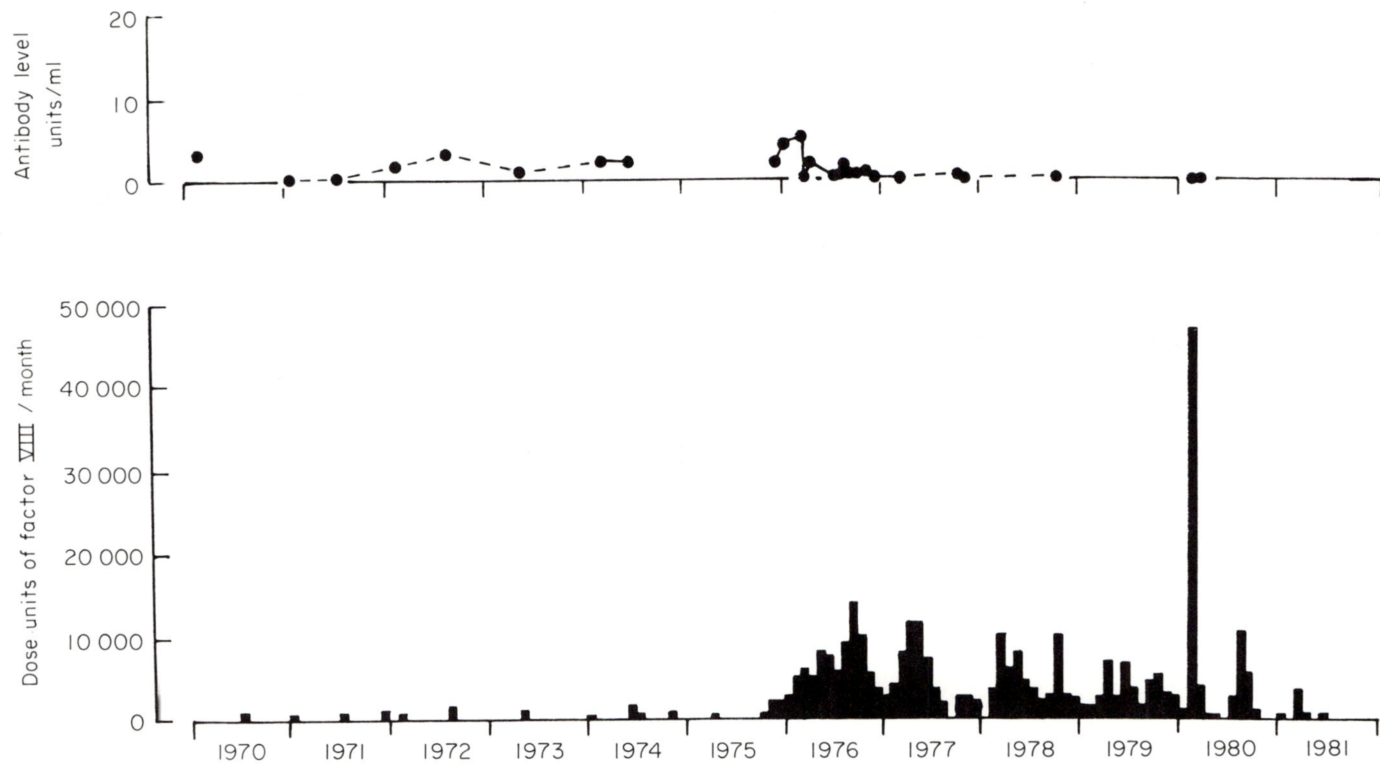

Fig. 36b. The increase and decrease in anti-VIII:C antibody in a haemophilia A patient observed for 11 years.

VIII:C may for a few days be nearly as good as that in patients who have no antibody (Table 19). In patients who have low titre antibodies the antibody may be neutralized by an excess of factor VIII:C and then the surplus appears as a plasma concentration of VIII:C. Table 20 shows the response to treatment by patients who have low titre anti-VIII:C antibodies.

Table 19. The treatment of patients whose antibodies have temporarily disappeared (from Rizza and Biggs 1973).

Patient	wt. kg	Pre* %	Post %	Dose u/kg	Response u/u/kg† %
1	20	0	47	27	1.74
2	62	3	18	16	0.93
		10	50	22	1.82
		9	50	22	1.86
		12	46	20	1.70
		10	40	23	1.30
		12	81	33	2.09
		18	48	17.5	1.71
		0	33	20	1.55
3	73	0	30	14.5	2.07
4	73	0	22	11.5	1.91
5	47	0	8	4.8	1.67
6	56	0	16	8.8	1.82
		13	45	16	2.00
7	73	0	40	27	1.48
		3	34	29	1.07
8	51	15	37	15	1.47
		0	23	25	0.92
		0	46	45	1.02
		4	62	61	0.95
		9	105	96	1.00
		22	80	33	1.75
		25	100	67	1.12
9	27	0	36	37	0.97
		4	18	13	1.08

* The pre-infusion factor VIII:C concentrations represent factor VIII remaining from a previous dose.
† The maximum possible response is about 2.44 u/u/kg; the response of most patients who have no anti-VIII:C antibodies varies from about 1.50–2.44 u/u/kg (Biggs 1978).

Table 20. The records of treatment of some patients who have low titre anti-factor VIII:C antibodies (Rizza and Biggs 1973).

Patient	wt. kg	Ab u/ml	Factor VIII:C Pre %	Post %	Dose u/kg	Response u/kg %
1	67	6P	0	0	90P	0
			0	3	180P	0
			0	7	110P	0.06
			0	107	110P	0.97
2	52	1.25H	0	43	95H	0.45
			1	57	57H	0.98
			3	54	75H	0.68
		2.8H	0	20	32H	0.62
		8.4H	0	24	42H	0.57
3	60	2.8H	0	6	27.5H	0.22
			0	14	38.5H	0.36
		1.25H	0	16	31.5H	0.51
		1.2H	0	13	32.5H	0.40
4	54	4.0H	0	5	24H	0.21
			0	8	12H	0.67
5	48	3.0H	0	7	21H	0.33
			0	8	23H	0.34
			0	8	21H	0.38
			0	9	16H	0.56

P = porcine factor VIII and H = Human factor VIII used in antibody assay. See notes to Table 18.

The treatment of patients who need surgery

The records of two patients who had surgical operations are shown in Figs 37 and 38. It will be seen that after initially large doses of factor VIII the antibody was neutralized and remained undetectable for 5–7 days when the response to treatment in each case was nearly normal. In both cases the initial antibody level was below 10 u/ml at the time of treatment. In one case (Fig. 37) treatment had been withheld for a year before the operation was undertaken in the hope that the antibody might disappear. In the other case (Fig. 38) a period of relatively frequent treatment had preceded the operation and neither patient had ever recorded antibody titres of over 50 u/ml. It must be emphasized that operations on patients who have antibodies are always dangerous and should be planned in immaculate detail. The antibody titre at the start should be as low as possible. The probable neutralizing dose of factor VIII:C should be calculated. One unit of VIII:C per unit of antibody, unit as defined by Rizza and

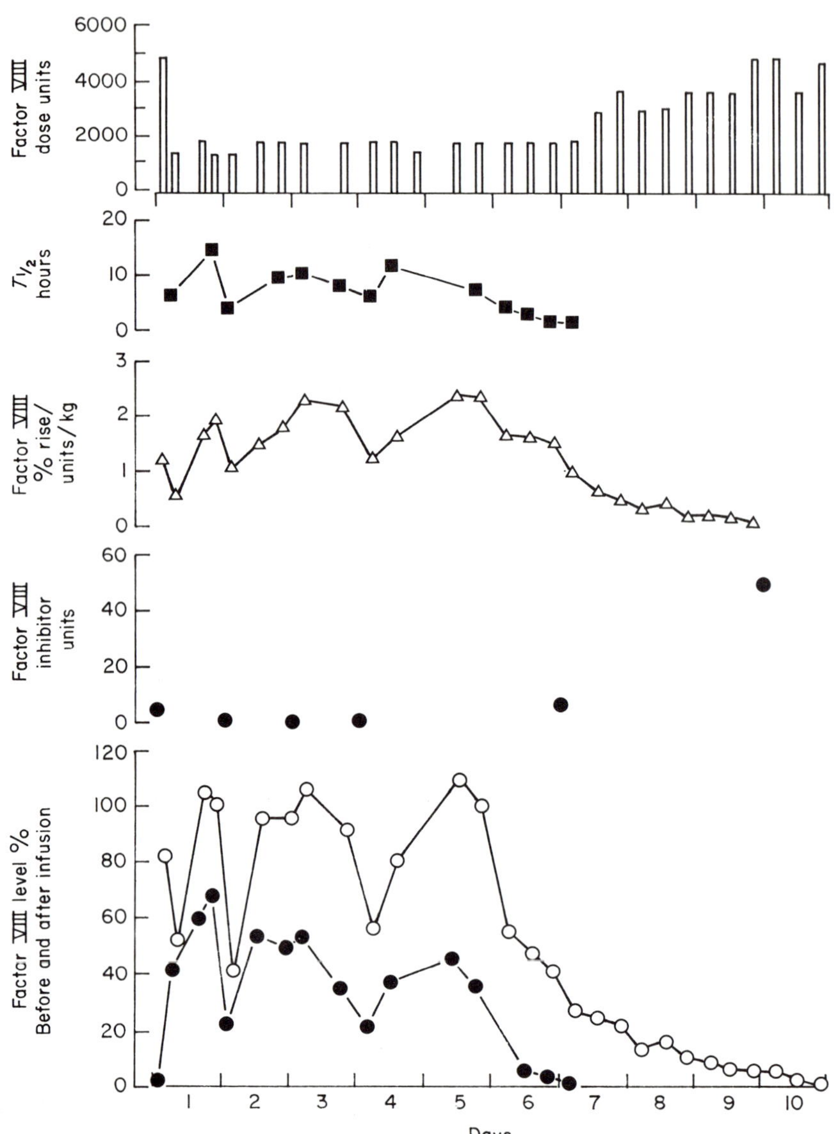

Fig. 37. The record of laboratory results for a haemophilia A patient, who had anti-VIII:C antibody, and who had an operation for invasive parotid tumour. The dose of VIII:C, the half-life ($T\frac{1}{2}$) of infused VIII:C, the response (% rise/units/kg), the plasma levels of VIII:C before and after infusion and the anti-VIII:C antibody levels are shown.

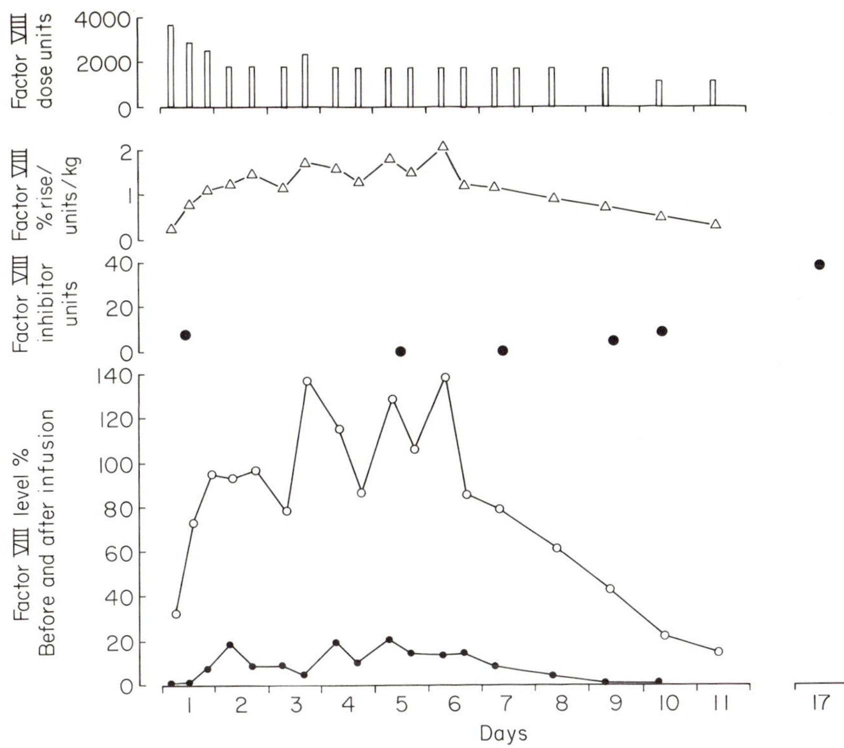

Fig. 38. Operation record for a patient having anti-VIII:C antibodies who had an operation for nasal polypectomy. The long-term record for this patient appears in Fig. 34b. The operation was carried out in 1979. The various measurements are the same as in Fig. 37.

Biggs (1973), is a minimum. Thus, for a patient weighing 30 kg, having an assumed plasma volume of 41 ml/kg and having an antibody level of 6 u/ml, the initial number of factor VIII units to be used would be:

$$30 \times 41 \times 6 = 7380$$

Allowing for a positive residual factor VIII:C level, one would probably use about 10 000 units. No factor VIII should be given until the day of operation, and thereafter the plasma factor VIII:C level should be kept as near to 100 per cent of normal as possible. In addition, tranexamic acid should be given to render the clots as permanent as possible.

In many patients the antibody is of much higher titre when tested with human VIII:C than when tested with bovine or porcine factor VIII. Should these preparations be available they may be useful in some emergencies for patients who have high titre anti-human VIII:C antibodies (Tables 20 and 21).

Table 21. The treatment of a patient having an acquired anti-VIII:C antibody (wt. 55 kg) using human (H) and porcine (P) factor VIII.

Day of treatment	Antibody u/ml		Factor VIII		
	P	H	Pre %	Post %	Dose u/kg
1	20	200	0	22	150P
			5	35	150P
2			6	43	75P
					75P
3			9	41	150P
					150P
4			16	32	45H
					45H
5	0	140+	7	15	36H
					44H
6	1		10	50	160P
					160P
7		200	7	80	220P
8					140P
9	10		5		140P
10	33	200			

P = porcine, H = human.

Treatment other than factor VIII:C for patients who have anti-factor VIII:C antibodies

Some batches of commercial factor IX concentrate contain a proportion of non-specific coagulant which will shorten the clotting time of most plasma samples including those containing anti-VIII:C antibodies. The exact replication of such material cannot be very reliable and various workers have used preparations from different companies and different batches to treat patients who have antibodies. The conclusions drawn are sometimes conflicting. Kurczynski and Penner (1974) and Lopaciuk and Ziemski (1979) report good results whereas Parry and Bloom (1978) and Dormandy and Sultan (1975) record no effect. Many of the reports concern the treatment of few episodes in few patients and give little detail about the criteria used to judge 'success' or 'failure' of treatment.

Since there is some evidence that the anti-factor VIII:C antibody may derive from a small clone of immunocytes it might seem reasonable to use immunosuppressive drugs to treat patients who have anti-factor VIII:C antibodies and promising results have been reported by Dormandy and Sultan (1975). The treatment has not been tried on any appreciable number of patients and most clinicians hesitate to use a potentially dangerous form of treatment for patients who have a life-long disability.

As previously noted for patients requiring operation, tranexamic acid may be beneficial in the treatment of haemorrhage in these patients. It probably acts by rendering haemostatic plugs more solid and long lasting.

Anti-VIII:C antibodies which arise in previously normal patients

A proportion of those patients who develop anti-factor VIII:C antibodies suffer from some variety of autoimmune disease such as rheumatoid arthritis, systemic lupus, penicillin allergy, hepatitis B antigenaemia, haemolytic anaemia, etc. (Green 1971, Lechner 1974, Green and Lechner 1981). A second group consists of women who develop the antibody following pregnancy. There are, in addition, a number of usually elderly patients who seem to develop the antibody with no obvious predisposing cause. The condition is extremely rare and the symptoms produced include massive bruising and muscle haematoma formation following minor trauma.

The kinetics of factor VIII destruction by these spontaneously occurring antibodies is usually of the complex variety described by Biggs *et al.* (1972b). This probably means that the antibody is less specific for the VIII:C site than is usual with haemophilia A patients who develop antibodies. It will also be remembered that a complex, VIII:CAb, is formed which retains some VIII:C activity. Immunologically the antibodies belong to the IgG4 or 5 subgroups and many contain predominantly one class of light chain. This last finding suggests a small clone type of antibody.

The treatment of patients who have spontaneously occurring anti-VIII:C antibodies

Previously normal patients who develop anti-factor VIII:C antibodies differ from haemophilia A patients in the obvious fact that these non-haemophilic patients are able to make their own factor VIII:C. Thus, if the antibody disappears, normal factor VIII levels are restored rapidly. The complex nature of the kinetics can also be helpful. In these patients some residual factor VIII:C activity often remains in the blood following treatment; this factor VIII:C is in the form of a complex with antibody which is less easily destroyed than free factor VIII:C. This complex may be accumulated by persistent treatment. The titre of antibody to animal factor VIII:C may be lower than that to human factor VIII:C and this may improve the prospects for treatment. A case record, reported by Rizza and Biggs (1973), is reproduced in Table 21.

Lechner (1974) and Green and Lechner (1981) record cases from the literature who were treated by immunosuppression. Of these, 12 had complete remission and 4 were improved. In the series reported by Green and Lechner (1981) 22 of 45 patients improved with corticosteroid therapy alone; 19 of 28 improved with combined corticosteroids and azathioprine and 37 of 80 patients improved on taking cyclophosphamide. It should be noted that 11 of 31 patients improved with no therapy. Nevertheless it would seem that immunosuppression may be valuable for patients who have acquired anti-VIII:C antibodies. The antibodies which follow pregnancy have a particular tendency to spontaneous improvement. Reports of patients treated with immunosuppression are also given by Rochon *et al.* (1971), Rizza *et al.* (1972), Allain, Vedrenne and Frommel (1973) and Mayer *et al.* (1977).

Exchange transfusion has been used but since most of the antibodies are of relatively high titre this treatment can only be of very limited effectiveness since the level of residual antibody after the exchange may remain too high for effective treatment using factor VIII.

REFERENCES

Abildgaard C.F., Vanderheiden J., Lindley A. & Rickles F. (1967) Studies of cross-reactivity of acquired factor VIII inhibitor activity in haemophilic plasma. *Thrombosis et Diathesis Haemorrhagica* **18**, 354–63.

Adelson E., Rheingold J.J., Parker O., Steiner M. & Kirby J.C. (1963) The survival of factor VIII (anti-hemophilic globulin) and factor IX (plasma thromboplastin component) in normal humans. *Journal of Clinical Investigation* **42**, 1040–7.

Allain J.P. & Frommel D. (1973) Antibodies to Factor VIII. I Variations in stability of antigen–antibody complexes in Hemophilia A. *Blood* **42**, 437–44.

Allain J.P., Vedrenne J. & Frommel D. (1973) Antibodies to Factor VIII. III Characterization of the immune response to iso- and heteroantigens in Hemophilia A. *Pathologie et Biologie* **21**, (Suppl.), 78.

Austen D.E.G. (1974) Factor VIII of small molecular weight and its aggregation. *British Journal of Haematology* **27**, 89–100.

Austen D.E.G. (1978) Factor VIII. In *The Treatment of Haemophilia A and B and von Willebrand's Disease*. Biggs R. (ed). Blackwell Scientific Publications, Oxford.

Austen D.E.G. (1979) The structure and function of factors VIII and IX. *Clinics in Haematology* **8**, 31–52.

Bangham D.R., Biggs R., Brozović M., Denson K.W.E. & Skegg J.L. (1971) A biological standard for measurement of blood coagulation factor VIII activity. *Bulletin of the World Health Organisation* **45**, 337–51.

Barrow E.M. & Graham J.B. (1972) Factor VIII (AHF) activity of small size produced by succinylating plasma. *American Journal of Physiology* **222**, 134–41.

Bennett B., Ratnoff O.D. & Levin J. (1972) Immunologic studies in von Willebrand's disease. Evidence that the antihemophilic factor (AHF) produced after transfusions lacks an antigen associated with normal AHF and the inactive material produced by patients with classic hemophilia. *Journal of Clinical Investigation* **51**, 2597–601.

Bennett E. & Huehns E.R. (1970) Immunological differentiation of three types of haemophilia and identification of some female carriers. *Lancet* **II**, 956–8.

Berglund G. (1962) Immunological studies of haemophilic plasma. *International Archives of Allergy and Applied Immunology* **22**, 1.

Biggs R. (1974) Jaundice and antibodies directed against Factors VIII and IX in patients treated for Haemophilia or Christmas disease in the United Kingdom. *British Journal of Haematology* **26**, 313–29.

Biggs R. (1977) Haemophilia treatment in the United Kingdom from 1969 to 1974. *British Journal of Haematology* **35**, 487–504.

Biggs R. (1978) *The Treatment of Haemophilia A and B and von Willebrand's disease.* Blackwell Scientific Publications, Oxford.

Biggs R., Austen D.E.G., Denson K.W.E., Rizza C.R. & Borrett R. (1972a) The mode of action of antibodies which destroy factor VIII. I Antibodies which have second-order concentration graphs. *British Journal of Haematology* **23**, 125–35.

Biggs R., Austen D.E.G., Denson K.W.E., Borrett R. & Rizza C.R. (1972b) The mode of action of antibodies which destroy factor VIII. II Antibodies which give complex concentration graphs. *British Journal of Haematology* **23**, 137–55.

Biggs R. & Bidwell E. (1959) A method for the study of antihaemophilic globulin inhibitors with reference to 6 cases. *British Journal of Haematology* **5**, 379–95.

Biggs R., Denson K.W.E. & Nossel H.L. (1964) A patient with an unusual circulating anticoagulant. *Thrombosis et Diathesis Haemorrhagica* **12**, 1–11.

Brinkhous K.M., Roberts H.R. & Weiss A.E. (1972) Prevalence of inhibitors in haemophilia A and B. *Thrombosis et Diathesis Haemorrhagica* (Suppl.) **51**, 315–20.

Cohn J. & Nielsen V.G. (1972) Development of circulating inhibitor directed against F.VIII in patients with Haemophilia A. *Scandinavian Journal of Haematology* **9**, 524–30.

Denson K.W.E., Biggs R., Haddon M.E., Borrett R. & Cobb K. (1969) Two types of haemophilia (A+ and A−); a study of 48 cases. *British Journal of Haematology* **17**, 163–71.

Dormandy K.M. & Sultan Y. (1975) The suppression of Factor VIII antibodies in Haemophilia. *Pathologie et Biologie* **23** (Suppl.), 17–23.

Dulbecco R., Vogt M. & Strickland A.G.R. (1956) A study of the basic aspects of neutralisation of two animal viruses, Western Equine Encephalitis Virus and Poliomyelitis Virus. *Virology* **2**, 162.

Feinstein D.I., Rapaport S.I. & Chong M.N.Y. (1969) Immunologic characterisation of 12 factor VIII inhibitors. *Blood* **34**, 85–90.

Frommel D. & Allain J.-P. (1977) Genetic predisposition to develop Factor VIII antibody in classic haemophilia. *Clinical Immunology and Immunopathology* **8**, 34–8.

Frommel D., Allain J.-P., Saint-Paul E., Bosser C., Noël B., Manucci P.M., Pannicucci F., Blombäck M., Prou-Wartelle O. & Muller J.Y. (1981) HLA antigens and factor VIII antibody in classic haemophilia. *Thrombosis and Haemostasis* **46**, 687–9.

Girma J.-P., Lavergne J.-M., Meyer D. & Larrieu M.-J. (1981) Immunoradiometric assay of factor VIII. Coagulant antigen using four human antibodies. Study of 27 cases of Haemophilia A. *British Journal of Haematology* **47**, 269–82.

Gralnick H.R., Abrell E. & Bagley J. (1971) Immunological studies of F.VIII (anti-haemophiliac globulin) in Haemophilia A. *Nature* (*New Biology*) **230**, 16–17.

Green D. (1971) Suppression of an antibody to factor VIII by a combination of factor VIII and cyclophosphamide. *Blood* **37**, 381–7.

Green D. & Lechner K. (1981) A survey of 215 non-haemophilic patients with inhibitors to factor VIII. *Thrombosis and Haemostasis* **45**, 200–3.

Griggs T.R., Cooper H.A., Webster W.P., Wagner R.H. & Brinkhous K.M. (1973)

Plasma aggregating factor (bovine) for human platelets: a marker study of antihemophilic and von Willebrand factors. *Proceedings of the National Academy of Sciences USA* **71**, 2087–90.

Hoyer L.W. & Breckenridge R.T. (1968) Immunologic studies of anti-hemophilic factor (AHF factor VIII): cross-reacting material in a genetic variant of Hemophilia A. *Blood* **32**, 962–71.

Hultin M.B., London F.S., Shapiro S.S. & Yount W.J. (1977) Heterogeneity of factor VIII antibodies. Further immunochemical and biologic studies. *Blood* **49**, 807–17.

Ikkala E. & Simonen O. (1971) Factor VIII inhibitors and the use of blood products in patients with Haemophilia A. *Scandinavian Journal of Haematology* **8**, 16–20.

Kaelin A.C. (1975) Sodium periodate modification of factor VIII procoagulant activity. *British Journal of Haematology* **31**, 349–59.

Kavanagh M.L., Wood C.N. & Davidson J.F. (1981) The immunological characterization of human antibodies to factor VIII isolated by immuno-affinity chromatography. *Thrombosis and Haemostasis* **45**, 60–4.

Kernoff P.B.A. (1974) The factor VIII-related antigen and antibodies to factor VIII. A thesis for the degree of Doctor of Medicine at the University of London.

Kurczynski E.M. & Penner J.A. (1974) Activated prothrombin concentrate for patients with factor VIII inhibitors. *New England Journal of Medicine* **291**, 164–7.

Laurell C.B. (1966) Quantitative estimation of proteins by electrophoresis in agarose gel containing antibodies. *Analytical Biochemistry* **15**, 45.

Lavergne J.-M., Meyer D. & Reisner H. (1976) Characterization of human antifactor VIII antibodies purified by immune complex formation. *Blood* **48**, 931–9.

Lazarchick J. & Hoyer L.W. (1978) Immunoradiometric measurement of the factor VIII procoagulant antigen. *Journal of Clinical Investigation* **62**, 1048–52.

Lechner K. (1974) Acquired inhibitors in non-hemophilic patients. *Haemostasis* **3**, 65.

Lee H., Tucker D. & Allain J.P. (1979) Rapid isolation and purification of antibody to factor VIII by protein A. *Thrombosis Research* **14**, 925–30.

Lopaciuk C.S. & Ziemski J.M. (1979) The treatment of patients with haemophilia A having antibodies to factor VIII. *Acta Haematologica Polska* **10**, 115.

Mayer C., Kalogjera V., Lieure C., Pauther J., Weisel M.-L. & Mayer S. (1977) Étude comparative d'un inhibiteur de factor VIII chez un malade non hémophile et chez un malade hémophile A gravis. *Semaine des Hôpitaux de Paris* **25–8**, 1511.

Mayer P.G., Noel G., Kalogjera V. & Waitz R. (1969) Les inhibiteurs faibles du facteur VIII chez les Hémophiles A. *Blut* **9**, 517–28.

Nilsson I.M. & Holmberg L. (1979) Von Willebrand's disease today. In *Clinics in Haematology.* Vol. 8:1. pp. 147–68. Rizza C.R. (ed.) W.B. Saunders Co., London.

Owen W.G. & Wagner R.H. (1972) Antihemophilic factor: separation of an active fragment following dissociation by salts or detergents. *Thrombosis et Diathesis Haemorrhagica* **27**, 502–15.

Parry D.H. & Bloom A.L. (1978) Failure of factor VIII inhibitor bypassing activity (Feiba) to secure haemostasis in haemophilic patients with antibodies. *Journal of Clinical Pathology* **31**, 1102–5.

Peake I.R. & Bloom A.L. (1978) Immunoradiometric assay of procoagulant factor VIII antigen in plasma and serum and its reduction in haemophilia. *Lancet* **I**, 473–5.

Piper W. & Schreier M.H. (1964) Über den immunologischen nachweis von Factor VIII-protein im bluterplasma und seine bedeutung für das verständnis der Hämophilie A. *Thrombosis et Diathesis Haemorrhagica* **11**, 423–43.

Pool J., Biggs R. & Miller R.G. (1976) The estimation of the number of binding sites for antibody on antigen molecules with reference to Factor VIII and its antibody. *Thrombosis and Haemostasis* **35**, 274–88.

Pool J. & Kaelin A.C. (1977) Absence of blocking antibody in non-inhibitor haemophilic plasma. *Thrombosis and Haemostasis* **38**, 717–20.

Rick M.E. & Hoyer L.W. (1973) Immunologic studies of anti hemophilic factor (AHF, Factor VIII) V. Immunologic properties of AHF subunits produced by salt dissociation. *Blood* **42**, 737–47.

Rizza C.R. & Biggs R. (1973) The treatment of patients who have factor VIII antibodies. *British Journal of Haematology* **24**, 65–82.

Rizza C.R., Edgcumbe J.O.P., Pitney W.R. & Child J.A. (1972) The treatment of patients having spontaneously occurring antibodies to antihaemophilic factor (factor VIII). *Thrombosis et Diathesis Haemorrhagica* **28**, 120–8.

Rizza C.R. & Matthews J.M. (1982) Effect of frequent factor VIII replacement on the level of factor VIII antibodies in haemophiliacs. *British Journal of Haematology* **52**, 1–13.

Rizza C.R. & Spooner R.J.D. (1983) Treatment of haemophilia and related disorders in Britain and Northern Ireland during 1976–80. *British Medical Journal* **286**, 929–33.

Rochon M., Neemeh J.-A., Goselin G. & Long L.-A. (1971) Inhibiteur anti-VIII cryptogénique. *L'Union Médical du Canada* **100**, 2353.

Roitt I. (1980) *Essential Immunology.* 4th edn. Blackwell Scientific Publications, Oxford.

Shanberge J.N. & Gore J. (1957) Studies on the immunologic and physiologic activities of antihemophilia factor (AHF). *Journal of Laboratory and Clinical Medicine* **50**, 945.

Shapiro S. (1967) The immunological character of acquired inhibitors of antihemophilic globulin (factor VIII) and the kinetics of their interaction with factor VIII. *Journal of Clinical Investigation* **46**, 147.

Shapiro S. (1978) Characterisation of factor VIII antibodies. *Annals of the New York Academy of Sciences* **3**, 350.

Strauss H.S. & Merler E. (1967) Characterization and properties of an inhibitor of Factor VIII in the plasma of patients with Hemophilia A following repeated transfusion. *Blood* **30**, 137–50.

Sultan Y. & Maisonneuve P. (1977) Incidence des inhibiteurs du F.VIII dans la population des hémophiles français. *Nouvelle Revue Française d'Hématologie* **213**, 12.

Thelin G.M. & Wagner R.H. (1961) Sedimentation of plasma antihemophilic factor. *Archives of Biochemistry and Biophysics* **95**, 70.

Uszynski L. (1966) The immunological properties of factor VIII (I) studies on the inhibitory activity of specific antisera to human antihemophilic globulin. *Thrombosis et Diathesis Haemorrhagica* **16**, 559–73.

Weiss H.J. & Kochwa S. (1970) Molecular forms of anti-haemophilic globulin in plasma, cryoprecipitate and after thrombin activation. *British Journal of Haematology* **18**, 89–100.

Weiss H.J., Phillips L.L. & Rosner W. (1972) Separation of sub-units of antihemophilic factor (AHF) by agarose gel chromatography. *Thrombosis et Diathesis Haemorrhagica* **27**, 212 19.

Chapter 11
Therapeutic Materials in the Management of Haemorrhagic Disorders

J. K. SMITH *and* T. J. SNAPE

It would be an over-simplification to claim that safe and potent concentrates of human coagulation factors have 'solved' all the problems of haemophilia. The management and support of individual sufferers remains complex in many cases, concentrates are not available for the less common deficiencies, and even well-established concentrates do not provide a perfect solution, carrying as they do certain hazards for some categories of patient. However, many younger haemophiliacs can look forward to a life with very little permanent joint and muscle damage and with confidence in the prompt relief of pain or restriction, often breaking a pattern of dependence set by earlier therapeutic regimes. Major surgery can now be contemplated in haemophiliacs rendered nearly 'normal' by infusions of the deficient factor for the necessary period.

Blood component therapy and plasma fractionation

Countries with a well-developed national blood transfusion service may separate half or more of their total whole blood intake into components such as red cell concentrate, platelet concentrate and fresh-frozen plasma. A small proportion of plasma is infused directly but, just as many transfusions of whole blood are now recognized as wasteful, it is becoming more common to prepare several concentrates from the plasma for treatment of different classes of patient. The use of whole plasma rather than a specific fraction now requires justification.

Some transfusion centres still prepare frozen cryoprecipitate in PVC bags for treatment of haemophilia, and in several European countries cryoprecipitate is collected and stabilized by freeze-drying at national centres. In the UK the local production of cryoprecipitate is diminishing quite rapidly in favour of comprehensive central fractionation of whole fresh-frozen plasma (FFP) providing several coagulation factors, immunoglobulins and albumin concentrates.

Plasma fractionation centres, whether organized as part of a national blood transfusion service as in the UK, or as purely commercial enterprises, are now formally regulated in most countries as one facet of the biological pharmaceutical industry. They must comply with strict manufacturing principles designed to ensure that successive batches of products are as homogeneous, safe and effective as possible in clinical use. The chemistry of plasma fractionation, although still central to the success of a range of products, is only one stage in the chain of manufacture which includes: procurement and quality control of plasma; procurement and quality control of reagents and materials; plasma processing under documented controlled conditions; control of hygiene in the processing environment; sterilization, aseptic dispensing and freeze drying; quality control of in-process and final products; correctly documented labelling, packing, inventory, dispatch and recall.

Every new concentrate developed by a fractionation centre or adapted from published methods may take months or years to become established in routine production or to fulfil criteria for clinical trial. Since very few readers will be in a position to produce concentrates for clinical use, we do not follow early editions in giving detailed processing instructions. Instead we will indicate how different intentions are reflected in the various principles of large-scale fractionation, and how these may affect the choice of a product for therapeutic use.

Plasma economy

The economy of plasma fractionation is dominated by the cost of plasma procurement, the yield of the most valued products (factor VIII and albumin) and the demand for these products. The yield of factor VIII in the vialled product seldom exceeds 20 per cent of the initial plasma content. On the other hand, the yield of albumin is over 70 per cent and the demand for albumin may have passed its peak. The demand for factor VIII is now the prime consideration in calculating the volume and quality of plasma required for national self-sufficiency in plasma products. There is a measure of agreement in the UK, qualified by considerations of plasma quality and yield of factor VIII, that the annual requirement is approximately 10 000 litres of FFP per million population. This greatly exceeds the demand for red cells, even if *all* blood were immediately separated and none used as whole blood.

Plasma from whole blood may need to be supplemented by plasma obtained from 'manual' or machine plasmapheresis (Rock, McCombe and Tittley 1981). In about one hour, 400–500 ml of plasma can be recovered and the cells returned to the donor, who may repeat the donation weekly. Plasmapheresis has been used for many years for the collection of valuable antibodies, e.g. from convalescent donors, and has been the main source of raw material for all commercial fractionation. As the cost of plasmapheresis equipment falls in relation to the value of factor VIII, this approach should provide national fractionators with extra plasma of a more consistent quality than that obtained after the diverse demands of component therapy programmes for platelet concentrates, red cells, etc.

Comprehensive central fractionation of plasma

Cellular components, cryoprecipitate for factor VIII and cryosupernatant for volume expansion can be derived very simply from a unit of whole blood in a closed system of interconnected plastic bags, but complete fractionation is usually more rewarding.

The aim of comprehensive fractionation should be to recover and stabilize all the proteins which are therapeutically useful, not only those which are overtly 'profitable'. Fractionators working as part of a national blood transfusion service, especially if they enjoy a monopoly in plasma, have an obligation to provide, as far as is practicable, therapeutic materials for even uncommon deficiencies and materials for experimental and diagnostic use.

From the first stage of blood collection to the removal of the last plasma protein (usually albumin), the methods used to remove successive components and fractions must be efficient, selective and present no obstacles to the recovery of the remaining valuable components. Exceptions are made to this principle, e.g. where the demand for a product is so small that it need not be removed from a large volume of plasma (e.g. factor VII) or the value of the plasma resides overwhelmingly in its content of a particular protein—e.g. 'hyperimmune' plasmas such as anti-D, anti-tetanus, etc. The major part of the fresh-frozen plasma collected in England and Wales in 1981 undergoes the central 'spine' of fractionation illustrated in Fig. 39.

Other valuable proteins may be recovered by insertion of other processes into the central spine. If factor VIII is not required, Cohn Fraction I, which is rich in *fibrinogen*, may be precipitated at 8 per cent ethanol concentration, replacing cryoprecipitate in the scheme. More than half the fibrinogen in plasma remains in cryosupernatant and can be recovered from this alternative source by a similar ethanol precipitation. Cohn Fraction I and cryoprecipitate both contain *fibronectin* and *factor XIII* but the demand for these proteins does not yet create serious conflict with factor VIII. It is possible to recover sufficient amounts of all these proteins without interfering with factor VIII recovery.

If *factor VII* is not recovered in the same eluate fraction as factors IX, II and X, as is the case after adsorption on to DEAE-cellulose, it may be selectively adsorbed from the factor IX-supernatant using DEAE-Sepharose, and eluted to give a separate concentrate of factor VII.

C1-esterase inhibitor can be selectively adsorbed from factor IX supernatant by DEAE-Sephadex, provided the supernatant is further diluted with water to reduce ionic strength.

Antithrombin III can be removed at almost any stage prior to ethanol

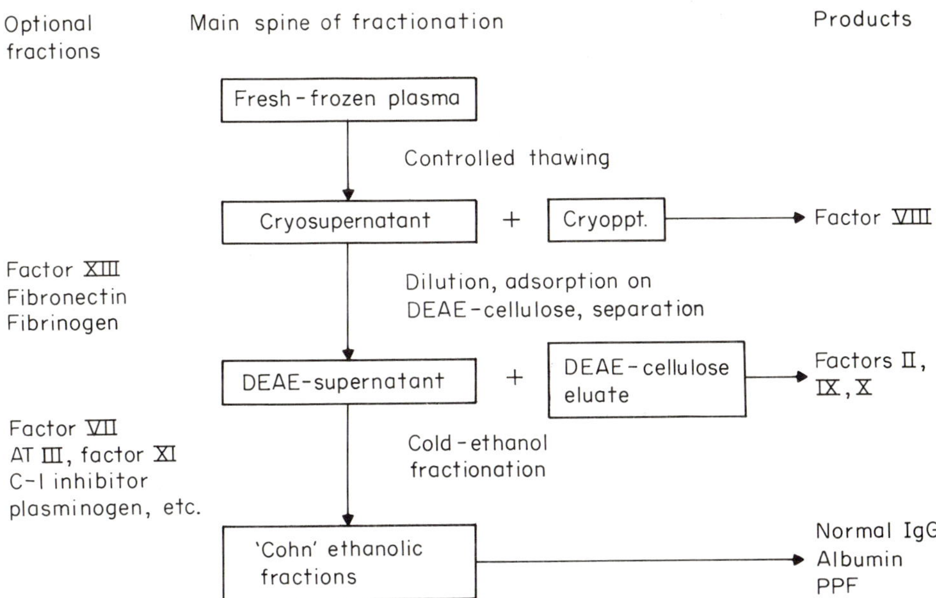

Fig. 39. A scheme for the comprehensive fractionation of plasma.

fractionation by batch adsorption on immobilized heparin. Alternatively, Fraction IV from Cohn ethanol fractionation yields useful amounts of antithrombin III.

Similarly, *plasminogen* may be adsorbed directly from plasma using immobilized lysine, or recovered from Cohn Fraction III.

The next few years are likely to see more exploitation of selective adsorption for specific proteins, including coagulation factors, protease inhibitors and other enzymes, before the potentially denaturing cold-ethanol stages of fractionation.

The quality control of coagulation factor concentrates

It is useful to distinguish between *quality control*, which may be defined as the procedure by which it is determined that a product conforms to a given specification, and *quality assurance*, which may be thought of as the definition and maintenance of a documented production procedure and environment such that a product could reasonably be expected to conform to that specification. *Quality assurance* is an integral part of blood component production, whether that production is carried out in a regional transfusion centre, as in the preparation of individual frozen cryoprecipitates from single plasma donations, or in the fractionation centre where thousands of plasma donations may be pooled to produce large batches of freeze-dried concentrates. *Quality control*, on the other hand, can only be effective if test procedures can be applied to representative samples from a batch, and the findings extended to cover the batch as a whole. This is clearly feasible for vials of freeze-dried concentrate from a single process batch, but not for individual cryoprecipitates—even those produced by a given operator in a single session. In the latter situation, *quality assurance* will be the only determinant of product quality (safety and efficacy).

It is possible to distinguish two levels of quality control. The first is that carried out 'in house' on the finished product prior to its release for clinical use. The second is the external (independent) assessment of the product carried out by the appropriate national control authority (in the UK, the National Institute for Biological Standards and Control, NIBSC) of the properties of samples of batches submitted to them by the manufacturer. One interface between these two levels of quality control is the monograph in the relevant pharmacopoeia.

The role of the pharmacopoeia

Pharmacopoeial monographs, as far as they exist, provide the manufacturer with a minimum specification for that product. This is best illustrated by an example, and Table 22 contains a summary of the requirements of British

Table 22. Pharmacopoeial requirements for 'Dried Factor VIII Fraction' (British Pharmacopoeia 1980 and Addendum 1981).

Properties of the reconstituted solution:	
Active factor concentration, iu/ml	$\not< 6$
Specific activity, iu/mg protein	$\not< 0.2$
Fibrinogen as per cent of total protein	$\not> 80\%$
Sodium ions, mmol/l	$\not> 200$
Citrate ions, mmol/l	$\not> 55$
Description of the product:	
Solubility time in water at 18–22°C, min.	$\not> 20$
Test of identity	Specific assay
pH	6.8–7.4
Loss on drying over P_2O_5 as per cent w/w	$\not> 0.5$
Biological safety tests:	
Pyrogen test in rabbits	Complies at $\not< 10$ iu/kg
Sterility	Complies
Abnormal toxicity in mice and guinea pigs	Complies at $\not< 75$ iu/kg
Estimated potency as per cent of stated potency	$\not< 80$, $\not> 125$
95 % confidence limits as per cent of stated potency	$\not< 64$, $\not> 156$

Pharmacopoeia 1980 (modified by the Addendum 1981) for Dried Factor VIII Fraction.

The limits specified in a pharmacopoeial monograph do not necessarily define an absolute minimum or maximum safe level. Rather they are achievable values agreed by a committee of 'experts' which would usually have been established as being safe in clinical practice. Thus the limit of 55 mmol/l is not based on citrate toxicity studies, but reflects the fact that factor VIII concentrates containing citrate at that level had a well-established record of safe clinical use at the time the monograph was first drafted (Blombäck and Nilsson 1958). Similarly, the specification of a maximum moisture content for freeze-dried factor VIII concentrate (as 'loss on drying over P_2O_5') does not necessarily define the optimum water content for such a product. The value of 0.5 per cent w/w is simply what was achievable by the freeze-drying technology available when the monograph was drawn up. In fact, the water content quoted is well below that at which water may be assumed to be 'free' to act as a solvent for enzymic reactions, or to allow microbial growth (Snape 1982) and it may be that a higher limit for 'loss on drying' would be acceptable, and might even confer advantages.

Since the pharmacopoeia specifications are regarded as minimum specifications, it is important that they should be achievable by all preparations of the type with an established record of clinical use—a monograph on a product would usually follow several years use of such a product type. The manufacturer may define a set of more rigorous 'in-house' limits for control purposes, but would be unlikely to define the product specification more restrictively than the pharmacopoeia required.

The product label

The pharmacopoeial monograph on a product also provides guidelines to the manufacturer on labelling. In respect of labelled potency the monographs 'Dried Factor VIII Fraction' and 'Dried Factor IX Fraction' require that, 'The estimated potency is not less than 80 per cent and not more than 125 per cent of the stated potency. The fiducial limits of error are not less than 64 per cent and not more than 156 per cent of the stated potency.' Generous as these limits may appear, problems of standardization of the factor VIII (and factor IX) assay, and systematic discrepancies between values returned by one- and two-stage assays for these factors, have led to significant disagreement between manufacturers' labelled value and values observed by experienced users (Austen, Rhymes and Rizza 1981, Barrowcliffe and Thomas 1981, Kasper 1981).

Other requirements for labelling include: the volume of water to be added, the concentration of protein, electrolytes and of added substances such as heparin, in the reconstituted solution; a warning in respect of the risks of hepatitis transmission; storage conditions and expiry date; a warning (which assumes microbial contamination on reconstitution) that the preparation should be used within three hours; a warning not to use the solution if a gel forms. The label also contains the product licence number, PL . . . . This refers to a document lodged with the licensing section of Medicines Division which defines the product manufacturing procedure and specification, and on the basis of which a product licence would have been granted.

Individual coagulation factor concentrates

Factor VIII concentrates

What matters most in choosing a factor VIII concentrate? Many clinicians with a wide experience of using many of the concentrates available would choose largely on cost, since all licensed products satisfy tests of safety and efficacy as required by the relevant pharmacopoeia or the national regulatory bodies—in the UK, Medicines Division of the Department of Health and Social Security.

From time to time individual manufacturers make specific claims for advances in product safety or clinical effectiveness, which may be associated with a change in cost. Such claims should be carefully evaluated by the user.

'Purity', defined as specific activity or units of factor VIII per milligram of total protein, is commonly used as an index to divide concentrates into three very broad categories from about 0.1 to 1.0 iu/mg. High purity concentrates have a specific activity exceeding 0.5 iu/mg protein and are used at a potency of 20–30 iu/ml; intermediate purity concentrates have a specific activity of 0.2–0.5 iu/mg and are used at a potency of 10–20 iu/ml; lower purity concentrates consist of frozen or freeze-dried cryoprecipitate, with a specific activity of 0.1–0.2 iu/mg and a potency of about 3–5 iu/ml. Not surprisingly, the yield of factor VIII from the original plasma drops dramatically as further purification stages are included in the preparation of a concentrate. Since 'pure' factor VIII would contain approximately 10 000 iu/mg protein, this classification is quite arbitrary and one must consider to what extent the preponderance of particular contaminating proteins is important to the therapeutic application of the preparation:

1   An increase in specific activity does not always correlate with a reduction in the time taken to redissolve the concentrate or the potency (units per ml solution) at which the concentrate can be redissolved and injected. For instance, minor contamination with a sticky protein such as lipoprotein might make resolution difficult whereas heavy contamination with albumin might improve the product's solubility.

2   Inert proteins such as albumin and fibrinogen may contribute to the remarkable stability of most factor VIII concentrates. Cofractionation of protease inhibitors such as antithrombin III may also be favourable. It is doubtful whether stability at room temperature for more than a few hours is of any therapeutic significance and such stability should not be confused with recovery or survival of factor VIII after infusion.

3   Although haemophiliacs have for many years been receiving massive doses of fibrinogen along with factor VIII, the increase in plasma fibrinogen levels during very intensive therapy has not been shown to be harmful.

4   Concentrates may contain varying concentrations of IgG haemagglutinins, not necessarily reflected in the overall 'specific activity', and these can cause haemolysis (Seeler 1972). The severity of haemolysis is dose-related but individuals vary in their sensitivity. With modern concentrates the problem should arise only when the haemophiliac receives many thousands of units of factor VIII per day. It is possible to obtain 'haemagglutinin-free' concentrates made from group AB plasma, or to supplement treatment with compatible cryoprecipitate.

5   All concentrates are occasionally implicated in minor reactions in the patient, e.g. flushing or transient headache. Quality control should ensure that frank pyrexial reactions are very rare. The clinician should be aware that a particular batch of concentrate may have an adverse effect on only one patient, and should not necessarily abandon a batch or stop using that type of concentrate on the basis of a single minor incident. Sensitivity to citrate ions or to low levels of vasoactive substances should be considered, since slow infusion often helps, but it is difficult to identify and implement quality control measures which would eliminate quite rare reactions.

6   Allergic reactions to either human or animal proteins may be much more serious. Such reactions are quite common with cryoprecipitate but are extremely rare with even intermediate concentrates.

7   'Purity' with respect to transmission of viral hepatitis is discussed below.

Claims for improved clinical effectiveness are almost invariably based on over-enthusiastic interpretation of too few infusions. Cross-over studies (e.g. Allain *et al.* 1980) which eliminate the large variation in response of different patients usually show no significant differences between cryoprecipitate and various types of concentrate, either in initial response or in the rate of decay of plasma factor VIII activity.

Methods of preparation of factor VIII concentrates

Virtually all current concentrates start from cryoprecipitate, since the starting plasma is always frozen at the collection centre to stabilize it during quality control, quarantine, transport, etc. and since cryoprecipitation interferes very little with the recovery of other valuable proteins.

Cryoprecipitate may be made in single satellite packs or bottles, although 6–12 individual cryoprecipitates may then have to be pooled for clinical use. A voluminous literature is devoted to consistent improvements in the yield of factor VIII by cryoprecipitation, mostly concerned with ensuring that factor VIII does not redissolve near the end of the thawing phase. Thaw-siphoning (Mason 1978) recognizes this problem and provides one solution, but is highly labour-intensive. The addition of low concentrations of ethanol (Newman *et al.* 1971), polyethylene glycol (Johnson, MacDonald and Brind 1979) or heparin (Rock *et al.* 1979) may improve the yield by selectively reducing the solubility of factor VIII in the critical temperature range, but additional unwanted proteins may also be precipitated. Calculating on the basis of a 200 ml plasma donation, single-pack cryoprecipitate of random blood group may routinely yield about 80 iu factor VIII. Its advantages over large-pool concentrate are: local availability (at least in theory); high initial yield of factor VIII; and a reduced risk of transmitting hepatitis virus. Some disadvantages are: labour-intensive preparation; difficulty in storage and preparation, especially for home therapy; inconsistent yields leading to over-prescription; compromises with ideal quality control, since a batch may be only one unit; and residual plasma proteins causing adverse reactions. The risk of reactions is reduced by centrifugation of the cryoprecipitate and by optional washing procedures which add to the complexity of preparation, and its convenience can be improved by freeze-drying, which is capital-intensive and tends to lead back to centralization. Most clinicians in the UK now prefer freeze-dried intermediate concentrate to cryoprecipitate, especially for home therapy. Large-scale thawing of 100–1000 kg lots of plasma now routinely approaches the primary yield of factor VIII achieved by conventional single-donor cryoprecipitation and, when the principles of controlled heat transfer are properly incorporated in process design, can comfortably exceed it (Foster *et al.* 1982). The final yield of factor VIII is reduced by additional purification stages and sampling for quality control. Table 23 summarizes the purpose of these stages and the losses sustained in a typical intermediate concentrate made from good quality FFP. In other variants, cold precipitation may be omitted or a similar improvement in solubility achieved by washing the cryoprecipitate (Wickerhauser, Mercer and Eckenrode 1978), the common feature of 'intermediate purity' concentrates being that the factor VIII is not further concentrated by reprecipitation.

The potency (15–20 iu/ml) and solubility of intermediate concentrates is sufficient for the treatment of the great majority of haemarthroses and haematomata. It should be possible to give over 10 000 iu per day of intermediate concentrate without circulatory overload. Where it is felt necessary to increase the potency of the infusion (as in saturation treatment of

Table 23. Aims of stages in the preparation of intermediate-purity factor VIII concentrate, and losses of coagulant activity.

Stage of preparations	Aim of stage	FVIII:C iu/kg FFP
Fresh-frozen plasma	Source of F.VIII from blood component programme	700–800
Large-scale cryoprecipitation and selective extraction	Provides crude concentrate of F.VIII with minimum effect on residual plasma. (Determines potency of concentrate.)	470
pH and temperature-controlled precipitation of unwanted proteins	Improves filtration and re-solution potency of product	360
Adsorption of unwanted coagulation factors, etc; adjustment of salts	Stabilizes F.VIII:C	330
Sterile filtration and dispensing into vials	Prepares solution for i.v. use	290
Freeze-drying	Stabilizes F.VIII:C for storage. Permits use at higher potency	260*

* A further 5–10 per cent of this yield, depending on batch size, is usually lost in control tests, etc. (Data from the best quality FFP fractionated at Blood Products Laboratory, Elstree during 1980.)

patients with inhibitors) or where there is an adverse response to intermediate concentrate or cryoprecipitate, it may be necessary to consider the use of a preparation of 'high purity'. Like intermediate concentrates, these are made from cryoprecipitate but usually include a further stage in which the factor VIII is reprecipitated and redissolved in small volume. There is invariably a large penalty in yield of factor VIII and therefore manufacturing cost. The precise methods are often commercial property, but sufficient is published to indicate some of the principles, e.g. reprecipitation of adsorbed cryoprecipitate extract with ethanol (Hershgold, Pool and Pappenhagen 1966); reprecipitation using polyethylene glycol and glycine (Brinkhous *et al.* 1968); heat denaturation and removal of fibrinogen (Heimburger *et al.* 1981); coprecipitation of factor VIII with cold insoluble globulin, using heparin (Rock and Palmer 1980).

Recent advances in chromatographic media and equipment point to future large-scale application of these more selective techniques; 'void volume' factor VIII from unmodified large-pore gel filtration media; adsorption of fibrinogen on immobilized heparin or silicate (Margolis and Rhoades 1979); separation of

FVIII:C from FVIII:RAg and fibrinogen on polyelectrolytes (Johnson *et al.* 1978); or on amino-acyl agarose (Austen 1979).

Replacement therapy in severe haemophilia A

Therapeutic regimes are discussed in Chapters 10 and 12.

All large-pool concentrates are designed for intensive therapy of severe haemophilia.

Replacement therapy in less severe deficiencies

Carriers of haemophilia and mildly affected haemophiliacs require only infrequent treatment and, after the maintenance of haemostasis, the main aim should be to avoid transmitting hepatitis in individuals who may not have the immunity of a multi-transfused severe haemophiliac. Until more effective screening can be adopted or better methods developed for inactivating viruses in factor VIII concentrates (see below), the use of small-pool concentrate such as cryoprecipitate should be considered. If a freeze-dried concentrate is preferred, those made from the plasma of unpaid donors are less likely to transmit non-A non-B hepatitis.

Similar arguments can be made for the treatment of von Willebrand's disease, although there is a trend towards more frequent and more liberal use of concentrates—238 treated patients used more than 1.4 million units of factor VIII in the UK in 1980. There is an additional incentive to use cryoprecipitate or intermediate purity concentrate. There are occasional reports that some concentrates of high purity fail to correct the bleeding tendency in von Willebrand's disease, at the dose calculated in relation to factor VIII coagulant activity of the concentrate (Green and Potter 1976). It is not clear why this should happen, since none of the commonly used concentrates has an unusual ratio of FVIIIR:Ag to FVIII:C (McCue *et al.* 1980), but FVIIIR:Ag may not reflect all the functions of the FVIII molecule important for functional activities, e.g. in platelet adhesion.

Methods of preparation of prothrombin complex (II, VII, IX, X) concentrates

These are made primarily for their factor IX content. Factors II, X and VII share the highly anionic characteristics of factor IX imposed by γ-carboxyglutamic acid residues, and they tend to occur in the same fractions.

Prothrombin complex may be adsorbed on to calcium phosphate from plasma collected in EDTA anticoagulant (Soulier and Steinbuch 1975). The usual citrate anticoagulants inhibit adsorption, and EDTA collection makes the blood unsuitable for recovery of red cells, factor VIII, etc. The adsorbed factors may be eluted using citrate buffers and further concentrated by ethanol precipitation. Other selective adsorbents, which are no longer used for clinical concentrates of factor IX, include barium sulphate and aluminium hydroxide.

Most manufacturers adsorb factors IX, II and X on a polysaccharide-based ion-exchanger. Ion-exchangers with a high charge density tend to adsorb factor VII also, offering opportunities to prepare four-factor concentrate or separate concentrates of factors II, IX and X and of factor VII. The advantages of alternative adsorption and elution techniques have been reviewed (Smith and Bidwell 1979). The risk of hepatitis or thromboembolic complications is not convincingly correlated with methods of adsorption and may be more dependent on the quality of the plasma and the particular eluate fractions selected for finishing to freeze-dried product.

In all three fractionation centres in the UK, cryoprecipitate supernatant is adsorbed batchwise with DEAE-cellulose, the 'loaded' ion-exchanger recovered by continuous centrifugation, and packed into a chromatographic column for highly selective frontal elution and concentration of the factor IX-rich fraction. The eluate may be further treated with PEG with the aim of reducing transmission of hepatitis and, incidentally, the concentration of unwanted coagulant activities (Johnson *et al.* 1976).

In the UK, factor VII is prepared separately from factors IX, II and X, taking advantage of its lower charge interaction with DEAE-cellulose (Dike *et al.* 1980). This concentrate does not require further purification stages and the factor VII is recovered wholly in the non-activated form.

Potential thrombogenicity of prothrombin complex concentrates

Thromboembolic complications have been reported as sequelae to the infusion of prothrombin complex concentrates. Kasper (1975), reviewing this problem, identified three groups of patients especially at risk. These were patients with liver dysfunction, neonates and patients undergoing major surgery.

Thromboembolic complications following the use of prothrombin complex concentrates to treat patients suffering liver dysfunction are now well-documented (Cederbaum and Roberts 1973, Blatt *et al.* 1974, Gazzard *et al.* 1974, Cederbaum, Blatt and Roberts 1976, Davey, Shashaty and Rath 1976) and will be considered in depth in the section 'Other uses of prothrombin complex concentrates'.

Waltl *et al.* (1973), reporting on the use of a four-factor concentrate (Immuno 'BEBULIN') to prevent intracranial haemorrhage in low birthweight infants, concluded that mortality in the treated group was at least as high as, and arguably higher than, in an untreated control group. Kasper (1975) also provided anecdotal evidence of other similar experiences suggesting that the use of prothrombin complex concentrates was not indicated in the treatment of neonates.

The circumstances surrounding the incidence of thromboembolic complications following the use of prothrombin complex concentrates to provide haemostatic cover for major surgery are more difficult to interpret. Although such complications have been reported (Kasper 1973, Steinberg and Dreiling 1973, Marchesi and Burney 1974, Machin and Miller 1978), it is not clear in most cases that the authors distinguished between complications directly ascribable to treatment with prothrombin complex concentrates and the rate of occurrence of such complications in patients undergoing similar surgical procedures without haemostatic cover. In contrast, Lane, Rizza and Snape (1975) and Bidwell *et al.* (1976) reported extensive use of factor IX concentrate type DE(1) in a range of clinical situations including major surgery, with only two confirmed reports of post-operative thromboembolic complications, both in situations where the patient might have been considered predisposed to thromboembolism.

There can be little doubt that the early high incidence of thromboembolic complications following the use, in North America, of these comparatively new concentrates, was due to particular preparations which contained high levels of activated factors (Kingdon *et al.* 1975). The contrasting long successful history of safe clinical use of factor IX concentrates in the UK (Bidwell *et al.* 1976) clearly indicated that safe prothrombin complex concentrates could be produced—although any preparation containing large quantities of factors II, IX and X will be hazardous if used incautiously. Intensive application, both to final product and products under development, of a range of *in vivo* and *in vitro* tests for potential thrombogenicity (Kingdon *et al.* 1975, White *et al.* 1977) has effectively eliminated the earlier type of activated concentrate, and the incidence of thromboembolic sequelae has been significantly reduced.

It is important to recognize, however, that prothrombin complex concentrates being used to treat factor IX deficiency, also contain high levels of factors II and X. In the type DE(1) concentrate, for example, IX, II and X are present at approximately 30, 45 and 25 iu or u/ml respectively. Given the longer half-disappearance time of prothrombin (about 72 h compared with 12–24 h for factor IX), the possibility of high plasma prothrombin concentrations should always be considered and monitored in a patient receiving repeated doses of a prothrombin complex concentrate.

Tests for activated factors in prothrombin complex concentrates

Thrombus formation is an *in vivo* phenomenon and as such cannot be properly simulated in an *in vitro* system. A number of animal models have been described, and the more important may be classified as follows:

1   Stasis thrombus (rabbit) model (Wessler, Reimer and Sheps 1959).

2   Non-stasis (dog) model (Cash *et al.* 1975, Hedner, Nillsson and Bergentz 1976).

3   Non-stasis (rabbit) model (Prowse and Williams 1980).

Unfortunately, the considerable technical difficulties involved in the application of these tests has resulted in most manufacturers relying upon *in vitro* tests to indicate potential thrombogenicity.

Prowse, Chirnside and Elton (1980) surveyed the available *in vitro* test systems, and attempted to define such correlations as existed between them. It is essential to bear in mind that each of these test systems is at best a test for one or more activated factors which might be assumed to be potentially thrombogenic. None of the tests has been sufficiently well characterized to be called an assay (even if the necessary dose-response relationship existed), and the relationship between the performance of concentrates in the test systems, and their record of clinical use, is at best circumstantial (Kingdon *et al.* 1975, White *et al.* 1977). It is therefore more appropriate to think of them as 'tests for activated factors' than as 'tests for potential thrombogenicity'. The more important test systems and some of their characteristics are outlined in Table 24.

The NAPTT test (Kingdon *et al.* 1975) is the test for activated factors required by BP 1980, the requirement being a clotting time in excess of 150 s, with a control clotting time in excess of 200 s. The test consists of measuring the partial thromboplastin time of non-contacted platelet-poor plasma in the presence and absence of the test preparation.

TGt_{50} and Xa generation tests (Sas *et al.* 1975, Pepper *et al.* 1977) involve measurement of the rate of generation of thrombin and factor Xa respectively, in a recalcified dilution of the sample. The XaGT is technically simpler than the TGt_{50} system, and has the advantage of being independent of the factor V and phospholipid content of the factor IX concentrates under test. No limit has been defined nationally or internationally for prothrombin complex concentrates in either of these tests.

The fibrinogen clotting time test, which involves measurement of the clotting time at 37°C of a mixture of the test sample and 0.4 per cent w/v fibrinogen solution, is essentially a test for thrombin. The WHO Technical Report '*Requirements for the collection, processing and quality control of human blood and blood products*' (1978) specifies a minimum clotting time for prothrombin complex concentrates of 6 h in this test system (equivalent to approximately 10^{-3} iu thrombin/ml. In practice, concentrates with at least ten times this level of thrombin (fibrinogen clotting time approximately 2.5 h) have been infused safely and it is unlikely that low levels of thrombin *per se* are important, except perhaps as indicators of previous activation.

In a recent study of *in vitro* test systems, Prowse and Pepper (1980) concluded that the NAPTT test mainly responds to factor IXa, whereas the

Table 24. Tests for 'potential thrombogenicity' of factor IX concentrates.

System	Description
NAPTT test	Determines the effect of dilutions of the test preparation on the partial thromboplastin time of non-contacted, platelet-poor plasma in the absence of surface activators. Sensitive principally to factor IXa (Prowse and Pepper 1980) but also responds to other activated factors of the intrinsic system.
TGt_{50} test	Provides a measure of the rate of thrombin generation in a recalcified dilution of the sample. Thrombin is detected by subsampling at intervals into fibrinogen solution and timing clot formation. Sensitive to a wide range of proteases, but may be controlled to an extent by levels of factor V and phospholipid in the sample, should these be limiting.
Xa generation test	Provides a measure of the rate of generation of factor Xa in a recalcified dilution of the sample. Factor Xa is detected by its esterolytic effect on the chromogenic substrate KABI S-2222. Sensitivity as for the TGt_{50} test, but the factor V and phospholipid content of the test sample are less important.
Fibrinogen clotting time test	Essentially a test/assay for thrombin.

TGt_{50} test (and by implication, therefore, the Xa generation test) was more sensitive to a wider range of proteases. Prowse, Chirnside and Elton (1980) concluded that a combination of the NAPTT and TGt_{50} (or XaGT) tests ought to be sufficient to demonstrate activation in factor IX concentrates. These two conclusions describe the current status of tests for activated factors quite well. Unfortunately, the relationship between the presence of low levels of activated factors and potential thrombogenicity is less well defined. Until such time, therefore, as clinical risk can be defined in terms of the particular properties of a concentrate (such as response in a test for activated factors), batch to batch consistency of all of the parameters determined, and an established history of safe and effective clinical use, must be the main criteria on which a concentrate is assessed.

Replacement therapy in congenital deficiency

CONGENITAL FACTOR IX DEFICIENCY

The use of prothrombin complex concentrates for this purpose in the UK was reviewed by Lane, Rizza and Snape (1975) and by Bidwell *et al.* (1976).

CONGENITAL FACTOR X DEFICIENCY

Fewer than ten factor X-deficient patients are known in the UK. If treatment must be too protracted to consider the use of fresh-frozen plasma or cryosupernatant, virtually any four-factor or three-factor prothrombin complex concentrate can be used for its content of factor X, but the expected benefits should be assessed against the increased hepatitis risk. The risk of thromboembolic complications may be at least as severe in factor X deficiency as in haemophilia B following infusion of concentrates (Blatt *et al.* 1974).

If there were sufficient incentive, factor X could be separated from other factors of the prothrombin complex by 'affinity' chromatography on immobilized heparin or dextran sulphate, but there has been no demand for such developments.

CONGENITAL FACTOR II DEFICIENCY

Like factor X deficiency, the very rare factor II deficiency may be treated with fresh-frozen plasma, cryosupernatant or prothrombin complex concentrates. There has been no demand for a separate concentrate of factor II, although this is technically feasible.

CONGENITAL FACTOR VII DEFICIENCY

Factor VII deficiency is not always accompanied by spontaneous bleeding but it may be necessary to provide cover up to at least 20 per cent of normal levels for surgery and in rare life-threatening episodes such as intracranial bleeding. Prophylaxis has been used but the short half-life of factor VII (3–4 h) militates against this in most cases.

Fresh-frozen plasma might be considered for a single treatment, but the short half-life of infused factor VII makes this unattractive. Prothrombin complex concentrates contain varying concentrations of factor VII. A factor VII concentrate containing clinically insignificant levels of factors II, IX and X is available in the UK.

Other uses of prothrombin complex concentrates

RAPID REVERSAL OF ANTICOAGULANT THERAPY

The anticoagulant effect of coumarin-type preparations is the result of reduced synthesis of vitamin K-dependent factors (II, VII, IX and X). Rapid reversal of the anticoagulant effect may be achieved by transfusion of fresh plasma or prothrombin complex concentrates. Plasma replacement therapy provides all four deficient factors but, since many of the patients involved have an underlying cardiovascular defect, circulatory overload may be a problem. The prothrombin complex concentrates most readily available in the UK (Edinburgh DEFIX and BPL/PFL factor IX type 9D) are three-factor concentrates with negligible factor VII content; if correction of the deficiency of factor VII is also desirable, a separate factor VII concentrate such as that described by Dike *et al.* (1980) must be given.

HAEMOSTATIC COVER OF PATIENTS UNDERGOING LIVER BIOPSY

In patients with acute or chronic liver disease, liver biopsy may be required to confirm a diagnosis or assess the progress of the disease state. The reduced levels of factors of the prothrombin complex reflected in the increased prothrombin time ratio of such patients has led many clinicians to believe that some form of replacement therapy is desirable. Kasper (1975), on the other hand, identified patients with liver dysfunction as one group of patients at increased risk of thromboembolic complications as sequelae to infusion of prothrombin complex concentrates, and thromboembolic complications in this group have been widely reported. The experience of Gazzard *et al.* (1974), using factor IX type 9D to correct the reduced levels of prothrombin complex factors in patients suffering fulminant hepatic failure, is relevant. The results, in nine patients thus treated, indicated that the concentrate not only failed to restore coagulation factors to acceptable levels, but also potentiated intravascular coagulation. The report by Green *et al.* (1975) of the successful use of prothrombin complex concentrates to provide haemostatic cover for patients undergoing liver biopsy describes the use of a now discontinued four-factor concentrate and must be interpreted with caution.

TREATMENT OF HAEMOPHILIA COMPLICATED BY FACTOR VIII INHIBITORS

The treatment of haemophilia complicated by inhibitors to factor VIII is discussed comprehensively elsewhere in this book, but the use of prothrombin complex concentrates for this purpose deserves special mention here. Efficacy has been claimed for preparations with little demonstrable activation (Abildgaard, Britton and Harrison 1976), controlled activated products such as

FEIBA (Lechner *et al.* 1978) and AUTOPLEX (Abilgaard, Penner and Watson-Williams 1981), spontaneously (i.e. accidentally) activated preparations such as the earlier batches of PROPLEX (Kurzcynski and Penner 1974) and KONYNE (Abildgaard, Britton and Harrison 1976) and for non-activated prothrombin complex concentrates deliberately activated before administration by the addition of calcium ions (Eckert and McVeagh 1975). Assessment of clinical effectiveness presents a major problem, and it is only recently that controlled clinical trials are being reported (Lusher *et al.* 1980).

It is generally assumed that the claimed effectiveness of these preparations is the result of activated factors bypassing the factor VIII requirement—and, therefore, the factor VIII inhibitors. Candidates for the activated factor have included a factor X-thrombin complex (Tishkoff 1977), modified or complexed Xa (Elsinger 1977) and activated factor VII (Seligsohn *et al.* 1979). Barrowcliffe, Kemball-Cook and Gray (1981) suggest that for preparations such as Immuno FEIBA which contain significant factor VIII activity, factor VIII complexed with and protected by phospholipid may also be important. It must be recognized, however, that all of these observations are extrapolations of *in vitro* studies to explain an (arguable) *in vivo* effect.

Replacement therapy for other deficiencies

FACTOR V DEFICIENCY

Factor V deficiency is rare and seldom results in spontaneous bleeding episodes. When treatment is necessary, fresh-frozen plasma should be given. Cryoprecipitation does not concentrate factor V. Patients may become refractory to whole plasma but at present there is no concentrate available. Factor V is very unstable in plasma and it can be satisfactorily purified only after the addition of protease inhibitors which are too toxic to consider for therapeutic concentrates (Dahlback 1980). Bolhuis *et al.* (1979) achieved considerable concentration of factor V from human cryosupernatant by precipitation with PEG and gel filtration, but activity is not well preserved during the freezing and drying necessary to maintain stable stocks of concentrate.

Combined factor V and VIII deficiency (Iverson and Bastrup-Madsen 1956) may be due to a deficiency of protein C inhibitor (Marlar and Griffin 1980). If this is confirmed, replacement therapy with the concentrated inhibitor might be feasible.

FACTOR XI DEFICIENCY

Not all factor XI-deficient patients have a bleeding tendency and bleeding does not necessarily correlate with the plasma level of factor XI. A poor response to infusion of factor XI should prompt an investigation of possible inhibitors.

The factor XI content should always be checked by assay of the batch of concentrate before infusion. Factor XI is adsorbed by immobilized heparin and may be recovered from plasma in the same way as antithrombin III. However, since the latter is usually pasteurized for clinical use, it should not be assumed that any concentrate of antithrombin III will contain useful factor XI activity.

FACTOR XIII DEFICIENCY

Since there is a relatively high incidence of life-threatening intracranial bleeds, some clinicians have preferred prophylaxis to episodic treatment. A factor XIII concentrate from human placenta has been used successfully for both modes of treatment (Losowski and Miloszewski 1977). Bleeding episodes are usually treated with plasma, or cryoprecipitate which is rich in factor XIII as well as factor VIII and fibrinogen, but some patients develop severe reactions to such treatment. A minor obstacle to the concentration of factor XIII from plasma is that cryoprecipitate, the most obvious source of factor XIII for the fractionator, is also required for factor VIII, but useful amounts of factor XIII can be removed from the cryosupernatant in the fibrinogen-rich Cohn Fraction I recovered by cold precipitation with 8 per cent ethanol at neutral pH. Factor XIII is relatively stable at temperatures which cause precipitation of fibrinogen. It can also be precipitated with neutral salts and with polyethylene glycol. Methods have been published for ion-exchange (Cooke and Holbrook 1974) and affinity chromatography of factor XIII (McDonagh *et al.* 1976) but these may not be necessary for a clinical concentrate. An alternative to the placental concentrates, a concentrate made from plasma as part of comprehensive fractionation, is now available in the UK. It has been possible to reduce the risk of transmitting hepatitis with a concentrate from pooled plasma by exploiting the stability of factor XIII at high temperatures. If, as seems likely, the risk of transmitting hepatitis can be overcome, the concentrate should be more convenient than plasma or cryoprecipitate infusions for prophylaxis and treatment of factor XIII deficiency.

There is some evidence that factor XIII concentrate promotes wound healing (Biel *et al.* 1971) and improves some symptoms in scleroderma (Delbarre, Godeau and Thivolet 1981).

FIBRINOGEN DEFICIENCY

Replacement therapy may still be indicated in DIC, particularly in obstetric cases, and in congenital afibrinogenaemia. Clinical demand for fibrinogen has fallen rapidly with increasing recognition of the risks of exacerbating consumption coagulopathies and of transmitting hepatitis to patients who require only a single treatment.

Since fibrinogen does not withstand treatments used to inactivate hepatitis viruses, fibrinogen from pooled plasma is now no longer produced in some countries. Cryoprecipitate contains approximately 200 mg fibrinogen per pack and could be used for its fibrinogen content even after factor VIII activity may have decayed. The use of single-donor or small-pool cryoprecipitate should always be considered before resorting to fibrinogen concentrates.

Large-pool concentrates containing more than 60 per cent clottable protein are derived from a cold-ethanol fraction, Cohn Fraction I. The plasma need not be fresh-frozen, and useful amounts of fibrinogen can be recovered even from cryosupernatant. The crude fraction is usually reworked by washing with glycine-citrate-ethanol buffers (Blombäck and Blombäck 1956). If required for a specific purpose, clottability may be increased to over 90 per cent by further reprecipitations or adsorptions of unwanted contaminants such as fibronectin, prothrombin complex, plasminogen, etc.

Fibrinogen for Isotopic Labelling, used in the diagnosis of thromboembolism, is prepared from small pools of plasma from specially 'accredited' donors, extensively screened to eliminate the risk of transmitting hepatitis.

Fibrinogen is now sometimes used in essentially topical applications in conjunction with thrombin, e.g. in sheathing of large nerves after surgery and removal of renal stones in a fibrin 'cast'.

THROMBIN

Thrombin is still used topically, e.g. on varices, gums, surgical incisions, etc., sometimes in conjunction with fibrinogen. *Thrombin must not be injected intravenously.* Thrombin is made from prothrombin concentrates, usually by activation with thromboplastin or venom, followed by ion-exchange or affinity chromatography.

FACTORS OF THE CONTACT PHASE

Deficiencies of factor XII, HMW kininogen (Fitzgerald factor, Flaujeac factor) or prekallikrein (Fletcher factor) are not associated with haemorrhagic problems. The major risk may be exsanguination for investigative purposes. No concentrates are available.

ANTITHROMBIN III

This serine esterase inhibitor has been used in congenital deficiency (Laharrague *et al.* 1980), DIC (Schipper *et al.* 1978), and pre-eclampsia (Buller *et al.*

1980). Potential uses include protection against thromboembolic complications sometimes associated with factor IX concentrates and replacement of the antithrombin III deficiency noted in the early stages of heparin therapy (Marciniak and Gockerman 1981). Congenital deficiency is often treated successfully with coumarin anticoagulants, but antithrombin III may be a useful adjunct during suspension of anticoagulant therapy for any reason.

Antithrombin III is present in Cohn Fraction IV, a 'waste' fraction from comprehensive ethanol fractionation, but much of the inhibitor has already combined with proteases and is not active. It may be adsorbed directly from cryosupernatant or factor IX supernatant on to heparin attached to an insoluble matrix (Wickerhauser, Williams and Mercer 1979). High salt concentrations necessary for elution may be reduced by ultrafiltration or gel filtration, and it is possible to pasteurize the product.

PLASMINOGEN

The use of plasminogen in thrombolysis, alone or in conjunction with streptokinase, has been disappointing (Kakkar, Sagar and Lewis 1975). New approaches to the selective delivery of plasmin are discussed in Chapter 17.

FIBRONECTIN

This protein, formerly called cold insoluble globulin, is thought to have important opsonic properties. Replacement therapy using cryoprecipitate in traumatized or septicaemic patients (Scovill *et al.* 1976) with very low fibronectin levels may result in greatly improved blood flow and oxygen-carrying capacity.

Although it is known that factor XIII catalyses the transglutamination of fibronectin, the role of fibronectin in normal or abnormal haemostasis is not yet understood. Haematologists should be aware that concentrates of fibronectin are being developed, and other plasma proteins with opsonic activity may be found.

C1-ESTERASE INHIBITOR

A concentrate of this inhibitor can be made by DEAE-Sephadex adsorption of diluted factor IX supernatant (Vogelaar, Brummelhuis and Krijen 1974). It may be useful in hereditary angio-neurotic oedema as an alternative to treatment with fibrinolytic inhibitors.

Transmission of viral hepatitis

Plasma fractions transmit very few infectious diseases. No bacteria pass the sterilizing filters universally used and most filter-passing viruses do not survive the freezing of plasma or even the gentle separation methods used for coagulation factor production. The most significant sources of infection are the hepatitis viruses (Seeff 1981). If a patient who has recently received blood products becomes jaundiced, it is not always easy to exclude non-viral causes or to identify the type of hepatitis virus responsible. For instance, the patient may have been recently infected non-parenterally with hepatitis A. Jaundice or other evidence of liver disease due to hepatitis B characteristically appears 7–25 weeks after the challenge. Positive diagnosis of hepatitis B is usually fairly straightforward on the basis of tests for specific viral antigens and specific antibodies developing during and after the period of active hepatitis. Non-A non-B hepatitis (NANBH) is still diagnosed by exclusion of other sources. Infection is often symptomless and detected only by elevation of serum enzymes, usually 2–16 weeks after challenge. Both type B and NANBH can be transmitted in plasma fractions and induce fatal fulminant hepatitis (Mathiesen *et al.* 1980) but such severe consequences are uncommon in multi-transfused patients.

Biopsies on regular recipients of blood products show evidence of liver damage (Mannucci *et al.* 1975), often without clinical symptoms but carrying a supposition of progress towards cirrhosis later in life. Liver damage is evident in approximately 10 per cent of hepatitis B patients and about half of those contracting NANBH. The latter may be particularly likely to develop chronic active hepatitis (Berman *et al.* 1979). At the very least, the risk inhibits many of the potential applications of blood products, e.g. of prothrombin complex in deficiencies other than haemophilia B.

Freeze-dried fibrinogen from large pools is now no longer made in the USA because the risk of transmitting hepatitis is considered to outweigh its potential benefits, even when properly used.

Approximately 70 per cent of severe haemophiliacs in most groups studied have shown laboratory or clinical evidence of having received a challenge from hepatitis B in blood products. The majority of hepatitis cases among haemophiliacs now seem to be associated with NANBH, possibly associated with more than one infective agent. In UK haemophiliacs alone, approximately 10–20 overt cases per year are now thought to be attributable to NANBH, of which approximately half may go on to suffer some degree of chronic liver disease. A number of approaches are being tried to reduce the risk of transmitting hepatitis with coagulation factor concentrates. If it is confirmed that Acquired Immune Deficiency Syndrome (AIDS) is transmitted by blood products, the approach to diminishing the risk may be similar to those described for NANBH.

1. Exclude virus-contaminated donations from fractionation

'Third generation' RIA tests can detect approximately 20 pg HBsAg/ml plasma, but blood screened in this way may still contain an infective dose of hepatitis B. Unfortunately, there is no screening test for NANBH and we must rely on diminishing the contribution from high-risk groups, for instance by recognizing the lower incidence of transmission from volunteer than from paid donors (Norkrans *et al.* 1981).

2. Reduce the probability of including virus in fractionation pools

For certain programmes it has been worthwhile to screen a small population of plasma donors more intensively than usual, including careful selection from well-known donors, serial estimation of amino-transferases, clinical surveillance and quarantining of plasma for more than three months as a final precaution.

The small-pool approach may be the best interim solution for infrequent users, but it is irrelevant to the needs of the majority of severe haemophiliacs who inevitably consume the product of many thousands of donations per year in some form. An alternative approach is being developed in the UK, based on the procurement of plasma batches from small panels of donors contributing to local programmes of automated plasmapheresis.

3. Inactivate any virus in whole plasma before fractionation

Viruses may be inactivated in the starting plasma by treatment with the virucidal agent β-propiolactone and u.v. radiation. Results from infusion of whole plasma so treated suggest that it does not transmit viral hepatitis of any sort and the sterilized plasma may be further fractionated to recover, for example, factors II, VII, IX and X. This process has not been used more widely because β-propiolactone is carcinogenic and mutagenic, and because plasma proteins are extensively modified by the treatment. Inactivation of hepatitis B virus is incomplete (Prince *et al.* 1980).

Alternative virucides are being assessed. Destruction of virus particles using detergents has been proposed. It would seem fruitful to explore the use of reagents which are more destructive to the organization and function of nucleic acids than of proteins.

4. Discriminate against hepatitis viruses during routine fractionation

The addition of concentrated human hepatitis B antibody to coagulation factor concentrates may neutralize residual virus, and has been successful in reducing hepatitis B transmission by factor IX concentrates (Tabor, Aronson and Gerety 1980). The difficulties here are to establish the effective excess antibody concentration; how to procure enough human antibody; and how to be sure that one is inactivating the virus rather than simply giving short-term passive protection. There is also a limit to the amount of IgG which can be given intravenously without risking adverse reactions.

Some of these difficulties could be reduced by solid-phase immunosorption of virus on insolubilized antibody, perhaps even non-human antibodies. The additional problems are the capacity of the adsorbent; the long contact period which may be necessary to reach equilibrium and which is inimical to unstable coagulation factors; potential leakage of the ligand; the concentrations of virus that may have to be removed and the difficulty of demonstrating that the product is no longer infective, even if markers such as HBsAg are reduced below detection limits.

Immunosorption methods are of course of little use for NANBH since we cannot yet quantitate either the infective agent or its antibody.

5. Remove virus semi-specifically at intermediate stages of production

We know nothing about the behaviour of NANBH during fractionation. What we know about hepatitis B is largely derived from following the HBsAg marker rather than the virus itself but some studies have attempted to follow other markers (Trepo *et al.* 1978). HBsAg is found in all coagulation factor concentrates from infected plasma, and all of these may transmit hepatitis B if the plasma is infected.

There are a number of published claims for the removal of HBsAg from concentrates, usually at an intermediate stage of production by semi-specific adsorbents such as polyelectrolytes or amino-acyl agarose. These claims have not yet been convincingly supported by animal or clinical trials.

Substantial removal of HBsAg from factor IX concentrates can be achieved by single or repeated precipitation of virus with PEG 4000, while the factor IX is kept in solution by manipulating ionic strength, pH, solvent components, etc. (Johnson *et al.* 1976). It is difficult to prove, even by following the HBsAg marker, that the process will work equally well at an undetectable but infective initial level of virus particles in the product. The approach is attractive because it might be applicable to viruses other than hepatitis B, e.g. non-A non-B hepatitis and possibly any infective agent transmitting AIDS.

6. Inactivate virus by heating solutions of products

Whole plasma and most isolated plasma proteins coagulate or otherwise denature when heated to 60°C for 10 h, the conditions found experimentally to destroy infectivity of hepatitis B virus. However, albumin preparations may be heated in the final container under the protection of fatty acids. Plasminogen can be heated under certain conditions and antithrombin III can be recovered in good yield in the presence of high concentrations of citrate ions (Holleman *et al.* 1977). Factor VIII can be pasteurized, protected by glycine and sucrose, and the product is said not to transmit hepatitis but the published yield of factor VIII is still uneconomic for routine production (Heimburger *et al.* 1981). Patients treated very infrequently may of course merit special consideration.

Other procedures, so far described only incompletely, include heating the concentrate in the freeze-dried state.

7. Vaccinate recipients of blood products against hepatitis viruses

A vaccine against hepatitis B promises to be very effective in some high-risk groups (Szmuness *et al.* 1980). However, it is questionable whether vaccination would be justified for, for example, carriers and very mild cases. There is no vaccine against non-A non-B hepatitis.

REFERENCES

Abildgaard C.F., Britton M. & Harrison J. (1976) Prothrombin complex concentrate (Konyne) in the treatment of hemophilic patients with factor VIII inhibitors. *Journal of Paediatrics* **88**, 200–5.

Abildgaard C.F., Penner J.A. & Watson-Williams W.J. (1981) Anti-inhibitor coagulant complex (Autoplex) for treatment of factor VIII inhibitors in hemophilia. *Blood* **56**, 978–84.

Allain J.P., Verroust F. & Soulier J.P. (1980) *In vitro* and *in vivo* characterisation of factor VIII preparations. *Vox Sanguinis* **38**, 68–80.

Austen D.E.G. (1979) The chromatographic separation of Factor VIII on aminohexyl sepharose. *British Journal of Haematology* **43**, 669–74.

Austen D.E.G., Rhymes I.R. & Rizza C.R. (1981) Factor VIII concentrates: what the label says. *Lancet* **II**, 1167.

Barrowcliffe T.W. & Thomas D.P. (1981) Factor VIII standardisation. *Lancet* **II**, 1342.

Barrowcliffe T.W., Kemball-Cook G. & Gray E. (1981) Factor VIII inhibitor bypassing activity: a suggested mechanism of action. *Thrombosis Research* **21**, 181–6.

Berman M., Alter H.J., Ishak K.G., Purcell R.H. & Jones E.A. (1979) The chronic sequelae of non-A non-B hepatitis. *Annals of Internal Medicine* **91**, 1–6.

Bidwell E., Dike G.W.R., Rizza C.R. & Snape T.J. (1976) Clinical use of factor IX concentrate. *Thrombosis and Haemostasis* **35**, 488–91.

Biel H., Bohn H., Ronneberger H. & Zwisler O. (1971) Speeding wound healing by factor XIII of blood clotting. *Drug Research* **21**, 1429–30.

Blatt P.M., Brinkhous K.M., Culp H.R., Krauss J.S. & Roberts H.R. (1976) Antihemophilic factor concentrate therapy in von Willebrand's disease. Dissociation of bleeding-time factor and ristocetin co-factor activities. *Journal of the American Medical Association* **236**, 2770–2.

Blatt P.M., Lundblad R.L., Kingdon H.S., McLean G. & Roberts H.R. (1974) Thrombogenic materials in prothrombin complex concentrates. *Annals of Internal Medicine* **81**, 766–70.

Blombäck B. & Blombäck M. (1956) Purification of human and bovine fibrinogen. *Arkiv for Kemi* **10**, 415–43.

Blombäck M. & Nilsson I.M. (1958) Treatment of hemophilia A with human antihemophilic globulin. *Acta Medica Scandinavica* **161**, 301–21.

Bolhuis P.A., Hakvoort T.B.M., Breederveld K., Mochtar L.A. & Ten Cate J.W. (1979) Isolation and partial characterization of human factor V. *Biochemica et Biophysica Acta* **578**, 23–30.

Brinkhous K.M., Shanbrom E., Roberts H.R., Webster W.P., Fekete L. & Wagner R.H. (1968) A new high-potency glycine precipitated antihemophilic factor (AHF) concentrate. *Journal of the American Medical Association* **205**, 613–17.

British Pharmacopoeia (1980) Addendum 1981.

Büller H.R., Weenink A.H., Treffers P.E., Kakle L.H., Otten H.A. & Ten Cate J.W. (1980) Severe antithrombin III deficiency in a patient with pre-eclampsia. Observations on the effect of human AT III concentrate transfusion. *Scandinavian Journal of Haematology* **25**, 81–6.

Cash J.D., Dalton R.G., Middleton S. & Smith J.K. (1975) Studies on the thrombogenicity of Scottish factor IX concentrate in dogs. *Thrombosis et Diathesis Haemorrhagica* **33**, 632–9.

Cederbaum A.I., Blatt P.M. & Roberts H.R. (1976) Intravascular coagulation with use of human prothrombin complex concentrates. *Annals of Internal Medicine* **84**, 683–7.

Cederbaum A.I. & Roberts H.R. (1973) Complications of the use of prothrombin complex concentrates in liver idsease. *Clinical Research* **21**, 92.

Cooke R.D. & Holbrook J.J. (1974) The calcium-induced dissociation of human plasma clotting factor XIII. *Biochemical Journal* **141**, 79–85.

Dahlback B. (1980) Human coagulation factor V purification and thrombin-catalyzed activation. *Journal of Clinical Investigation* **66**, 583–91.

Davey R.J., Shashaty G.G. & Rath C.E. (1976) Acute coagulopathy following infusion of prothrombin complex concentrate. *American Journal of Medicine* **60**, 719–22.

Delbarre F., Godeau P. & Thivolet J. (1981) Factor XIII treatment for scleroderma. *Lancet* **II**, 204.

Dike G.W.R., Griffiths D., Bidwell E., Snape T.J. & Rizza C.R. (1980) A factor VII concentrate in therapeutic use. *British Journal of Haematology* **45**, 107–18.

Eckert H. & McVeagh P. (1975) Activated PPSB in the treatment of a patient with haemophilia and antibodies to factor VIII. *Medical Journal of Australia* **2**, 675–7.

Elsinger F. (1977) Preparations with factor VIII inhibitor bypassing activity. In *Proceedings of the Workshop on Inhibitors of Factors VIII and IX*. Facultas-Verlag, Vienna.

Foster P.R., Dickson A.J., McQuillan T.A., Dickson I.H., Keddie S. & Watt J.G. (1982) Control of large-scale plasma thawing for recovery of cryoprecipitate factor VIII. *Vox Sanguinis* **42**, 180–9.

Gazzard B.G., Lewis H.L., Ash G., Rizza C.R., Bidwell E. & Williams R. (1974) Coagulation factor concentrate in the treatment of the haemorrhagic diathesis of fulminant hepatic failure. *Journal of the British Society of Gastroenterology—GUT* **15**, 993–8.

Green G., Poller L., Dymock I.M. & Thompson J.M. (1975) Use of factor-VII-rich prothrombin complex concentrate in liver disease. *Lancet* **I**, 1311.

Green D. & Potter E.V. (1976) Failure of AHF concentrate to control bleeding in von Willebrand's disease. *American Journal of Medicine* **60**, 357–60.

Gunson H.H., Bidwell E., Lane R.S., Wensley R.T. & Snape T.J. (1978) Variables involved in cryoprecipitate production and their effect on factor VIII activity. *British Journal of Haematology* **43**, 287–95.

Hedner U., Nilsson I.M. & Bergentz S.E. (1976) Studies on the thrombogenic activities in two prothrombin complex concentrates. *Thrombosis and Haemostasis* **42**, 1022-32.

Heimburger N., Schwinn H., Gratz P., Kumpe G. & Herchenhan B. (1981) A factor VIII concentrate, highly purified and heated in solution. *Haemostasis* **10** (Suppl. 1), 204.

Heimburger N., Schwinn H., Kumpe G. & Herchenhan B. (1977) Factor VIII concentrates—progress in development. *Pharmazeutische Zeitung* **122**, 1382–6.

Hershgold E.J., Pool J.G. & Pappenhagen A.R. (1966) A potent antihaemophilic globulin concentrate derived from a cold insoluble fraction of human plasma: characterisation and further data on preparation and clinical trial. *Journal of Laboratory and Clinical Medicine* **67**, 23–32.

Holleman W.H., Coen L.J., Capobianco J.O. & Barlow G.H. (1977) Isolation of human antithrombin III by affinity chromatography on heparin agarose. *Thrombosis and Haemostasis* **38**, 201 (Abstract).

Iverson T. & Bastrup-Madsen P. (1956) Congenital familial deficiency of factor V (para-haemophilia) combined with deficiency of antihaemophilic globulin. *British Journal of Haematology* **2**, 265-75.

Johnson A.J., Macdonald B.E. & Brind J. (1979) Enhanced yield of antihaemophilic factor and von Willebrand factor by cryoprecipitation with polyethylene glycol. *Vox Sanguinis* **36**, 72–6.

Johnson A.J., Macdonald B.E., Semar M., Fields J.E., Schuck J., Lewis C. & Brind J. (1978) Preparation of the major plasma fractions by solid-phase polyelectrolytes. *Journal of Laboratory and Clinical Medicine* **92**, 194–209.

Johnson A.J., Semar M., Newman J., Harris R.B., Brandt D., Middleton S. & Smith J. (1976) Removal of hepatitis B surface antigen (NB Ag) from plasma fractions. *Journal of Laboratory and Clinical Medicine* **88**, 91–101.

Kakkar V.V., Sagar S. & Lewis M. (1975) Treatment of deep-vein thrombosis with intermittent streptokinase and plasminogen infusion. *Lancet* **ll**, 674–6.

Kasper C.K. (1973) Postoperative thromboses in hemophilia B. *New England Journal of Medicine* **289**, 160.

Kasper C.K. (1975) Clinical use of factor IX concentrates: report on thrombo-embolic complications. *Thrombosis et Diathesis Haemorrhagica* **33**, 640–4.

Kasper C.K. (1981) Problems with the potency of factor VIII concentrate. *New England Journal of Medicine* **305**, 50–1.

Kingdon H.S., Lundblad R.L., Veltkamp J.J. & Aronson D.L. (1975) Potentially thrombogenic materials in factor IX concentrates. *Thrombosis et Diathesis Haemorrhagica* **33**, 617–31.

Kurzcynski E.M. & Penner J.A. (1974) Activated prothrombin concentrate for patients with factor VIII inhibitors. *New England Journal of Medicine* **291**, 164–7.

Laharrague P., Bierme R., Cerene A., Boucays A. & Massip P. (1980) Antithrombin III: Substitutive treatment of the hereditary deficiency. *Thrombosis and Haemostasis* **43**, 72.

Lane J.L., Rizza C.R. & Snape T.J. (1975) A five-year experience of the use of factor IX type DE(1) concentrate for the treatment of Christmas disease at Oxford. *British Journal of Haematology* **30**, 435–46.

Lechner K., Nowotny C., Krinninger B., Zegner M. & Deutsch E. (1978) Effect of treatment with activated prothrombin complex concentrate (FEIBA) on factor VIII-antibody level. *Thrombosis and Haemostasis* **40**, 478–85.

Losowski M.S. & Miloszewski K.J.A. (1977) Annotation: Factor XIII. *British Journal of Haematology* **37**, 1–5.

Lusher J.M., Shapiro S.S., Palascak J.E., Rao A.V., Levine P.H., Blatt P.M. and the Hemophilia Study Group (1980) Efficacy of prothrombin-complex concentrates in hemophiliacs with antibodies to factor VIII. A multicenter therapeutic trial. *New England Journal of Medicine* **303**, 421–5.

McCue M.J., Broissoit A.D., Marmer D.J. & Head D.R. (1980) Von Willebrand factor (VIII$_{VWF}$) in lyophilized factor VIII concentrates. *American Journal of Hematology* **9**, 39–42.

McDonagh J., Waggoner W.G., Hamilton E.G., Hindenach B. & McDonagh R.P. (1976) Affinity chromatography of human plasma and platelet factor XIII on organo-mercurial agarose. *Biochimica et Biophysica Acta* **446**, 345–57.

Machin S.J. & Miller B.R. (1978) Thrombosis and factor IX concentrates. *Lancet* I, 1367.

Mannucci P.M., Capitanio A., Del Ninno E., Colombo M., Pareti F. & Ruggeri Z.M. (1975) Asymptomatic liver disease in haemophiliacs. *Journal of Clinical Pathology* **28**, 620–4.

Marchesi S.L. & Burney R. (1974) Prothrombin complex concentrates and thromboses. *New England Journal of Medicine* **290**, 403–4.

Marciniak E. & Gockerman J.P. (1981) Kinetics of elimination of Antithrombin III concentrate in heparinized patients. *British Journal of Haematology* **48**, 617–25.

Margolis J & Rhoades P. (1979) Preparation of stable intermediate-purity factor VIII concentrate with a note on high-purity factor VIII. *Vox Sanguinis* **36**, 369–74.

Marlar R.A. & Griffin J.H. (1980) Deficiency of protein C inhibitor in combined Factor V/VIII deficiency. *Journal of Clinical Investigation* **66**, 1186.

Mason E.C. (1978) Thaw-siphon technique for production of cryoprecipitate concentrate of factor VIII. *Lancet* **2**, 15.

Mathiesen L.R., Skinoj P., Nielsen J.O., Purcell R.H., Wong D. & Ranek L. (1980) Hepatitis type A, B, and non-A non-B in fulminant hepatitis. *Gut* **21**, 72–7.

Newman J., Johnson A.J., Karpatkin M.H. & Puszkin S. (1971) Methods for the production of clinical effective intermediate and high purity factor VIII concentrates. *British Journal of Haematology* **21**, 1–20.

Norkrans G., Widell A., Teger-Nilsson A.-C., Kjellman H., Frosner G. & Iwarson S. (1981) Acute hepatitis non-A, non-B following administration of factor VIII concentrates. *Vox Sanguinis* **41**, 129–33.

Pepper D.S., Banhegyi D., Howie A. & Cash J.D. (1977) *In vitro* thrombogenicity tests of factor IX concentrates. *British Journal of Haematology* **36**, 573–83.

Prince A.M., Stephan W., Brotman B. & van den Ende M.S. (1980) Evaluation of the effect of β-propiolactone/ultra violet irradiation (BPL/UV) treatment of source plasma on hepatitis transmission by factor IX complex in chimpanzees. *Thrombosis and Haemostasis* **45**, 138–42.

Prowse C.V., Chirnside A. & Elton R.A. (1980) *In vitro* thrombogenicity tests of factor IX concentrates. 1. A survey of available assays. *Thrombosis and Haemostasis* **42**, 1355–67.

Prowse C.V. & Pepper D. (1980) *In vitro* tests of the potential thrombogenicity of factor IX concentrates: inhibition and characterisation studies of NAPTT, TGt50 and PF3 moieties. *Thrombosis Research* **20**, 49–8.

Prowse C.V. & Williams A.E. (1980) A comparison of the *in vitro* and *in vivo* thrombogenic activity of factor IX concentrates using stasis (Wessler) and non-stasis rabbit models. *Thrombosis and Haemostasis* **44**, 81–6.

Rock G.A., Cruickshank W.H., Tackaberry E.S. & Palmer D.S. (1979) Improved yields of factor VIII from heparinised plasma. *Vox Sanguinis* **36**, 294–300.

Rock G.A., McCombe N. & Tittley P. (1981) A new technique for the collection of plasma: machine plasmapheresis. *Transfusion* **21**, 241–6.

Rock G.A. & Palmer D.S. (1980) Intermediate purity factor VIII utilising a cold-insoluble globulin technique. *Thrombosis Research* **18**, 551–6.

Sas G., Owens R.E., Smith J.K., Middleton S. & Cash J.D. (1975) *In vitro* spontaneous thrombin generation in human factor IX concentrates. *British Journal of Haematology* **31**, 25–35.

Schipper H.G., Jenkins C.S.P., Kahle L.H. & Ten Cate J.W. (1978) Antithrombin-III transfusion in disseminated intravascular coagulation. *Lancet* **I**, 854–6.

Scovill W.A., Saba T.M., Kaplan J.E. *et al.* (1976) Deficits in reticuloendothelial humoral control mechanisms in patients after trauma. *Journal of Trauma* **16**, 898–904.

Seeff L.B. (1981) Post-transfusion hepatitis. In *Haemophilia*, Seligsohn U., Rimon A. & Horoszowski H. (eds), pp. 131–9. Castle House Publications, Wells, Kent.

Seeler R.A. (1977) Haemolysis due to anti-A and anti-B with intensive therapy in haemophilia. In *Unsolved Therapeutic Problems in Haemophilia*. US DHEW Publication No. (NIH) 77-1089, p. 113.

Seligsohn U., Kasper C.K., Osterud B. & Rapaport S.I. (1979) Activated Factor VII: presence in factor IX concentrates and persistence in the circulation after infusion. *Blood* **53**, 828–37

Smith J.K. & Bidwell E. (1979) Therapeutic materials used in the treatment of coagulation defects. In *Clinics in Haematology*. Vol. 8:1. pp. 183–206. Rizza C.R. (ed.) W.B. Saunders Co., London.

Snape T.J. (1982) The development of a system for the control of coagulation factor concentrates for clinical use. Ph.D. thesis, University of London.

Soulier J.P. & Steinbuch M. (1975) La fraction coagulante P.P.S.B. *La Nouvelle Presse Médicale* **4**, 836, 2581–4.

Steinberg M.H. & Dreiling B.J. (1973) Vascular lesions in hemophilia B. *New England Journal of Medicine* **289**, 592.

Szmuness W., Harley E.J., Ikram H. & Stevens C.E. (1978) Sociodemographic aspects of the epidemiology of hepatitis B. In *Viral Hepatitis*. Vyas G.N., Cohen S.N. & Schmidt R. (eds). pp. 297-320. Franklin Institute Press, Philadelphia.

Tabor E., Aronson D.L. & Gerety R.J. (1980) Removal of hepatitis-B-virus infectivity from factor-IX complex by hepatitis-B immune-globulin. Experiments in chimpanzees. *Lancet* **II**, 68–9.

Tishkoff G.H. (1977) Factor IX concentrate to treat factor VIII inhibitor: biochemical studies on its mode of action. In *Proceedings of the Workshop on Inhibitors of Factors VIII and IX*. Facultas-Verlag, Vienna.

Trepo C., Hantz O., Jacquier M.F., Nemoz G., Cappel R. & Trepo D. (1978) Different dates of hepatitis B virus markers during plasma fractionation. A clue to the infectivity of blood derivatives. *Vox Sanguinis* **35**, 143–8.

Urbaniak S.J. & Cash J.D. (1977) Blood replacement therapy. *British Medical Bulletin* **33**, 273–82.

Vogelaar E.F., Brummelhuis H.G.J. & Krijnen H.W. (1974) Large-scale preparation of human C1 esterase inhibitor for clinical use. *Vox Sanguinis* **26**, 118–27.

Waltl H., Kurz R., Mitterstieler G., Fodisch H.J., Hohenauer L. & Rossler H. (1973) Intracranial haemorrhage in low-birthweight infants and prophylactic administration of coagulation-factor concentrate. *Lancet* I, 1284.

Wessler S., Reimer S.M. & Sheps M.C. (1959) Biologic assay of a thrombosis-inducing activity in human serum. *Journal of Applied Physiology* **14**, 943–6.

White G.C., Roberts H.R., Kingdon H.S. & Lundblad R.L. (1977) Prothrombin complex concentrates: potentially thrombogenic materials and clues to the mechanism of thrombosis *in vivo*. *Blood* **49**, 159–70.

WHO Technical Report (1960) Requirements for biological substances. 6. General requirements for the sterility of biological substances. *World Health Organisation Technical Report Series*, No. 200. WHO, Geneva.

WHO Technical Report (1978) Requirements for the collection, processing and quality control of human blood and blood products. *World Health Organization Technical Report Series*, No. 626, Annex 1. WHO, Geneva.

Wickerhauser M., Mercer J.E. & Eckenrode J.W. (1978) Development of large-scale fractionation methods. *Vox Sanguinis* **35**, 18–31.

Wickerhauser M., Williams C. & Mercer J. (1979) Development of large scale fractionation methods. VII. Preparation of Antithrombin III concentrates. *Vox Sanguinis* **36**, 281–93.

Appendix 1

Sources of less common concentrates

Most national fractionation centres or commercial fractionators provide coagulation factor concentrates of factor VIII and of factor IX (usually with factors II, X and VII). This appendix suggests *possible* sources of less common concentrates which may not be available from the clinician's usual supplier. Entries in brackets indicate that the product is at the development stage, may be available for clinical use only under certain conditions, or may not be produced routinely.

Product	Supplier
Factor VIII, 'haemagglutinin-free'	6
Factor VIII, pasteurized	1, 2, 3
Factor VIII, porcine	10
Factor IX activated, for treatment of factor VIII inhibitors	6, 8
Factor IX, treated with β-propiolactone	4
Factor IX, reprecipitated with PEG	2
Factor VII	1, 6
Factor XIII	3 (1)
Factor XI	(1)
Fibrinogen	1, 7
Antithrombin III	7 (1)
Plasminogen	11 (7)
C1-esterase inhibitor	5 (2)
Thrombin (topical)	1
Fibronectin	9 (1)

List of suppliers

1   Blood Products Laboratory, Elstree, Herts/ Plasma Fractionation Laboratory, Churchill Hospital, Oxford.

2   Scottish National Blood Transfusion Service, Protein Fractionation Centre, Edinburgh.

3   Behringwerke AG, Marburg/Lahn.

4   Biotest-Serum-Institut, Frankfurt am Main.

5   Central Laboratory of the Netherlands Red Cross, Amsterdam.

6   Immuno, Vienna.

7   Kabi AB, S-11287 Stockholm.

8   Hyland Division, Travenol Laboratories, Costa Mesa, California.

9   New York Blood Center, New York.

10   Speywood Laboratories, Bingham Nottingham.

11   Choay Laboratories, Paris.

12   Cutter Laboratories, Berkeley, California.

Chapter 12
The Management of Patients with Coagulation Factor Deficiencies

C. R. RIZZA *and* J. M. MATTHEWS

Inherited deficiencies

Deficiencies of blood coagulation factors may be inherited or acquired. In the case of inherited deficiencies of blood coagulation factors the patient usually lacks only one factor whereas in acquired deficiency states several factors are usually affected. A typical example of an inherited deficiency is the deficiency of factor VIII seen in haemophilia. Deficiencies of factors II, VII, IX and X as seen in patients with liver disease or in patients receiving coumarin-type anticoagulants are probably the commonest form of acquired coagulation factor deficiencies. In inherited deficiencies treatment usually requires the intravenous transfusion of the missing clotting factor although in certain patients with factor VIII deficiency it is possible to raise the level of circulating factor VIII by the administration of 1-deamino-8-D-arginine vasopressin (DDAVP). It has been claimed also that factor VIII encapsulated in liposomes (Hemker *et al.* 1980) or bound to chylomicra (Paulssen and van Pelt 1981) administered by the oral route is effective in bringing about a small but useful increase of the level of factor VIII in the blood. This observation is interesting and important but still awaits confirmation.

In the case of acquired coagulation factor deficiency, replacement therapy may have an important part to play but other measures may be of equal or greater importance, such as the administration of vitamin K or the medical or surgical treatment of some underlying disorder.

Principles of replacement therapy

Haemophilia is the commonest of the severe inherited bleeding disorders. Because of this, most of what is known about factor replacement has been acquired from observation of haemophiliacs over many years and from the use of many different therapeutic preparations in the treatment of haemorrhages of differing severity. From these observations it has been possible to lay down some basic principles of treatment. These principles apply to haemophilia and Christmas disease, and probably also to the management of patients deficient

273

in factors II, VII, X, V, XI and XIII. In the latter group the small numbers of patients affected make it difficult to gain much information about the level of the different factors required for haemostasis.

The aim of replacement therapy in coagulation factor deficiencies is to raise the plasma concentration of the relevant clotting factor by means of intravenous transfusion to a level which will bring about haemostasis and to maintain an adequate level for as long as is necessary to allow wound healing. The level of factor required will depend on the site, severity, and type of lesion being treated, and may be different in the different deficiency states. The levels of the different clotting factors thought to be required for haemostasis along with some other properties of those factors are shown in Table 25. These levels should be regarded as only rough guides.

Haemostasis and the level of factor VIII in the blood

The severity of clinical manifestations in haemophilia is inversely related to the level of factor VIII in the blood; the severely affected patients who suffer from spontaneous haemorrhages into muscles and joints are generally found to have factor VIII levels less than 1 iu/dl whereas patients who are clinically more mildly affected usually have factor VIII levels above 1 or 2 iu/dl. This relationship between haemostasis and level of factor VIII is shown in Table 26. As might be expected, severe and extensive injuries require higher levels of factor VIII to control bleeding than do minor injuries (Table 27). Also, haemorrhages endangering important structures such as the trachea, major

Table 25. Some *in vivo* characteristics of blood coagulation factors.

Factor	Minimum plasma concentration required for haemostasis in surgery (u/dl)	Immediate recovery in circulation (expressed as % of amount transfused)	Half-life of transfused factor
II	40	40–50	3 days
V	15	80	12 hours
VII	10	80	4–6 hours
VIII	>40	60–80	8–12 hours
IX	>40	40–50	12–24 hours
X	10	50	2 days
XI	30	90–100	2–3 days
XIII	1–5	50–100	? 6–10 days
Fibrinogen	50 mg/dl	50	4–6 days

Table 26. Relationship of plasma factor VIII level to the severity of bleeding manifestation.

Plasma level of factor VIII (iu/dl)	Bleeding manifestations
>40	None
20–40	Tendency to bleed after major injury. Often not diagnosed
5–20	Bleeding after minor injury and surgery
1–5	Severe bleeding after minor injury. Occasional haemarthroses and 'spontaneous' bleeding
<1	Severe haemophilia. Spontaneous haemarthroses and muscle haemorrhages. Joint ankylosis and crippling

blood vessels or nerves require intensive treatment, with the level of the factor being *maintained* above 40–50 per cent of normal.

Materials used for the treatment of haemophilia

There are numerous human factor VIII-containing preparations, as well as one factor VIII concentrate prepared from pig blood, now available for the treatment of haemophilia. The blood products used for the treatment of

Table 27. Approximate levels of factor VIII required for haemostasis in different circumstances.

Lesion	Plasma concentration of factor VIII (iu/dl)	Initial dose of factor VIII (iu/kg body weight)
Minor bleeding spontaneous or otherwise into joints muscles and other sites	15–20 (8–10)	8–10
Severe bleeding episodes. minor surgery	20–40 (10–20)	10–20
Major surgery	80–100 (40–50)	40–50

Figures in brackets represent approximate level of factor VIII 12 hours after transfusion.

bleeding disorders are described in detail in Chapter 11 and will be discussed here only briefly.

WHOLE BLOOD

Factor VIII coagulant activity is relatively unstable at +4°C so that stored whole blood contains variable and often low levels of the factor. Moreover, in most circumstances it is not possible to administer whole blood sufficiently rapidly to achieve a haemostatic level of factor VIII. Whole blood therefore should not be used as a means of replacing factor VIII but should be reserved for the treatment of blood loss.

PLASMA

Plasma separated from blood within 12 to 18 hours of collection and stored at −20°C to −40°C for up to three months was used widely until the middle 1960s for the treatment of bleeding. It proved particularly useful for those types of lesions which required factor VIII levels of less than 20 per cent of normal for haemostasis. More severe haemorrhages and in particular bleeding after surgery were not easily controlled by plasma therapy since it was rarely possible, because of the large volume required, to achieve a sufficiently high level of factor VIII in the patient's blood.

CRYOPRECIPITATE

Cold-precipitated plasma proteins are rich in factor VIII activity (Pool, Hershgold and Pappenhagen 1964) and in 1965 Pool and Shannon reported the successful use of cryoprecipitate in the treatment of haemophilic bleeding. Numerous reports confirmed this work and cryoprecipitate has since been used widely to treat haemophiliacs who are bleeding or about to undergo surgery. The material may be given by intravenous transfusion using a drip set or by injection using a syringe. The main drawbacks to its use are the variability in factor VIII content from pack to pack (although this may not be so important in large pooled doses), the need for storage in a refrigerator at −20°C to −40°C which is an important disadvantage to its use in home therapy, and difficulty of reconstitution, which may result in loss of material left behind in the plastic bag. On the other hand, the method of preparation is simple and can be carried out at most blood transfusion centres without the need for expensive equipment and the yield of factor VIII from the starting plasma is higher than with the semi-purified lyophilized concentrates. Allergic and other reactions following the administration of cryoprecipitate are uncommon but more common than with freeze-dried factor VIII. Cryoprecipitate is still widely used in the world but is being superseded by freeze-dried preparations. Cryoprecipitate as well as plasma may sometimes be used for the treatment of mildly affected haemophiliacs and carriers who are infrequently treated and in whom donor exposure should be kept to a minimum.

Lyophilized human factor VIII

Human factor VIII in freeze-dried form is now widely available for the treatment of haemophilia. In the UK factor VIII is prepared at the Blood Products Laboratory, Elstree, at the Plasma Fractionation Laboratory in Oxford and at the Protein Fractionation Centre in Edinburgh. The material prepared by these laboratories is of intermediate purity and is dispensed in glass bottles each containing approximately 230–260 iu factor VIII, to be reconstituted in sterile distilled water. In addition to these National Health Service products there are at present several commercial preparations available in the UK, some of high purity, others of intermediate purity. In our experience the intermediate purity factor VIII is satisfactory for the management of most types of bleeding in the majority of patients, but there may be an important place for the high purity VIII preparations in the treatment of patients requiring large amounts of factor VIII in a small volume: for example, in patients with antibody to factor VIII. Lyophilized factor VIII has the advantage of being supplied in bottles which contain a known amount of factor VIII which has undergone rigid quality control. The most important drawback to the use of large pool freeze-dried concentrate is the risk of transmitting hepatitis. In addition there are fears that the use of large pool concentrates may in some way bring about impaired immunity in frequently transfused patients. Reactions following transfusion of this material are extremely rare.

LYOPHILIZED ANIMAL FACTOR VIII

At present the only freeze-dried preparation of animal factor VIII is of porcine origin. Bovine and porcine factor VIII preparations for therapeutic use were first prepared by Bidwell (1955a,b) and were used successfully by the Oxford group for the management of haemophiliacs undergoing surgery at a period when there was insufficient human factor VIII (Macfarlane, Biggs and Bidwell 1954, Macfarlane *et al.* 1957). These early preparations were valuable in the treatment of patients but had some important side-effects, namely, thrombocytopenia, allergic and pyrogenic reactions, development of resistance to treatment, and increased incidence of factor VIII antibodies. Bovine and porcine factor VIII-related antigen causes aggregation of human platelets *in vitro* (Forbes and Prentice 1973, De Gaetano *et al.* 1974) and this is probably the mechanism whereby these materials cause thrombocytopenia when injected into haemophiliacs. The resistance seen in many patients after 7–10 days of treatment with the early materials is still not explained and was characterized by a progressive fall in the patient's post-transfusion factor VIII response associated sometimes with increasingly severe allergic type reactions. The poor factor VIII response in resistant patients did not seem to be due to the development of antibodies to factor VIII:C since these antibodies could not be demonstrated using *in vitro* tests. Moreover, a patient resistant to one animal preparation still responded to the other animal factor VIII preparation and to human factor VIII.

The porcine factor VIII available today* has few of the above drawbacks (Kernoff and Tuddenham 1981). The method of manufacture results in a material rich in factor VIII:C but containing very little factor VIII-related antigen. The absence of thrombocytopenia with this newer preparation is thought to be due to its very low content of factor VIII-related antigen.

Because of the easy availability of potent preparations of human factor VIII, the porcine factor VIII is at present used mainly for patients who have factor VIII antibodies in their blood and especially when the antibody is less active against porcine factor VIII than against human factor VIII.

CALCULATION OF DOSAGE

Most of the human factor VIII preparations in use today, when administered by intravenous injection, bring about an increase of factor VIII in the circulation of approximately 2.0 iu per cent per 1 iu of dose per kg, body weight. Factor IX concentrate produces a rise of about 1 iu%/iu/kg. Thus the factor VIII level in a patient who weighs 70 kg and receives 700 iu of human factor VIII (10 iu/kg) should increase by about 20 iu per cent. The dose for any other desired increase of factor VIII may easily be calculated. A useful formula for calculating factor VIII dosage is:

$$\text{dose required (iu)} = \frac{\text{wt. (kg)} \times \text{desired increase iu\%}}{2.0}$$

In the case of factor IX concentrate, for 2.0 substitute 1.0.

When using this formula it is important to remember that the units used for expressing the dose must be the same as those used for expressing the level in the patient's plasma. This is particularly important with regard to factor IX where the international unit is considerably different from the unit expressed as a percentage of average normal plasma. In our laboratory 100 iu per cent factor VIII ≡ 125 per cent average normal and 100 iu per cent factor IX ≡ 167 per cent average normal.

* Speywood Laboratories Ltd, Ash Road, Wrexham Industrial Estate, Wrexham, Clwyd, UK.

Treatment of specific lesions

Bleeding into muscles and joints is the commonest feature of severe haemophilia and 80–90 per cent of all factor VIII used each year at the Oxford Centre is for treatment of bleeding into those sites. The treatment of bleeding involving the locomotor system is therefore of great importance in the management of haemophilia and will be discussed here in some detail.

Bleeding into joints

Bleeding into joints produces pain, swelling, and limitation of movement in the joint and in the long-term, if not adequately treated, results in degenerative changes in the joint, ankylosis, and crippling. By giving factor VIII as soon as possible after the onset of bleeding the pain, swelling and limitation of movement are minimized and hopefully the chronic arthropathy which is such a characteristic feature of inadequately treated haemophilia will become less common. The majority of severely affected patients are at present receiving episodic or 'on demand' treatment, that is, treatment is not given until bleeding occurs and is then given as soon as possible. With large amounts of commercially prepared factor VIII now available a small but increasing number of patients are receiving prophylactic doses several times a week. The aim of this form of treatment is to maintain a low level of factor VIII in the patient's blood at all times and thereby prevent spontaneous bleeding.

If treated promptly within 30–60 minutes most minor haemarthroses will respond rapidly (within 4–8 hours) to a single dose of factor VIII of 7–10 iu/kg and movement of the limb can be encouraged within a few hours thereafter. More severe haemarthroses, especially those caused by obvious injury, will usually require a larger initial dose, for example 10–25 iu/kg. This dose should be repeated daily for several days until it is clear that bleeding has been controlled and joint function is improving. In addition to factor VIII replacement the more severe painful haemarthroses may need to be immobilized in the position of maximum comfort. A simple well fitting padded plaster of Paris backslab lightly bandaged on to the limb is usually sufficient. An analgesic may also be required to enable the patient to sleep during the first night; paracetamol or dihydrocodeine should be tried in the first instance. With very painful haemarthroses it may be necessary to give more powerful drugs such as dextromoramide or pethidine for a day or two. Aspirin preparations should be avoided. With the above treatment the pain of a severe haemarthrosis usually diminishes within 6–12 hours. After two or three days it is often desirable to change the plaster of Paris backslab to allow the limb to take up a more normal position which is then held and protected for a few days longer in a new plaster. Exercises are started as soon as the joint is pain-free and in a reasonable position, and a removable splint may be used to protect the joint until adequate joint and muscle function returns.

The 'optimum' dosage of factor VIII for the treatment of acute haemarthroses is still being widely debated. Practice varies considerably from country to country and from centre to centre in the same country, depending on the personal views of the doctor and patient as well as on the availability of factor VIII. In one report a single dose of 8–12 iu/kg body weight administered promptly after onset of symptoms has been found effective in controlling 100 per cent of early spontaneous haemorrhages in joints (Ashenhurst, Langehennig and Seeler 1977). Similar results were reported by Penner, Kelly and Boutaugh (1977) who found that a dose of factor VIII of 7–9 iu/kg body weight if administered early was effective in the management of 90 per cent of mild to moderate haemorrhagic episodes. For more severe episodes large doses were required, doses of 15–17 iu/kg being effective in only 50 per cent of severe joint haemorrhages. Aronstam and his colleagues (1980) have carried out a double-blind controlled trial comparing factor VIII doses of 7, 14 and 28 iu/kg in the treatment of knee, ankle and elbow haemarthroses. They concluded that the highest dose (28 iu/kg) did not appear to offer any advantage over doses of 7 or 14 iu/kg for any site of bleeding and they thought that knee bleeds in which there was any restriction of movement required dosage of 14 iu/kg as did the more severe haemorrhages into ankles and elbows. Much higher doses have been recommended by Allain (1979) who suggested that a dose of approximately 30 iu/kg is required to achieve 99 per cent success with treatment. Clearly a great deal of work is still needed to define the optimum dose level for the treatment of haemarthroses. Such studies are extremely difficult for a variety of reasons and the results are affected by numerous factors, for example the state of the joint and synovial membrane before onset of bleeding, the degree of trauma which caused the bleeding, the timing of dose after injury or onset of symptoms, and the 'success rate' sought. Furthermore, the definition of effectiveness or success of treatment is notoriously difficult and relies on the assessment by doctor and patient of changes in joint swelling, joint movement and pain over a given period of time. We have found that provided the dose is given within 15–30 minutes of onset of symptoms a dose of 10 iu/kg of factor VIII will be effective in more than 85–90 per cent of haemarthroses and no further dose will be required. Should there be no improvement within 6–12 hours of this first dose or should the pain become more severe a second dose of 20–30 iu/kg is given and this is repeated daily until the haemarthrosis resolves. The timing of the dose is probably as important as the size of the dose. A tense haemarthrosis which has developed rapidly or has resulted from delay in treatment will remain painful, stiff and swollen for several days no matter how much factor VIII is given. As will be discussed later it is hoped that home therapy will allow prompt treatment of haemarthroses and in time reduce the degree of joint damage. It must be stressed that the patient will get little benefit from having home treatment if he works or goes to school several miles from home and puts off treating a haemorrhage until he returns home some hours later. Patients who are able to administer their own doses should make some arrangement to keep stocks of the factor at work or at school and to have access to a first aid room or sick room where they can treat themselves at the first sign of bleeding.

Bleeding into muscles

Treatment of haemorrhage into a muscle is similar to that of haemarthrosis but in our experience muscle haemorrhage shows a tendency to recur if the limb is exercised too vigorously too soon. Remobilization should be cautious and accompanied by fairly aggressive treatment with factor VIII.

Bleeding into the iliacus muscle is particularly important since a large proportion of such haemorrhages cause pressure on the femoral nerve on that side with loss of sensation down the front of the thigh and more important, loss of quadriceps function with instability of the knee joint. During the acute phase of the haemorrhage there is usually severe pain in the iliac fossa made worse by any movement of the thigh and a palpable mass within the rim of the pelvis. Haematoma in the psoas muscle is much less common but in this case the patient may lose a considerable volume of blood into the muscle and may be shocked as a consequence of this and the associated severe pain and muscle spasm. In severe iliacus and psoas haematomas, in addition to treating with factor VIII (40–50 iu/kg body weight) and blood replacement as required, it is sometimes desirable to immobilize the part by means of a plaster of Paris hip spica extending from the subcostal margin to enclose the foot on the affected side and leaving the lower leg and foot on the unaffected side free. Once the patient has been placed in such a spica, there is usually rapid diminution of pain and muscle spasm. As the haematoma resolves the spica is removed and the patient starts cautiously exercising in bed, progressing to hydrotherapy and then to walking. Throughout this period of mobilization the patient is treated with factor VIII in a daily dosage of 10–20 iu/kg body weight immediately before he starts exercising.

Chronic haemophilic arthropathy

Repeated bleeding into joints if not treated adequately eventually leads to joint destruction with limb deformity, crippling and chronic pain. Treatment of patients at this stage of the condition should be aimed at reducing pain and improving joint function, and this requires close collaboration with ortho-paedic surgeons and physiotherapists. Forms of treatment which may prove useful are as follows:

1   Physiotherapy.
2   Stabilizing the joint by splinting.
3   Conservative procedures such as reversed dynamic slings aimed at correcting a flexion deformity.
4   Analgesics.
5   Corrective surgical procedures.

PHYSIOTHERAPY

The value of physiotherapy depends largely on the extent to which the joint is damaged and disorganized. A joint with minimal structural changes may gain considerable benefit from exercises aimed at improving the range of movement and increasing muscle bulk and power. This is particularly important with regard to the knee joint where a powerful quadriceps femoris muscle is crucial for joint function and stability. Having been taught the appropriate exercises by an experienced physiotherapist the patient is then encouraged to carry out the exercises himself at home several times each day. Exercises carried out twice a week at the physiotherapy department and thereafter forgotten are useless. If an element of muscle spasm is present ice packs applied to the area before physiotherapy may facilitate progress. In the case of severely damaged joints where the articular surfaces have been destroyed and there are fixed flexion contractures, physiotherapy seems to be of less benefit. As in advanced rheumatoid arthritis and osteoarthritis there is little hope of regaining any degree of normal function although some improvement may be obtained by improving muscle power about the joint.

SPLINTING

Joints which are unstable or damaged and subject to recurrent bleeding may be supported and protected by means of a metal caliper, particularly where the knee and ankle on the same side are affected. Patients dislike such appliances and if possible they should be avoided as they are clumsy, heavy and unsightly. There are now more acceptable forms of splinting made of light plastic which can be worn under the patient's clothes. These can be moulded to fit the particular limb and may be articulated and fitted with a locking device in the region of the joint to allow the limb to bend when sitting or during physiotherapy. The Yates' splint (Yates 1963) for the ankle is often of benefit in the management of recurrent bleeding into that joint as are firm boots lacing above the ankle. Cinch knee support may be of value in providing support for an unstable knee.

REVERSED DYNAMIC SLINGS

Stein and Dickson (1975) have described a system of dynamic slings for the treatment of fixed flexion contracture of the knee. In contractures of less than a year's duration the method is often rapidly effective over a few days, is free of complications and requires minimal or no factor VIII replacement.

Reconstructive orthopaedic surgery

Sometimes pain is insufficiently controlled by analgesic drugs or by measures such as immobilization with splints or other appliances. Consideration must then be given to the possibility of relieving pain by surgical means. In the case of the hip joint, total hip replacement is a proven and effective procedure in haemophiliacs. Management of painful arthropathy of the knee is more difficult and although a procedure such as patellectomy may improve function, some cases, particularly those with a very restricted range of movement may require arthrodesis of the joint. The place of knee arthroplasty in haemophilia is still undetermined particularly in the younger more active patient. The same is true of arthroplasty of the ankle and elbow.

ANALGESICS

The control of chronic pain can be extremely difficult. Various analgesic drugs have been tried but none is entirely satisfactory for long-term use. Drugs such as paracetamol, pentazocine and dihydrocodeine are not always effective so that there may sometimes be a need to give potentially addictive drugs such as dextromoramide, pethidine and other narcotic analgesics. It is still too early to say if the recently introduced analgesic drug, buprenorphine (Temgesic) which can be taken under the tongue will be of any value. Non-steroidal anti-inflammatory drugs such as ibuprofen (Brufen) may prove of value in some patients. To suit a particular patient it may be necessary to try a number of different drugs and each patient should explore with his doctor the alternative medications which are available, keeping in mind the dangers of addiction which accompany the more potent analgesics. Aspirin, and other anti-inflammatory agents such as indomethacin, phenylbutazone, and oxy-phenbutazone should be avoided because of the risk of gastrointestinal haemorrhage and their effect in impairing platelet function.

Haematuria

Bleeding from the renal tract is much less common than bleeding into muscles and joints. Most severely affected haemophiliacs will have experienced at least one episode before adulthood. Haematuria in haemophiliacs is usually painless and not associated with injury, urinary infection or demonstrable pathology in the urogenital tract. The condition may resolve promptly after administration of a few doses of factor VIII at 10–15 iu/kg. In other instances it is difficult to treat and may show little response to treatment with large doses of factor VIII. Many episodes stop spontaneously. If the haematuria is slight, the patient is encouraged to increase his fluid intake and to continue his routine activities but to avoid any unnecessary exertion. With this simple treatment many episodes will stop within 7–10 days. If bleeding is heavy and in particular if it is associated with clotting in the renal tract and with severe abdominal pain, it may be necessary to give large doses of factor VIII, 20–25 iu/dl, daily or twice daily. The patient shuld be encouraged to drink as much as possible before and after treatment to maintain a good diuresis and thereby reducing the risk of formation of bulky clots following transfusion of factor VIII. Obstruction of the renal pelvis by clot may be the reason for abrupt cessation of heavy haematuria. This obstruction, given time, usually clears itself. Pethidine may be required for renal colic. Antifibrinolytic agents should not be given. If haematuria persists the urinary tract should be investigated in case there is some underlying remediable cause for the bleeding.

Cerebral haemorrhage

Intracranial bleeding in haemophilia is not common but may follow some quite trivial head injury. Any haemophiliac who sustains a blow to the head sufficient to cause unconciousness or giddiness, headache, vomiting or visual symptoms should be admitted to hospital for at least 24 hours for observation of his neurological state and should receive factor VIII replacement. A dose of 40–50 iu/kg should be given after admission and a similar dose given 12 hours later. Should signs of intracranial bleeding appear, the necessary investigations to determine the site of the haemorrhage should be carried out, followed by any surgery that is required. Adequate doses of factor VIII should be given for those procedures.

Dental management

It is a regrettable fact that in the UK caries is still a major problem in the population and many people eventually come to require extraction of decayed teeth. Haemophiliacs are similarly affected but because of the problems and expense of haemophilia treatment strenuous efforts should be made to encourage the patient to take care of his teeth from a very early age. Twice or thrice daily brushing should be encouraged, preferably using a toothpaste containing fluoride. The child should be taught the dangers of eating too many sweets, biscuits, and other foods containing much fine flour or sugar and should be encouraged to make three-monthly or six-monthly visits to his local dentist for inspection of his teeth and gums and to have any conservative treatment that may be required. Dental fillings and scaling can usually be carried out without any factor replacement but if the minor gum trauma which sometimes results from scaling does produce troublesome bleeding a dose of factor may be given. In young children it is often possible to carry out cavity fillings without the use of local anaesthesia or at most using interpapillary infiltration of the gum. Inferior dental nerve block is dangerous in haemophilia and should not be carried out without adequate factor replacement before the procedure. Should conservative dental care fail it may become necessary to extract carious teeth. The following regimen of management has been followed at this Centre for more than ten years with excellent results. The procedure is essentially that described by Walsh *et al.* (1971). Having tested the patient's blood and made sure that antibodies to factor VIII are not present, the patient is given on the morning of operation a dose of factor VIII sufficient to raise his blood factor level to 50 iu per cent. At the same time he is given intravenously tranexamic acid 8 mg/kg diluted in 25–30 ml saline. The extraction is carried out under general anaesthesia with endotracheal intubation. Thereafter the patient continues to take 14 mg/kg tranexamic acid three times a day and penicillin three times a day six-hourly by mouth for ten days. Following extraction the gums are not stitched unless cavities gape unduly and dental splints are not used. No further factor replacement is given unless bleeding takes place and this is rare. Patients who live within 20–30 miles of the Centre usually go home two to four days after the operation depending on the number of teeth removed and the degree of local trauma caused during extraction. Patients who live a long way from a Centre and especially those in whom many teeth, including the 3rd molars, have been removed are encouraged to remain in hospital for five to seven days.

Major surgery

The carrying out of major surgery in a haemophiliac requires close collaboration between surgeon, physician, and laboratory staff. With potent preparations of factor VIII and IX now available it is possible to carry out any surgical procedure that the patient may need. Standard surgical techniques should be used and the surgeon should not modify or limit his procedure just because the patient is a haemophiliac.

Before surgery on a haemophiliac it is essential that his blood is tested for the presence of antibodies to factor VIII and that his medical records are studied to make sure that he has not had antibodies in the past. This latter point is particularly important when dealing with patients who are infrequently seen or have been referred from another Centre. In most instances the finding of antibodies would be a contraindication to surgery.

A transfusion of factor VIII sufficient to raise the patient's plasma level of the factor to 80–100 iu per cent is given immediately before surgery. Assays are carried out immediately after the dose and four to six hours later to ascertain the level of the factor in his blood. Further doses are given according to the assay results obtained. It is usually necessary to give factor replacement three times in the first 24 hours and 12-hourly thereafter, to maintain the factor VIII level above 40 iu per cent. This regimen of treatment is continued until wound healing is well advanced and there is little risk of haemorrhage, at which time the dosage may be reduced to daily doses.

Home treatment

As mentioned above, bleeding into joints and muscles should be treated as soon as possible after onset of symptoms. In view of the delay often encountered by patients travelling to hospital for transfusion therapy, many centres throughout the world now encourage the patients to be treated at home (Rabiner and Telfer 1970, Lazerson 1972, Le Quesne *et al.* 1974, Levine 1974, Rizza and Spooner 1977, Jones *et al.* 1978). The dose may be administered by the patient himself or by his wife or in the case of a child may be administered by his parents. In some cases the dose is given by the general practitioner but in our experience this is not very common. Criteria for inclusion of a patient on home therapy may vary slightly from centre to centre but usually include some or all of the following:

1   The patient should be severely affected so that the risk of bleeding for little reason is present.
2   The patient should be sufficiently intelligent and competent to follow instructions.
3   The patient should have good veins.
4   The patient should have a relative or doctor who is prepared to give doses promptly or he must be able to administer the dose to himself.

These requirements are very broad and will be modified by different Centres in individual patients according to circumstances. For example, patients who bleed infrequently may, if they live a long way from a Centre or in an isolated area, be encouraged to treat themselves at home. Some patients who have antibodies to factor VIII may also find home treatment of value. At present 12 of our patients who have antibodies to factor VIII treat themselves at home.

With regard to the minimum age for starting home therapy, this depends very much on the child and his mother and the relationship between the two. In general, we do not encourage home therapy in boys less than six years of age although we have several children who started at the age of four to five years without problems. There seems to be no upper age limit for starting home treatment.

Having decided to start a patient on home treatment he, or the relative who is to give the dose, is trained at the Centre in the technique of venepuncture and is shown how to reconstitute the dose using aseptic technique. Thereafter, the relative or the patient administers doses under the supervision of a doctor and only when this is seen to be done competently is home treatment allowed. The time taken to learn the necessary techniques varies very much from person to person but on average six treatment sessions are usually sufficient. The patient is then given a box containing freeze-dried factor VIII, filter needles, butterfly needles, syringes, distilled water, cotton wool, swabs and forms for keeping records of doses given and the reasons for giving the doses. The patients on home therapy are encouraged to telephone the Centre if they have any problems or doubts about treatment particularly in the early months on home treatment. With regard to the types of haemorrhage treated at home we advocate that only minor bleeding into a joint or muscle should be treated by the patient at home without hospital supervision since this is the type of haemorrhage which is often controlled by a single dose of 7–10 iu/kg. In the case of more severe haemorrhage, especially after injury, the patient is advised to give himself a dose two or three times larger than his usual dose as soon as possible and then to attend the Centre for examination, further replacement therapy or orthopaedic or other specialist treatment if it is required. A similar procedure should be followed if the patient suffers unusual pain, for example, severe headache especially following head injury or abdominal pain, or notices bleeding from the gut or elsewhere which may be potentially serious.

An important aspect of home treatment is regular follow-up at the out-patient clinic. We arrange to see young children every three to six months and adults are seen every six months. At the follow-up clinic the patient undergoes a general clinical examination, particular attention being paid to the state of joints and muscles. Joint movements are measured and restrictions of function discussed in relation to capacity for activities at home, school or work. The state of the patient's veins is noted. Clinical evidence of liver or renal disease and of AIDS is sought and the blood pressure is measured. The factor VIII usage, bleeding episodes suffered, and any arthritic or analgesic problems are discussed and the educational, work and social background is reviewed. Blood samples are taken for general haematological examination, liver function tests, and to check for the presence of HBs Ag, HBs Ab and factor VIII antibody.

At present 145 patients attending the Oxford Centre are receiving treatment at home and many of these have been on home therapy for more than eight years. There seems little doubt that attendance at work and school has been improved by home therapy and that the patients and their families are happier when on home therapy, and all benefit socially. Because of the general upward trend in the use of factor VIII in the UK it is difficult to assess to what extent home therapy results in increased usage of factor VIII. From our own experience it would seem that soon after the commencement of home therapy most patients use significantly more factor VIII than before but within

12–18 months the usage falls to a level which is only 15–20 per cent greater than that before home therapy (Rizza and Spooner 1977, Rizza, Biggs and Spooner 1978).

With regard to cost, Ingram and his associates (1979) in a small collaborative study found home therapy resulted in a clear saving when the cost of staff time spent with the patients and patients' travel costs were estimated. There was also a saving when costs borne by the community, wages lost and leisure time lost were calculated.

Finally, the important question of the effectiveness of home therapy in delaying or preventing joint damage and long-term crippling has still to be assessed. Children who have been on home therapy from a very early age are still relatively few in number and as the oldest of these will be no more than 10–11 years of age it is probably too early to decide whether or not the joints have been spared. Moreover, it is difficult to obtain a group of similarly affected boys for comparison since most severely affected children are likely to be on home treatment. Comparison retrospectively with similar age groups before the use of home therapy is probably not valid because of the major change in treatment and therapeutic material which took place during that period. Recent work suggests that despite early replacement therapy progressive joint changes may still occur in severely affected haemophiliacs although the process may be delayed (Helske *et al.* 1982).

The management of haemophilia complicated by factor VIII antibodies

Approximately 6 per cent of all haemophiliacs develop antibodies to factor VIII. This is a serious complication of their condition since the antibodies destroy transfused factor VIII and as a consequence control of bleeding may be very difficult. The presence of antibodies does not in our experience result in more frequent bleeding but when bleeding does occur it may persist longer, be more severe, and do more damage because of the poor factor VIII response following transfusion. The management of such patients is one of the outstanding problems in the treatment of haemophilia.

Views on the management of bleeding in patients with factor VIII antibodies have changed during the past ten years. In 1973, when writing for the previous edition of this book, our approach along with that of many others was to withhold factor VIII replacement except for major life-endangering haemorrhages and to treat minor bleeding into muscles and joints with ice packs, splinting, and analgesics. This approach to treatment was based on the fact that the administration of factor VIII usually resulted in an increase in the level of antibody after five to six days which made effective factor VIII therapy very difficult if the patient then suffered some major accident or serious bleeding. By withholding treatment and allowing the antibody to remain at a low level, we were ensuring that it would be possible to give the patient four to seven days' effective replacement therapy should he suffer serious injury. This view which was partly decided by shortage of factor VIII supplies has changed during the past ten years and factor VIII replacement as well as other forms of treatment are now used in the management of patients with antibodies (Table 28).

Table 28. Treatment of haemophiliacs with factor VIII antibodies.

1   Factor VIII—human or porcine
2   Prothrombin complex concentrate—activated or non-activated
3   Plasmapheresis
4   Immunosuppressive therapy
5   Various combinations of two or more of the above forms of treatment
6   Antifibrinolytic drugs

Factor VIII replacement

Factor VIII of human and animal origin has been used with varying degrees of success depending on the titres of antibody encountered and their relative activities against human and porcine factor VIII. With low levels of antibody, short-lived, but perhaps haemostatic, levels of factor VIII can be achieved with factor VIII. In our experience this is usually possible if the antibody level is less than 10–15 New Oxford units and depending on the reaction kinetics of the particular antibody (see Chapter 10). Once the antibody level rises much above this the likelihood of achieving any measurable level of factor VIII in the patient's blood becomes much less. But the failure to find factor VIII activity in post-transfusion samples does not mean that there was not a significant level of factor VIII in the patient's blood during or immediately after the transfusion since the delay in transporting the post-transfusion sample to the laboratory for testing would be sufficient to allow the antibody to destroy any factor VIII present. Factor VIII replacement has been our preferred method of treatment for the past eight years and is used to treat all bleeding episodes in haemophiliacs who have antibodies. The dosage ranges from 20–70 iu/kg daily, twice or thrice daily and varies from patient to patient depending on the level of his antibody, the severity of bleeding and our knowledge of the patient's previous clinical response to treatment. The part affected is immobilized when necessary and when practicable to minimize disturbance to haemostasis.

Brackmann and his colleagues (Brackmann and Gormsen 1977, Brackmann 1981, Brackmann and Egli 1981) have recently described the use of very large doses of factor VIII combined with a prothrombin complex concentrate (Factor Eight Inhibitor Bypassing Activity—FEIBA) in the treatment of patients with antibody. Factor VIII and FEIBA were given daily or twice daily in a dosage of 75–100 iu/kg body weight and 40–60 iu/kg body weight respectively over many months. This regimen of treatment was maintained until the level of antibody fell to less than 0.5 u/ml. Thereafter both FEIBA and factor VIII doses were gradually reduced. Using this form of treatment Brackmann and his associates were able to suppress the antibody even in patients with antibody levels of more than 1000 units. Clearly this method of treatment is very expensive and in the UK with factor VIII at its current price (5–6p/unit) the cost of one month's treatment for a man weighing 70 kg could be of the order of £20 000 for the factor VIII alone. Also it remains to be seen if there are any long-term risks to the patient receiving such high doses of factor VIII.

Stenbjerg *et al.* (1982) have found that prolonged administration of relatively low doses of factor VIII resulted in a reduction in the level of antibody. They used doses of factor VIII of 3–90 u/kg body weight per week. Our experience in a study of 24 patients (Rizza and Matthews 1982) is similar to theirs. In seven patients with low levels of antibody the antibody disappeared during the course of frequent factor VIII replacement over 1–3 years. In a further six patients with higher levels of antibody the anamnestic response became less and the maximum level of antibody fell significantly. In the remaining 11 patients, the majority of whom were less frequently treated, the antibody level showed little change.

Prothrombin complex concentrates

A most interesting and potentially valuable material for the treatment of patients with factor VIII antibody was reported by Breen and Tullis (1969) and Fekete and his colleagues (1972). These workers found that a preparation of prothrombin complex concentrate (factors II, VII, IX and X) which had become activated during manufacture was effective in controlling haemorrhage in haemophiliacs with antibody. Since these early observations similar claims have been made by other workers using other activated prothrombin complex preparations (Penner and Kelly 1975, Buchanan and Kevy 1978). In addition, some workers have found that non-activated prothrombin complex concentrates are also of value in treatment (Lusher *et al.* 1980). Recently, double-blind controlled trials have shown that activated prothrombin complex concentrates are slightly but significantly more effective than placebo or non-activated concentrates in controlling 'closed' haemorrhages in patients with factor VIII antibody (Lusher *et al.* 1980, Sjamsoedin *et al.* 1981). Similar trials comparing the effect of prothrombin complex concentrates with factor VIII concentrate have not yet been carried out. The activated prothrombin complex concentrates are thought to act by bypassing the site of factor VIII in the clotting cascade reaction. The active agent or agents have still not been defined and assay of the activity in the concentrate depends on the ability of the material to shorten the whole blood clotting time or the partial thromboplastin time of factor VIII- deficient or antibody-containing blood or plasma.

Plasmapheresis

Plasma exchange has long been recognized to be of value in the management of certain patients with factor VIII antibodies (Strauss 1969). The introduction of continuous-flow cell centrifuge equipment has made this form of treatment more practicable and allows exchange of large volumes of plasma. Edson and his associates (1973) carried out two plasma exchanges during a three-week period in combination with cyclophosphamide, corticosteroids and EACA for the successful treatment of a patient undergoing surgery for subdural haematoma. Pintado and his colleagues (1975) used plasmapheresis combined with immunosuppressive therapy for the treatment of a large sublingual haematoma in an elderly patient with an acquired factor VIII antibody. More recently, Cobcroft, Tamagnini and Dormandy (1977) carried out plasma exchange to prepare a patient for elective dental surgery and Slocumbe *et al.* (1981) employed plasma exchange, four times daily, along with factor VIII replacement in the successful management of two patients with antibodies who had undergone surgery. The latter authors from their experience concluded that plasma exchange should be carried out daily as long as there is a risk of bleeding and that large doses of factor VIII should be given immediately after the exchange. This form of treatment has a part to play in the management of dangerous bleeding in patients with antibodies to factor VIII or in the preparation of such patients for unavoidable surgery. A detailed protocol for plasmapheresis is given by Slocumbe *et al.* (1981).

Immunosuppressive drugs

Corticosteroids, ACTH, azathioprine and cyclophosphamide have all been used alone or in various combinations to try to suppress factor VIII antibodies. Although there have been several reports of success with immunosuppressive drugs the consensus now is that these drugs have little part to play in the treatment of haemophiliacs with antibodies (Hruby and Schulman 1973, Dormandy and Sultan 1975, Hultin *et al.* 1976,

Treatment of Christmas disease

In general, the principles governing replacement therapy in Christmas disease are the same as those for haemophilia. Approximately the same blood levels of factor IX as of factor VIII are required for haemostasis in the different lesions (Table 29). Factor IX is more stable *in vitro* than factor VIII and even after storage at $+4°C$ for several weeks whole blood still contains 80–90 per cent of its original content of factor IX (Geratz and Graham 1960). In addition to this stability *in vitro*, factor IX has a half-life in the patient's circulation of 18–30 hours (Biggs and Denson 1963). Unfortunately, these two advantages are to some extent offset by the relatively poor recovery of factor IX in the patient's blood following transfusion compared to factor VIII. Bleeding in Christmas disease as in haemophilia affects mainly the joints and muscles. In addition to giving factor IX transfusions it is often necessary to seek the aid of the orthopaedic surgeon in the management of acute joint haemorrhages as well as in the management of chronic arthropathy.

Table 29. Approximate levels of factor IX required for haemostasis in different circumstances.

Lesion	Plasma concentration of factor IX iu/dl	Initial dose of factor IX iu/kg body weight
Minor spontaneous bleeding into joints and muscles— minor injuries to mucous membranes of mouth and nose	8–16	8–16
Severe bleeding into joint or muscle	16–32	16–32
Major surgery	40–60	40–60

Materials used for the treatment of Christmas disease

Although fresh-frozen plasma may be used for the treatment of minor bleeding episodes, it is of little value in the management of major bleeding or for treating patients undergoing surgery. With a dose of plasma of 12–15 ml/kg body weight the patient's factor IX level should rise by 12–15 per cent of normal. Factor IX concentrates are now widely used for the treatment of Christmas disease and in the UK factor IX concentrate prepared by National Health Service Fractionation Laboratories is the only material at present used. The material is clinically effective and is used for the day-to-day management of bleeding episodes and for treating patients undergoing surgery.

Some other measures used in the treatment of haemophilia and Christmas disease

With the introduction of potent and effective preparations of factor VIII and IX for transfusion therapy many agents which in the past played an important part in treatment are now little used. Local applications of coagulants and other substances such as Russell's viper venom, thrombin, adrenaline and fibrin foam are only of temporary value and are at best first aid measures.

ANTIFIBRINOLYTIC AGENTS

Inhibitors of fibrinolysis have been used for nearly 20 years in the management of haemophilic bleeding. The rationale of their use is that they make formed clots less susceptible to dissolution by the body's fibrinolytic enzymes and thereby help to maintain haemostasis.

Epsilon-aminocaproic acid (EACA, Epsikapron) and tranexamic acid (AMCHA, Cyklokapron) are the two drugs which have been most widely used. The latter is preferred as it causes less gastrointestinal upset, giddiness and postural hypotension than EACA.

Antifibrinolytic drugs have been used in the treatment of haemophilia in four ways:
1   For the treatment of haematuria.
2   As a prophylactic agent to prevent bleeding into muscles and joints.
3   As an adjunct to factor replacement in dental surgery and other forms of surgery.
4   In the management of bleeding from superficial injuries and those affecting mucous membranes of the mouth and nose.

There have been several reports of the successful use of EACA in the management of haematuria in haemophiliacs (Barkhan 1964, Tsevrenis and Mandalaki 1965) but there is a high incidence of clot colic and renal obstruction following the use of inhibitors of fibrinolysis (Stark *et al.* 1965, Van Itterbeek, Vermylen and Verstraete 1968, Hilgartner 1975). Because of this, antifibrinolytic drugs are contraindicated in haemophiliacs suffering from haematuria unless it is certain that bleeding originates from the bladder, prostate or urethra.

With regard to spontaneous bleeding into muscles and joints there is very little evidence to suggest that inhibitors of fibrinolysis prevent bleeding. Four controlled trials, two of EACA and two of tranexamic acid, have been carried out (Gordon *et al.* 1965, Strauss, Kevy and Diamond 1965, Bennett, Ingram and Inglish 1973, Rainsford, Jordan and Hall 1973). In only one of these trials (Rainsford, Jordan and Hall 1973) was there a significant reduction in spontaneous bleeding episodes while tranexamic acid was being taken. The other studies showed no significant effect.

The value of antifibrinolytic drugs in the management of haemophiliacs undergoing dental extractions is now well established. Reid and his associates (1964) gave EACA before and after dental extraction with beneficial effect and similar results were reported by Cooksey, Perry and Raper (1966) and Tavenner (1968). Double-blind studies have shown conclusively that EACA (Walsh *et al.* 1971) and tranexamic acid (Forbes *et al.* 1972) are useful adjuncts to transfusion therapy in patients undergoing dental extractions and their use leads to a significant saving of factors VIII and IX.

Oral bleeding apart from that following dental extraction is seen quite commonly in young haemophiliacs and usually arises from injuries to the tongue, gums, lips or frenulum. Because the injury is often very small and because of the distress caused by venepuncture in young children, it may be justified to give, in the first place, a short trial of antifibrinolytic drugs in an attempt to control the bleeding. This is particularly worthwhile in less severely affected patients. Corrigan (1972) has described the successful use of combined EACA and factor replacement therapy to control bleeding from the mouth not associated with dental extraction.

Inhibitors of fibrinolysis have been used in patients undergoing a variety of orthopaedic operation (Storti *et al.* 1972) with apparent benefit. The place of antifibrinolytic drugs in other forms of surgery is not clear. We have always avoided these drugs in haemophiliacs undergoing thoracic or abdominal surgery for fear that any haemorrhage into the closed cavities might result in troublesome insoluble clots. On the other hand, we have used either EACA or tranexamic acid along with factor replacement in patients undergoing operations such as repair of inguinal hernia, haemorrhoidectomy, stripping of varicose veins, and adenotonsillectomy as well as in orthopaedic operations such as arthrodesis, tendon lengthening and total hip replacement.

1-DEAMINO-8-D-ARGININE VASOPRESSIN (DDAVP)

DDAVP is a synthetic derivative of vasopressin but without the visceral and vasoactive effects of the latter drug. When infused intravenously into normal individuals, mildly affected haemophiliacs or certain patients with von Willebrand's disease, it brings about an increase in the level of factor VIII complex in the blood (Mannucci, Ruggeri and Capitano 1977, Mannucci *et al.* 1977, Ludlam *et al.* 1980). Similar effects are obtained when the material is taken by the intranasal route in the form of 'snuff' (Mannucci *et al.* 1981). It should be noted that DDAVP brings about no increase in the level of factor VIII in severely affected haemophiliacs.

When transfused into mildly affected haemophiliacs in a dose of 0.4–0.5 μg/kg there is a four- to six-fold increase in the level of factor VIII:C which may be sufficient to enable major surgery to be carried out without excessive bleeding (Mannucci, Ruggeri and Capitano 1977, Mannucci *et al.* 1977). Because of the concomitant release of plasminogen activator following infusion of DDAVP (Gader, Da Costa and Cash 1973), it is wise to administer tranexamic acid at the same time. Experience so far suggests that the drug has a small but useful place in the treatment of mildly affected haemophiliacs, carriers of haemophilia with low levels of factor VIII and some patients with von Willebrand's disease. Such patients, because of the mildness of their disease, are infrequently transfused and are therefore particularly at risk of developing hepatitis following transfusion of factor VIII concentrates.

Side-effects of the drug include tachycardia and flushing which may be related to speed of administration. Water retention occurs following administration of the drug so that a careful watch must be kept on the patient's fluid balance and fluid intake restricted if necessary. It is probably wise not to give the drug to patients who suffer from hypertension or have a history suggestive of coronary artery disease. Some patients show a diminishing factor VIII response to DDAVP following several days of treatment. This should be borne in mind when planning to use the drug to cover any procedure in which wound healing is prolonged.

CORTICOSTEROIDS

There have been several reports on the value of steroids in the treatment of haemophilia. Here again, as with many trials of therapeutic agents in haemophilia, many of the studies were not adequately controlled or involved only small numbers of patients. Abildgaard, Simone and Schulman (1965) and Gourdeau and Denton (1968) have reported on the effect of corticosteroids in the management of haematuria and in both studies benefit was found. In a double-blind study of prednisolone compared with placebo in patients with haematuria no benefit was found by Rizza *et al.* (1977).

With regard to spontaneous bleeding, Bennett and Ingram (1967) carried out a double-blind controlled study of prednisolone in low dosage, 2.5 mg 8-hourly for adults and 1 mg 8-hourly for children, and found that the incidence of bleeding was reduced in children but not in adults. Nevertheless they concluded that this form of treatment is not to be recommended since the benefit to the patient is slight compared with the potential hazards of long-term prednisolone therapy.

FEMALE SEX HORMONES

The taking of the contraceptive pill, which is a mixture of oestrogenic and progestogenic hormones, has been found to raise the level of factor VIII in normal women (Egeberg and Owren 1963) and in carriers of haemophilia (Schiffman and Rapaport 1966). The use of these preparations in the treatment of haemophilia has been described by Ozsoylu and Corbacioglu (1967). In this latter study, eight out of ten haemophiliacs showed some improvement in bleeding tendency. The development of gynaecomastia in all and behavioural changes in two of the patients would seem a strong contraindication to the use of those hormones in the management of haemophilia.

von Willebrand's disease

Bleeding in von Willebrand's disease is due to a deficiency of the factor VIII complex and the cornerstone of treatment is factor replacement by means of transfusion of material containing the factor VIII complex. Following transfusion of this material the patient with von Willebrand's disease shows an increase of factor VIII:C in his blood which is often greater and more persistent than one would expect from the size of the dose (Nilsson, Blombäck and von Francken 1957) (Fig. 40). Because of the prolonged increase of factor VIII:C after transfusion, it may be possible to maintain haemostatic levels of the factor by giving transfusions daily or every second day. Fresh-frozen plasma, cryoprecipitate and certain intermediate purity freeze-dried concentrates have all been shown to be effective in controlling bleeding (Biggs and Matthews 1963, Bennett and Dormandy 1966, Perkins 1967). There are several reports that highly purified factor VIII preparations are not as effective as the intermediate purity concentrates or cryoprecipitate in correcting the abnormal bleeding time in von Willebrand's disease in spite of a post-transfusion increase of factor VIII:C, factor VIII-related antigen, and ristocetin cofactor activity (Perkins 1967, Blatt *et al.* 1976, Nilsson and Hedner 1977).

For many years now we have treated von Willebrand's disease patients, including those undergoing surgery, with an intermediate purity factor VIII concentrate prepared by National Health Service Fractionation Laboratories. Following transfusion of this material some patients have shown a temporary correction of the bleeding time whereas others have not (Biggs and Matthews 1963); moreover, the same person often showed different bleeding time responses on different occasions. Irrespective of whether the bleeding time was corrected or not the patients did not bleed excessively during or after surgery. It is our experience that, providing the level of factor VIII:C is maintained above 40–50 per cent of normal and close attention is paid to achieving haemostasis by local measures at the time of surgery, bleeding is not a problem.

Antibodies to the factor VIII complex occasionally arise in patients with severe von Willebrand's disease who have received repeated transfusion of blood products (Stratton *et al.* 1975, Egeberg and Blombäck 1976, Mannucci

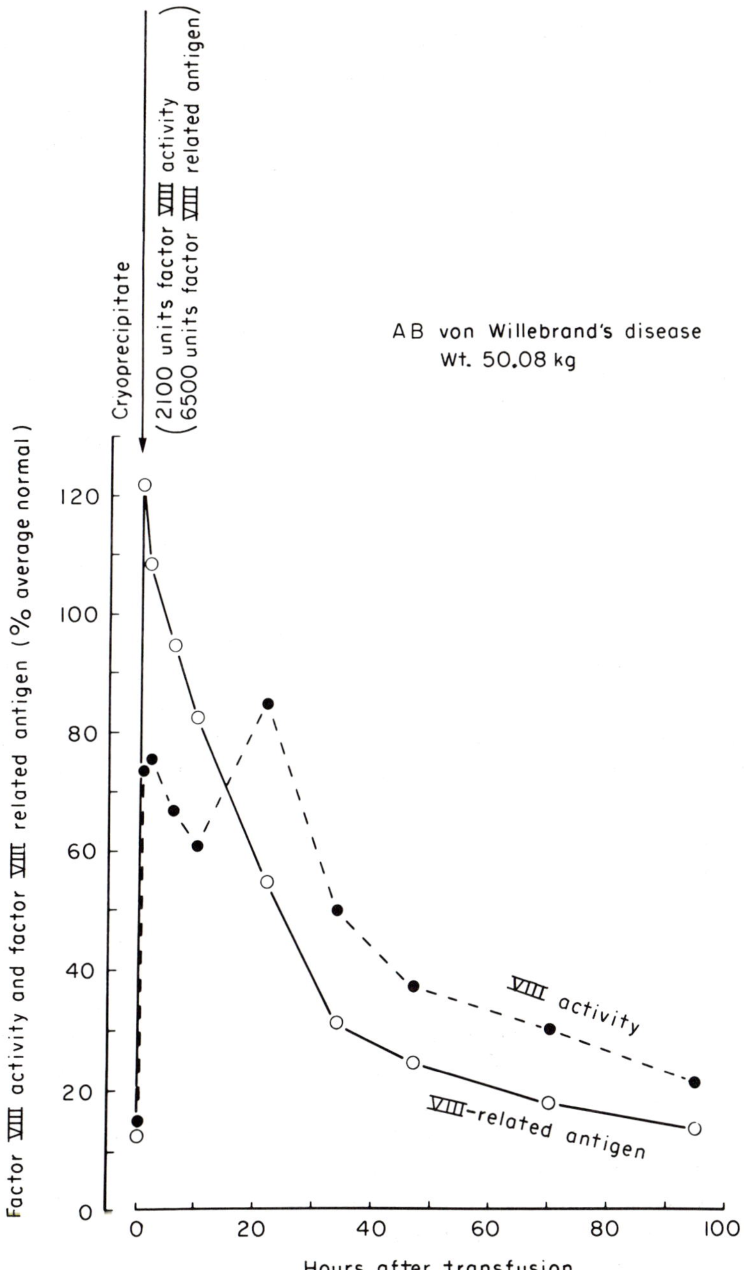

Fig. 40. Transfusion response in a patient with von Willebrand's disease treated with cryoprecipitate.

et al. 1976). The antibodies seem to be directed mainly against the high molecular weight component of the factor VIII complex and affect, in particular, the platelet-related activities. The effect of the antibody on the low molecular weight coagulant component is less marked. Occasionally the antibodies are precipitating antibodies (Mannucci *et al.* 1976) and in these cases transfusion of factor VIII-containing material causes severe reactions in the patient presumably due to antigen-antibody complexes.

Other agents used in the treatment of von Willebrand's disease

As in haemophilia, antifibrinolytic agents are sometimes of value in encouraging haemostasis in patients with von Willebrand's disease. Epsilon-aminocaproic acid (EACA) and tranexamic acid (AMCHA) have both been used in the treatment of patients undergoing dental extraction and have been found useful in the treatment of menorrhagia. Menorrhagia may also be effectively treated by means of oestrogen–progestogen mixtures. These hormones cause an increase in the level of factor VIII complex in the blood but their mode of action in controlling menorrhagia in von Willebrand's disease is more likely to be due to their local effect on the uterus.

As mentioned above, administration of DDAVP to normal subjects, mildly affected haemophiliacs and patients with the less severe forms of von Willebrand's disease brings about an increase in the level of factor VIII complex in the blood. Because of this, the drug has found a place in the management of patients with von Willebrand's disease (Mannucci *et al.* 1977).

The management of congenital deficiencies of factors I, II, V, VII, X, XI, XII and XIII

Congenital deficiencies of the above clotting factors are very rare compared with deficiencies of factors VIII and IX (see Chapter 7). As a consequence, experience in their management is limited. The principles of treatment are much the same as those for haemophilia but taking into account the different levels of the different factors required for haemostasis and the different half-life of the various factors. Bleeding into muscles and joints should, in addition, be treated by the appropriate orthopaedic procedures as in haemophilia and Christmas disease.

Fibrinogen (factor I)

A plasma fibrinogen level of approximately 100 mg/100 ml is usually sufficient to bring about haemostasis. Since the half-life of transfused fibrinogen is of the order of four to six days, haemostatic levels for major surgery can be achieved and maintained by transfusing 10–15 ml/kg of fresh-frozen plasma or 8–16 g of freeze-dried fibrinogen every three to four days. Prophylactic treatment with fibrinogen may be thought necessary in severely affected patients but the dangers of transmitting hepatitis must be borne in mind as well as the risk of stimulating formation of antibodies to fibrinogen (Ingram, McBrien and Spencer 1966, Egbring *et al.* 1971).

Factor II (prothrombin) VII and X

Bleeding in patients with congenital deficiencies of factor II, VII or X can be treated by transfusion of fresh-frozen plasma or prothrombin complex concentrate rich in those factors. Vitamin K has no part to play in the treatment of those congenital deficiencies.

The level of prothrombin required for haemostasis is approximately 40 per cent of normal. This level cannot be easily achieved with fresh-frozen plasma unless the patient's basic level is 20 per cent of normal or more. It is therefore wise if bleeding is severe to use one of the freeze-dried concentrates rich in prothrombin.

In the case of factor VII, relatively low levels of the order of 5–10 per cent of normal would seem to be sufficient for haemostasis. Bleeding following surgical procedures occasionally occurs but is rarely serious (Ratnoff 1960, Marder and Shulman 1964, Strauss 1965, Yorke and Mant 1977). We have under our care a patient with less than 1 per cent factor VII who, despite receiving no replacement therapy, underwent tonsillectomy without bleeding excessively.

Views on the need for factor VII replacement before major surgery vary but it is probably wise to administer one of the above concentrates to severely affected patients before surgery and to repeat the dose two or three times a day for several days after surgery (Fig. 41). Patients severely affected with factor VII deficiency may suffer from recurrent haemarthroses like haemophiliacs, and like haemophiliacs may develop severe joint damage and subsequent crippling.

Bleeding into joints may be controlled by transfusions of fresh-frozen plasma in a dosage of 10–15 ml/kg body weight or by administration of prothrombin complex concentrate or factor VII concentrate (Dike *et al.* 1980).

The patient with congenital factor X deficiency may be treated with transfusions of fresh-frozen plasma or prothrombin complex concentrate which contains factor X. Because of the relatively long half-life of transfused factor X in the blood it is usually easy to achieve and maintain a haemostatic level.

Factor XI

Bleeding due to deficiency of this factor can usually be controlled by

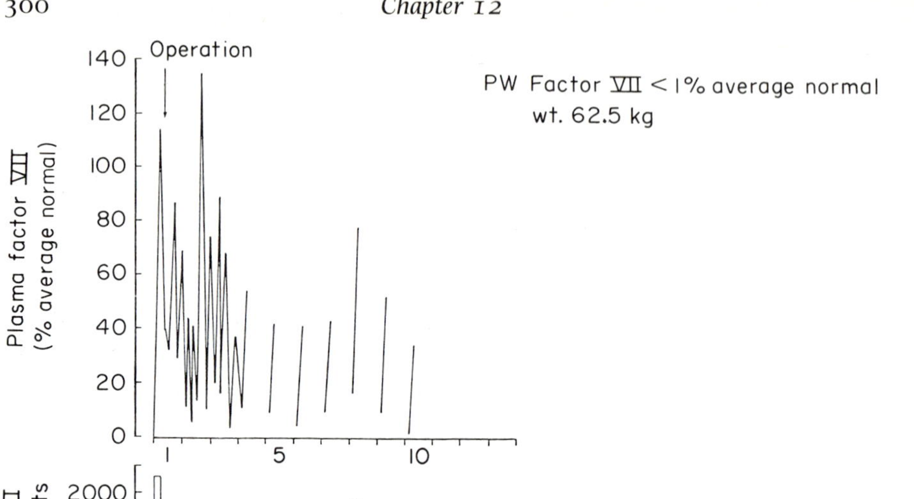

Fig. 41. Plasma factor VII levels before and after transfusion of factor VII concentrate in a patient with severe congenital factor VII deficiency. Surgery for total hip replacement was carried out without bleeding complications. The patient had a past history of repeated haemarthroses involving elbows shoulders and knees.

transfusion of fresh-frozen plasma. For very severe bleeding or for major surgery it is desirable to raise the patient's factor XI level to at least 40 per cent of normal (Nossel *et al.* 1966). This can be achieved by transfusing plasma in a dose of 10–15 ml/kg body weight. Because of the long half-life, approximately 60 hours, it is possible thereafter to maintain haemostatic levels by giving infusions of 10–15 ml plasma/kg body weight twice or three times in the week. The severity of bleeding symptoms in factor XI deficiency patients does not correlate well with the severity of the factor XI deficiency as assessed by *in vitro* testing. There are no concentrated preparations of factor XI available although Bick, Adams and Radack (1974) have found that certain batches of commercial prothrombin complex concentrates contain sufficient factor XI to make them useful for the management of severely affected patients undergoing major surgery. The risk of transmitting hepatitis with such concentrates must be carefully weighed against the potential advantages to the patient.

Factor V

The level of factor V required for haemostasis is thought to be of the order of

10–15 per cent of normal and at these levels it has been found possible to carry out major surgery without excessive bleeding (Borchgrevink and Owren 1961). Following transfusion of fresh-frozen plasma, approximately 80 per cent of the transfused activity is detected in the patient's plasma and the half-life is approximately 12 hours (Mellinger and Duckert 1971). The latter authors noted, however, that in the post-operative period the recovery of factor V in the circulation fell to approximately 50 per cent of that expected, which is similar to the figure obtained by Rush and Ellis (1965). There are at present no concentrated preparations of factor V available but, because of the relatively low levels of factor V required for haemostasis, it is possible to achieve those levels by means of transfusion of fresh or fresh-frozen plasma.

Factor XIII

Deficiency of this factor can lead to a severe bleeding disorder. Fortunately, only a low level of factor XIII is required for haemostasis; levels of 2–3 per cent of normal (Duckert, Jung and Shmerling 1961) will usually prevent bleeding even after major surgery. Walls and Losowski (1969) have shown that as little as 175 ml of plasma will control haemorrhage in an adult patient following dental extraction. Moreover, the half-life of transfused factor XIII is of the order of 12 days (Miloszewski and Losowski 1970, Lorand, Losowski and Miloszewski 1980) so that replacement therapy need be given only infrequently. The urea solubility test may remain normal for 2–3 weeks after the infusion of 1 litre of fresh-frozen plasma into an adult and this can result in the diagnosis being missed in a recently transfused patient. Fresh plasma, fresh-frozen plasma and cryoprecipitate are all effective in the treatment of factor XIII deficiency. More recently a factor XIII concentrate prepared from placenta has proved useful (Miloszewski and Losowski 1975).

The majority of patients with factor XIII deficiency experience severe bleeding symptoms and in particular are at risk of intracranial haemorrhage (Lorand, Losowski and Miloszewski 1980). Because of this, it is probably wise to give prophylactic treatment with plasma, cryoprecipitate or factor XIII concentrate. The latter is particularly convenient to use because of its potency, low dose volume and freedom from allergic reactions. A dose of 2–3 ampoules every 6–8 weeks will usually allow the patient to lead a normal unrestricted life (Miloszewski and Losowski 1975, Lorand, Losowski and Miloszewski 1980).

FACTOR XII

Congenital deficiency of factor XII is characterized by marked impairment of blood coagulation *in vitro*. Despite this, the majority of patients described have suffered no haemorrhagic symptoms even after major surgery (Ratnoff and Colopy 1955, Ramot *et al.* 1956, Ratnoff, Busse and Sheon 1968).

Treatment of acquired deficiencies of blood clotting factors

Acquired disorders of blood coagulation factors usually involve more than one coagulation factor and usually result from some underlying disease process. Treatment of the coagulation factor deficiency therefore requires management of the underlying disease as well as factor replacement when necessary.

Deficiency of factor II, VII, IX and X is probably the most common acquired coagulation defect and is seen clinically in haemorrhagic disease of the newborn and in patients who are suffering from vitamin K deficiency, liver disease or who are taking coumarin-type anticoagulant drugs.

In babies at risk of developing haemorrhagic disease of the newborn, a single dose of 0.5–1.0 mg phytonadione (Konakion) administered parenterally shortly after birth will prevent the fall in coagulation factors. If bleeding should occur, a further dose of phytonadione should be given and the use of factor replacement by fresh-frozen plasma at a dose of 12 ml/kg should be considered.

If the coagulation defect is due to vitamin K deficiency, as for example in coeliac disease or obstruction of the common bile duct, treatment is relatively easy. A dose of 10–20 mg of vitamin K_1 (Konakion) given by the intravenous or intramuscular route will usually bring about an increase in the levels of the clotting factors and correction of the prothrombin time within 6–12 hours. Other measures to correct the underlying cause may also be necessary. If the patient is bleeding severely and more urgent treatment is required, fresh-frozen plasma should be given in a dose of 10–15 ml/kg body weight. Because of the risks of transmitting hepatitis viruses, prothrombin complex concentrates are best not used in such cases unless there are strong contraindications to the use of plasma, for example, allergy to plasma or danger of circulatory overloading in a patient with cardiac failure.

The coagulation factor deficiency seen in chronic liver disease is due mainly to hepatocellular dysfunction with only a small element of biliary obstruction and vitamin K malabsorption. Because of this, the administration of vitamin K has little effect in correcting the deficiency of factor II, VII, IX and X. In patients who are suffering severe haemorrhage as a consequence of their liver disease or who require liver biopsy or some other surgical procedure, it may be necessary to raise the level of clotting factor in the blood by means of transfusion. Fresh-frozen plasma is the material of choice in such patients. A dose of 10–15 ml/kg body weight should raise the concentration of the factors sufficiently to maintain haemostasis. If there is a significant degree of thrombocytopenia, platelet transfusions may also be required. Even with repeated transfusions of fresh-frozen plasma, it is often not possible in patients with liver disease to raise the blood clotting factors to the normal level. The reason for this is not known. Prothrombin complex concentrates should not be used since they may precipitate diffuse intravascular clotting (Ménaché 1976) especially in patients with fulminating hepatitis (Gazzard *et al.* 1974). Fresh-frozen plasma in addition to containing factor II, VII, IX and X has the advantage of containing fibrinogen, factor V and antithrombin III, all of which may be reduced or altered in liver disease as a consequence of impaired synthesis, or increased consumption if disseminated intravascular clotting is present. Depending on the site of bleeding, other measures may be found of use. For example, balloon tamponade or the injection of vasopressin may be of value in controlling bleeding from oesophageal varices and antifibrinolytic agents may prevent clot lysis at sites of injury (Ratnoff 1977).

Patients receiving oral anticoagulants occasionally require to have the effects of the drug reversed either because of bleeding or because of the need for surgery. When there is no urgency and when there is no intention of reinstituting anticoagulant therapy, reversal is best achieved by withdrawing the drug and giving vitamin K_1 by mouth, or by the parenteral route (5–10 mg). Larger doses of vitamin K will make the patient resistant to subsequent anticoagulant treatment for two weeks or more. Should the patient be bleeding severely or require emergency surgery, rapid reversal of the anticoagulant effect can be brought about by giving a transfusion of fresh-frozen plasma or a prothrombin complex concentrate. Here again fresh-frozen plasma is probably the treatment of choice unless the patient is in severe cardiac failure, when the transfusion of a large volume of plasma may be contraindicated. It should be noted that some prothrombin complex concentrates contain factors II, IX and X but no factor VII and, therefore, do not correct completely the coagulation factor defect or the prolonged prothrombin time.

Should serious bleeding occur during treatment with heparin, administration of the drug should be stopped and blood replacement given if required. If bleeding is due to massive overdosage, it may be necessary, in addition, to administer protamine to reverse the action of the heparin. The standard procedure is to administer 1 mg of protamine sulphate for every 100 units of heparin calculated to be in the patient's circulation. Alternatively, the heparin content of the patient's plasma can be titrated *in vitro* against protamine sulphate and the appropriate dose of protamine sulphate calculated.

Treatment of patients who have spontaneous inhibitors of factor VIII

An inhibitor to a blood coagulation factor may occur in previously normal people and bring about a severe haemorrhagic disorder. Factor VIII is by far the most commonly affected factor. Inhibitors acting against factor I, V, IX, XI, XII and XIII have also been described.

The treatment of haemorrhage in patients with spontaneously occurring antibodies to factor VIII is generally very difficult since transfused factor VIII is rapidly destroyed by the antibody in the patient's blood. As in the case of classical haemophilia with antibodies to factor VIII a variety of therapeutic measures have been tried. Clinical benefit has been reported following the use of corticosteroids (Ellis, Handley and Taylor 1959, Horowitz and Fujimoto 1962). On the other hand, the antibody has been found to develop in patients during the course of corticosteroid therapy for dermatitis (Cook, Anderson and Gamble 1962). We have seen two patients who developed factor VIII antibodies while receiving prednisolone, one for rheumatoid arthritis and the other for severe bronchial asthma.

Immunosuppressive drugs have been used with or without concomitant factor VIII replacement and the results have been encouraging (Sherman, Goldstein and Sise 1969, Green 1971, Rizza *et al.* 1972, Hultin *et al.* 1976). In a recent survey of 215 non-haemophilic patients with inhibitors to factor VIII Green and Lechner (1981) found that in 11 of 31 patients receiving no therapy apart from transfusion of blood or factor VIII concentrate, the inhibitor disappeared after being present for an average of 14 months. Corticosteroids were thought to be effective in abolishing the inhibitor in 22 of 45 patients in whom those were the only drugs used. Twenty-eight patients received azathioprine as well as corticosteroids and in 19 the inhibitor declined or disappeared during treatment. Eighty patients received cyclophosphamide along with prednisolone and in 37 there was a satisfactory response. The above study suggests that the inhibitor disappears relatively infrequently without treatment and that each of the drug therapies used seems to give more benefit than no treatment.

When faced with life-endangering bleeding in patients with spontaneous inhibitor to factor VIII, our policy is to give large doses of human factor VIII concentrate (50–70 iu/kg body weight) once or twice daily for 5–10 days along with cyclophosphamide 100 mg daily which is continued for 6–12 months or until the antibody disappears or there is evidence of bone marrow depression. Porcine factor VIII may prove of value if the antibody shows little activity against it.

Acquired inhibitors to other coagulation factors are extremely rare and hence little is known about their management. A detailed review of cases has been carried out by Shapiro and Hultin (1975) and it would seem that acquired inhibitors of factors V, IX and XI occasionally disappear during treatment with corticosteroids and immunosuppressive drugs such as cyclophosphamide or azathioprine. Inhibitors to factor XIII do not seem to be influenced by these drugs.

Management of disseminated intravascular coagulation (DIC)

The management of the condition requires, where possible, the effective treatment of the underlying condition as well as treatment of the haemostatic and thrombotic complications. For example, in acute DIC associated with abruptio placentae, in addition to treating the severe haemorrhage and shock every effort should be made to empty the uterus as quickly as possible.

The treatment of the DIC condition will to some extent be governed by the mode of presentation but broadly speaking will consist of the following:

1 Supportive therapy and correction of shock by administration of whole blood, electrolytes or oxygen where necessary.

2 When bleeding is severe, it should be assumed that blood coagulation factors and platelets are depleted. Replacement therapy should be instituted immediately and if necessary before the results of laboratory tests are known.

Fresh-frozen plasma contains all the necessary coagulation factors as well as providing volume and is probably the treatment of choice. Cryoprecipitate is an excellent source of factor VIII and fibrinogen and should be used where deficiencies of these factors are severe. Fibrinogen concentrates, once widely used, are less used now because of the dangers of transmitting hepatitis and also because of fear of 'adding fuel to the DIC'. If thrombocytopenia is severe and thought to be contributing significantly to the haemostatic defect, transfusions of platelet concentrates should be given.

The place of heparin in the management of DIC is still in dispute. The administration of heparin is justified usually on the grounds that some attempt must be made to halt the process of coagulation factor consumption and to prevent or minimize the deposition of microclots. The arguments for this approach are based mainly on laboratory experiments and theoretical considerations. A review of the literature suggests that heparin therapy may have some part to play in DIC associated with infection, with disseminated malignancy and with the chronic DIC associated with intra-uterine fetal death (Minna, Robboy and Colman 1974, Sharp 1977). Its use is contraindicated when the main risk to the patient is severe haemorrhage since the giving of heparin would make bleeding worse. If heparin therapy is to be given, it should be administered by continuous infusion in a dosage of 5–15 u/kg body weight per hour. The effect on the DIC process can be monitored by carrying out platelet count and measurement of levels of FDP and fibrinogen in the blood.

In addition to laboratory studies it is important to assess the patient's clinical condition at regular and frequent intervals and to look for signs of haemorrhage. Inhibitors of fibrinolysis such as tranexamic acid seem to have very little part to play in the management of DIC (Ratnoff 1969). Their use should be considered only in those very rare patients in whom the DIC has triggered a massive and excessive fibrinolytic response with resultant haemorrhage.

Oral anticoagulant drugs are of little value in the management of DIC. The place of antiplatelet drugs such as aspirin, sulphinpyrazone and dipyridamole is still not clear.

Complications of transfusion therapy

Blood coagulation factor replacement therapy may be occasionally accompanied by unwanted side-effects. Those such as pyrogenic and allergic reactions may appear during or shortly after the transfusion; others such as post-transfusion hepatitis do not occur until several weeks or months after the transfusion. So far, these complications have not been considered a contraindication to treatment especially when dealing with patients suffering from a severe coagulation disorder. The recent concern about acquired immune deficiency state in haemophiliacs and the possible role of lyophilized factor VIII concentrates in the development of the condition has led some workers to reassess the use of those concentrates in haemophilia management.

Circulatory overload

This is a well-recognized complication of treatment with whole plasma especially if large volumes are transfused rapidly. Transfusion of 10–15 ml/kg body weight given over a period of 30–45 minutes is usually well tolerated providing there is no cardiovascular abnormality. Volumes of more than two litres per day are rarely tolerated for more than two or three days even by fit, young adults. Should it be necessary to give such large volumes of plasma, it may be useful to give 40 mg frusemide intravenously at the time of transfusion. Hypervolaemia is practically never seen when concentrates of coagulation factor are used unless the concentrates are of low potency, so that large volumes must be used.

Pyrogenic and allergic reactions

Occasionally the transfusion of plasma or blood coagulation factor concentrate is complicated by a 'reaction'. These reactions vary in their severity and are most commonly seen with plasma, less so with cryoprecipitate and rarely with the freeze-dried concentrates at present available.

Probably the commonest reaction is that seen when a factor concentrate is transfused too rapidly. Most haemophiliacs, if given factor VIII concentrate rapidly, will complain of flushing of the face, pounding of the head and tingling of the skin. To the observer the patient is obviously flushed with suffusion of the conjunctivae. On stopping the infusion or decreasing the rate of administration this type of reaction settles within 1–2 minutes and the infusion can then be continued at a slower rate without further upset. Other reactions which may be seen during or within a few hours of transfusion include backache, headache, rigor, tightness of the chest sometimes with wheezing, urticaria and itching. Occasionally the patient may feel nauseated and vomit. On very rare occasions the reaction may be very severe with pulmonary oedema and death (Kernoff *et al.* 1972).

The mechanism of the above reactions has in some cases been elucidated. The presence of white cell antibodies in the recipient's plasma is probably the commonest cause of non-haemolytic febrile transfusion reactions. It has been shown that other blood components such as gammaglobulin may cause reactions of the type described above (Fudenberg *et al.* 1964, Vyas, Perkins and Fudenberg 1968). Mild reactions can usually be controlled by stopping or slowing down the transfusion and by administering 10 mg of chlorpheniramine maleate intravenously. In the case of more severe reactions the transfusion material should be immediately changed to normal saline and hydrocortisone 100 mg given intravenously. Adrenaline as a 1/1000 solution administered subcutaneously may also be required, especially if bronchospasm is marked.

Patients who have experienced a severe reaction should be observed carefully during subsequent transfusions. A proportion will have no further reaction but some will continue to have reactions. For these patients, a search should be made to find the therapeutic material which gives least trouble and this should then be used for all future transfusions. In these patients an antihistamine preparation may also be given before giving a dose of factor VIII.

Post-transfusion hepatitis

Viral hepatitis is now regarded as the most important complication of coagulation factor replacement therapy. Patients who suffer from severe bleeding disorders are given from an early age large amounts of blood products prepared from large pools of plasma (2000–5000 donations). There seems little doubt that the use of such materials greatly increases the risk of transmitting hepatitis to the recipients. Patients who have previously been infrequently transfused, such as mildly affected haemophiliacs, carriers of haemophilia and patients with von Willebrand's disease seem to be particularly at risk of developing hepatitis following their first transfusions of coagulation factor concentrates (Kasper and Kipnis 1972). Liver biopsy has been carried out in several studies and these show a significant incidence of chronic active hepatitis amongst haemophiliacs (Lesesne *et al.* 1977, Mannucci *et al.* 1978, Spero *et al.* 1978).

Screening each donation of blood and each batch of therapeutic concentrate for hepatitis B antigen has, without doubt, reduced the incidence of infection with this agent. Even so, with the most sensitive radioimmunoassays available, low but potentially infectious amounts of hepatitis B virus may remain undetected. The situation is further complicated by the fact that many cases of hepatitis now seen in haemophiliacs are due to neither the hepatitis A virus nor the hepatitis B virus. There are as yet no specific tests for non-A non-B hepatitis. The diagnosis must be made by a process of exclusion when a patient with acute viral hepatitis shows no serological evidence of infection with hepatitis A virus, hepatitis B virus, cytomegalovirus or Epstein–Barr virus. Attempts to remove the hepatitis B virus infectivity from labile blood products by solid phase immunoadsorption using anti-HBs and by polyethlene glycol precipitation of hepatitis B virus have been on the whole unsuccessful (Gerety, Hoofnagle and Barker 1980). However, Tabor, Aronson and Gerety (1980) were able to neutralize the infectivity of hepatitis B virus in a factor IX concentrate by means of a high titre anti-HBs. Early efforts to reduce infectivity using ultraviolet light or β-propiolactone were also unsuccessful (Murray *et al.* 1955, Barker and Murray 1971). Recent work suggests that it is possible to render prothrombin complex concentrate non-infective by means of β-propiolactone without destroying the coagulation factor activity (Stephan *et al.* 1981).

Another approach to the problem of prevention of hepatitis B is to immunize patients at risk at an early age. Studies with a vaccine prepared from formalin-inactivated HBs Ag particles have given encouraging results in a high-risk population of homosexual men in the USA (Szmuness *et al.* 1980). Hepatitis B immunoglobulin has been found valuable for prophylaxis after accidental exposure to the virus but its place in the management of haemophiliacs is uncertain. One might justifiably use it in a mildly affected patient who was about to receive a factor concentrate for the first time.

With regard to non-A non-B hepatitis, there is at present no vaccine available and the value of normal immunoglobulin is unclear.

Acquired immune deficiency syndrome (AIDS)

During 1980 and 1981, the Centres for Disease Control, Atlanta, Georgia became aware of an increase in the number of reports of serious opportunistic infections and Kaposi's sarcoma among homosexual men in the USA. In these cases there were none of the known predisposing causes of immunosuppression such as treatment with steroids, cytotoxic drugs, and malignancy (*Mortality and Morbidity Weekly Reports* 1982a,b). The syndrome is associated with abnormalities of cell-mediated immunity and has proved fatal in approximately 40 per cent of cases. In addition to homosexuals, this condition has also been observed in heroin addicts, Haitians, and in a small number of haemophiliacs (*Mortality and Morbidity Weekly Reports* 1982c). Immunological studies in patients affected show impaired lymphocyte responsiveness to mitogens and a relative and absolute increase in suppressor T cells compared to helper T cells. The pathogenesis of the syndrome is still not known but the epidemiology is consistent with a blood-borne transmissible agent. Two recent reports (Lederman *et al.* 1983, Menitove *et al.* 1983) have shown impaired tests of cell-mediated immunity in otherwise healthy haemophiliacs treated with lyophilized factor VIII. The abnormalities seen were qualitatively similar to those seen in patients suffering from AIDS but quantitatively less severe. In the latter studies haemophiliacs treated with cryoprecipitate behaved like the normal healthy male controls.

The possibility that lyophilized large pool factor VIII concentrates may induce the AIDS syndrome is of great importance in haemophilic care and it has been suggested that although the evidence is still sparse it may be necessary to stop using lyophilized factor VIII concentrates and revert to the use of cryoprecipitate (Desforges 1983). On the other hand, it has been suggested (*Lancet* 1983) that the evidence at present available does not provide a strong enough argument for a change of treatment policy. We agree with the latter view. Clearly all patients receiving lyophilized factor VIII must be closely observed for signs of development of illness due to impaired immunity. If it transpires that AIDS is due to a transmissible agent, it will be all the more urgent for the new factor VIII concentrates which have been treated by pasteurization or β-propriolactone to be evaluated in haemophiliacs with regard to induction of immunosuppression as well as transmission of hepatitis.

Haemolysis

Most factor VIII concentrates contain small amounts of blood group isoagglutinins. These are not usually of any clinical significance when conventional doses of the factor are given but when large doses are given over a period of days or weeks in patients whose blood group is A or B, haemolysis may occur (Rosati *et al.* 1972, Seeler 1972, Orringer 1976). This situation may arise particularly in patients who have antibodies to factor VIII and who consequently require large doses of factor VIII. Some patients who are receiving large doses of factor VIII have often bled or have just undergone surgery so that the diagnosis of the haemolytic reaction may be missed. Progressive anaemia and mild fever should draw attention to the possibility of haemolysis. Examination of the blood usually shows spherocytosis and a positive direct antiglobulin test. The condition rapidly reverses itself when factor VIII replacement is stopped. Recent work (Smith *et al.* 1980) shows that factor VIII concentrate prepared from cryoprecipitate obtained from single donations of plasmas unselected for A, B, and O groups contains significantly less anti-A than concentrate prepared from cryoprecipitates of mixed pools of plasma.

Thromboembolic complications

Thromboembolism and death have been reported following the administration of certain batches of prothrombin complex concentrates (Kasper 1973, Marchesi and Burney 1974, Kasper 1975, Campbell, Neff and Bowdler 1977). Patients particularly at risk seemed to be the newborn, patients with liver disease and patients with Christmas disease undergoing surgery. However, even patients with uncomplicated Christmas disease occasionally suffered thrombotic episodes following transfusion of these concentrates. Although all prothrombin complex concentrates are potentially thrombogenic, the majority of thromboembolic episodes in patients with Christmas disease have been associated with the use of certain batches of commercial concentrates made in the USA. The experience with these latter concentrates contrasts with the apparent safety over many years of prothrombin complex concentrates made in Europe (Lane, Rizza and Snape 1975, Bidwell *et al.* 1976, Prowse and Cash 1981). Activated factors have been sought in prothrombin complex concentrates using a variety of clotting tests but these tests are not specific or quantitative and it is still not known for certain which factor or factors are responsible for causing thrombosis. On the basis of work carried out in animal models the International Committee on Thrombosis and Haemostasis has recommended the addition of heparin to all prothrombin complex concentrates to give a concentration of heparin of 5–10 iu/ml in the dose when reconstituted for use (Ménaché and Roberts 1975). Whether or not the addition of heparin reduces the risk of thromboembolism in human beings is not known.

In conclusion, prothrombin complex concentrates should be administered with care and circumspection at all times. Unless there are very pressing clinical reasons, they should not be used in the newborn or in patients suffering from liver disease but reserved for the management of Christmas disease. The material should be given immediately after reconstitution and on no account should it be left standing at room temperature for any length of time before it is given to the patient. The dose should be given by slow intravenous injection. Even in patients who have undergone surgery and require repeated injections it is wise, we think, to perform separate venepunctures for each dose to be given. Should it be necessary to insert an indwelling intravenous catheter for giving factor, this catheter should be used only for the administration of factor IX. On no account should other blood products or other drugs be administered by the same catheter. The hazards of adding drugs to intravenous fluids have been well reviewed (Engel 1972).

REFERENCES

Abildgaard C.F., Simone J.V. & Schulman I. (1965) Steroid treatment of hemophilic hematuria. *Journal of Pediatrics* **66**, 117.

Allain J.P. (1979) Dose requirement for replacement therapy in hemophilia A. *Thrombosis and Haemostasis* **42**, 825–31.

Aronstam A., Wassef M., Choudhury D.P., Turk P.M. & McLellan D.S. (1980) Double-blind controlled trial of three dosage regimes in treatment of haemarthroses in haemophilia A. *Lancet* **I**, 169–79.

Ashenhurst AB., Langehennig P.L. & Seeler R.A. (1977) Early treatment of bleeding episodes with 10 u/kg of factor VIII. *Blood* **50**, 181–2.

Barker L.F. & Murray R. (1971) Relationship of virus dose to incubation time of clinical hepatitis and time of appearance of hepatitis-associated antigen. *American Journal of Medical Sciences* **263**, 27–33.

Barkhan P. (1964) Haematuria in a haemophilic treated with E-aminocaproic acid. *Lancet* **II**, 1061.

Bennett A.E. & Ingram G.I.C. (1967) A controlled trial of long-term steroid treatment in haemophilia. *Lancet* **I**, 967–70.

Bennett A.E., Ingram G.I.C. & Inglish P.J. (1973) Antifibrinolytic treatment in haemophilia: A controlled trial of prophylaxis with tranexamic acid. *British Journal of Haematology* **24**, 83–8.

Bennett E. & Dormandy K. (1966) Pool's cryoprecipitate and exhausted plasma in the treatment of von Willebrand's disease and factor XI deficiency. *Lancet* **II**, 731.

Bick R.L., Adams R. & Radack K. (1974) Surgical hemostasis with a factor XI-containing concentrate. *Journal of the American Medical Association* **229**, 163–5.

Bidwell E. (1955a) The purification of bovine antihaemophilic globulin. *British Journal of Haematology* **I**, 35–45.

Bidwell E. (1955b) The purification of antihaemophilic globulin from animal blood. *British Journal of Haematology* **I**, 386–9.

Bidwell E., Rizza C.R., Dike G.W.R. & Snape T.J. (1976) Clinical use of factor IX concentrates. *Thrombosis and Haemostasis* **35**, 488–91.

Biggs R. & Denson K.W.E. (1963) The fate of prothrombin and factor VIII, IX and X transfused to patients deficient in these factors. *British Journal of Haematology* **9**, 532–47.

Biggs R. & Matthews J.M. (1963) The treatment of haemorrhage in von Willebrand's disease and the blood level of factor VIII. *British Journal of Haematology* **9**, 203–14.

Blatt P.M., Brinkhous K.M., Culp II.R., Krauss J.S. & Roberts H.R. (1976) Antihemophilic factor concentrate therapy in von Willebrand's disease. Dissociation of bleeding time factor and ristocetin cofactor activities. *Journal of the American Medical Association* **236**, 2770–2.

Borchgrevink C.F. & Owren P.A. (1961) Surgery in a patient with factor V (proaccelerin) deficiency. *Acta Medica Scandinavica* **170**, 743–6.

Brackmann H.H. (1982) The treatment of inhibitor against factor VIII by continuous treatment with factor VIII and activated prothrombin complex concentrates. In

Activated Prothrombin Complex Concentrates. Mariani G., Russo M.A. & Mandelli F. (eds). Praeger Publishers, New York.

Brackmann H.H. & Egli H. (1981) Treatment of haemophilia patients with antibodies. In *Hemophilia.* Seligsohn U., Rimon A. & Horoszowski H (eds). Based on Symposia held during the XIIIth Congress of the World Federation of Hemophilia. Tel Aviv, Israel 1979. Castle House Publications, Wells, Kent.

Brackmann H.H. & Gormsen J. (1977) Massive factor VIII infusion in haemophiliac with factor VIII inhibitor, high responder. *Lancet* II, 933.

Breen F.A. & Tullis J.L. (1969) Prothrombin complex concentrates in treatment of Christmas disease and allied disorders. *Journal of the American Medical Association* **208**, 1848–52.

Buchanan G.R. & Kevy S.V. (1978) Use of prothrombin complex concentrates in hemophiliacs with inhibitors. *Pediatrics* **62**, 767–74.

Campbell E.W., Neff S. & Bowdler A.J. (1976) Therapy with factor IX concentrate resulting in DIC and thromboembolic phenomena. *Transfusion* **18**, 94–7.

Cobcroft R., Tamagnini G. & Dormandy K.M. (1977) Serial plasmapheresis in a haemophiliac with antibodies to factor VIII. *Journal of Clinical Pathology* **30**, 763–5.

Cook J.V., Anderson J.B. & Gamble W.S. (1962) Circulating factor VIII anticoagulant in bullous dermatitis. *Archives of Internal Medicine* **110**, 511.

Cooksey M.W., Perry C.B. & Raper A.B. (1966) Epsilon-aminocaproic acid therapy for dental extractions in haemophiliacs. *British Medical Journal* II, 1633–4.

Corrigan J.J. (1972) Oral bleeding in hemophilia: Treatment with epsilon-aminocaproic acid and replacement therapy. *Journal of Pediatrics* **80**, 124–8.

de Gaetano G., Donati M.B. & Vermylen J. (1974) Evidence that human platelet aggregating activity in porcine plasma is a property of von Willebrand factor. *Thrombosis et Diathesis Haemorrhagica* **32**, 549–53.

Desforges J.F. (1983) AIDS and preventive treatment in hemophilia. *New England Journal of Medicine* **308**, 94–5.

Dike G.W.R., Bidwell E. & Rizza C.R. (1972) The preparation and clinical use of a new concentrate containing factor IX, prothrombin and factor X and of a separate concentrate containing factor VII. *British Journal of Haematology* **22**, 469–90.

Dike G.W.R., Griffiths D., Bidwell E., Snape T.J. & Rizza C.R. (1980) A factor VIII concentrate for therapeutic use. *British Journal of Haematology* **45**, 107–18.

Dormandy K.M. & Sultan Y. (1975) The suppression of factor VIII antibodies in haemophilia. *Pathologie et Biologie* (Paris) **23** (Suppl.), 17–23.

Duckert F., Jung E. & Shmerling D.H. (1961) A hitherto undescribed congenital haemorrhagic diathesis probably due to fibrin stabilizing factor deficiency. *Thrombosis et Diathesis Haemorrhagica* **5**, 179–86.

Edson J.R., McArthur J.R., Branda R.F., McCullough J.J. & Chou S.N. (1973) Successful management of a subdural hematoma in a hemophiliac with an antifactor VIII antibody. *Blood* **41**, 113–22.

Egberg N. & Blombäck M. (1976) On the characterization of acquired inhibitors to ristocetin induced platelet aggregation found in patients with von Willebrand's disease. *Thrombosis Research* **9**, 527–31.

Egbring R., Egli J., Andrassy K. & Meyer-Lindenberg J. (1971) Diagnostische und therapeutische Probleme bei congenitaler Afibrinogenamie. *Blut* **22**, 175–201.

Egeberg O. & Owren P.A. (1963) Oral contraception and blood coagulability. *British Medical Journal* I, 220–1.

Ellis H., Handley D.A. & Taylor K.B. (1959) Surgery in a patient with an acquired circulating anticoagulant. *Lancet* I, 1167.

Engel G. (1972) Addition of drugs to intravenous fluids. *Drug Intelligence and Clinical Pharmacy* **6**, 145–8.

Fekete L.F., Holst S.L., Peetom F. & Deveber L.L. (1972) 'Auto' factor IX concentrate: A new therapeutic approach to treatment of hemophilia A patients with inhibitors. *14th International Congress of Hematology, Sao Paulo, Brazil.* Abstract No. 295.

Forbes C.D., Barr R.D., Reid G., Thomson C., Prentice C.R.M., McNichol G.P. & Douglas A.S. (1972) Tranexamic acid in control of haemorrhage after dental extraction in haemophilia and Christmas disease. *British Medical Journal* **II**, 311–13.

Forbes C.D. & Prentice C.R.M. (1973) Aggregation of human platelets by purified porcine and bovine antihaemophilic factor. *Nature* **241**, 149.

Fudenberg H.H., Stiehm E.R., Franklin E.C., Meltzer M. & Frangione B. (1964) Antigenicity of hereditary human gamma globulin (Gm) factor—biological and biochemical aspects. *Cold Harbour Symposium on Quantitative Biology* **29**, 463–72.

Gader A.M.A., Da Costa J. & Cash J.D. (1973) A new vasopressin analogue and fibrinolysis. *Lancet* **II**, 1417–18.

Gazzard B.G., Lewis M.L., Ash G., Rizza C.R., Bidwell E. & Williams R. (1974) Coagulation factor concentrate in the treatment of the haemorrhagic diathesis of fulminant hepatic failure. *Gut* **15**, 993–8.

Geratz J.D. & Graham J.B. (1960) Plasma thromboplastin component (Christmas factor, factor IX) levels in stored human blood and plasma. *Thrombosis et Diathesis Haemorrhagica* **4**, 376–88.

Gerety R.J., Hoofnagle J.H. & Barker L.F. (1980) Hepatitis associated with hemophilia treatment. In *Treatment of Bleeding Disorder with Blood Components.* Mammen E.F., Barhart M.I., Lusher J.M. & Walsh R.T. (eds). pp. 199–215. Reviews of Hematology, Vol. 1. Westbury, New York, PJD Publication.

Gordon A.M., McNicol G.P., Dubber H.H.L., McDonald G.A. & Douglas A.S. (1965) Clinical trial of epsilon aminocaproic acid in severe haemophilia. *British Medical Journal* **I**, 1632–5.

Gourdeau R. & Denton R.L. (1970) Steroids and hemophilia. In *The Hemophiliac and his World. Proceedings, 5th Congress of the World Federation of Hemophilia, Montreal 1968.* Bibliotheca Haematologica; No. 34, 65–8. Karger, Basel/New York.

Green D. (1971) Suppression of an antibody to factor VIII by a combination of factor VIII and cyclophosphamide. *Blood* **37**, 381–7.

Green D. (1972) Circulating anticoagulants. *Medical Clinics of North America* **56**, 145–51.

Green D. & Lechner K. (1981) A survey of 215 non-haemophilic patients with inhibitors to factor VIII. *Thrombosis and Haemostasis* **45**, 200–3.

Helske T., Ikkala E., Myllylä G., Nevanlinna H.R. & Rasi V. (1982) Joint involvement in patients with severe haemophilia A in 1975–59 and 1978–79. *British Journal of Haematology* **51**, 643–7.

Hemker H.C., Hermens W.T.H., Muller A.D. & Zwaal R.F.A. (1980) Oral treatment of haemophilia A by gastrointestinal absorption of factor VIII entrapped in liposomes. *Lancet* **I**, 70–1.

Hilgartner M.W. (1975) Use of antifibrinolytic agents in hemophilia. In *Handbook of Hemophilia*, Part II. Brinkhous K.M. & Hemker H.C. (eds). pp. 689–99. Excerpta Medica, Amsterdam.

Horowitz H.I. & Fujimoto M.M. (1962) Acquired hemophilia due to a circulating anticoagulant. *American Journal of Medicine* **33**, 501.

Hruby M.A. & Schulman I. (1973) Failure of combined factor VIII and cyclophosphamide to suppress antibody to factor VIII in hemophilia. *Blood* **42**, 919–23.

Hultin M.B., Shapiro S.S., Bowman H.S., Gill F.M., Andrews A.T., Martinez J., Eyster M.E. & Sherwood W.C. (1976) Immunosuppressive therapy of factor VIII inhibitors. *Blood* **48**, 95–108.

Ingram G.I.C., Dykes S.R., Creese A.L., Mellor P., Swan A.V., Kaufert J., Rizza C.R., Spooner R.J.D. & Biggs R.(1979) Home treatment in haemophilia: clinical, social and economic advantages. *Clinical and Laboratory Haematology* **1**, 13–27.

Ingram G.I.C., McBrien D.J. & Spencer H. (1966) Fatal pulmonary embolus in congenital fibrinopenia. Report of two cases. *Acta Haematologica* **35**, 56–62.

International Multi-Centre Trial (1975) Prevention of fatal post-operative preliminary embolism by low doses of heparin. *Lancet* **II**, 45–51.

Jones P., Fearns M., Forbes C. & Stuart J. (1978) Haemophilia A home therapy in the United Kingdom 1975–76. *British Medical Journal* **I**, 1447–50.

Kasper C.K. (1973) Post-operative thromboses in hemophilia B. *New England Journal of Medicine* **289**, 160.

Kasper C.K. (1975) Thromboembolic complications. *Thrombosis et Diathesis Haemorrhagica* **33**, 640–4.

Kasper C.K. & Kipnis S.A. (1972) Hepatitis and clotting factor concentrates. *Journal of the American Medical Association* **221**, 510.

Kernoff P.B.A., Durrant I.J., Rizza C.R. & Wright F.W. (1972) Severe allergic pulmonary oedema after plasma transfusion. *British Journal of Haematology* **23**, 777–81.

Kernoff P.B.A. & Tuddenham E.G.D. (1981) Reaction to low-molecular-weight porcine factor VIII concentrates. *British Medical Journal* **283**, 381–2.

Kim H.C., Saidi P., Ackley A.M., Bringelsen K.A. & Gocke D.J. (1980) Prevalence of type B and non-A, non-B hepatitis in hemophilia: relationship to chronic liver disease. *Gastroenterology* **79**, 1159–64.

Lancet (1983) Acquired immunodeficiency in haemophilia. Leading Article **I**, 745.

Lane J.L., Rizza C.R. & Snape T.J. (1975) A five year experience of the use of factor IX type DE(1) concentrate for the treatment of Christmas disease at Oxford. *British Journal of Haematology* **30**, 435–46.

Lazerson J. (1972) Hemophilia home transfusion program: effect on school attendance. *Journal of Pediatrics* **81**, 330–2.

Lederman M.M., Ratnoff O.D., Scillian J.J., Jones P.K. & Schacter B. (1983) Impaired cell-mediated immunity in patients with classic hemophilia. *New England Journal of Medicine* **308**, 79–83.

Le Quesne B., Britten M.I., Maragaki C. & Dormandy K.M. (1974) Home treatment for patients with haemophilia. *Lancet* **II**, 507–9.

Lesesne H.R., Morgan J.E., Blatt P.M., Webster W.P. & Roberts M.R. (1977) Liver biopsy in hemophilia A. *Annals of Internal Medicine* **86**, 703–7.

Levine P.H. (1974) Efficacy of self-therapy in hemophilia. *New England Journal of Medicine* **291**, 1381–4.

Leyvraz P.F., Richard J., Bachmann F., van Melle G., Treyvaud J.M., Livio J.J. & Candadjis G. (1983) Adjusted versus fixed-dose subcutaneous heparin in the prevention of deep-vein thrombosis after total hip replacement. *New England Journal of Medicine* **309**, 954–8.

Lorand L., Losowski M.S. & Miloszewski K.J.M. (1980) Human factor XIII: Fibrin stabilizing factor. In *Progress in Hemostasis and Thrombosis*, Vol. 5. Spaet T.H. (ed.). Grune & Stratton, New York.

Ludlam C.A., Peake I.R., Allen N., Davies B.L., Furlong R.A. & Bloom A.L. (1980) Factor Factor VIII and fibrinolytic response to deamino-8-D-arginine vasopressin in normal subjects and dissociate response in some patients with haemophilia and von Willebrand's disease. *British Journal of Haematology* **45**, 499–511.

Lusher J.M., Shapiro S., Palascak J.E., Rao A.V., Levine P.H. & Blatt P.M. and the Hemophilia Study Group (1980) Efficacy of prothrombin-complex concentrates in hemophiliacs with antibodies to factor VIII: A multi center therapeutic trial. *New England Journal of Medicine* **303**, 421–5.

Macfarlane R.G., Biggs R. & Bidwell E. (1954) Bovine antihaemophilic globulin in the treatment of haemophilia. *Lancet* **II**, 985.

Macfarlane R.G., Mallam P.C., Witts L.J., Bidwell E., Biggs R., Fraenkel G.J., Honey G.E. & Taylor K.B. (1957) Surgery in haemophilia. The use of animal antihaemophilic globulin and human plasma in thirteen cases. *Lancet* **II**, 251.

Mannucci P.M., Canciani M.T., Rota L. & Donovan B.S. (1981) Response of factor VIII/von Willebrand factor to DDAVP in healthy subjects and patients with haemophilia A and von Willebrand's disease. *British Journal of Haematology* **47**, 283–93.

Mannucci P.M., Meyer D., Ruggeri Z.M., Koutts J., Ciavarella N. & Lavergne J.-M. (1976) Precipitating antibodies in von Willebrand's disease. *Nature* **262**, 141–2.

Mannucci P.M., Ronchi G., Rota L. & Colombo M. (1978) A clinico-pathological study of liver disease in haemophiliacs. *Journal of Clinical Pathology* **31**, 779–83.

Mannucci P.M., Ruggeri Z.M. & Capitanio A. (1977) DDAVP in haemophilia. *Lancet* **II**, 1171–2.

Mannucci P.M., Ruggeri Z.M., Pareti F.I. & Capitanio A. (1977) 1-deamino-8-D-arginine vasopressin: a new pharmacological approach to the management of haemophilia and von Willebrand's disease. *Lancet* **I**, 869–72.

Mant M.J., Thong K.L., Birtwhistle R.V., O'Brien B.D., Hammond G.W. & Grace M.G. (1977) Haemorrhagic complication of heparin therapy. *Lancet* **I**, 1133–5.

Marchesi S.L. & Burney R. (1974) Prothrombin-complex concentrates and thrombosis. *New England Journal of Medicine* **290**, 403–4.

Marder V.I. & Shulman N.R. (1964) Clinical aspects of congenital factor VIII deficiency. *American Journal of Medicine* **37**, 182–94.

Melliger E.J. & Duckert F. (1971) Major surgery in a subject with factor V deficiency. *Thrombosis et Diathesis Haemorhagica* **25**, 438–46.

Ménaché D. (1976) Report of the Task Force on the clinical use of factor IX concentrates. *Thrombosis and Haemostasis* **35**, 748–50.

Ménaché D. & Roberts H.R. (1975) Summary report and recommendations of task force members and consultants. *Thrombosis et Diathesis Haemorrhagica* **33**, 645–7.

Menitove J.E., Aster R.H., Casper J.T., Lauer S.J., Gottschall J.L., Williams J.E., Gill J.C., Wheeler D.V., Piaskowski V., Kirchner R. & Montgomery R.R. (1983) T-lymphocyte subpopulations in patients with classic hemophilia treated with cryoprecipitate and lyophilized concentrates. *New England Journal of Medicine* **308**, 83–6.

Miloszewski K. & Losowski M.S. (1970) The half-life of factor XIII *in vivo*. *British Journal of Haematology* **19**, 685–90.

Miloszewski K. & Losowski M.S. (1975) Factor XIII concentrate in the long-term management of congenital factor XIII deficiency. *Thrombosis et Diathesis Haemorrhagica* **34**, 323 4.

Minna J.D., Robboy S.J. & Colman R.W. (1974) *Disseminated Intravascular Coagulation in Man.* Charles C. Thomas, Springfield, Illinois.

Mortality and Morbidity Weekly Reports (1982a) Update on Kaposi's sarcoma and opportunistic infections in previously healthy persons—United States. **31**, 294–301.

Mortality and Morbidity Weekly Reports (1982b) Opportunistic infections and Kaposi's sarcoma among Haitians in the United States. **31**, 353–61.

Mortality and Morbidity Weekly Reports (1982c) Pneumocystis carinii pneumonia among persons with hemophilia A. **31**, 365–7.

Murray, R., Oliphant J.W., Tripp J.T., Hamphil B., Ratner F., Diefenbach W.C.L. & Geller H. (1955) Effect of ultraviolet radiation on the infectivity of icterogenic plasma. *Journal of the American Medical Association* **157**, 8–14.

Nilsson I.M., Blombäck M. & von Francken I. (1957) On an inherited autosomal hemorrhagic diathesis with antihemophilic globulin (AHG) deficiency and prolonged bleeding time. *Acta Medica Scandinavica* **159**, 35–57.

Nilsson I.M. & Hedner U. (1977) Characteristics of various factor VIII concentrates used in treatment of haemophilia A. *British Journal of Haematology* **37**, 543–57.

Nossel H.L., Niemetz J., Mibashan R.S. & Schulze W.G. (1966) The measurement of factor XI (Plasma Thromboplastin antecedent). Diagnosis and therapy of the congenital deficiency state. *British Journal of Haematology* **12**, 133–44.

Orringer E.P., Koury M.J., Blatt P.M. & Roberts H.R. (1976) Hemolysis caused by factor VIII concentrates. *Archives of Internal Medicine* **136**, 1018–20.

Ozsoylu S. & Corbacioglu B. (1967) Oral contraceptives for haemophiliacs. *Lancet* **I**, 1001.

Paulssen M.M.P. & van Pelt B.C. (1981) Oral treatment of haemophilia A by factor VIII bound chylomicra. *Lancet* **I**, 1310.

Penner J.A. & Kelly P.E. (1975) Management of patients with factor VIII or IX inhibitors. *Seminars in Thrombosis and Hemostasis* **I**, 386–99.

Penner J.A., Kelly P.E. & Boutaugh M. (1977) Lower doses of factor VIII for hemophilia. *New England Journal of Medicine* **297**, 401.

Perkins H.A. (1967) Correction of the hemostatic defects in von Willebrand's disease. *Blood* **30**, 375–80.

Pintado T., Taswell H.F. & Bowie E.J.W. (1975) Treatment of life-threatening hemorrhage due to acquired factor VIII inhibitor. *Blood* **46**, 535–41.

Pool J.G., Hershgold E.J. & Pappenhagen A.R. (1964) High potency antihaemophilic factor prepared from cryoglobulin precipitate. *Nature* **203**, 312.

Pool J.G. & Shannon A.E. (1965) Production of high-potency antihemophilic globulin in a closed bag system. *New England Journal of Medicine* **273**, 1443–7.

Prowse C.V. & Cash J.D. (1981) The use of factor IX concentrates in man: a 9-year experience of Scottish concentrates in the South-East of Scotland. *British Journal of Haematology* **47**, 91–104.

Rabiner S.F. & Telfer M.C. (1970) Home transfusion for patients with hemophilia A. *New England Journal of Medicine* **283**, 1011–15.

Rainsford S.G., Jouhar A.J. & Hall A. (1973) Tranexamic acid in the control of spontaneous bleeding in severe haemophilia. *Thrombosis et Diathesis Haemorrhagica* **30** 272–9.

Ramot B., Singer K., Kelber P. & Zimmerman H.I. (1956) Hageman factor (HF) deficiency. *Blood* **II**, 745.

Ratnoff O.D. (1960) *Bleeding Syndromes: A Clinical Manual.* p. 72. Charles C. Thomas, Springfield, Illinois.

Ratnoff O.D. (1969) Epsilon aminocaproic acid—a dangerous weapon. *New England Journal of Medicine* **280**, 1124–5.

Ratnoff O.D. (1977) The haemostatic defects of liver disease. In *Haemostasis: Biochemistry, Physiology and Pathology.* Ogston D. & Bennett B. (eds). John Wiley & Sons, London.

Ratnoff O.D., Busse R.J. & Sheon R.P. (1968) The demise of John Hageman. *New England Journal of Medicine* **279**, 760–1.

Ratnoff O.D. & Colopy J.E. (1955) A familial hemorrhagic trait associated with a deficiency of a clot promoting fraction of plasma. *Journal of Clinical Investigation* **34**, 602.

Reid W.O., Lucas O.M., Francisco J., Geisler P.J. & Erslev A.J. (1964) The use of epsilon-amino caproic acid in the management of dental extraction in the hemophiliac. *American Journal of Medical Science* **248**, 184–8.

Rizza C.R., Biggs R. & Spooner R.J.D. (1978) Home therapy. In *The Treatment of Haemophilia A and B and von Willebrand's disease*. Biggs R. (ed.). Blackwell Scientific Publications, Oxford.

Rizza C.R., Edgcumbe J.O.P., Pitney W.R. & Child J.A. (1972) The treatment of patients having spontaneously occurring antibodies to antihaemophilic factor (factor VIII). *Thrombosis et Diathesis Haemorrhagica* **28**, 120–8.

Rizza C.R., Kernoff P.B.A., Matthews J.M., McLennan C.R. & Rainsford S.G. (1977) A comparison of coagulation factor replacement with and without prednisolone treatment of haematuria in haemophilia and Christmas disease. *Thrombosis and Haemostasis* **37**, 86–90.

Rizza C.R. & Matthews J.M. (1982) Effect of frequent factor VIII replacement on the level of factor VIII antibodies in haemophiliacs. *British Journal of Haematology* **52**, 13–24.

Rizza C.R. & Spooner R.J.D. Home treatment of haemophilia and Christmas disease: five years' experience. *British Journal of Haematology* **37**, 53–66.

Rosati L.A., Barnes B., Oberman H.A. & Penner J.A. (1970) Hemolytic anemia due to anti-A in concentrated antihemophilic factor preparations. *Transfusion* **10**, 139–41.

Rush B. & Ellis H. (1965) The treatment of patients with factor V deficiency. *Thrombosis et Diathesis Haemorrhagica* **14**, 74–82.

Schiffman S. & Rapaport S.I. (1966) Increased factor VIII levels in suspected carriers of hemophilia A taking contraceptives by mouth. *New England Journal of Medicine* **275**, 599.

Schleider M.A., Nachman R.L., Jaffe E.A. & Coleman M. (1976) A clinical study of the lupus anticoagulant. *Blood* **48**, 499–509.

Seeler R.A. (1972) Hemolysis due to anti-A and anti-B in factor VIII preparations. *Archives of Internal Medicine* **130**, 101–3.

Shapiro S.S. & Hultin M. (1975) Acquired inhibitors to the blood coagulation factor. *Seminars in Thrombosis and Hemostasis* **1**, 336–85.

Sharp A.A. (1977) Diagnosis and management of disseminated intravascular coagulation. *British Medical Bulletin* **33**, 265–72.

Sherman L.A., Goldstein M.A. & Sise H.S. (1969) Circulating anti-coagulant (anti-factor VIII) treated with immunosuppressive drugs. *Thrombosis et Diathesis Haemorrhagica* **21**, 249.

Sjamsoedin L.J.M., Heijnen L., Mauser-Bunschoten E.P., Van Geijlswijk J.L., van Houwelingen H., van Asten P. & Sixma J.J. (1981) The effect of activated prothrombin-complex concentrate (FEIBA) on joint and muscle bleeding in patients with hemophilia A and antibodies to factor VIII. *New England Journal of Medicine* **305**, 717–21.

Slocumbe G.W., Newland A.C., Colvin M.P. & Colvin B.T. (1981) The role of intensive plasma exchange in the prevention and management of haemorrhage in patients with inhibitors to factor VIII. *British Journal of Haematology* **47**, 577–85.

Smith J.K., Bowell P.J., Bidwell E. & Gunson H.H. (1980) Anti-A haemagglutinins in factor VIII concentrates. *Journal of Clinical Pathology* **33**, 954–7.

Spero J.A., Lewis J.H., Van Thiel D.H., Hasibe U.T.E. & Rabin B.S. (1978) A symptomatic structural liver disease in hemophilia. *New England Journal of Medicine* **298**, 1373–8.

Stark S.N., White J.G., Langer L. & Krivit W. (1965) Epsilon-aminocaproic acid therapy as a cause of intrarenal obstruction in haemophiliacs. *Scandinavian Journal of Haematology* 2, 99–107.

Stein H. & Dickson R.A. (1975) Reversed dynamic slings for knee flexion contractures in the haemophiliac. *Journal of Bone and Joint Surgery* 57A, 282.

Stenbjerg S. & Jørgensen J., Tauris P. & Slottun T. (1982) Low dose factor VIII for the treatment of hemophilia with inhibitors. In *Activated Prothrombin Complex Concentrates*. Mariani G., Russo M.A. & Mandelli F. (eds). Praeger Publishers, New York.

Stephan W., Kotitschke R., Prince A.M. & Brotman B. (1981) Long-term tolerance and recovery of β-propiolactone-ultraviolet (B-PL-UV) treated PPSB in chimpanzees. *Thrombosis and Haemostasis* 46, 511–14.

Storti E., Ascari E., Turpini R., Molinari E., Camba G. & Pettene A. (1972) Epsilon-aminocaproic acid for synovectomy in haemophilic patients. *Acta Haematologica* 47, 146–56.

Stratton R.D., Wagner R.H., Webster W.P. & Brinkhous K.M. (1975) Antibody nature of circulating inhibitor of plasma von Willebrand factor. *Proceedings of the National Academy of Sciences of the USA* 72, 4167–71.

Strauss H.S. (1965) Surgery in patients with congenital factor VII deficiency (congenital hypoproconvertinemia). *Blood* 25, 325–34.

Strauss H.S. (1969) Acquired circulating anticoagulants in hemophilia. *New England Journal of Medicine* 281, 866–73.

Strauss H.S., Kevy S.B. & Diamond L.K. (1965) Ineffectiveness of prophylactic epsilon amino caproic acid in severe hemophilia. *New England Journal of Medicine* 273, 301–4.

Szmuness W., Stevens C.E., Harley E.J., Zang E.A., Oleszko W.R., William D.C., Sadovsky R., Morrison J.M. & Kellner A. (1980) Hepatitis B vaccine: demonstration of efficacy in a controlled clinical trial in a high-risk population in the United States. *New England Journal of Medicine* 303, 833–41.

Tabor E., Aronson D.L. & Gerety R.J. (1980) Removal of hepatitis-B-virus infectivity from factor IX complex by hepatitis-B immune globulin. *Lancet* II, 68–70.

Tavenner R.W.H. (1968) Epsilon amino-caproic acid in the treatment of haemophilia and Christmas disease with special reference to the extraction of teeth. *British Dental Journal* 124, 19–22.

Tsverenis H. & Mandalaki T. (1965) Haematuria in a haemophiliac treated with epsilon amino caproic acid. *Lancet* (letter) I, 610.

Van Itterbeek H., Vermylen J. & Verstraete M. (1968) High obstruction of urine flow as a complication of the treatment with fibrinolysis inhibitor of haematuria in haemophiliacs. *Acta Haematologica* 39, (4), 237–42.

Vyas G.N., Perkins H.A. & Fudenberg H.H. (1968) Anaphylactoid transfusion reactions associated with anti-IgA. *Lancet* II, 312–15.

Walls W.D. & Losowski M.S. (1969) Congenital deficiency of plasma factor XIII. *Coagulation* I, 111–18.

Walsh P.N., Rizza C.R., Matthews J.M., Eipe J., Kernoff P.B., Coles M.D., Bloom, A.L., Kaufman B.M., Beck P., Hanahan C.M. & Biggs R. (1971) Epsilon-amino caproic acid therapy for dental extractions in haemophilia and Christmas disease: a double-blind controlled trial. *British Journal of Haematology* 20, 463–75.

Yates G.A. (1963) Light-weight aesthetic orthopaedic appliances. *Orthopaedics* I, 153–62.

Yorke A.J. & Mant M. (1977) Factor VII deficiency and surgery. Is preoperative replacement therapy necessary? *Journal of the American Medical Association* 238, 424–5.

Chapter 13
Functional Physiology of Platelets

G. V. R. BORN, NICOLA A. BEGENT
and N. J. CUSACK

Physiological haemostasis depends on the following sequence of processes:

1   Contraction of the injured blood vessel.

2   Adhesion and aggregation of platelets which block the injured vessel with a haemostatic plug.

3   Coagulation of the blood plasma around and behind the plug.

The contribution of each of these processes to produce the haemostatic effect varies in different types of blood vessel and under different physiological conditions. The overall result of their operation is the closure of wounds in injured vessels with the prevention of further bleeding. When one or more of these processes is defective, an injury tends to cause abnormally prolonged and severe bleeding.

The purpose of this chapter is to describe the role of the platelets in these three processes. The essential feature of this role is the rapid metamorphosis by which solitary platelets circulating through normal vessels are piled together into clumps containing millions of them within a few seconds of the slightest vascular injury. The ease with which this change can be induced makes it more astonishing that the blood is normally free of platelet clumps than that they should be the main cause of acute thrombosis in diseased arteries.

Platelets in the contraction of injured vessel

When a blood vessel is injured, any smooth muscle in the wall rapidly contracts. The effect of this on the vessel depends on the amount of muscle present and on the type of injury. A muscular arteriole contracts much more than a thin-walled venule. When an artery is severed, the muscle all around the vessel contracts so that the vessel becomes constricted symmetrically and may be closed. After a partial cut the wound edges retract which may slow the loss of blood but may also accelerate it.

The rapidity with which platelets collect in a wounded vessel, and their comparatively large content of a potent vasoconstrictor, 5-hydroxytryptamine or *serotonin* (Rand and Reid 1951), led to the suggestion that the rapid release of this amine caused or contributed to the observed vasoconstriction. This suggestion has been tested experimentally in two main ways as follows:

1   by microscopic observation of injured small vessels, and
2   by comparing the bleeding time in animals with and without 5-hydroxy-
tryptamine in their platelets.

Contraction of small injured vessels

When a cut is made into the small vein at the edge of the rat meso-appendix,
the injured vessel rapidly constricts and so does the accompanying artery
(Zucker 1947). This was taken to indicate the diffusion of a vasoconstrictor
substance, presumably 5-hydroxytryptamine, from platelets adhering in the
injured vein to the artery. Another possible cause would be the diffusion of
noradrenaline released from the injured tissues. This interesting observation
should be investigated further.

The effect of 5-hydroxytryptamine on the bleeding time

The evidence from bleeding time estimations is conflicting. When 5-hydroxy-
tryptamine was almost wholly removed from platelets *in vivo* by giving
reserpine to rabbits, rats and guinea-pigs, the bleeding time was not altered
significantly (Shore *et al.* 1956). Similarly, when reserpine was used clinically
in man, no relation was found between the 5-hydroxytryptamine content of
platelets and the bleeding time, nor did such people bleed excessively after
accidental injuries. On the other hand, administration of a specific antagonist
to 5-hydroxytryptamine for several days caused the bleeding time to be
prolonged (O'Brien 1963); this observation may, however, have explanations
other than that platelet serotonin is involved in haemostasis.

Platelets of several mammalian species, including man, contain adrenaline
although in lower concentrations than 5-hydroxytryptamine (Born, Hornykiewicz and Stafford 1958, Markwardt 1967); whether they contain noradrenaline also is not certain. The arterioles of many tissues, including skin,
are constricted by adrenaline so that its release from adhering platelets could
contribute to vascular constriction. This possibility is supported by the
demonstration that adrenaline, like 5-hydroxytryptamine, is released from
human platelets by thrombin, probably from cytoplasmic organelles in which
the amines are accumulated (Born and Smith 1970); however, the amounts of
adrenaline released in this way are much smaller than those of 5-hydroxytryp-
tamine.

Another way in which platelets could contribute to vasoconstriction is by
the contraction of the platelet plug which adheres in an injured vessel (see
below); this contribution has, however, not yet been demonstrated directly.

Platelets in the formation of a haemostatic plug

Normal spontaneous haemostasis depends mainly on the formation of a haemostatic plug which fills any gaps in the continuity of an injured vessel and covers it like a capsule. At first this haemostatic plug consists only of platelets which have somehow been arrested in their circulation by the injury. A fundamental problem is, therefore, the nature of the signal from the injury site to the platelets.

Contact with a vascular lesion causes a remarkably rapid change in platelets which makes them adhere and cause other platelets chancing to touch them to adhere also. Thus the formation of a haemostatic plug involves first *adhesion* of platelets to other tissues, followed very rapidly by the *aggregation* of platelets to each other. Initially the platelets adhere loosely to each other so that the plasma and cells continue to pass out of the vessel. Within a few minutes the platelets become packed much more closely, indeed almost as closely as is theoretically possible (Born and Hume 1967) so that the plug becomes more effective in its haemostatic function. The mechanism of platelet aggregation is probably different in these two phases (see below); whether either mechanism is also responsible for the initial adhesion of platelets to an abnormal vessel wall is still uncertain.

Platelet adhesion

Platelets do not adhere to normal endothelial cells but do adhere to gaps between endothelial cells, even when the gaps are produced in normal vessels by the action of pharmacological agents (Tranzer and Baumgartner 1967). The gaps expose vascular basement membrane to which platelets apparently tend to adhere. Whether this tendency has any physiological or pathological significance is not yet known. In small venules, histamine and some other vasoactive agents cause contraction of the endothelial cells with the appearance of gaps between them (Majno, Shea and Leventhal 1969). These gaps presumably account for the great increase in the permeability of these vessels to proteins and other constituents of plasma in inflammation. The adhesion of platelets in such gaps might have the effect of diminishing vascular permeability.

When a blood vessel is injured, the exposed subendothelial tissues are covered by a layer of adhering platelets. This adhesion is so rapid (Hugues 1953) that its mechanism provides interesting problems. The probability of a platelet adhering presumably increases with both the closeness and the duration of contact between the platelets and the site. These parameters have to be related to biochemical mechanisms capable of providing sufficient attraction to hold a platelet against the sheer force of the flowing blood. No forces are known which could attract platelets towards an adhesion site over distances greater than a few tens of nanometres. That means that adhesion depends on collision and poses the problem in another way, i.e. what is the collision rate between circulating platelets and vessel wall and what fraction of the collisions is successful in making platelets stick? Measurements of successful collisions have provided estimates of the adhesiveness of other cell types *in vitro* (Curtis 1967) and could be made with platelets; but *in vivo* the problem is much more complicated.

As might be expected on the basis of the foregoing, the trauma required to make platelets adhere to a vessel may be extremely slight; indeed, the question has still to be answered as to what constitutes the least abnormality for adhesion to occur. Even the loss of some of the net negative surface charge on intact endothelium with a consequent diminunition of the normal electrostatic repulsion of platelets, accomplished *in vivo* by perfusing vessels with *neuraminidase* to remove accessible sialic acids, suffices to induce adhesion (Görög, Schraufstätter and Born 1982). Platelets have been found to adhere in endothelial gaps in apparently normal venules situated at some distance from an experimentally injured vessel (Fig. 42). The application of adenosine 5′-diphosphate (ADP) in small amounts by iontophoresis on to the outside of an apparently undamaged venule in the hamster cheek pouch causes the adhesion of platelets in the lumen within a few seconds (Begent and Born 1970); there are no gaps between the endothelial cells and the cell membranes look intact on electron micrographs, so that the amount of applied ADP reaching the inside of the vessel must be very small indeed. The platelets which adhere are rapidly covered by others and a mural thrombus of platelets forms with an exponential increase in volume. The first-order rate constant of this increase depends, within limits, on the blood flow velocity in a characteristic manner which can be explained on the single assumption that it takes platelets a certain time (about 0.3 s) to change from a non-adhesive into an adhesive state (Richardson 1973). This assumption is compatible with evidence, summarized below, indicating that this change requires a rapid alteration in the shape of platelets.

When small vessels are injured mechanically, thermally or electrically, mural thrombi do not form unless the site has been denuded of endothelium. Which tissue constituents, normally separated from circulating platelets by intact endothelium, could bring about their adhesion when a lesion makes contact possible? The answers depend on inferences from *in vitro* experiments. These have shown that the adhesiveness of platelets is markedly increased by several substances which are present in normal vessel wall; they include collagen fibres, the catecholamines adrenaline and noradrenaline and particularly ADP, a constituent of all cells which tends to be increased by any form of cellular injury. Recently it has been demonstrated directly *in vivo* that blood

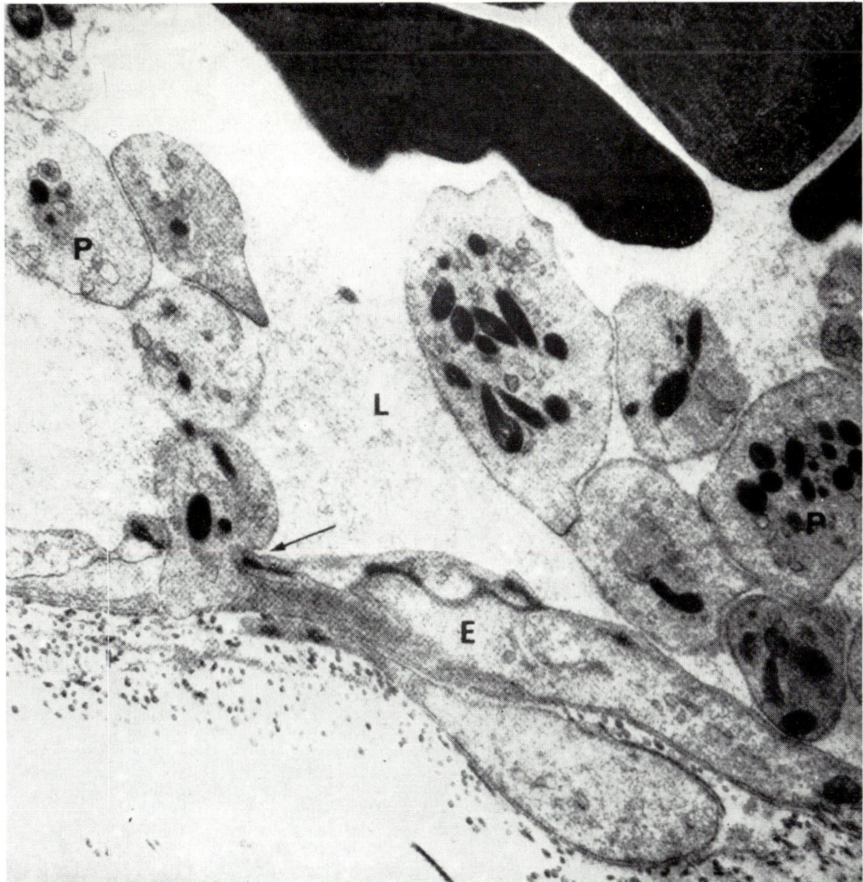

Fig. 42. Part of the wall of a small vein in a hamster shows a group of platelets (P) in the lumen (L). One platelet occupies an intercellular gap (arrows) in the endothelium (E). (× 24 000. From French 1967.)

emerging from punctured arteries contains ADP derived from the vessel wall in sufficient quantities to induce platelet aggregation (Born and Kratzer 1982). Another potent agent is thrombin, the formation of which is initiated at injury sites by tissue thromboplastin. The effects of all these substances on the platelets, at least *in vitro*, depends primarily on ADP and secondarily on the generation of thromboxanes. *In vivo*, this implies than when a circulating platelet is thrown into contact with collagen it induces the platelet to adhere until these mechanisms (see below) come into play; this apparently happens in a very short time indeed, probably within a few milliseconds. As activation of platelets in indicated by adhesiveness, the change to an adhesive state presumably involves one or more constituents of the platelet surface membrane, in particular the exposure of receptors for fibrinogen (Born and Cross 1964).

In vitro platelet aggregability is correlated with the binding of radiolabelled fibrinogen (Peerschke *et al.* 1980). The activation time may be defined, therefore, as the interval between the encounter of platelets with an activating agent and their ability to react with plasma fibrinogen (Born and Richardson 1980). *In vivo* experiments suggest also that the process is potentiated *in vivo* by the effects of the other agents such as thromboxanes and phospholipids which may be released or produced at the same time. There is evidence that an agent, probably ADP, is released from the erythrocytes in amounts large enough to activate the platelets (Born, Bergquist and Arfors 1976, Born and Wehmeier 1979). On the other hand, the effectiveness of this and other agents is diminished by the blood flow which dilutes them and washes them away.

What happens then is determined in different vessels by their blood flow. In a large artery, e.g. the aorta, in which flow is fast, an area from which endothelium is removed is covered by only a single layer of platelets (Fig. 43);

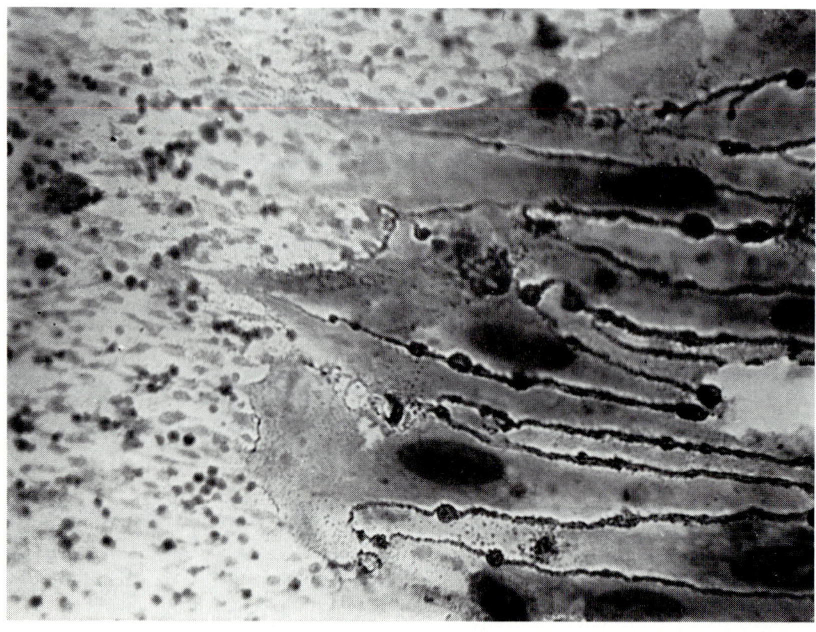

Fig. 43. The edge of endothelium 24 hours after scraping it in the abdominal aorta in a rabbit. In the upper half of the picture is the surface from which endothelium was removed. The small round objects are platelets adhering to the denuded surface. The endothelial cells below are apparently extending a cytoplasmic film over the denuded area. Häutchen preparation. Silver nitrate and Verhoeff. ($\times$ 800. From Poole, Sanders and Florey 1958.)

these are gradually replaced by granulocytes. In a *small* artery, in which the blood flow is much slower, similar damage to endothelium is followed by adhesion of platelets not only to the denuded area but also to each other until the aggregates may block the lumen and so arrest the blood flow altogether (Fig. 44). This difference can be explained by assuming that fast blood flow removes agents released from the damaged wall before their concentration is sufficient to affect platelets, even those that come in contact with the lesion, and that the shear forces are so great that they overcome the forces making for adhesion; and that neither of these effects operate in smaller vessels with slower flow. This explanation still requires experimental verification; but the repeated, exponential growth of platelet thrombi on injury sites of rabbit

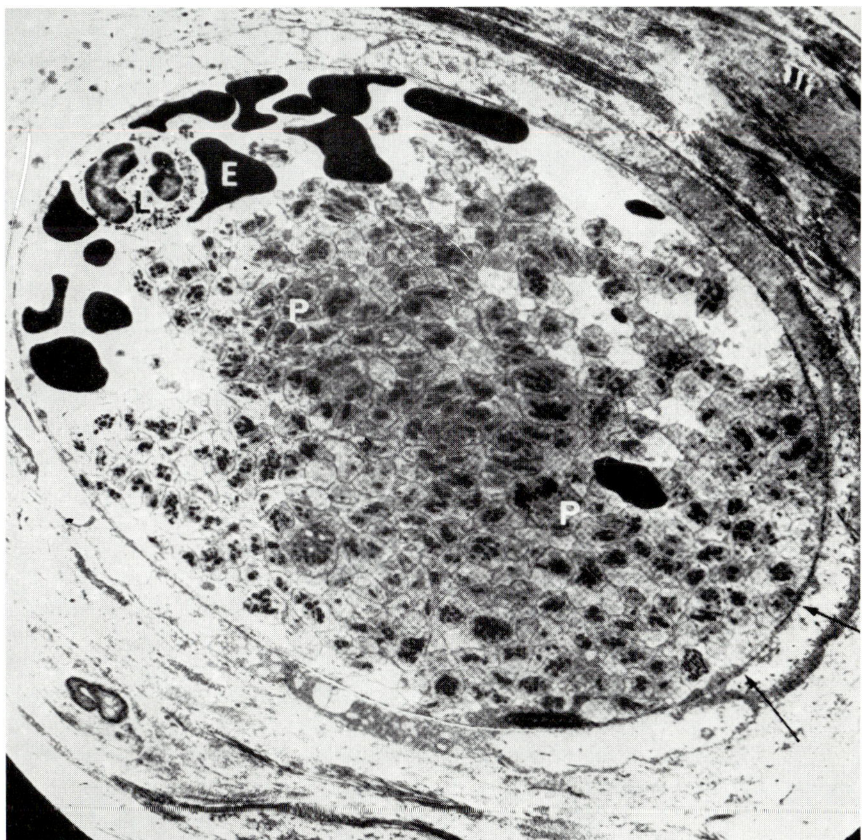

Fig. 44. A thrombus in a small artery in a hamster cheek pouch consisting predominantly of platelets (P). A few erythrocytes (E) and a single leucocyte (L) are seen at its edge. The endothelium is missing at the site of injury (arrows). PTA stain. (× 3000. From French 1967.)

arterioles (Afors, Cockburn and Gross 1975) suggests that the high wall shear rates in these vessels is not in itself sufficient to prevent activated platelets from adhering and aggregating. Both flow velocity distribution in, and the geometry of, a vessel are major determinants in platelet thrombogenesis (Baumgartner 1973) as in haemostasis (Born 1977).

Platelet aggregation

The adhesion of platelets to each other is called *platelet aggregation* unless the reaction is immunological when it is called *platelet agglutination*. After an injury to all but the largest blood vessels, adhesion of platelets to the damaged wall is followed very rapidly by the formation of platelet aggregates on top of the adhering layer. The initial adhesion process cannot be validly imitated outside the living vessel so that the mechanism is difficult to investigate experimentally. The process of aggregation, on the other hand, can be observed *in vitro* by various methods in which it appears to operate much as *in vivo*. Much more is known, therefore, about aggregation than about adhesion (for review see CIBA Symposium, 1975).

The method which has provided most information about aggregation (Born 1962a,b) is a simple adaptation of the turbidimetric technique commonly used for measuring growth rates of microorganisms or enzymic reactions in heterogeneous systems. The method depends on the continuous measurement of changes in optical density of a suspension of platelets, either in plasma or in physiological saline solutions. When platelets aggregate the optical density decreases and when the aggregates disperse the optical density increases. This has made possible quantitative measurements of the aggregation process and provided much information about its mechanism and about promoting and inhibiting agents (for reviews see Born 1970a,b, Mills 1969, Mustard and Packham 1970).

AGGREGATING AGENTS

In vitro, human platelets are caused to aggregate by adenosine 5'-diphosphate (ADP), adrenaline, 5-hydroxytryptamine, thrombin, collagen, vasopressin, arachidonic acid and its metabolites, and platelet activating factor (PAF), as well as by several other agents less immediately relevant to haemostasis. Platelets of other mammalian species are also aggregated by some of these agents but not all of them are active in all species (Mills 1970). Each agent reacts initially with some kind of receptor site specific for it on the outer membrane of the platelets which thereupon undergo rapid changes in their morphology. The initial reaction apparently induces the local formation and/or release of ADP and it may be this which causes the changes in surface properties of platelets resulting in their aggregation. The evidence for this is as follows:

1 The demonstration of the release of ADP from platelets by the other agents.

2 The inhibition of aggregation by enzymes which remove ADP from the plasma.

3 Inhibition by specific antagonists of the effect of ADP (for review see Haslam and Cusack 1981).

Because aggregation by collagen and thrombin involves ADP, it is convenient to describe the effects of added ADP on platelets and then to point out any differences in the effects of the other agents.

Effects of ADP

CHANGE IN SHAPE

When suspensions of platelets in plasma are stirred, the record of optical density shows small, nearly uniform oscillations. When ADP is added, the oscillations disappear almost immediately; at the same time there is a rapid increase in the optical density of the plasma, amounting to a decrease of a few per cent in light transmission (Fig. 45). The optical changes indicate the first and, possibly, the only effect of ADP itself on platelets, namely to change their shape from smooth discs to spheres with pseudopodia of varying lengths protruding from the surface (Macmillan and Oliver 1965). This effect, already referred to when describing platelet adhesion *in vivo*, has some interesting properties (Born 1970b):

1 It appears to be due to a reaction between ADP and a specific receptor on the platelet surface; the reaction does not require the cofactors calcium ions and fibrinogen, which are required for subsequent aggregation.

2 It is associated with a net movement of sodium into the platelets, reminiscent of the effect of depolarizing agents such as acetyl choline on excitable cells (Feinberg *et al.* 1975).

3 It is very rapid and has an extraordinarily high temperature coefficient suggesting an underlying reaction with a high activation energy such as, for example, the extrusion of hydrophilic structures through a lipid membrane, as might happen during the appearance of the long thin pseudopodia or spikes (Born 1970b).

4 Some substances closely related to ADP inhibit the effect. Thus adenosine triphosphate (ATP) and adenosine cause inhibition but their modes of action differ. ATP competes with ADP at its receptor (Macfarlane and Mills 1975) whereas inhibition by adenosine depends on its activation of adenylate cyclase in the platelet membrane (Mills and Smith 1972, Mills 1974).

5 The change in shape is accompanied not by a change in volume of the

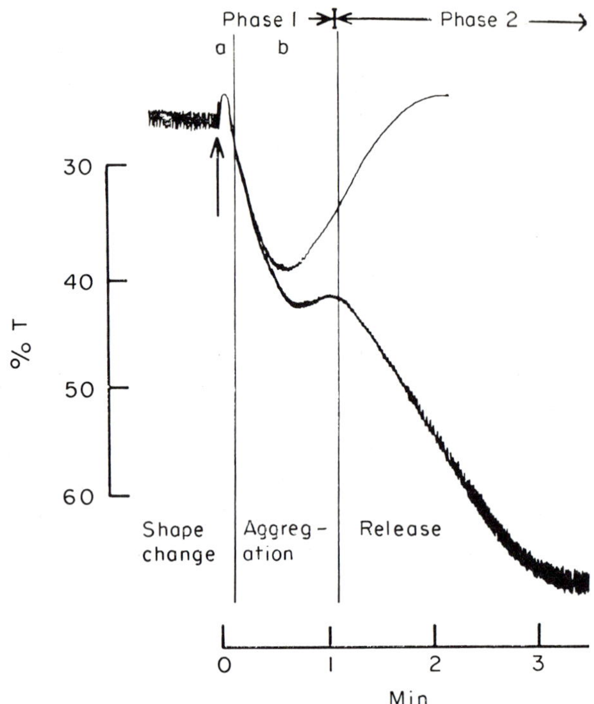

Fig. 45. Diagram of the pen-recorded changes in the optical density of human platelet-rich plasma following the addition of ADP at the arrow. See text.

Abscissa: time in min.

Ordinate: optical density as percentage light transmission, increasing downwards. (Drawn by D.C.B.Mills.)

platelets (Born 1970b) but by a remarkable increase in the ratio of surface to volume up to three-fold (Born *et al.* 1972). The rapidity of this increase and the biosynthetic sluggishness of platelets indicate that the additional surface consists not of newly formed but newly shaped structures.

Indirect support for this conclusion is provided by some rearrangement of the contents of the platelets which can be seen on electromicrographs. A bundle of microtubules which encircles the platelets just beneath their outer membrane appears contracted and the cytoplasmic granules become concentrated within it (White 1968).

The change in shape is brought about by the other endogenous aggregating agents except, apparently, by collagen; it is interesting that this is the only agent which causes aggregation to begin after a considerable lag period.

The functional significance of the rapid change in shape is not yet certain. The pseudopodial extensions increase the effective collision diameter of the platelets so that the function of the shape-change could well be to increase the probability of contact between platelets in the flowing blood and a lesion in the vessel wall. The negative charge density on a cell surface is decreased at the tips of thin pseudopodia or cytoplasmic extrusions, so that such extrusions diminish the effect of electrostatic repulsion between cells and increase the effect of other forces making for adhesion (Bangham 1964, Born 1972a).

FIRST PHASE OF AGGREGATION

The optical effect of the shape-change is followed by an effect in the opposite direction, i.e. an increase in light transmission which is usually also much larger (Fig. 45). This part of the record is the resultant of several simultaneous processes in which single platelets adhere to each other to form small aggregates and to aggregates already formed, and in which small aggregates adhere to each other to form larger ones. The stages in which the aggregates are small, i.e. containing less than ten platelets, are passed through very rapidly and throughout this phase the platelets adhere to each other loosely (Born and Hume 1967) (Fig. 46). The looseness is also seen on electron microscope pictures of small platelet aggregates adhering to injured vessels *in vivo*. These initial events in aggregation can be accounted for by a simple mathematical model (Cronberg 1970).

DISAGGREGATION

The first phase of aggregation by ADP, just described, is completely reversible and the dispersion of the aggregates is shown by an increase in the optical density of the plasma (Fig. 45). With platelets from man, cat and guinea-pig, aggregation reverses spontaneously when caused by low concentrations of ADP; higher concentrations may induce the second phase of aggregation (see below) which obscures and delays disaggregation. In other species, e.g. rat and rabbit, the second phase never occurs so that disaggregation can be observed even after ADP is added at comparatively high concentrations. Disaggregation is caused by the following:

1 The breakdown of ADP in plasma by enzymic reactions which simultaneously produce inhibitory derivatives (see below).
2 A change in the platelets whereby the effectiveness of ADP on them is diminished.

The rate of disaggregation is controlled by the development of a refractory state of the platelets towards ADP and by the rate at which ADP is removed from plasma by enzymic reactions. Nothing is known yet about the cause of the refractoriness of platelets to ADP. In plasma, ADP is broken down by two enzymes; which of these predominates depends on the ADP concentration. At

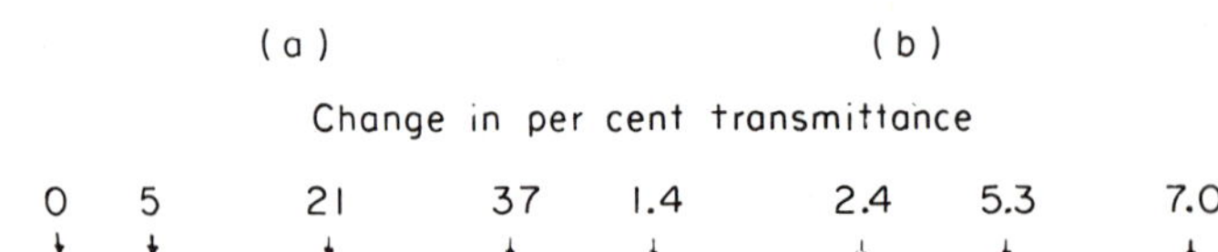

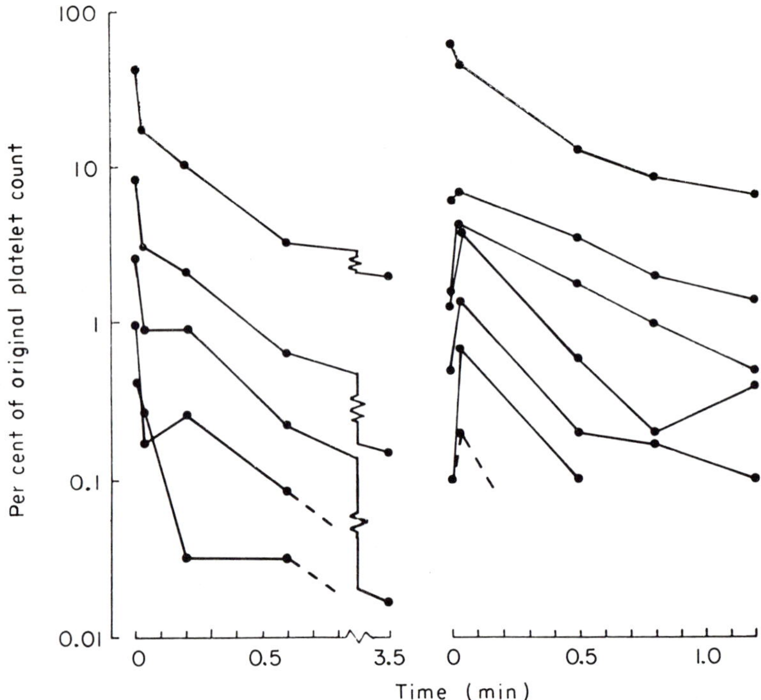

Fig. 46. Platelets countable as singles, doubles (× 2), triples (× 3) and so on related to change in light transmission and time after adding ADP.

(a) Using high concentration of ADP. The top line gives the number of platelets countable as singles and the lines from above down indicate aggregates of two, three, four and five platelets.

(b) Using a low concentration of ADP. Aggregation proceeds more slowly than in (a) and transitory increase in small aggregates is seen (from Born and Hume 1967).

high concentrations (above 100 μM) the rate of removal is determined by adenylate kinase which converts two molecules of ADP to one of AMP and one of ATP; thus the enzyme catalyses not only the inactivation of the antagonist ADP but also the formation of ATP which antagonizes aggregation by ADP (Born 1962b). This enzyme is present in high concentrations in most cells including erythrocytes; therefore, adenylate kinase activity in plasma *in vitro* depends mainly on leakage of the enzyme from red cells (Haslam and Mills 1967). Low concentrations of ADP (1–5 μM) which cause reversible platelet aggregation are removed mainly by a specific ADPase which hydrolyses ADP to AMP and inorganic phosphate. This enzyme has a high affinity for ADP and is inhibited by the reaction product AMP but not by adenosine. The activity of this enzyme in human plasma is low and independent of haemolysis (Mills 1966); its source has not been established.

SPECIFICITY FOR ADP

Aggregation of platelets by ADP is highly specific (Gaarder *et al.* 1961). Other naturally occurring nucleotides are inactive except 3'-deoxy adenosine diphosphate and guanosine diphosphate which have less than 10 per cent of the potency of ADP. On the other hand, some synthetic derivatives, viz. 2-chloroadenosine 5'-diphosphate and 2-azidoadenosine 5'-diphosphate, are up to ten times more potent than ADP itself (Gough, Maguire and Michal 1969, Cusack and Born 1977). Contamination by ADP accounts for aggregation activities of ATP (Haslam 1968) and adenosine tetraphosphate (Harrison and Brossmer 1976) preparations; ATP (Born 1962b) and adenosine tetraphosphate (Harrison and Brossmer 1976) are indeed competitive inhibitors.

ESSENTIAL COFACTORS

At least two other substances are essential for aggregation by ADP, viz. ionized calcium and fibrinogen (Born and Cross 1964, Cross 1964). The velocity of aggregation increases with the concentration of calcium up to about 1 mM; higher concentrations inhibit aggregation. Therefore, plasma containing EDTA as anticoagulant cannot be used for investigating platelet aggregation whereas citrate in the concentration which is usually added interferes little.

Fibrinogen, also, is essential for physiological aggregation of platelets in plasma. *In vitro*, aggregation velocity increases with fibrinogen concentration. Association of fibrinogen to the platelet takes place immediately after the addition of ADP, and dissociation occurs if platelets disaggregate (Mustard *et al.* 1978). Binding of radiolabelled fibrinogen to platelets depends on calcium and correlates with the extent of aggregation (Maguerie, Plow and Edgington 1979). Platelets from patients with Glanzmann's thrombasthenia, which do not aggregate in response to ADP, do not bind fibrinogen (Bennett and Vilaire 1979). In patients with congenital afibrinogenaemia, platelet aggregation is greatly slowed but not abolished (Inceman, Caen and Bernard 1966); the reason seems to be that, even in the severest cases, some fibrinogen remains associated with the platelets themselves. This may also explain why the almost total removal of fibrinogen from plasma of patients treated with Malayan pit

 Chapter 13

viper venom does not affect platelet aggregation by ADP or by thrombin (Sharp *et al.* 1968). There is experimental evidence that some other plasma proteins, particularly Hageman factor and gamma globulins, can substitute for fibrinogen as cofactor *in vitro* (Bang, Heidenreich and Trygstad 1972). Whether this observation is relevant to the process *in vivo* is uncertain.

POTENTIATING AGENTS

Aggregation of platelets by ADP is potentiated by *potassium* ions (Born and Cross 1964, Born and Schraufstätter 1982) but neither these nor sodium ions are essential.

The effect of ADP is greatly increased by *adrenaline* (Ardlie, Glew and Schwartz 1966), even in very low concentrations. This potentiation shows itself both as an acceleration of primary aggregation and as a diminution in the ADP concentration required to initiate the second phase of aggregation in which aggregating substances are released from the platelets. These observations are given clinical significance by the appearance of such concentrations of adrenaline in the plasma of people during stress who, as is well known, are particularly liable to suffer from arterial occlusion by platelet thrombi (see Born 1967). Adrenaline also potentiates aggregation by thrombin and by collagen (Thomas 1968) but these effects may, at least in part, represent potentiation of ADP which these agents release from platelets.

SECOND PHASE OF AGGREGATION AND THE RELEASE REACTION

The optical method resulted in the discovery that critical concentrations of ADP added to citrated plasma of man (Macmillan 1966) or guinea-pig (Constantine 1966) at 37°C cause two distinct phases of decrease in the optical density (Fig. 45). The second phase is associated with the release of ADP from the platelets themselves so that its concentration in the plasma may increase up to seven times (Mills, Robb and Roberts 1968). Other substances released at the same time include ATP and 5-hydroxytryptamine in proportions which vary in different species, as well as platelet factor 3 which accelerates coagulation of plasma (Hardisty and Hutton 1966), and products of arachidonate metabolism. This release action can be induced also by thrombin (Grette 1962) or adrenaline, and the latter diminishes the concentrations of all other agents needed to initiate the reaction.

The decrease in optical density during this phase of aggregation is caused by the contraction of aggregates already formed rather than by the formation of larger aggregates (Fig. 47). There is evidence that this contraction also occurs *in vivo* where it presumably increases the effectiveness of the platelet plug as a barrier against further blood loss.

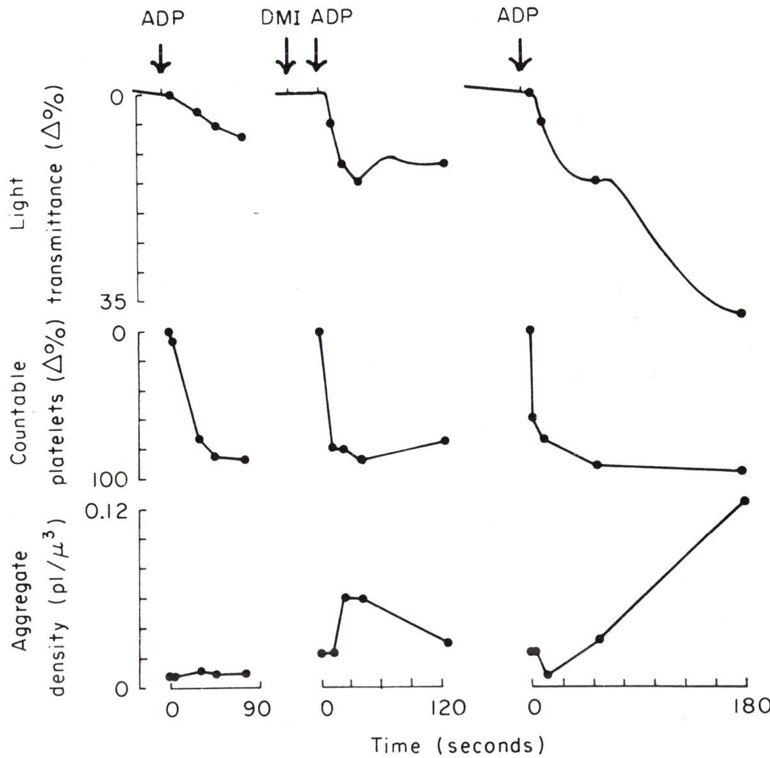

Fig. 47. Simultaneous determination during platelet aggregation by ADP of light transmission (top, percentage change); countable platelets, i.e. single platelets together with those in aggregates containing from 2–8 platelets (middle, percentage change); and the mean density of all platelet aggregates (bottom, expressed as platelets per μ^3). In (a), beginning of first phase only; in (b), complete first phase, the second phase being inhibited by desmethylimipramine (DMI); and in (c), during both phases (from Born and Hume 1967).

INHIBITION OF PLATELET AGGREGATION

The successive responses of platelets to ADP and to the other agents can be inhibited by a variety of means. The photometric method has been particularly successful in the discovery of substances capable of preventing or reversing aggregation. Further research may provide a drug effective against platelet thrombosis without, at the same time, interfering with the haemostatic function of platelets. That this can be achieved in principle was shown by infusing adenosine intravenously into rabbits in which it accelerated the dispersal of intravascular platelet thrombi without prolonging the bleeding time (Born, Honour and Mitchell 1964).

From the preceding descriptions it is clear that inhibition of the initial shape-change should also prevent both phases of aggregation; inhibition of the first phase should also prevent the second phase; and that inhibition of the second phase without inhibition of the first ought to arrest the growth of platelet aggregates. All these possibilities have been demonstrated experimentally.

Platelet aggregation can be inhibited irreversibly or reversibly. *Irreversible inhibition* is produced by exposing platelets to grossly unphysiological conditions or to inhibitors of metabolism; these effects are of little interest. More interesting is the irreversible inhibition produced by acetylsalicylic acid; this will be discussed later.

Reversible inhibition can be achieved by conditions which cause no significant damage to the platelets, shown by normal functions *in vitro* and/or by normal survival *in vivo*. Thus, platelet aggregation is inhibited reversibly by (1) lowering the temperature; (2) lowering the pH by not more than about 1 unit; (3) removing or inactivating the cofactors in plasma; (4) eliminating ADP or the aggregating agents from plasma; (5) antagonizing the effects of ADP or of the other aggregating agents by specific inhibitors; and (6) the inactivation or deficiency of specific receptors on the platelets.

TEMPERATURE

The remarkable dependence of the shape-change on temperature has already been described. The velocity of the first phase of aggregation also diminishes with temperature but not so markedly (Born and Cross 1963a). As for the release reaction, it is difficult to induce at all except at 37°C although it has apparently happened at 25°C (Born and Cross 1963b).

pH

The shape-change is not affected by pH between about 6 and 9 (Born 1970a). Reversible aggregation is fastest at about pH 7.8 and is inhibited below pH 6.3. This inhibition may be caused by increased competition of hydrogen ions for the sites required for calcium ions in aggregation. It is interesting that the low pH diminishes the rate at which platelets *lose* their aggregability; this is the reason why platelets are collected into acid media when they have to be preserved for transfusions (Aster and Jandl 1964).

Plasma cofactor deficiences or inactivation have already been considered (see above).

ELIMINATION OF ADP AND OF OTHER AGGREGATING AGENTS

When enzymes which remove ADP are added to plasma its effects are diminished or abolished; indeed, such an enzyme system was used to demonstrate aggregation by ADP released from platelets by other agents (Haslam 1964). It is of great interest, therefore, that infusion of the combination creatine phosphate with *creatine kinase*, which specifically converts ADP to ATP, into rats or rabbits causes their bleeding times to be increased several fold (Zawilska, Born and Begent 1982). Similar observations have not been made with the other agents but the response of platelets to adrenaline or 5-hydroxytryptamine must depend in part on the rate of their inactivation in the plasma. Aggregation by collagen *in vitro* can be inhibited by denaturing the protein by blocking the ε-amino groups of its lysine residues (Wilner, Nossel and LeRoy 1968) and by a synthetic nonapeptide having an amino acid sequence related to the binding site of collagen for platelets (Legrand *et al.* 1980).

INHIBITORS

The change in shape and first phase of aggregation caused by ADP are inhibited specifically by a number of related nucleotides. These nucleotides include ATP (Born 1962b) and a number of synthetic analogues of AMP and ATP (Cusack and Hourani 1982). Inhibition by other naturally occurring nucleotides is much weaker; whether AMP inhibits at all is still controversial. The kinetics of inhibition by ATP suggests that it competes with ADP for the surface receptor (Macfarlane and Mills 1975). It is reasonable to assume that the mode of action of all inhibitory nucleotides is similar, and that the phosphate group prevents their penetration through the cell membrane.

Particularly interesting is the inhibition by adenosine and by several closely related synthetic nucleosides, particularly 2-chloroadenosine and 5′-N-ethylcarboxamidoadenosine which are up to ten times more potent than adenosine itself (Born 1964, Cusack and Hourani 1981). Inhibition by these substances increases considerably in the first few minutes after their addition to platelet-rich plasma, and the uptake of adenosine by platelets can be almost completely prevented by certain other drugs without diminishing its inhibitory action on aggregation (Born and Mills 1969). Inhibition by adenosine of aggregation induced by ADP has non-competitive kinetics, and is non-specific; adenosine also inhibits aggregation by other agents including adrenaline, 5-hydroxytryptamine and thrombin. A similar inhibition of aggregation by prostaglandin E$_1$ was shown to be mediated by *adenylate cyclase* and is associated with increases in the concentration of cyclic 3′,5′-AMP within the platelets (Haslam and Taylor 1971). Inhibition by adenosine is also associated with increased concentrations of cyclic 3′,5′-AMP and is apparently mediated by an external adenosine receptor. This receptor is coupled to *adenylate cyclase* and is distinct from the ADP receptor that mediates aggregation (Mills and Smith 1971, Haslam and Rosson 1975). Support for this role for cyclic

$3',5'$-AMP comes from the observation that platelet aggregation is inhibited by substances which inhibit *cyclic $3',5'$-AMP phosphodiesterase* (Mills and Smith 1971).

The adenosine analogues that inhibit platelet aggregation produce vasodilation with undesirable hypotension (Born *et al.* 1965). The nucleotide 2-methylthioadenosine $5'$-monophosphate has no significant vasodilator effect (Michal, Maguire and Gough 1969); this reopens the possibility that a compound related to ADP may possess the properties required from an inhibitor for clinical use.

The second phase of agregation and the concomitant release reaction are powerfully inhibited by certain drugs which have no effect on primary aggregation. They are phenothiazine and imipramine derivatives (Mills and Roberts 1967) and non-steroidal anti-inflammatory drugs including phenyl-butazone (Evans *et al.* 1967) and acetylsalicylic acid or aspirin.

Platelets and prostaglandins

That platelets are affected by prostaglandins was first observed about 15 years ago (Kloeze 1967) as inhibitions of aggregation by prostaglandins E_1 and E_2. It was then demonstrated (Smith and Willis 1970, 1971) that thrombin causes human platelets to produce prostaglandins E_2 and F_2 and that aspirin inhibits this biosynthesis. Arachidonic acid, a 20-carbon fatty acid which is the principal component of cellular phospholipids and the precursor of the bisenoic prostaglandins (MacIntyre 1981) also induces platelet aggregation and concomitantly the biosynthesis of prostaglandins E_2 and F_2 (Silver *et al.* 1973). On this evidence for the involvement of prostaglandins in platelet function, subsequent research has concentrated on the role of arachidonic acid and its derivatives in the activation of platelets.

Prostaglandins are not stored in platelets, but synthesized *de novo* following any stimulus which activates phospholipidase A_2 to cleave arachidonic acid from membrane phospholipids. Arachidonic acid is then metabolized by two enzyme systems present in platelet membranes. *Lipoxygenase* saturates double bonds to form several hydroxy or hydroperoxy arachidonic acids (Walker *et al.* 1980) whose biological activity has not been fully elucidated. *Cyclooxygenase* (also known as *prostaglandin synthetase*) converts arachidonic acid to the unstable cyclic endoperoxides prostaglandin G_2 and then to prostaglandin H_2 which is transformed non-enzymatically to prostaglandins E_2, D_2 and $F_{2\alpha}$, as well as a 17-carbon hydroxy-acid and malondialdehyde (Moncada 1982). Platelets contain an enzyme *thromboxane synthetase* which converts prosta-glandin H_2 to thromboxane A_2. Thromboxane A_2 is extremely labile ($T_{\frac{1}{2}} = 30$ s) being rapidly and spontaneously broken down to the stable, inactive thromboxane B_2. Radioimmunoassay of thromboxane B_2 gives an indication of thromboxane A_2 production.

Thromboxane A_2 is a potent vasoconstrictor and one of the most potent naturally occurring aggregators of platelets. The mechanism by which thromboxane A_2 and prostaglandins G_2 and H_2 activate platelets is not fully understood.

The *cyclooxygenase* of platelets catalyses the formation of stable prostaglandins known as D_2, E_2 and $F_{2\alpha}$; they are all vasoactive. Prostaglandin $F_{2\alpha}$ has little effect on platelets; prostaglandin E_2 induces whereas prostaglandin D_2 inhibits platelet aggregation.

Vessel walls contain little or no *thromboxane synthetase* but another enzymic activity which converts cyclic endoperoxides to a labile ($T_{\frac{1}{2}} = 2$–3 min) substance, prostaglandin I_2, now commonly known as prostacyclin (Moncada and Vane 1979). Prostacyclin is the most potent inhibitor of platelet aggregation known so far, and a potent vasodilator. Like adenosine and prostaglandin E_1, prostacyclin acts by stimulating *adenylate cyclase* thereby increasing the concentration of cyclic 3′,5′-adenosine monophosphate (cAMP) in platelets (Moncada 1982). Prostacyclin is rapidly broken down to 6–oxo-prostaglandin $F_{1\alpha}$ which is inactive, stable, and can be quantified by radioimmunoassay.

Sensitive bioassays indicate that the arterial blood of rabbits does not contain sufficient prostacyclin to affect platelet function (Haslam and McClenaghan 1981). Similarly, human blood contains 6-oxo-prostaglandin $F_{1\alpha}$ at such low concentrations as to exclude the possibility of prostacyclin having a physiological function in the circulation (Blair *et al.* 1982). These and other results (Smith *et al.* 1978) would appear to dispose of the claim that prostacyclin is a circulating hormone (Moncada *et al.* 1978). Instead, prostacyclin, like other prostaglandins, appears under pathological conditions when vascular cells are damaged. At concentrations higher than those required to inhibit aggregation (Higgs *et al.* 1978) prostacyclin inhibits the adhesion of platelets to vascular endothelium. This has been put forward as the explanation for the anti-thrombogenic properties of normal blood vessels (e.g. Moncada and Vane 1981). That, however, is unlikely to be correct, for at least two reasons. Firstly, the non-adhesion of platelets to normal endothelium is due mainly to electrostatic repulsion between the excess negative charges which are present on the surfaces of both these and on all other cells; interestingly, the density of these charges on endothelium exceeds that on other cells by one or two orders of magnitude (Görög and Born 1982). Secondly, thrombosis, particularly in coronary or carotid arteries, is initiated by sudden major events affecting the vessel wall (see, for example, Born, Görög and Kratzer 1981), most commonly haemorrhage into an atheromatous lesion (see, for example, Davies and Thomas 1981). The unpredictability of such events is evidence against the dependence of thrombotic platelet aggregation on the presence or absence of endothelial prostacyclin.

The synthesis of prostaglandins in tissues is inhibited by acetylsalicylic acid (aspirin) and similar non-steroidal anti-inflammatory agents. Aspirin acetylates cyclooxygenase and this inhibits the enzyme irreversibly for the lifespan of the platelets. As cyclooxygenase is responsible for forming the endoperoxides which are precursors of thromboxane and prostacyclin, aspirin inhibits the formation of both. The possibility that aspirin might become an effective antithrombotic drug by decreasing the production of thromboxane A_2 by platelets was put in question by the discovery of prostacyclin, the formation of which is also inhibited by aspirin. Inhibition of vascular cyclooxygenase disappears more rapidly than inhibition of platelet cyclooxygenase because vascular cells, unlike platelets, can synthesize new enzyme. Therefore, efforts are still being made to find a dosage schedule for aspirin which would inhibit the production of thromboxane A_2 but not of prostacyclin (Moncada 1982, de Gaetano, Cerletti and Bertele 1982).

If thrombogenecity did depend on opposing effects of endogenous prostaglandin derivatives, it might be expected that specific inhibitors of thromboxane synthetase might be effective anti-thrombotic drugs. Such inhibitors have been synthesized and are being tested in animals and man. Agents such as 13-aza-prostanoic acid (Le Breton *et al.* 1979) which do not inhibit thromboxane synthesis but block thromboxane receptors competitively, represent another possible way of antagonizing the aggregating effect of thromboxane on platelets.

Changes in vessel walls such as occur during atherosclerosis can alter the local prostacyclin production. Production of prostacyclin by vessel walls is decreased in rabbits fed an atherogenic diet (Gryglewski *et al.* 1978) and human atherosclerotic plaques generate very little prostacyclin (Angelo, Myshievlec and de Gaetano 1978). However, the hypothesis that prostacyclin is responsible for the non-thrombogenicity of normal blood vessel walls does not account for important clinical, pathological and experimental facts. Thus, arterial thrombosis does not occur continually on all atherosclerotic lesions. Most thrombi are associated with rupture of an atherosclerotic plaque with haemorrhage and exposure of platelets to constituents of the wall beneath the endothelium (Davies and Thomas 1981). In artificial blood vessels which cannot produce prostacyclin, platelets do not form thrombi except where the blood flow is grossly turbulent. Experimentally, platelets from an aspirin-treated animal remain haemostatically effective in a thrombocytopenic animal with non-aspirin-treated blood vessels (Dejana, Barbieri and de Gaetano 1980). Indeed, it is now known that the haemostatic aggregation of platelets depends less on thromboxane and probably other prostaglandin derivatives than on adenosine 5′-diphosphate (ADP) (Born and Kratzer 1982, Zawilska, Born and Begent 1982).

Recently, interest has grown in the effect of diet on the incidence of vascular diseases prevalent in Western society. Epidemiological studies have shown that Eskimos and the Japanese have a low incidence of ischaemic heart disease, and it has been postulated that this is because these peoples consume more fish than Europeans and North Americans, in whom the incidence is high. The predominant polyunsaturated fatty acid in lipid fractions of blood from Eskimos is eicosapentaenoic acid (20:5, ω3) rather than arachidonic acid (eicosatetranoic acid, 20:4, ω6) which predominates in blood from Danish control subjects (Dyerberg *et al.* 1978). Marine lipids contain a high proportion of eicosapentaenoic acid, whereas animal fats and plant oils contain mainly arachidonic acid and its precursor, linoleic acid (18:2, ω6) (Goodnight *et al.* 1982). Much work is in progress to elucidate the mechanism by which diets rich in the ω3 series of lipids could act protectively against cardiovascular diseases (Dyerberg *et al.* 1978, Thorngren, Shafi and Born 1983).

High concentrations of thrombin or collagen are still able to aggregate platelets that have been treated with agents that remove released ADP and that block the formation of thromboxanes (Kinlough-Rathbone *et al.* 1977). The search for a mediator of this third pathway of aggregation led to the identification of platelet-activating factor (PAF) (Chignard *et al.* 1980), a low molecular weight phospholipid which is also secreted by leucocytes during immunological challenge (Benveniste *et al.* 1979, Demopoulos, Pinckard and Hanahan 1979). Synthetic PAF, viz. 1-o-octadecyl-2-acetyl-*sn*-glyceryl-3-phosphorylcholine, is an extraordinarily potent aggregating agent, for even nanomolar concentrations can induce aggregation of rabbit platelets, although human platelets seem less responsive (Chesney *et al.* 1982). Whether PAF is involved in physiological haemostasis is still uncertain.

Platelets in the coagulation of plasma

The involvement of platelets in physiological coagulation has been established experimentally by removing them from normal plasma and clinically by their deficiency in certain diseases. If blood is collected with great care to avoid surface contact, and platelet-free plasma is prepared by high-speed centrifuging, the clotting time of the plasma after surface contact is much longer than when it contains platelets. Even when only a few platelets are present, as in most cases of thrombocytopenia, the conversion of prothrombin is incomplete (Quick 1947). Clearly the platelets provide something which greatly accelerates the coagulation of plasma.

PLATELET FACTOR 3

The material responsible for this acceleration is called platelet factor 3 and consists of phospholipoprotein. It has not yet been purified sufficiently to establish whether the activity is associated with particular molecular species. The main lipid components are the phosphatides of serine, ethanolamine and inositol, but there are also smaller amounts of the other lipids.

Phospholipoproteins with platelet factor 3 activity are present in all fractions of platelets but most are in the surface membrane and the cytoplasmic organelles. Intact normal platelets accelerate coagulation very much less than platelets that are damaged or in the process of aggregating (Hardisty and Hutton 1966). Aggregation by different agents accelerates the clotting time of plasma by Russell's viper venom in proportion to the velocity and magnitude of the aggregation. Inhibition of aggregation by adenosine causes proportional inhibition of the accelerated clotting. Adenosine inhibits the first phase of aggregation so that this phase changes the platelet surface sufficiently to expose phospholipoprotein with factor 3 activity which is normally masked; indeed, this may happen as early as the initial change in shape.

The second phase of aggregation is associated with the release of platelet factor 3 activity, probably as phospholipoprotein micelles of very small size. Inhibition of the release reaction by phenothiazines halts the increase in the factor 3 activity of platelets but does not reverse it.

The mechanism by which platelet phospholipoproteins accelerate coagulation is discussed in Chapter 4. In the form of micelles they provide optimal conditions for the activation of plasma factors which are bound to the micelles by ionic calcium (Cross 1962). Thus, the micelles accelerate the conversion of prothrombin to thrombin by concentrating the reagents involved in the reaction, viz. prothrombin, activated factor X and factor V (Esnouf and Macfarlane 1968).

OTHER PLATELET FACTORS

At least four other platelet factors can influence plasma coagulation *in vitro* (for review, see Verstraete 1966). Some of these are probably identical with well-defined plasma factors which are known to be absorbable by platelets. Thus, *platelet factor 1* is probably plasma factor V and *platelet factor 5* is probably fibrinogen with which it is antigenically identical. *Platelet factor 4* antagonizes the effect of heparin. The factor is a basic lipoprotein of low molecular weight and is quite distinct from platelet factor 3. During the release phase of platelet aggregation factor 4 activity is released into the plasma. Its functional significance is uncertain but the anticoagulant effectiveness of heparin is increased in patients suffering from thrombocytopenia. Apart from factor 3, the other platelet factors do not seem to be involved in coagulation associated with physiological haemostasis; but they may account, partly or wholly, for the formation of pathological clots in veins, the walls of which appear normal but in which the blood flow has diminished or stopped (Macfarlane *et al.* 1975).

PLATELETS IN CLOT RETRACTION

When plasma clots in the presence of platelets, the coagulum soon begins to shrink until it occupies only one-quarter or less of its original volume; at the same time clear serum is expressed. The mechanism of clot retraction has been much investigated (for review, see Budtz-Olsen 1951). Retraction does not occur in the absence of platelets, and their concentration determines the extent of retraction over a wide range; clearly, therefore, platelets are essential for the process. The platelets must be viable, i.e. metabolically intact; inhibition of their energy metabolism, particularly of glycolysis, prevents clot retraction (Lüscher 1956). The reason is that retraction depends on a reaction between ATP in platelets and their contractile protein thrombasthenin (Bettex-Galland and Lüscher 1961). In human plasma, retraction is associated with the disappearance of about half of the ATP in the platelets and with a corresponding increase of inorganic phosphate in the plasma (Born 1958). Presumably, in analogy with muscular contraction, the ATP is used in reactions which bring about the changes in shape of the platelets on which the mechanics of clot retraction depend. The pseudopodial protrusions become attached to the fibres of fibrin which are pulled together when the pseudopodia subsequently contract. If the work done during clot retraction is, however distantly, associated with the breakdown of ATP there is more than enough for it in the platelets (Born and Esnouf 1961).

The function of clot retraction is uncertain. Like the contraction of a platelet aggregate, the retraction of a clot in a wounded vessel would promote haemostasis if the walls of the vessel were pulled together to narrow the lumen. Retraction of a coagulation thrombus could prevent the complete occlusion of a vessel and promote its reopening to the flow of blood.

REFERENCES

Afors K.-E., Cockburn J.S. & Gross J.F. (1976) Measurement of growth rate of laser-induced intravascular platelet aggregation and the influence of blood flow velocity. *Microvascular Research* 11, 79.

Al-Mondhiry H., Marcus A. & Spaet T.H. (1969) Acetylation of human platelets by aspirin. *Federation Proceedings* 28, 576.

Ardlie N.G., Glew G. & Schwartz C.J. (1966) Influence of catecholamines on nucleotide-induced platelet aggregation. *Nature (London)* **212**, 415.

Angelo V.M., Myshieviec M.B. & de Gaetano G. (1978) Defective fibrinolytic and prostacyclin-like activity in human atheromatous plaques. *Thrombosis and Haemostasis* **39**, 535–6.

Astor R.H. & Jandl J.H. (1964) Platelet sequestration in man. I. Methods. *Journal of Clinical Investigation* **43**, 843.

Bang N.V., Heidenreich R.O. & Trygstad C.W. (1972) Plasma protein requirements for human platelet aggregation. *Annals of the New York Academy of Sciences* **201**, 280.

Bangham A.D. (1964) The adhesiveness of leucocytes with special reference to the zeta potential. *Annals of the New York Academy of Sciences* **116**, 945.

Baumgartner H.R. (1973) The role of blood flow in platelet adhesion, fibrin deposition, and formation of mural thrombi. *Microvascular Research* **5**, 167.

Begent N. & Born G.V.R. (1970) Growth rate *in vivo* of platelet thrombi produced by iontophoresis of adenosine diphosphate as a function of mean blood flow velocity. *Nature (London)* **227**, 926.

Bennett J.S. & Vilaire G. (1979) Exposure of fibrinogen receptors by ADP and epinephrine. *Thrombosis and Haemostasis* **36**, 343–56.

Benveniste J., Tence M., Varenne P., Bidault J., Boullet C. & Polonsky J. (1979) Semi-synthèse et structure proposée du facteur activant les plaquettes (P.A.F.): PAF-acether, un alkyl ether analogue de la lysophosphatidylcholine. *Comptes Rendus de l'Académie des Sciences Series D*, **289**, 1037–40.

Bettex-Galland M. & Lüscher E.F. (1961) Thrombasthenin—a contractile protein from thrombocytes. Extraction from human blood platelets and some of its properties. *Biochimica et Biophysica Acta* **49**, 536.

Blair I.A., Barrow S.E., Waddell K.A., Lewis P.J. & Dollery C.T. (1982) Prostacyclin is not a circulating hormone. *Prostaglandins* **23**, 579–89.

Born G.V.R. (1958) Changes in the distribution of phosphorus in platelet rich plasma during clotting. *Biochemical Journal* **68**, 695.

Born G.V.R. (1962a) Quantitative investigations into the aggregations of blood platelets. *Journal of Physiology* **162**, 67P.

Born G.V.R. (1962b) Aggregation of blood platelets by adenosine diphosphate and its reversal. *Nature (London)* **194**, 927.

Born G.V.R. (1964) Strong inhibition by 2-chloroadenosine of the aggregation of blood platelets by adenosine diphosphate. *Nature (London)* **202**, 95.

Born G.V.R. (1967) Recent research on thrombosis. In *Current Medical Research*, p. 45. HMSO, London.

Born G.V.R. (1970a) The functional physiology of blood platelets. *Symposia of the Zoological Society of London* No. 27, 75.

Born G.V.R. (1970b) Observations on the change in shape of blood platelets brought about by adenosine diphosphate. *Journal of Physiology (London)* **209**, 487.

Born G.V.R. (1972a) Current ideas on the mechanism of platelet aggregation. *Annals of the New York Academy of Sciences* **201**, 4.

Born G.V.R. (1972b) Platelet aggregation and cyclic AMP. In *Effects of Drugs on Cellular Control Mechanisms*. Rabin B.R. & Freedman R.B. (eds)., p. 237. Macmillan, London.

Born G.V.R. (1977) Fluid-mechanical and biochemical interactions in haemostasis. *British Medical Bulletin* **33**, 193–7.

Born G.V.R., Bergquist D. & Arfors K.-E. (1976) Evidence for inhibition of platelet activation in blood by a drug effect on erythrocytes. *Nature* **259**, 233–5.

Born G.V.R. & Cross M.J. (1963a) The aggregation of blood platelets. *Journal of Physiology* **168**, 178.

Born G.V.R. & Cross M.J. (1963b) Effect of adenosine diphosphate on the concentration of platelets in circulating blood. *Nature (London)* **197**, 974.

Born G.V.R. & Cross M.J. (1964) Effects of inorganic ions and of plasma proteins on the aggregation of blood platelets by adenosine diphosphate. *Journal of Physiology* **170**, 397.

Born G.V.R. & Esnouf M.P. (1961) The breakdown of phospholipids and of other phosphorus compounds during coagulation of platelet-rich plasma. In *Blood Platelets*. Johnson S.A., Monto R.W., Rebuck J.W. & Horn R.C. (eds). pp. 365–81. Little, Brown & Co., Boston.

Born G.V.R., Foulks J., Michal F. & Sharp D.E. (1972) Reversal of the rapid morphological reaction of platelets. *Journal of Physiology* **225**, 27.

Born G.V.R., Görög P. & Kratzer M.A.A. (1981) Aggregation of platelets in damaged vessels. *Philosophical Transactions of the Royal Society, Series B* **294**, 241–50.

Born G.V.R., Haslam R.J., Goldman M. & Lowe R.D. (1965) Comparative effectiveness of adenosine analogues as inhibitors of blood platelet aggregation and as vasodilators in man. *Nature (London)* **205**, 678.

Born G.V.R., Honour A.J. & Mitchell J.R.A. (1964) Inhibition by adenosine and by 2-chloroadenosine of the formation and embolization of platelet thrombi. *Nature (London)* **202**, 761.

Born G.V.R., Hornykiewicz O. & Stafford A. (1958) The uptake of adrenaline and nonadrenaline by blood platelets of the pig. *British Journal of Pharmacology and Chemotherapy* **13**, 411.

Born G.V.R. & Hume M. (1967) Effects of the numbers and sizes of platelet aggregates on the optical density of plasma. *Nature (London)* **215**, 1027.

Born G.V.R. & Kratzer M.A.A. (1982) Source of adenine nucleotides responsible for haemostatic platelet aggregation. *Journal of Physiology* **324**, 52P–53P.

Born G.V.R. & Mills D.C.B. (1969) Potentiation of the inhibitory effect of adenosine on platelet aggregation by drugs that prevent its uptake. *Journal of Physiology* **202**, 41P.

Born G.V.R. & Richardson P.D. (1980) Activation time of blood platelets. *Journal of Membrane Biology* **57**, 87–90.

Born G.V.R. & Schraufstätter I. (1982) Influence of external Na and K on platelet aggregability. *Journal of Physiology* **326**, 38P–39P.

Born G.V.R. & Smith J.B. (1970) Uptake, metabolism and release of ^{3}[H]-adrenaline by human platelets. *British Journal of Pharmacology* **39**, 765.

Born G.V.R. & Wehmeier A. (1979) Inhibition of platelet thrombus formation by chlorpromazine acting to diminish haemolysis. *Nature* **282**, 212–13.

Budtz-Olsen O.E. (1951) *Clot Retraction*. Blackwell Scientific Publications, Oxford.

Chesney C.M., Pifer D.D., Byers L.W. & Muirhead E.E. (1982) Effect of platelet-activating factor (PAF) on human platelets. *Blood* **59**, 582–5.

Chignard M., Le Covedic J.P., Vargaftig B.B. & Benveniste J. (1980) Platelet-activating factor (PAF-Acether) secretion from platelets: effect of aggregating agents. *British Journal of Haematology* **46**, 455.

CIBA Foundation Symposium No. 35 on *Biochemistry and Pharmacology of Platelets*. Elliott K.M. & Knight J. (eds). Associated Scientific Publishers, Amsterdam.

Constantine J.W. (1966) Aggregation of guinea-pig platelets by adenosine diphosphate. *Nature (London)* **210**, 162.

Cronberg S. (1970) A mathematical model for optical platelet aggregation test. *Acta Medica Scandinavica* **525**, (Suppl.) 49.

Cross M.J. (1962) The nature of the thromboplastin activity appearing during the clotting of pig's plasma. *Thrombosis et Diathesis Haemorrhagica* **8**, 472.

Cross M.J. (1964) Effect of fibrinogen on the aggregation of platelets by adenosine diphosphate. *Thrombosis et Diathesis Haemorrhagica* **12**, 524.

Curtis A.S.G. (1967) *The Cell Surface: Its Molecular Role in Morphogenesis.* Academic Press, London.

Cusack N.J. & Born G.V.R. (1977) Effects of photolysable 2-azido analogues of adenosine, AMP and ADP on human platelets. *Proceedings of the Royal Society, Series B* **197**, 515–20.

Cusack N.J. & Hourani S.M.O. (1981) 5′-N-Ethylcarboxamidoadenosine: a potent inhibitor of human platelet aggregation. *British Journal of Pharmacology* **72**, 443–7.

Cusack N.J. & Hourani S.M.O. (1982) Adenosine diphosphate antagonists and human platelets: no evidence that aggregation and inhibition of stimulated adenylate cyclase are mediated by different receptors. *British Journal of Pharmacology* **76**, 221–7.

Davies M.J. & Thomas T. (1981) The pathological basis and microanatomy of occlusive thrombus formation in human coronary arteries. *Philosophical Transactions of the Royal Society, Series B* **294**, 225–9.

de Gaetano G., Cerletti C. & Bertele V. (1982) Pharmacology of anti platelet drugs and clinical trials on thrombosis prevention: a difficult link. *Lancet* **II**, 974–7.

Dejana E., Barbieri B. & de Gaetano G. (1980) 'Aspirinated' platelets are haemostatic in thrombocytopenic rats with 'nonaspirinated' vessel walls—evidence from an exchange transfusion model. *Blood* **56**, 959–62.

Demopoulos C.A., Pinckard R.N. & Hanahan D.J. (1979) Platelet-activating factor. Evidence for 1-o-alkyl-2-acetyl-*sn*-glyceryl-3-phosphorylcholine as the active component (a new class of lipid chemical mediators). *The Journal of Biological Chemistry* **19**, 9355–8.

Dyerberg J., Bang H.O., Stoffersen E., Moncada S. & Vane J.R. (1978) Eicosapentaenoic acid and prevention of thrombosis and atherosclerosis? *Lancet* **II**, 117–19.

Esnouf M.P. & Macfarlane R.G. (1968) Enzymology and the blood clotting mechanism. In *Advances in Enzymology.* Nord F.F. (ed). **30**, 255.

Evans G., Packham M.A., Nishizawa E.E. & Mustard J.F. (1967) The effect of platelet-collagen reaction and blood coagulation on haemostasis. *Journal of Clinical Investigation* **46**, 1053.

Feinberg H., Scorer M., LeBreton G.C. & Born G.V.R. (1974) ADP induction of ^{22}Na uptake by platelets. *Circulation* **50**, 1059.

French J.E. (1967) Blood platelets: morphological studies on their properties and life cycle. *British Journal of Haematology* **13**, 595.

Gaarder A., Jonsen J., Laland S., Hellem A. & Owren P.A. (1961) Adenosine diphosphate in red cells as a factor in the adhesiveness of human blood platelets. *Nature (London)* **192**, 531.

Goodnight Jr. S.H., Harris W.S., Conner W.E. & Illingworth D.R. (1982) Polyunsaturated fatty acids, hyperlipidemia and thrombosis. *Arteriosclerosis* **2**, 87–113.

Görög P. & Born G.V.R. (1982) Increased uptake of circulating low-density lipoproteins and fibrinogen by arterial walls after removal of sialic acids from their endothelial surface. *British Journal of Experimental Pathology* **63**, 447–51.

Görög P., Schraufstätter I. & Born G.V.R. (1982) Effect of removing sialic acids from endothelium on the adherence of circulating platelets in arteries *in vivo*. *Proceedings of the Royal Society, Series B* **214**, 471–80.

Gough G., Maguire M.H. & Michal F. (1969) 2-Chloroadenosine 5′-phosphate and 2-chloroadenosine 5′-diphosphate, pharmacologically active nucleotide analogues. *Journal of Medicinal Chemistry* **12**, 494.

Grette K. (1962) Studies on the mechanism of thrombin-catalysed haemostatic reactions in blood platelets. *Acta Physiologica Scandinavica* **56** (Suppl. 195), 5.

Gryglewski R.J., Dembinska-Kiec A., Chylkowski A. & Gryglewska T. (1978) Prostacyclin and thromboxane A_2 biosynthesis capacities of heart, arteries and platelets at various stages of experimental atherosclerosis in rabbits. *Atherosclerosis* **31**, 385–94.

Hardisty R.M. & Hutton R.A. (1966) Platelet aggregation and the availability of platelet factor 3. *British Journal of Haematology* **12**, 764.

Harrison M.J. & Brossmer R. (1976) Inhibition of ADP-induced platelet aggregation by adenosine tetraphosphate. *Thrombosis and Haemostasis* **36**, 388–411.

Haslam R.J. (1964) Role of adenosine diphosphate in the aggregation of human blood-platelets by thrombin and by fatty acids. *Nature (London)* **202**, 765.

Haslam R.J. (1968) Biochemical aspects of platelet function. In *Proceedings of the 12th Congress of the International Society for Haematology*, New York, p. 198.

Haslam R.J. & Cusack N.J. (1981) Blood platelet receptors for ADP and for adenosine. In *Purinergic Receptors: Receptors and Recognition Series B*, Vol. 12. Burnstock G. (ed.) pp. 221–85. Chapman & Hall, London.

Haslam R.J. & McClenagham M.D. (1981) Measurement of circulating prostacyclin. *Nature* **292**, 364–6.

Haslam R.J. & Mills D.C.B. (1967) The adenylate kinase of human plasma, erythrocytes and platelets in relation to the degradation of adenosine diphosphate in plasma. *Biochemical Journal* **103**, 773.

Haslam R.J. & Rosson G.M. (1975) Effects of adenosine cyclic 3′,5′-monophosphate in human blood platelets in relation to adenosine incorporation and platelet aggregation. *Molecular Pharmacology* **11**, 528–44.

Haslam R.J. & Taylor A. (1971) Role of cyclic 3′,5′-adenosine monophosphate in platelet aggregation. In *Platelet Aggregation*. Caen J. (ed.), pp. 85–93. Masson, Paris.

Higgs E.A., Moncada S., Vane J.R., Caen J.P., Michel H. & Tobelem G. (1978) Effect of prostacyclin (PGI_2) on platelet adhesion to rabbit arterial endothelium. *Prostaglandins* **16**, 17–22.

Hugufs J. (1953) Contribution a l'étude des facteurs vasculaires et sanguins dans l'hémostase spontanée. *Archives of International Physiology* **61**, 565.

Inceman S., Caen J. & Bernard J. (1966) Aggregation, adhesion and viscous metamorphosis of platelets in congenital fibrinogen deficiencies. *Journal of Laboratory and Clinical Medicine* **68**, 21.

Kinlough-Rathbone R.L., Packham M.A., Reimers H.J., Cazenave J.P. & Mustard J.F. (1977) Mechanisms of platelet shape change, aggregation and release induced by collagen, thrombin, or A23187. *Journal of Laboratory and Clinical Medicine* **90**, 707–19.

Kloeze J. (1967) Influence of prostaglandins on platelet adhesiveness and platelet aggregation. In *Nobel Symposium 11. Prostaglandins.* Bergstrom S. & Samuelson B. (eds). pp. 24–52. Almquist and Wiksell, Stockholm.

Kloeze J. (1969) Influence of prostaglandins on ADP-induced platelet aggregation. *Acta Physiologica Pharmacologica Neerlandica* **15**, 50.

LeBreton G.C., Venton D.L., Enke S.E. & Halushka P.V. (1979) 13-Azoprostanoic acid: a specific antagonist of the human blood thromboxane/endoperoxide receptor. *Proceedings of the National Academy of Sciences of the USA* **76**, 4097–101.

Legrand Y.L., Karniguian A., Le Francier P., Fauvel F. & Caen J.P. (1980) Evidence that a collagen-derived nonapeptide is a specific inhibitor of platelet-collagen interaction. *Biochemical and Biophysical Research Communications* **96**, 1579–85.

Lüscher E.F. (1956) Glukose als Cofactor-bei der Retraktion des Blutgerinnsels. *Experientia* **12**, 294.

Macfarlane D.E. & Mills D.C.B. (1975) The effect of ATP in platelets: evidence against the central role of released ADP in primary aggregation. *Blood* **46**, 309–20.

Macfarlane D.E., Walsh P.N., Mills D.C.B., Holmsen H. & Day H.J. (1975) The role of thrombin in ADP induced platelet aggregation and release: a critical evaluation. *British Journal of Haematology* **30**, 457.

MacIntyre D.E. (1981) Platelet prostaglandin receptors. In *Platelets in Biology and Pathology-2.* Gordon J.L. (ed.) pp. 211–47. Elsevier-North Holland Publications, Amsterdam.

Macmillan D.C. (1966) Secondary clumping effect in human citrated platelet-rich plasma produced by adenosine diphosphate and adrenaline. *Nature (London)* **211**, 140.

Macmillan D.C. & Oliver M.F. (1965) The initial changes in platelet morphology following the addition of adenosine diphosphate. *Journal of Atherosclerosis Research* **5**, 440.

Maguerie G.A., Plow E.F. & Edgington T.S. (1979) Human platelets possess an inducible and saturable receptor specific for fibrinogen. *The Journal of Biological Chemistry* **254**, 5357–63.

Majno G., Shea S.M. & Leventhal M. (1969) Endothelial contraction induced by histamine-type mediators. *Journal of Cell Biology* **3**, 647.

Markwardt F. (1967) Studies on the release of biogenic amines from blood platelets. In *Biochemistry of Blood Platelets.* Kowalski E. & Niewiarowski S. (eds). p. 105. Academic Press, London & New York.

Michal F., Maguire M.H. & Gough G. (1969) 2-methylthioadenosine-5′-phosphate: a specific inhibitor of platelet aggregation. *Nature (London)* **222**, 1073.

Mills D.C.B. (1966) The breakdown of adenosine diphosphate and of adenosine triphosphate in plasma. *Biochemical Journal* **98**, 32P.

Mills D.C.B. (1969) Platelet aggregation. In *The Biological Basis of Medicine.* Bittar E.E. & Bittar N. (eds). Vol. 3. Academic Press, London.

Mills D.C.B. (1970) Platelet aggregation and platelet nucleotide concentration in different species. *Symposia of the Zoological Society of London.* No. **27**, 75.

Mills D.C.B. (1974) Factors influencing the adenylate cyclase system in human blood platelet. In *Platelets and Thrombosis.* Sherry S. & Scriabine A. (eds). pp. 45–67. University Park Press, Baltimore.

Mills D.C.B., Robb I.A. & Roberts G.C.K. (1968) The release of nucleotides, 5-hydroxytryptamine and enzymes from human blood platelets during aggregation. *Journal of Physiology* **195**, 715.

Mills D.C.B. & Roberts C.G.K. (1967) Membrane active drugs and the aggregation of human blood platelets. *Nature (London)* **214**, 35.

Mills D.C.B. & Smith J.B. (1971) The influence on platelet aggregation of drugs that affect the accumulation of adenosine 3':5'cyclic monophosphate in platelets. *Biochemical Journal* **121**, 185.

Mills D.C.B. & Smith J.B. (1972) The control of platelet responsiveness by agents that influence cyclic AMP metabolism. *Annals of the New York Academy of Sciences* **201**, 391.

Moncada S. (1982) Biological importance of prostacyclin. *British Journal of Pharmacology* **76**, 3–31.

Moncada S., Korbut R., Bunting S. & Vane J.R. (1978) Prostacyclin is a circulating hormone. *Nature* **273**, 767–8.

Moncada S. & Vane J.R. (1979) Pharmacology and endogenous roles of prostaglandin endoperoxides, thromboxane A$_2$ and prostacyclin. *Pharmacological Reviews* **30**, 292–331.

Moncada S. & Vane J.R. (1981) Prostacyclin: biosynthesis, actions and clinical potential. *Philosophical Transactions of the Royal Society, Series B* **294**, 305–29.

Mustard J.F. & Packham M.A. (1970) Factors influencing platelet function: adhesion, release, and aggregation. *Pharmacological Review* **22**, 97.

Mustard J.F., Packham M.A., Kinlough-Rathbone R.L., Perry D.W. & Regoeczi E. (1978) Fibrinogen and ADP-induced platelet aggregation. *Blood* **52**, 453–66.

O'Brien J.R. (1963) An *in vitro* trial of an anti-adhesive drug. *Thrombosis et Diathesis Haemorrhagica* **9**, 120.

Peerschke E.I., Zucker M.B., Grant R.A., Egan J.J. & Johnson M.M. (1980) Correlation between fibrinogen binding to human platelets and platelet aggregability. *Blood* **55**, 841–7.

Poole J.C.F., Sanders A.G. & Florey H.W. (1958) The regeneration of aortic endothelium. *Journal of Pathology and Bacteriology* **75**, 133.

Quick A.J. (1947) Studies on the enigma of the hemostatic dysfunction of hemophilia. *American Journal of Medical Science* **214**, 272.

Rand M. & Reid G. (1951) Source of serotonin in serum. *Nature (London)* **168**, 385.

Richardson P.D. (1973) Effect of blood flow velocity on growth rate of platelet thrombi. *Nature (London)* **245**, 103.

Sharp A.A., Warren B.A., Paxton A.M. & Allington M.J. (1968) Anticoagulant therapy with a purified fraction of Malayan pit viper venom. *Lancet* I, 493.

Shore P.A., Pletscher A., Tomich E.G., Kuntzman R. & Brodie B.B. (1956) Release of blood platelet serotonin by reserpine and lack of effect on bleeding time. *Journal of Pharmacology and Experimental Therapeutics* **117**, 232.

Silver M.J., Smith J.B., Ingerman C. & Kocsis J.J. (1973) Arachidonic acid induced human platelet aggregation and prostaglandin formation. *Prostaglandins* **4**, 863–75.

Smith J.B., Ogletree M.L., Lefer A.M. & Nicolaou K.C. (1978) Antibodies which antagonise the effects of prostacyclin. *Nature* **274**, 64–5.

Smith J.B. & Willis A.L. (1970) Formation and release of prostaglandins in response to thrombin. *British Journal of Pharmacology* **40**, 545P.

Smith J.B. & Willis A.L. (1971) Aspirin selectively inhibits prostaglandin formation in human platelets. *Nature (London)* **231**, 235–7.

Thomas D.P. (1968) The role of platelet catecholamines in the aggregation of platelets by collagen and thrombin. *Experimental Biology and Medicine* 3, 129.

Thorngren M., Shafi S. & Born G.V.R. (1983) Quantification of blood from skin bleeding time determinations: effects of fish diet or acetylsalicyclic acid. *Haemostasis* (in press).

Tranzer J.P. & Baumgartner H.R. (1967) Filling gaps in the vascular endothelium with blood platelets. *Nature (London)* 216, 1126.

Vermylen J., Chamone D.A.F. & Verstraete M. (1979) Stimulation of prostacyclin release from vessel wall by BAYg6575, an antithrombotic compound. *Lancet* I, 518–20.

Verstraete M. (1966) Antithrombin. In *Diffuse Intravascular Clotting.* Transactions of the Conference of the International Committee on Haemostasis and Thrombosis. Brinkhous K.M., Wright I.S., Duckert F., Koller F. & Streuli F. (eds). p. 385. Schattauer, Stuttgart.

Walker I.C., Jones R.L., Kerry P.J. & Wilson N.H. (1980) An epoxy-hydroxy product from arachidonate. *Advances in Prostaglandins and Thromboxane Research* 6, 107–10.

White J.G. (1968) Fine structural alterations induced in platelets by adenosine diphosphate. *Blood* 31, 604.

Wilner G.D., Nossel H.L. & Leroy E.C. (1968) Aggregation of platelets by collagen. *Journal of Clinical Investigation* 47, 2616.

Zawilska K.M., Born G.V.R. & Begent N.A. (1982) Effect of ADP-utilising enzymes on the arterial bleeding time in rats and rabbits. *British Journal of Haematology* 50, 317–25.

Zucker M.B. (1947) Platelet agglutination and vasoconstriction as factors in spontaneous hemostasis in normal thrombocytopoenic, heparinized and hypoprothrombinaemic rabbits. *American Journal of Physiology* 148, 275.

Chapter 14
Disorders of Platelet Function

R. M. HARDISTY

Platelets not only play an essential role in the arrest of haemorrhage after injury, but are also required for maintenance of the integrity of apparently uninjured vessels. Thus platelet defects, whether of number or function, are typically characterized by spontaneous purpuric lesions as well as by a long bleeding time. In thrombocytopenic states without evidence of functional abnormality of the platelets, a fairly close inverse correlation exists between the bleeding time and the platelet count (Harker and Slichter 1972), while in disorders of platelet function the bleeding time is usually disproportionately prolonged. Careful study of such functional disorders has contributed much to our understanding of the physiology of haemostasis, and of the relative clinical importance of the steps leading to the formation of a haemostatic plug. As in the case of the blood coagulation mechanism, it is the genetic disorders which have so far provided the clearest information, since the site of the defect can be more closely defined in them than in most of the acquired disorders, which often involve more than one aspect of platelet function. The latter group, on the other hand, is much more commonly encountered in clinical practice: disturbances of platelet function are seen in a wide range of diseases, and may be caused by many different classes of drugs. Whether abnormally reactive platelets are ever a cause of thrombotic states, and to what extent interference with platelet function can prevent thrombosis, are considered in Chapters 15 and 18. The present chapter is confined to those conditions in which defective platelet function may contribute to a haemorrhagic state.

INHERITED DISORDERS OF PLATELET FUNCTION

A bleeding tendency may result from genetically determined abnormalities affecting any of the steps leading to the formation of a haemostatic plug—adhesion to vascular connective tissues, aggregation, thromboxane synthesis, secretion of the contents of storage organelles, or the contribution of platelets to blood coagulation. While severe defects of adhesion and aggregation tend to cause more serious bleeding symptoms than the other types of abnormality, all are characterized by superficial bruising, a tendency to mucous membrane bleeding and prolonged post-traumatic haemorrhage. The various disorders cannot therefore be distinguished from each other on this basis, and depend for their diagnosis on associated clinical features, hereditary pattern and the results of laboratory tests. Defective platelet function may result not only from primary platelet abnormalities but also from hereditary disorders of the connective tissues with which they normally react (e.g. Ehlers–Danlos and Marfan's syndromes) or of plasma proteins necessary for their interaction, as in von Willebrand's disease and afibrinogenaemia. This chapter, however, is confined to disorders of the platelets themselves.

All the hereditary disorders of platelet function which have yet been well characterized can be classified (Table 30) into three groups: defects of the plasma membrane, of the storage organelles, and of the prostaglandin endoperoxide/thromboxane system. The first group encompasses disorders of adhesion, aggregation and blood coagulation, but the other types of disorder are all chiefly characterized by a failure of the release reaction.

Membrane abnormalities

Bernard–Soulier syndrome

This autosomal recessive disorder, first described by Bernard and Soulier (1948), is characterized by a variable degree of thrombocytopenia with giant

Table 30. Inherited disorders of platelet function.

Defects of the plasma membrane:
   Bernard–Soulier syndrome
   Thrombasthenia
   Membrane procoagulant defect
Deficiency of storage organelles:
   Dense-body deficiency (δ-SPD)
      Hermansky–Pudlak syndrome
      Wiskott–Aldrich syndrome
      Chediak–Higashi syndrome
      Thrombocytopenia with absent radii
      Idiopathic
   α-Granule deficiency (α-SPD)
      Gray platelet syndrome
   Deficiency of dense bodies and α-granules ($\alpha\delta$-SPD)
Defects involving the prostaglandin-endoperoxide pathway:
      Cyclooxygenase deficiency
      Thromboxane synthetase deficiency
      Failure to respond to thromboxane
Miscellaneous

---

platelets, which often show a wide variation in size and appearance on a stained film. The bleeding time is disproportionately prolonged relative to the platelet count, and the severity of the bleeding symptoms is likewise greater than might be expected from the degree of thrombocytopenia. Superficial bruises and ecchymoses, often without obvious cause, are usually first seen during infancy or early childhood, and mucosal bleeding is common. The clinical severity varies between one patient and another, and cannot be closely correlated with the results of laboratory investigations.

LABORATORY FINDINGS AND PATHOGENESIS

Besides the features mentioned above, Bernard and Soulier (1948) drew attention to the normal clot retraction and defective prothrombin consumption. More recently, Bernard–Soulier platelets have been shown to be defective in their ability to agglutinate in response to bovine factor VIII (Bithell, Parekh and Strong 1972, Caen *et al.* 1976) or to human factor VIII–von Willebrand factor (VIII–VWF) and ristocetin (Caen and Levy-Toledano 1973, Howard, Hutton and Hardisty 1973). They aggregate and secrete normally, on the other hand, in response to ADP, adrenaline and collagen, and appear to adhere normally to particulate collagen *in vitro*.

The reaction of platelets with ristocetin and factor VIII–VWF appears to be an *in vitro* analogue of their adhesion to subendothelium in the presence of VIII–VWF: Weiss *et al.* (1974a) showed that Bernard–Soulier platelets were defective in their ability to adhere to the subendothelium of rabbit aorta, but not in their capacity for aggregation at sites where they did adhere. They suggested that this might be due to the lack of a membrane receptor for VIII–VWF. Meanwhile, the observation of Gröttum and Solum (1969) that Bernard–Soulier platelets had a low sialic acid content and a reduced mobility provided independent evidence in favour of a membrane abnormality, and this was confirmed by Nurden and Caen (1975), who demonstrated a specific deficiency of the sialic acid-rich glycoprotein (GP) I complex in the membrane. This abnormality has since been shown to involve both glycocalicin (GP Is), a readily proteolysed component of the GP I complex, which is undetectable in Bernard–Soulier platelets, and GP Ib (Solum, Hagen and Sletbakk 1980), a more stable component from which glycocalicin is probably derived, which is either reduced in amount or absent (Jamieson *et al.* 1979, Hagen *et al.* 1980). The GP I complex is evidently essential for the reaction of platelets with VIII–VWF, and thus for both adhesion to subendothelium and agglutination by ristocetin; it is probably the site of a factor VIII receptor.

Nachman, Jaffe and Weksler (1977) raised an antibody in rabbits which reacted with a platelet membrane protein of similar molecular weight to GP I, and showed that it inhibited the agglutination of normal platelets by ristocetin, and an antibody developing in a patient with the Bernard–Soulier syndrome after multiple platelet transfusions (Degos *et al.* 1977) had the same effect. This latter antibody, which was evidently directed against components of the GP I complex (Tobelem *et al.* 1979), also inhibited the adhesion of normal platelets to subendothelium, but not their aggregation by ADP or thrombin. Bernard–Soulier platelets themselves, on the other hand, have been found to have a partial defect of thrombin-induced aggregation and a reduced number of thrombin binding sites (Ganguly 1977, Jamieson and Okumura 1978). Since there is evidence that the missing binding sites are located on the glycocalicin (Okumura, Hasitz and Jamieson 1978), it seems likely that the site recognized by the antibody is on the more stable (GP Ib) part of the complex. The receptor for quinine- and quinidine-dependent antibodies, which is not expressed on Bernard–Soulier platelets (Kunicki, Johnson and Aster 1978), is evidently also located on GP Ib of normal platelets (Kunicki *et al.* 1981c).

The thrombocytopenia of the Bernard–Soulier syndrome is at least partly due to a shortened platelet survival. This seems likely to be another result of the membrane glycoprotein abnormality, as perhaps is also the impaired coagulant activity of the platelets, first described in terms of defective prothrombin consumption, and subsequently shown to be associated with a failure to bind and activate plasma factor XI (Walsh *et al.* 1975).

The chief laboratory findings in the Bernard–Soulier syndrome are contrasted with those in thrombasthenia (see below) in Table 31.

Table 31. Laboratory findings in the Bernard–Soulier syndrome and thrombasthenia.

	BSS	Thrombasthenia
Platelet count	↓	N
Adhesion to subendothelium	↓	N
ADP:		
Shape change	↓	N
Release	N	Nil
Aggregation	N	Nil
Thrombin:		
Release	N	N
Aggregation	↓	Nil
Ristocetin agglutination	↓↓	N
Platelet fibrinogen	↑	↓
Platelet VIIIR:Ag	↑	↓
Membrane glycoprotein deficiency	I	IIb/IIIa

N = Normal.

DIAGNOSIS

The haemorrhagic features of the Bernard–Soulier syndrome are no different from those of thrombasthenia or other inherited platelet disorders, and the diagnosis rests on the results of laboratory tests. The combination of a long bleeding time and giant platelets suggests the diagnosis, which may be strengthened by evidence of autosomal recessive inheritance. Confirmation depends on the demonstration of defective ristocetin agglutination of the patient's platelets, not corrected by normal plasma (Fig. 48). Other diagnostic features are shown in Table 32. It should be remembered that giant platelets may be seen in other thrombocytopenic states, particularly when megakaryo-

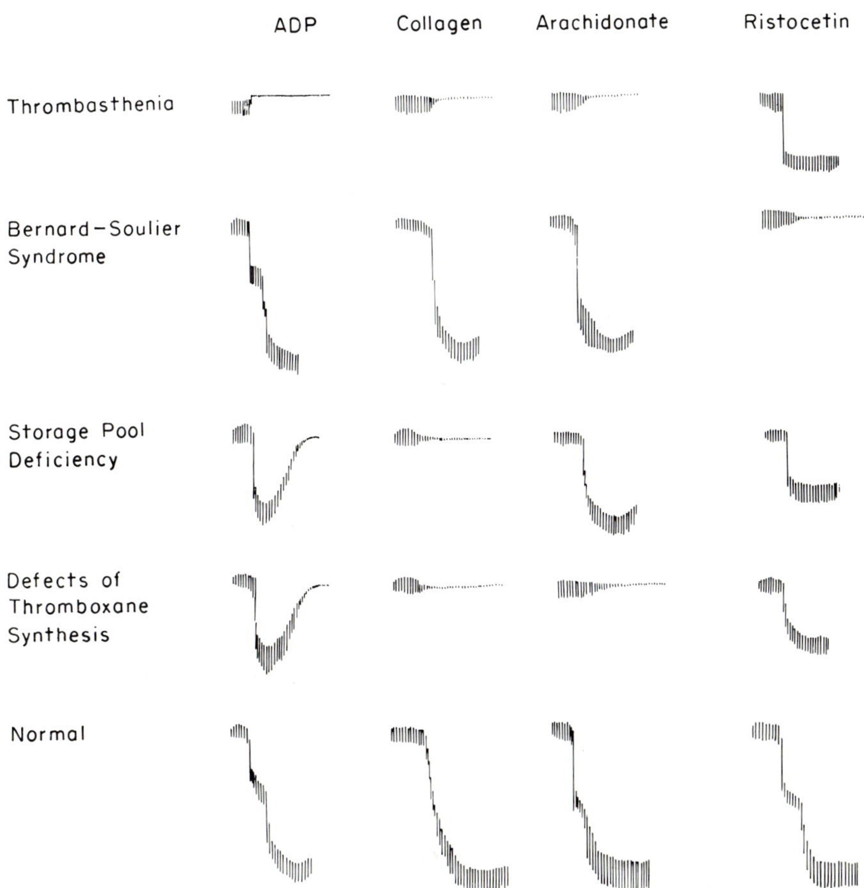

Fig. 48. Aggregation patterns in platelet disorders, in response to ADP, collagen, arachidonate and ristocetin.

Table 32. Hereditary disorders of platelet function: diagnosis.

	Platelet count	Platelet size	Platelet aggregation				Release of 5HT/ADP by thrombin	Heredity	Associated abnormalities
			ADP	Collagen	Arachidonic acid	Ristocetin			
Thrombasthenia	N	N	O	O	O	(1)	N	Autosomal recessive	
Bernard–Soulier syndrome	↓ (or N)	↑	N	N	N	O	N or ↓	Autosomal recessive	
Hermansky–Pudlak syndrome	N	N	(1)	↓	N	(1)	↓	Autosomal recessive	Albinism. Pigmented macrophages in bone marrow
Storage-pool disease	N	N or ↓	(1)	↓	N (or ↓)	(1)	↓	Autosomal dominant	
Wiskott–Aldrich syndrome	↓	↓	↓	↓			↓	X-borne recessive	Eczema. Recurrent infections
Chediak–Higashi syndrome	N or ↓	N	(1)	↓			↓	Autosomal recessive	Partial albinism. Recurrent infections. Lysosomal abnormality of granulocytes
Gray platelet syndrome	↓	↑	↓	↓	N	N	↓	Autosomal dominant	
Defects of thromboxane synthesis and response	N	N	(1)	↓	↓		↓	?	

(1) First phase aggregation only.   N = Normal.

cytopoiesis is greatly increased, but this is not associated with defective ristocetin agglutination.

DETECTION OF HETEROZYGOTES

Heterozygotes are clinically unaffected and have no detectable abnormality of platelet function, but may possibly have reduced amounts of the GP I complex in their platelet membranes. Tobelem *et al.* (1976) obtained results on presumed heterozygotes intermediate between those given by normal and Bernard–Soulier platelets in agglutination tests with their naturally occurring antibody (see above), and similar immunological or other methods of measuring GP I may provide a means of carrier detection.

MANAGEMENT

Superficial bleeding can usually be adequately controlled by local measures, but platelet transfusions are necessary for the control of major bleeds and the prevention of serious surgical haemorrhage. Corticosteroids have no place in treatment, but splenectomy, though a hazardous undertaking, has sometimes resulted in partial amelioration of symptoms through a reduction in the degree of thrombocytopenia. It cannot be expected to be of more than limited benefit, however, and should not be undertaken lightly. Serious menorrhagia may require the suppression of menstruation.

Thrombasthenia (Glanzmann's disease)

Glanzmann (1918) was the first to describe a hereditary bleeding disorder due to an abnormality of platelet function: his criteria were defective clot retraction and abnormal light microscopy, and he named the condition 'hereditary haemorrhagic thrombasthenia'. The term thrombasthenia, or Glanzmann's disease, is now applied to an autosomal recessive trait resulting in a moderately severe bleeding tendency, and characterized by a greatly prolonged bleeding time, normal platelet count and morphology, and defective clot retraction. Besides these, the essential diagnostic feature is a complete failure of the platelets to aggregate in response to any concentration of ADP, adrenaline, 5-hydroxytryptamine, collagen or thrombin (Hardisty, Dormandy and Hutton 1964, Caen *et al.* 1966, Zucker, Pert and Hilgartner 1966). The clinical features are indistinguishable from those of the Bernard–Soulier syndrome (see p. 351), and vary somewhat in severity between one patient and another, although the defect of aggregation is always absolute. Caen (1972) divided his patients into two groups on the basis of platelet fibrinogen and clot retraction: type I, in which the defect of each of these was profound, was clinically more severe than the relatively rarer type II, in which they were only moderately reduced.

LABORATORY FINDINGS AND PATHOGENESIS (Table 31)

In contrast to the absolute defect of aggregation referred to above, thrombasthenic platelets agglutinate normally in response to bovine factor VIII (Caen *et al.* 1966) or ristocetin (Howard and Firkin 1971). This pattern of *in vitro* responses is thus in direct contrast to that of Bernard–Soulier platelets, and correlates with the observation that thrombasthenic platelets adhere normally to subendothelium (Tschopp, Weiss and Baumgartner 1975) and to collagen fibres *in vitro* (Zucker, Pert and Hilgartner 1966), but do not aggregate in response to these stimuli. Unlike adhesion to connective tissue, adhesion to glass, or retention in a glass-bead column, being largely dependent on an intact aggregation mechanism, is severely defective in thrombasthenia. Although thrombasthenic platelets fail to aggregate or to alter their electrophoretic mobility (Hampton and Hardisty 1967) in response to ADP and other agonists, they evidently do not lack membrane receptors for them. Thus they bind ADP normally (Legrand and Caen 1976, 1978), undergo a normal shape change on exposure to ADP (Zucker, Pert and Hilgartner 1966), and not only bind thrombin normally but secrete 5HT normally in response to it (White, Workman and Lundblad 1978). Malmsten *et al.* (1977) have also shown that thromboxane synthesis occurs normally in response to thrombin or arachidonic acid, though not in response to ADP or collagen, which evidently only mediate this process as a secondary effect of aggregation (Charo, Feinman and Detwiler 1977).

Following the original observation of Nurden and Caen (1974), it is now well established (Phillips and Agin 1977, Hagen and Solum 1979, Jamieson *et al.* 1979) that the platelets of thrombasthenic patients are deficient in two closely associated membrane glycoproteins, designated GP IIb and IIIa. The exact relationship between these two glycoproteins remains to be resolved: they form a single precipitin line with both xenogeneic and allogeneic antibodies, from which the two separate components can be resolved by SDS-polyacrylamide gel electrophoresis (Hagen *et al.* 1980). The glycoprotein deficiency has been found to be complete in type I, but only partial (about 15 per cent of normal) in type II thrombasthenia, although the failure of aggregation is absolute in each case (Hagen *et al.* 1980).

Meanwhile, thrombasthenic platelets have been shown to have a defect of exposure of fibrinogen receptors in response to ADP and other aggregating agents (Bennett and Vilaire 1979, Mustard *et al.* 1979, Peerschke, Grant and Zucker 1979), and to fail to bind fibronectin in response to thrombin (Ginsberg *et al.* 1981). Like the glycoprotein deficiency, the failure of fibrinogen binding is only partial in type II thrombasthenia (Lee *et al.* 1981), suggesting that the receptor is located on the GP IIb/IIIa complex, but that the aggregation defect is not entirely attributable to the failure of fibrinogen binding (though the defect of clot retraction may be). The observation of Kunicki *et al.* (1981b) that the association of the two glycoproteins is reversible and calcium-dependent suggests a possible mechanism for the role of calcium ions in platelet aggregation. Although the proposal of Gerrard *et al.* (1979) that GP IIIa was identical with α-actinin has not withstood critical re-examination, there is evidence that actin becomes associated with the GP IIb and IIIa of normal platelets following thrombin-induced aggregation (Phillips, Jennings and Williams 1980), and that this reaction is defective in thrombasthenic platelets (George and Morgan 1981). This failure of association of actin with the membrane may underline the defect of clot retraction. Glycoprotein IIIa has been shown to be the site of the Pl[A1] (Zw[a]) platelet-specific alloantigens, which are partially or wholly deleted in thrombasthenia (Kunicki and Aster 1978, 1979, Van Leeuwen *et al.* 1979).

Other abnormalities of thrombasthenic platelets include low levels of factor VIII-related antigen (Howard, Montgomery and Hardisty 1974), severe impairment of platelet factor-3 availability (Hardisty, Dormandy and Hutton 1964) resulting from the aggregation defect (Hardisty and Hutton 1966), and a defect of activation of factors XII and XI (Walsh 1972). The last of these was found to be more closely correlated with clinical severity than the aggregation defect.

As in the case of the Bernard–Soulier syndrome, an antibody developing in response to multiple transfusions in a thrombasthenic patient has proved a useful means of studying interrelationships between the various platelet abnormalities. It appears to be directed against the GP IIb/IIIa complex (Hagen *et al.* 1980), and has been found to inhibit aggregation and clot retraction, but not adhesion to subendothelium, ristocetin-induced agglutination, ADP binding or shape change of normal platelets (Caen *et al.* 1977, Levy-Toledano *et al.* 1978).

DIAGNOSIS

Diagnosis depends on demonstration of the characteristic defect of aggregation (Table 32, Fig. 48). Complete failure of aggregation in response to any concentration of ADP is virtually pathognomonic of thrombasthenia.

DETECTION OF HETEROZYGOTES

Heterozygotes are symptomless and have no demonstrable abnormality of platelet function, but their platelets have reduced amounts of the GP IIb/IIIa

complex, detectable either biochemically (Kunicki *et al.* 1981a) or immunologically (Degos *et al.* 1975, McEver, Baenziger and Majerus 1980).

MANAGEMENT

Platelet transfusions provide the only logical approach to the management of
major bleeding episodes. Local haemostatic measures will usually suffice to
control minor superficial bleeds. Severe menorrhagia may call for the use of
anovulatory drugs.

Isolated platelet procoagulant defect

Platelet factor-3 availability, in response to stimulation of the platelets by
kaolin or ADP, is profoundly reduced in thrombasthenia and often somewhat
diminished in defects of the release reaction (Hardisty and Hutton 1967, Weiss
1967a), presumably as a result of the defective aggregation (Hardisty and
Hutton 1966), but until recently no primary defect of procoagulant activity of
the platelets had been convincingly described. Weiss *et al.* (1979a) studied a
patient who had suffered from a moderately severe bleeding disorder since
her teens, whose only demonstrable abnormality was a defect of platelet
procoagulant activity, in the presence of normal aggregation and secretion
and a consistently normal bleeding time. Prothrombin consumption was
reduced and platelet factor-3 availability, which was consistently below
normal, was not restored to normal by lysing the platelets, as occurs in
aggregation defects. These abnormalities were probably due to a diminished
number of factor-V binding sites on the platelet membrane, leading to impaired
binding of factor Xa (Miletich *et al.* 1979). A defect of activation of the contact
system by platelet-rich plasma was also observed, but no abnormality of
membrane phospholipids or proteins could be demonstrated. Surgical haemostasis was effectively achieved by means of platelet transfusion. There was no
family history and no detectable abnormality of the patient's parents' platelets,
so that the genetic basis of the disorder remains in doubt.

Deficiency of storage organelles

Since the original observations of Hardisty and Hutton (1967) and Weiss
(1967a), it has been widely recognized that certain bleeding disorders are due
to defects, whether hereditary or acquired, of secretion of the contents of
platelet granules. These may be divided into deficiencies of the granules
themselves, and defects affecting the intracellular mechanisms, including the
prostaglandin endoperoxide–thromboxane pathway, which are necessary for
the secretory process. Both types of abnormality give rise to mild bleeding

disorders, less severe than the disorders of membrane function discussed above. They seldom require any special therapeutic measures except in the case of surgery or serious accidental injury, when platelet transfusions may be indicated. Somewhat surprisingly, however, Gerritsen, Akkerman and Sixma (1978) claimed that the bleeding time of patients with storage pool deficiency (see below) could be shortened, and surgical bleeding controlled, by cryoprecipitate, though the platelet abnormalities remained unaffected. Mielke, Levine and Zucker (1981) obtained similar results with a short course of prednisone to cover surgery in a miscellaneous group of patients with defective platelet aggregation, some of whom probably had storage pool deficiency.

Deficiencies of platelet storage organelles may be divided into those affecting only the dense bodies, those in which both these types of organelle are deficient and the very rare isolated deficiency of α-granules. Weiss *et al.* (1979b) have suggested that these should be described, under the general name of storage pool deficiency (SPD), as δ-SPD, $\alpha\delta$-SPD and α-SPD respectively. They are described separately below.

Dense-body deficiency (δ-SPD)

LABORATORY FINDINGS

The bleeding time is often moderately prolonged, and routine tests of platelet aggregation reveal the characteristic pattern of results shown in Fig. 48 and Table 32: an absent or greatly reduced response to collagen and rapid reversal after initial normal aggregation with ADP, but a relatively normal response to arachidonate, which serves to distinguish the condition from disorders of thromboxane synthesis. Uptake of serotonin (5HT) commences rapidly but soon reaches saturation at a low level, and secretion of 5HT and adenine nucleotides from the platelets in response to thrombin or collagen is severely impaired. The distribution of adenine nucleotides within the platelet is equivalent to that of the metabolic pool alone of normal platelets, with a proportionately greater reduction of ADP than ATP and a high ATP:ADP ratio (Hardisty, Mills and Ketsa-Ard 1972, Pareti, Day and Mills 1974, Weiss *et al.* 1974b). The deficiency of dense bodies can be demonstrated by means of electron microscopy (White *et al.* 1971, Weiss and Ames 1973) or by fluorescence microscopy of mepacrine-treated platelets (Rendu *et al.* 1978, 1979b). Lorez *et al.* (1979), using both these methods, demonstrated the presence of atypical dense bodies as well as a reduction in their total number. The releasable pool of platelet calcium, which is also situated in the dense bodies, is correspondingly deficient (Lages *et al.* 1975). Although the conversion of arachidonic acid to endoperoxides and thromboxane A_2 is normal, at least some patients with SPD have a defect of activation of phospholipase A_2, leading to diminished liberation of arachidonic acid by ADP, collagen and adrenaline in addition to the dense-body deficiency (Rendu *et al.* 1978, Minkes, Joist and Needleman 1979, Weiss and Lages 1981).

CLINICAL ASSOCIATIONS

δ-SPD occurs in a variety of hereditary bleeding disorders with associated clinical features, and may also be inherited as a separate entity, in which only the platelets are involved. The latter condition has been termed *storage pool disease*: autosomal dominant inheritance has been demonstrated in several of the families involved. Amongst the other syndromes of which δ-SPD forms a part, the *Hermansky–Pudlak syndrome* is the best studied with regard to the platelet defect. This is an autosomal recessive trait comprising oculocutaneous albinism of the tyrosinase-positive variety, the platelet disorder and the presence of pigmented macrophages in the bone marrow and throughout the reticulo-endothelial system. Pulmonary fibrosis and inflammatory bowel disease may result from involvement of macrophages in the lung and intestine (Davies and Tuddenham 1976, Garay *et al.* 1979). The platelet disorder has been well characterized by White *et al.* (1971), Hardisty, Mills and Ketsa-Ard (1972) and others. Heterozygotes are clinically unaffected, but in a large Dutch family they were found to have low platelet 5HT levels (Gerritsen *et al.* 1977).

Deficiency of platelet dense bodies has also been observed in the Wiskott–Aldrich syndrome (Gröttum *et al.* 1969), the syndrome of thrombocytopenia with absent radii (Day and Holmsen 1972) and the Chediak-Higashi syndrome (Buchanan and Handin 1976, Boxer *et al.* 1977). In all of these, however, the bleeding tendency is chiefly attributable to the thrombocytopenia.

Alpha-δ-SPD

Weiss *et al.* (1979b) studied 18 patients with SPD—seven with the Hermansky–Pudlak syndrome and 11 with platelet defects only. Amongst the latter group they found four with δ-SPD, and seven (from three families) with both ultrastructural and biochemical evidence of some degree of deficiency of α-granules as well as of dense bodies. These patients' platelets were deficient in platelet factor 4, β-thromboglobulin, fibrinogen and platelet-derived growth factor, all of which are stored in the α-granules, as well as in ADP and 5HT. There were no obvious clinical differences between the two groups. Weiss and Lages (1981) found that patients with $\alpha\delta$-SPD, in contrast to those with δ-SPD, had a defect of both aggregation and malonyldialdehyde production in response to arachidonic acid, perhaps suggesting that one or more α-granule constituents play a part in the conversion of arachidonic acid to its active metabolites.

Gray platelet syndrome (α-SPD)

This is a very rare autosomal dominant trait, described in Swiss and Dutch families (Hemmeler 1958, Kurstjens *et al.* 1968, Libanska *et al.* 1975) under the name of 'hereditary hypogranular thrombocytopenia' and subsequently in an American boy by Raccuglia (1971), who called it the 'gray platelet syndrome' from the appearance of platelets on electron microscopy. The platelets are moderately reduced in number, large, vacuolated and with greatly reduced cytoplasmic granulation. The defect has been shown on both ultrastructural and biochemical grounds to be confined to the α-granules; mitochondria, dense bodies, peroxisomes and lysosomes are present in normal numbers (White 1979, Gerrard *et al.* 1980). A partial defect of aggregation and release has been observed in response to collagen, thrombin and ADP, suggesting a role—at present unexplained—for α-granule constituents in these reactions. Despite the thrombocytopenia and the functional abnormality of the platelets, the reported cases have been clinically only mildly affected.

Defects of thromboxane synthesis and response

The commonest cause of failure of platelet secretion in clinical practice is the ingestion of aspirin or other drugs which inhibit the synthesis of prostaglandin endoperoxides and thromboxane A_2 from arachidonic acid (see p. 368). A number of patients have been studied in whom a similar type of abnormality appears to have resulted from a constitutional defect, unrelated to drug ingestion, and this condition has therefore been described as 'aspirin-like defect' (Weiss and Rogers 1972, Pareti, Day and Mills 1974). In most of the cases originally so described, the actual mechanism of the defect was not accurately defined, but more recently the platelets of some such patients have been shown to have defects either of the enzymes involved in the endo-peroxide–thromboxane synthetic pathway, or of response to preformed thromboxane A_2. Thus naturally occurring deficiencies of cyclooxygenase (Malmsten *et al.* 1975, Lagarde *et al.* 1978) and thromboxane synthetase (Defreyn *et al.* 1981) have been described, and in a number of patients a similar pattern of subnormal aggregation and secretion has been shown to be due to a defective response to thromboxane A_2 in the presence of normal thromboxane synthesis (Lages *et al.* 1981, Samama *et al.* 1981, Wu *et al.* 1981). All these defects result in an impairment of aggregation and secretion in response to collagen and arachidonate, and of the second phase of aggregation induced by ADP or adrenaline. The distinction between them depends on detailed examination of the synthesis of prostaglandin endoperoxides and their derivatives by the platelets, and of their response to preformed endoperoxides and thromboxane A_2. They can all be distinguished from δ-SPD by their normal platelet nucleotide content and 5HT uptake. The chief difficulty in diagnosis is to exclude aspirin ingestion as the cause of the platelet abnormality.

Although most patients described with these disorders have had a mild bleeding tendency first noticed in early childhood, few family studies have been performed and, except for the case of Defreyn *et al.* (1981) there is little direct evidence that the conditions are genetically determined.

Miscellaneous hereditary disorders

Epstein's syndrome is an autosomal dominant trait in which mild thrombocytopenia with giant platelets is associated with Alport's syndrome of hereditary nephritis and nerve deafness. Epstein *et al.* (1972) reported defects of platelet aggregation and secretion in response to ADP and collagen, and this was confirmed by Bernheim *et al.* (1976) but disputed by Eckstein, Filip and Watts (1975). The bleeding tendency is presumably chiefly attributable to the thrombocytopenia.

Defective 5HT uptake by the platelets has been described in Down's syndrome (Boullin and O'Brien 1971) but these children do not suffer from a bleeding disorder. Although defects of platelet function have been reported in various hereditary connective tissue disorders (e.g. Ehlers–Danlos and Marfan's syndromes, osteogenesis imperfecta), the bleeding tendency in these conditions is more likely to be due to the abnormality of the connective tissue itself.

Diagnosis of hereditary disorders

The diagnosis of a hereditary disorder of platelet function is suggested by a life-long history of multiple superficial bruises, prolonged bleeding after superficial injuries, and perhaps apparently spontaneous haemorrhage into the skin or from mucous membranes. The nature of the haemorrhagic lesions themselves does not distinguish one platelet disorder from another or any of them from von Willebrand's disease, for example, but clues to a more specific diagnosis may come from the genetic pattern or from associated clinical features characteristic of particular syndromes (Table 32). The characteristic laboratory pointers to a defect of platelet function are a long bleeding time and a normal (or possibly moderately reduced) platelet count: this combination indicates the need for platelet function tests, as may a strongly suggestive clinical history even in the absence of a prolonged bleeding time. von Willebrand's disease can be excluded by appropriate investigations of the factor VIII complex, and tests of aggregation by ADP, collagen, arachidonic acid and ristocetin will serve to identify most of the recognized types of platelet abnormalities: typical aggregation patterns are shown in Fig. 48. Other confirmatory investigations in particular circumstances may include measurement of platelet size by means of an electronic particle sizer (see Table 32), electron microscopy, content and secretion of dense-body and α-granule constituents, platelet coagulant activities, clot retraction, endoperoxide and thromboxane synthesis and surface membrane glycoproteins. In practice, these special investigations are seldom necessary for routine diagnostic purposes, though they may help to identify and explain new and unusual disorders.

ACQUIRED DISORDERS OF PLATELET FUNCTION

Platelet function may be disturbed in a wide range of diseases, and by the action of several different classes of drugs. The platelet abnormalities in many of the conditions listed in Table 33 are less well defined than in the hereditary platelet disorders, and even the degree to which they contribute to the bleeding tendency may be in doubt, since other defects of the haemostatic mechanism not infrequently coexist.

Table 33. Causes of acquired platelet dysfunction.

Uraemia
Bartter's syndrome
Myeloproliferative disorders
Acute leukaemias, preleukaemic states
Dysproteinaemias
Chronic hypoglycaemia
Liver disease
Immune or mechanical damage to platelets from:
    Autoimmune disorders
    Disseminated intravascular coagulation
    Heart disease
    Cardiopulmonary bypass
    Burns
Scurvy
Drugs (see Table 34)

Uraemia

Although defects of coagulation and thrombocytopenia may contribute to the bleeding tendency in some cases, defective platelet function is evidently the chief cause of haemostatic failure in uraemia. The bleeding time is often prolonged even in the presence of a relatively normal platelet count, and other reported evidence of platelet dysfunction includes defects of platelet retention in glass-bead columns, platelet factor-3 availability and clot retraction (Castaldi, Rozenburg and Stewart 1966, Salzman and Neri 1966, Horowitz *et al.* 1967, Rabiner and Hrodek 1968). Many different patterns of platelet aggregation have been reported in such patients, ranging from complete normality to severe defects of either the first or second phase of ADP-induced aggregation. Ballard and Marcus (1972) suggested that these inconsistencies might be partly attributable to lack of standardization of calcium concentrations in the platelet-rich plasma samples studied. There is general agreement, however, that the platelet abnormalities, whatever their cause—and indeed the long bleeding time and the bleeding tendency itself—can be corrected by haemodialysis or peritoneal dialysis (Stewart and Castaldi 1967), suggesting that they are due to inhibitory plasma components. Early candidates for this role included urea (Eknoyan *et al.* 1969, Davies *et al.* 1972), guanidinosuccinic acid (Horowitz *et al.* 1970) and phenolic acids (Rabiner and Molinas 1970); more recently, Remuzzi *et al.* (1977, 1978) have presented evidence that the inhibitory substance may be prostacyclin (PGI_2), produced in excess by vessel walls of patients in renal failure. Matthias and Palinski (1977) and Remuzzi *et al.* (1978) have also observed a reduced rate of synthesis of prostaglandin endoperoxides in the platelets of uraemic patients, suggesting that their aggregation defect may be due to an imbalance between PGI_2 and thromboxane synthesis.

Apart from these effects of chronic renal failure on the platelets, many renal diseases are associated with abnormalities of platelet function related to their underlying pathogenic mechanisms. The complex roles of platelets and vascular tissues in the pathogenesis of renal disease have formed the subject of a recent symposium (Remuzzi, Mecca and de Gaetano 1980).

Bartter's syndrome

This is a rare metabolic disorder associated with hyperplasia of the renal juxtaglomerular apparatus and characterized by hypokalaemic alkalosis, hyper-reninaemia, aldosteronism, increased excretion of urinary prostaglandins and normal blood pressure (Bartter *et al.* 1976). The defective platelet aggregation which has been observed (Stoff *et al.* 1978) seems likely to be due to over-production of prostacyclin (Gullner *et al.* 1979) or a more stable related substance (Stoff *et al.* 1979); it is improved by indomethacin.

Myeloproliferative disorders

Both haemorrhagic symptoms and arterial thromboses are frequent complications of this group of disorders, and both may occur in the same patient—usually, but not exclusively, in association with a raised platelet count. Typical symptoms of the bleeding disorder are large superficial ecchymoses, epistaxis and gastrointestinal haemorrhage; thrombosis most commonly occurs in peripheral arteries of the limbs or in cerebral arteries.

Many different abnormalities of platelet function have been described in these patients, and none of them can be regarded as especially characteristic of any one of the myeloproliferative disorders: similar defects have been observed in patients with essential thrombocythaemia, polycythaemia vera, chronic granulocytic leukaemia and myelofibrosis. Secondary thrombocytosis, in contrast to essential thrombocythaemia, seldom results in either a bleeding tendency or a demonstrable defect of platelet function (McClure *et al.* 1966, Ginsburg 1975).

Amongst the platelet abnormalities which have been described, the commonest is a failure of aggregation in response to adrenaline or noradrenaline (Spaet *et al.* 1969, Cardamone *et al.* 1972, Neemeh *et al.* 1972, Adams, Schultz and Goldberg 1974), which has been shown to be due to a deficiency of α-adrenergic receptors on the platelet membrane (Kaywin *et al.* 1978). Defects of secretion in response to other inducing agents are also frequently seen, however, and may have a multiple pathogenesis: storage pool deficiency has been described in many such patients (Gerrard *et al.* 1978, Rendu *et al.* 1979a, Russell *et al.* 1981), and defects of arachidonic acid metabolism (Keenan *et al.* 1977, Jubelirer *et al.* 1980) and response to thromboxane A_2 (Okuma, Takayama and Uchino 1982) have also been observed. Bolin, Okumura and Jamieson (1977) and Vainer and Bussel (1977) have described altered distribution of membrane glycoproteins in the platelets of patients with various types of myeloproliferative disorder, but these were not correlated with the defect of aggregation or secretion. In general, the results of laboratory tests (e.g. Zucker and Mielke 1972, Keenan *et al.* 1977) have only relatively seldom been found to correlate well with clinical evidence of bleeding. The incidence of thrombosis, on the other hand, has been found to correlate with laboratory evidence of hyperaggregability of the platelets (Preston *et al.* 1974, Wu 1978). One possible explanation for such hyperaggregability (Cooper *et al.* 1978, Cooper and Ahern 1979) is the resistance of platelets from these patients to the inhibitory action of prostaglandin D_2, due to the loss of specific membrane receptors, while another (Okuma and Uchino 1979) might be an increased sensitivity to aggregation by arachidonic acid, associated with a deficiency of lipoxygenase activity.

The bleeding tendency and the platelet functional defects usually respond to myelosuppressive therapy, and improvement has even followed venesection in polycythaemia vera (Berger *et al.* 1973). Aspirin and dipyridamole have been used successfully in the management of thrombotic episodes in thrombocythaemia.

Acute leukaemias and preleukaemic states

Bleeding in the acute leukaemias is usually due to thrombocytopenia, but defects of platelet function may also contribute during the overt disease as well as in preleukaemic states. Defects of aggregation and secretion have been attributed to storage pool deficiency and a defect of adenine nucleotide metabolism (Cowan, Graham and Baunach 1975), a reduction of thrombin binding sites in the membrane (Ganguly, Sutherland and Bradford 1978), and a defect of thromboxane A_2 activity (Russell, Keenan and Bellingham 1979).

Dysproteinaemias

The haemostatic abnormalities observed in this group of diseases also include disorders of coagulation and fibrinolysis, but defects of platelet function and hyperviscosity seem to be the most closely correlated with clinical bleeding (Perkins, McKenzie and Fudenberg 1970, Lackner 1973). Defects of platelet retention in glass-bead columns, platelet factor-3 availability, aggregation and adhesion to connective tissues have all been described, and all are presumably due to the inhibitory effect of the paraprotein, which apparently acts by coating the platelet and collagen surfaces. Like the long bleeding time with which they are often associated, the platelet defects can be corrected by plasmapheresis.

Chronic hypoglycaemia

A mild haemorrhagic tendency, characterized by superficial bruising, epistaxis and prolonged bleeding after trauma, and by a long bleeding time, forms part of the syndrome resulting from glycogen storage disease type I (glucose-6-phosphatase deficiency), and also occurs in fructose-1, 6-diphosphatase deficiency. The defect of platelet aggregation and nucleotide release which has been observed in such patients (Czapek *et al.* 1973, Corby, Putnum and Green 1974) is not a direct result of the underlying hereditary metabolic defect, but is evidently due to a defect of platelet nucleotide synthesis (Hutton, Macnab and Rivers 1976). This is secondary to the chronic hypoglycaemia, which itself results from the hereditary enzyme defect in the liver cells. Continuous intravenous administration of glucose restores the capacity of the platelets to synthesize ATP, and so gradually corrects the haemostatic defect.

Liver disease

Haemostatic failure in liver disease is usually chiefly due to coagulation defects, but thrombocytopenia and disorders of platelet function, including defective aggregation in response to ADP and thrombin, are also sometimes seen; though the impairment of aggregation has been found to parallel prolongation of the thrombin time, the suggestion that it is due to low molecular-weight fibrinogen degradation products (Thomas 1972) has been disputed (Solum *et al.* 1973, Ballard and Marcus 1976).

Miscellaneous causes of platelet dysfunction

Evidence continues to accumulate that a variety of forms of injury to circulating platelets, whether mechanical or immune, may induce the 'release reaction' *in vivo*, and so result in a depletion of dense-body contents—an acquired storage pool deficiency. Amongst the conditions in which this mechanism has been thought to contribute to a haemorrhagic tendency are autoimmune disorders (Zahavi and Marder 1974, Karpatkin and Lackner 1975), disseminated intravascular coagulation (Pareti *et al.* 1976), valvular heart disease and cardiopulmonary bypass surgery (Beurling-Harbery and Galvan 1978) and severe burns (Hourdillé *et al.* 1981). A similar mechanism may account for the defective ADP-induced aggregation observed in patients with sickle-cell disease during vaso-occlusive crises (Stuart, Stockman and Oski 1974).

Other conditions in which less well-defined abnormalities of platelet function have been observed include scurvy (Wilson, McNicol and Douglas 1967) infectious mononucleosis (Clancy, Jenkins and Firkin 1971), congenital heart disease (Maurer *et al.* 1972), vitamin B_{12} deficiency (Levine 1973) and homozygous β-thalassaemia (Stuart 1979).

Drug-induced defects of platelet function

Various classes of drugs are known to interfere with platelet function: some of them are used as potential antithrombotic agents on account of their antiplatelet effects, while others may cause bleeding symptoms as a side-effect of their use for other purposes: acetylsalicylic acid (aspirin) falls into both these groups. Others again, including tricyclic antidepressants, antihistamines, phenothiazines and general and local anaesthetics, can be used to inhibit various aspects of platelet function *in vitro* but do not significantly impair haemostasis at pharmacological dosage. The present account is confined to those (Table 34) which may cause bleeding as a side-effect. It is essential, before performing platelet function tests in the course of investigating a

Table 34. Drugs which may cause bleeding through interference with platelet function.

Acetylsalicylic acid
Other non-steroidal anti-inflammatory agents:
    Indomethacin
    Sulphinpyrazone
    Phenylbutazone
Dextrans
Heparin
Penicillins, cephalosporins

---

possible bleeding tendency, to ensure that the patient has not taken any drugs which may have interfered with platelet function during the preceding 7–10 days.

ACETYLSALICYLIC ACID (ASPIRIN)

Aspirin has long been known to prolong the bleeding time when taken at ordinary pharmacological dosage, and to provoke bleeding in some patients; its use is contraindicated in patients with known bleeding disorders. This effect is due to its inhibition of the enzyme cyclooxygenase, leading to a failure of endoperoxide and thromboxane synthesis by the platelets (Smith and Willis 1971, Vane 1971), and of prostacyclin (PGI_2) synthesis by the vascular endothelium. Aspirin inhibits platelet cyclooxygenase irreversibly by acetylation (Roth, Stanford and Majerus 1975), and the effect of a single pharmacological dose (300–900 mg) can be detected for up to a week or more— throughout the lifespan of the platelets exposed to it. The effect on the endothelial cell enzyme, however, is incomplete and relatively short-lived, so that the net result may be to shift the balance of synthesis in favour of PGI_2 and away from thromboxane A_2. Aspirin-treated platelets fail to aggregate or to secrete normally in response to arachidonic acid or collagen and typically show no second-phase aggregation with ADP or adrenaline. Other non-steroidal anti-inflammatory drugs, including indomethacin, sulphinpyrazone and phenylbutazone, have a similar but less prolonged effect, and some of them (unlike aspirin itself) have also been claimed to inhibit platelet adhesion to subendothelial structures (Cazenave *et al.* 1974).

DEXTRANS

These, given at clinical dosage, have been shown to prolong the bleeding time and to inhibit PF3 availability, retention in glass-bead columns and collagen-induced aggregation (Bygdeman and Eliasson 1967, Weiss 1967b). These effects, which are dose-related and are more pronounced with HMW dextrans, reach a maximum 4–8 hours after the end of an infusion. It has been suggested that the inhibitory effect may be due to refractoriness following transitory aggregation by the dextran (Evans and Gordon 1974).

HEPARIN

Some heparin preparations inhibit platelet aggregation and secretion, probably inducing a refractory state after partial activation by the heparin itself (Zucker 1977). Salzman *et al.* (1980) have shown that the anticoagulant effect of heparin from porcine intestinal mucosa can be dissociated from the platelet aggregating effect.

PENICILLINS AND CEPHALOSPORINS

McClure *et al.* (1970) observed purpuric bleeding in patients receiving carbenicillin in high dosage, and found that the drug prolonged the bleeding time and impaired ADP-induced platelet aggregation. Several other penicillins have been found to have a similar effect, penicillin G and ampicillin being more active in this respect than ticarcillin or methicillin (Brown *et al.* 1975, 1966); cephalosporins have also been incriminated (Natelson *et al.* 1976). Adhesion to collagen-coated surfaces and subendothelium has been shown to be inhibited *in vitro* by both these types of antibiotic, as well as aggregation and secretion, and it has been suggested that they act by coating the platelet surface (Cazenave *et al.* 1977). They produce bleeding symptoms only when given in very high dosage, particularly to patients in renal failure, whose platelet function may already be defective and in whom clearance of the drug is impaired.

REFERENCES

Adams T., Schultz L. & Goldberg L. (1974) Platelet function abnormalities in the myeloproliferative disorders. *Scandinavian Journal of Haematology* **13**, 215–24.

Ballard H.S. & Marcus A.J. (1972) Primary and secondary platelet aggregation in uraemia. *Scandinavian Journal of Haematology* **9**, 198–203.

Ballard H.S. & Marcus A.J. (1976) Platelet aggregation in portal cirrhosis. *Archives of Internal Medicine* **136**, 316–19.

Bartter F.C., Gill J.R., Frolich J.C., Bowden R.E., Hollifield J.W., Radfar N., Keiser H.R., Oates J.A., Seyberth H. & Taylor A.A. (1976) Prostaglandins are overproduced by the kidneys and mediate hyperreninemia in Bartter's syndrome. *Transactions of the Association of American Physicians* **89**, 77–91.

Bennett J.S. & Vilaire G. (1979) Exposure of platelet fibrinogen receptors by ADP and epinephrine. *Journal of Clinical Investigation* **64**, 1393–401.

Berger S., Aledort L.M., Gilbert H.S., Hanson J.P. & Wasserman L.R. (1973) Abnormalities of platelet function in patients with polycythemia vera. *Cancer Research* **33**, 2683–7.

Bernard J. & Soulier J.P. (1948) Sur une nouvelle variété de dystrophie thrombocytaire hémorrhagipare congénitale. *Semaine des Hôpitaux de Paris* **24**, 3217–23.

Bernheim J., Dechavanne M., Byron P.A., Lagarde M., Colon S., Pozet N. & Traeger J. (1976) Thrombocytopenia, macrothrombocytopathia, nephritis and deafness. *American Journal of Medicine* **61**, 145–50.

Beurling-Harbury G. & Galvan C.A. (1978) Acquired decrease in platelet secretory ADP associated with increased postoperative bleeding in post-cardiopulmonary bypass patients and in patients with severe valvular heart disease. *Blood* **52**, 13–23.

Bithell T.C., Parekh S.J. & Strong R.R. (1972) Platelet function in the Bernard–Soulier syndrome. *Annals of the New York Academy of Sciences* **201**, 145–60.

Bolin R.B., Okumura T. & Jamieson G.A. (1977) Changes in distribution of platelet membrane glycoproteins in patients with myeloproliferative disorders. *American Journal of Hematology* **3**, 63–71.

Boullin D.J. & O'Brien R.A. (1971) Abnormalities of 5-hydroxytryptamine uptake and binding by blood platelets from children with Down's syndrome. *Journal of Physiology* **212**, 287–97.

Boxer G.J., Holmsen H., Robkin L., Bang N.U., Boxer L.A. & Baehner R.L. (1977) Abnormal platelet function in Chediak-Higashi syndrome. *British Journal of Haematology* **35**, 521–33.

Brown C.H. III, Bradshaw M.W., Natelson E.A., Alfrey C.P. & Williams T.W. (1976) Defective platelet function following the administration of penicillin compounds. *Blood* **47**, 949–56.

Brown C.H. III, Natelson E.A., Bradshaw M.W., Alfrey C.P. & Williams T.W. Jr (1975) Study of the effects of ticarcillin on blood coagulation and platelet function. *Antimicrobial Agents and Chemotherapy* **7**, 652–7.

Buchanan G.R. & Handin R.I. (1976) Platelet function in the Chediak–Higashi syndrome. *Blood* **47**, 941–8.

Burch J.W., Baenziger N.L., Stanford N. & Majerus P.W. (1978) Sensitivity of fatty acid cyclooxygenase from human aorta to acetylation by aspirin. *Proceedings of the National Academy of Sciences of the USA* **75**, 5181–4.

Bygdeman S. & Eliasson R. (1967) Effect of dextrans on platelet adhesiveness and aggregation. *Scandinavian Journal of Clinical and Laboratory Investigation* **20**, 17–23.

Caen J. (1972) Glanzmann thrombasthenia. In *Clinics in Haematology*. Vol. 1:2. pp. 383–92. O'Brien J.R. (ed.). W.B. Saunders, London.

Caen J.P., Castaldi P.A., Leclerc J.C., Inceman S., Larrieu M.J., Probst M. & Bernard J. (1966) Congenital bleeding disorders with long bleeding time and normal platelet count. I. Glanzmann's thrombasthenia (report of 15 patients). *American Journal of Medicine* **41**, 4–26.

Caen J.P. & Levy-Toledano S. (1973) Interaction between platelets and von Willebrand factor provides a new scheme for primary haemostasis. *Nature (New Biology)* **244**, 159–60.

Caen J.P., Michel H., Tobelem G., Bodevin E. & Levy-Toledano S. (1977) Adhesion and aggregation of human platelets to rabbit subendothelium. A new approach for investigation: specific antibodies. *Experimentia* **33**, 91–3.

Caen J.P., Nurden A.T., Jeanneau C., Michel H., Tobelem G., Levy-Toledano S., Sultan Y., Valensi F. & Bernard J. (1976) Bernard–Soulier syndrome—a new platelet glycoprotein abnormality. Its relationship with platelet adhesion to subendothelium and with the factor VIII von Willebrand protein. *Journal of Laboratory and Clinical Medicine* **87**, 586–96.

Cardamone J.M., Edson J.R., McArthur J.R. & Jacob H.S. (1972) Abnormalities of platelet function in the myeloproliferative disorders. *Journal of the American Medical Association* **221**, 270–3.

Castaldi P.A., Rozenberg M.C. & Stewart J.H. (1966) The bleeding disorder of uraemia. *Lancet* **II**, 66–9.

Cazenave J.P., Guccione M.A., Packham M.A. & Mustard J.F. (1977) Effects of cephalothin and penicillin G on platelet function *in vitro*. *British Journal of Haematology* **35**, 135–52.

Cazenave J.P., Packham M.A., Guccione M. & Mustard J.F. (1974) Inhibition of platelet adherence to a collagen-coated surface by non-steroidal anti-inflammatory drugs, pyrimido-pyrimidine and tricyclic compounds, and lidocaine. *Journal of Laboratory and Clinical Medicine* **83**, 797–806.

Charo I.F., Feinman R.D. & Detwiler T.C. (1977) Interrelations of platelet aggregation and secretion. *Journal of Clinical Investigation* **60**, 866–73.

Clancy R., Jenkins E. & Firkin B. (1971) Platelet defect of infectious mononucleosis. *British Medical Journal* **IV**, 646–8.

Cooper B. & Ahern D. (1979) Characterization of the platelet prostaglandin D_2 receptor. Loss of prostaglandin D_2 receptors in platelets of patients with myeloproliferative disorders. *Journal of Clinical Investigation* **64**, 586–90.

Cooper B., Schafer A.I., Puchalsky D. & Handin R.I. (1978) Platelet resistance to prostaglandin D_2 in patients with myeloproliferative disorders. *Blood* **52**, 618–26.

Corby D.G., Putnum C.W. & Greene H.L. (1974) Impaired platelet function in glucose-6-phosphatase deficiency. *Journal of Pediatrics* **85**, 71–6.

Cowan D.H., Graham R.C. & Baunach D. (1975) The platelet defect in leukemia, platelet ultrastructure, adenine nucleotide metabolism, and the release reaction. *Journal of Clinical Investigation* **56**, 188–20.

Czapek E.E., Deykin D. & Salzman E.W. (1973) Platelet dysfunction in glycogen storage disease type I. *Blood* **41**, 235–47.

Davies B. & Tuddenham E.G.D. (1976) Familial pulmonary fibrosis associated with oculocutaneous albinism and platelet function defect. *Quarterly Journal of Medicine* **45**, 219–32.

Davies J.W., McField J.R., Phillips P.L. & Graham B.A. (1972) Effects of exogenous urea, creatinine, and guanidinosuccinic acid on human platelet aggregation *in vitro*. *Blood* **39**, 388–97.

Day H.J. & Holmsen H. (1972) Platelet adenine nucleotide 'storage pool deficiency' in thrombocytopenic absent radii syndrome. *Journal of the American Medical Association* **221**, 1053–4.

Defreyn G., Machin S.J., Carreras L.O., Vergera Daudon M., Chamone D.A.F. & Vermylen J. (1981) Familial bleeding tendency with partial platelet thromboxane synthetase deficiency: reorientation of cyclic endoperoxide metabolism. *British Journal of Haematology* **49**, 29–41.

Degos L., Dautigny A., Brouet J.C., Colombani M., Ardaillou N., Caen J.P. & Colombani J. (1975) A molecular defect in thrombasthenic platelets. *Journal of Clinical Investigation* **56**, 236–40.

Degos L., Tobelem G., Lethielleux P., Levy-Toledano S., Caen J. & Colombani J. (1977) A molecular defect in platelets from patients with Bernard–Soulier syndrome. *Blood* **50**, 899–903.

Eckstein J.D., Filip D.J. & Watts J.C. (1975) Hereditary thrombocytopenia, deafness, and renal disease. *Annals of Internal Medicine* **82**, 639–45.

Eknoyan G., Wacksman S.J., Glueck H.I. & Will J.J. (1969) Platelet function in renal failure. *New England Journal of Medicine* **280**, 677–81.

Epstein C.J., Sahud M.A., Piel C.F., Goodman J.R., Bernfield M.R., Kushner J.H. & Ablin A.R. (1972) Hereditary macrothrombocytopathia, nephritis and deafness. *American Journal of Medicine* **52**, 299–310.

Evans R.J. & Gordon J.L. (1974) Mechanisms of the antithrombotic action of dextran. *New England Journal of Medicine* **290**, 748.

Ganguly P. (1977) Binding of thrombin to functionally defective platelets: a hypothesis on the nature of the thrombin receptor. *British Journal of Haematology* **37**, 47–51.

Ganguly P., Sutherland S.B. & Bradford H.R. (1978) Defective binding of thrombin to platelets in myeloid leukaemia. *British Journal of Haematology* **39**, 599–605.

Garay S.M., Gardella J.E., Fazzini E.P. & Goldring R.M. (1979) Hermansky-Pudlak syndrome: pulmonary manifestations of a ceroid storage disorder. *American Journal of Medicine* **66**, 737–47.

George J.N. & Morgan R.K. (1981) Glanzmann's thrombasthenia: deficient association of actin with the platelet membrane following thrombin-induced secretion. *Thrombosis Research* **22**, 503–6.

Gerrard J.M., Phillips D.R., Rao G.H.R., Plow E.F., Walz D.W., Ross R., Harker L.A. & White J.G. (1980) Biochemical studies of two patients with the gray platelet syndrome. Selective deficiency of platelet alpha granules. *Journal of Clinical Investigation* **66**, 102–9.

Gerrard J.M., Schollmeyer J.V., Phillips D.R. & White J.G. (1979) α-Actinin deficiency in thromboasthenia: possible identity of α-actinin and glycoprotein III. *American Journal of Pathology* **94**, 509–23.

Gerrard J.M., Stoddard S.F., Shapiro R.S., Coccia P.F., Ramsay N.K.C., Nesbit M.E., Rao G.H.R., Krivit W. & White J.G. (1978) Platelet storage pool deficiency and prostaglandin synthesis in chronic granulocytic leukaemia. *British Journal of Haematology* **40**, 597–607.

Gerritsen S.M., Akkerman J.W.N., Nijmeijer B., Sixma J.J., Witkop C.J. & White J. (1977) The Hermansky–Pudlak syndrome: evidence for a lowered 5-hydroxytryptamine content in platelets of heterozygotes. *Scandinavian Journal of Haematology* **18**, 249–56.

Gerritsen S.M., Akkerman J.W.N. & Sixma J.J. (1978) Correction of the bleeding time in patients with storage pool deficiency by infusion of cryoprecipitate. *British Journal of Haematology* **40**, 153–60.

Ginsberg M., Chediak J., Lightsey A. & Plow E.F. (1981) Thrombasthenic platelets do not bind plasma fibronectin. *Thrombosis and Haemostasis* (Abstract) **46**, 84.

Ginsburg A.D. (1975) Platelet function in patients with high platelet counts. *Annals of Internal Medicine* **82**, 506–11.

Glanzmann E. (1918) Hereditäre hämorrhagische Thrombasthenie. Ein Beitrag zur Pathologie der Blutplättchen. *Jahrbuch der Kinderheilkunde* **88**, 1–42.

Gröttum K.A., Hovig T., Holmsen H., Abrahamsen A.F., Jeremic M. & Seip M. (1969) Wiskott–Aldrich syndrome: qualitative platelet defects and short platelet survival. *British Journal of Haematology* **17**, 373–88.

Gröttum K.A. & Solum N.O. (1969) Congenital thrombocytopenia with giant platelets: a defect in the platelet membrane. *British Journal of Haematology* **16**, 277–90.

Gullner H-G., Cerletti C., Bartter F.C., Smith J.B. & Gill J.R. Jr (1979) Prostacyclin overproduction in Bartter's syndrome. *Lancet* **II**, 767–9.

Hagen I., Nurden A., Bjerrum O.J., Solum N.O. & Caen J. (1980) Immunochemical evidence for protein abnormalities in platelets from patients with Glanzmann's thrombasthenia and Bernard–Soulier syndrome. *Journal of Clinical Investigation* **65**, 722–31.

Hagen I. & Solum N.O. (1979) Further studies of the protein composition and surface structure of normal platelets and platelets from patients with Glanzmann's thrombasthenia and Bernard–Soulier syndrome. *Thrombosis Research* **13**, 845–55.

Hampton J.R. & Hardisty R.M. (1967) Platelet electrophoretic mobility in thrombasthenia. *Nature (London)* **213**, 400.

Hardisty R.M., Dormandy K.M. & Hutton R.A. (1964) Thrombasthenia: studies on three cases. *British Journal of Haematology* **10**, 371–87.

Hardisty R.M. & Hutton R.A. (1966) Platelet aggregation and the availability of platelet factor 3. *British Journal of Haematology* **12**, 764–76.

Hardisty R.M. & Hutton R.A. (1967) Bleeding tendency associated with 'new' abnormality of platelet behaviour. *Lancet* **I**, 983–4.

Hardisty R.M., Mills D.C.B. & Ketsa-Ard K. (1972) The platelet defect associated with albinism. *British Journal of Haematology* **23**, 679–92.

Harker L.A. & Slichter S.J. (1972) The bleeding time as a screening test for evaluation of platelet function. *New England Journal of Medicine* **287**, 155–9.

Hemmeler G. (1958) Thrombopathie familiale. *Schweizerische Medizinische Wochenschrift* **88**, 1018–19.

Horowitz H.I., Cohen B.D., Martinez P. & Papayoanou M.F. (1967) Defective ADP-induced platelet factor 3 activation in uremia. *Blood* **30**, 331–40.

Horowitz H.I., Stein I.M., Cohen B.D. & White J.G. (1970) Further studies on the platelet inhibitory effect of guanidinosuccinic acid: its role in uremic bleeding. *American Journal of Medicine* **49**, 336–45.

Hourdillé P., Bernard P., Belloc F., Radet A., Sanchez R. & Boisseau M.R. (1981) Platelet abnormalities in thermal injury. Study of platelet-dense bodies stained with mepacrine. *Haemostasis* **10**, 141–52.

Howard M.A. & Firkin B.G. (1971) Ristocetin: a new tool in the investigation of platelet aggregation. *Thrombosis et Diathesis Haemorrhagica* **26**, 362–9.

Howard M.A., Hutton R.A. & Hardisty R.M. (1973) Hereditary giant platelet syndrome: a disorder of a new aspect of platelet function. *British Medical Journal* **II**, 586–8.

Howard M.A., Montgomery D.C. & Hardisty R.M. (1974) Factor VIII-related antigen in platelets. *Thrombosis Research* **4**, 617–24.

Hutton R.A., Macnab A.J. & Rivers R.P.A. (1976) Defect of platelet function associated with chronic hypoglycaemia. *Archives of Disease in Childhood* **51**, 49–55.

Jaffe E.A. & Weksler B.B. (1979) Recovery of endothelial cell prostaglandin production after inhibition by low doses of aspirin. *Journal of Clinical Investigation* **63**, 532–5.

Jamieson G.A. & Okumura T. (1978) Reduced thrombin binding and aggregation in Bernard–Soulier platelets. *Journal of Clinical Investigation* **61**, 861–4.

Jamieson G.A., Okumura T., Fishback B., Johnson M.M., Egan J.J. & Weiss H.J. (1979) Platelet membrane glycoproteins in thrombasthenia, Bernard–Soulier syndrome and storage pool disease. *Journal of Laboratory and Clinical Medicine* **93**, 652–60.

Jubelirer S.J., Russell F., Vaillancourt R. & Deykin D. (1980) Platelet arachidonic acid metabolism and platelet function in ten patients with chronic myelogenous leukemia. *Blood* **56**, 728–31.

Karpatkin S. & Lackner H.L. (1975) Association of antiplatelet antibody with functional platelet disorders. Autoimmune thrombocytopenic purpura, systemic lupus erythematosus and thrombopathia. *American Journal of Medicine* **59**, 599–604.

Kaywin P., McDonough M., Insel P.A. & Shattil S.J. (1978) Platelet function in essential thrombocythemia. Decreased epinephrine responsiveness associated with a deficiency of platelet α-adrenergic receptors. *New England Journal of Medicine* **299**, 505–9.

Keenan J.P., Wharton J., Shepherd A.J.N. & Bellingham A.J. (1977) Defective lipid peroxidation in myeloproliferative disorders; a possible defect of prostaglandin synthesis. *British Journal of Haematology* **35**, 275–83.

Kunicki T.J. & Aster R.H. (1978) Deletion of the platelet-specific alloantigen Pl^{A1} from platelets in Glanzmann's thrombasthenia. *Journal of Clinical Investigation* **61**, 1225–31.

Kunicki T.J. & Aster R.H. (1979) Isolation and immunologic characterization of the human platelet alloantigen Pl^{A1}. *Molecular Immunology* **16**, 353–60.

Kunicki T.J., Johnson M.M. & Aster R.H. (1978) Absence of the platelet receptor for drug-dependent antibodies in the Bernard–Soulier syndrome. *Journal of Clinical Investigation* **62**, 716–19.

Kunicki T.J., Pidard D., Cazenave J-P., Nurden A.T. & Caen J.P. (1981a) Inheritance of the human platelet alloantigen Pl^{A1}, in Type I Glanzmann's thrombasthenia. *Journal of Clinical Investigation* **67**, 717–24.

Kunicki T.J., Pidard D., Rosa J-P. & Nurden A.T. (1981b) The formation of Ca^{++}-dependent complexes of platelet membrane glycoproteins IIb and IIIa in solution as determined by crossed immunoelectrophoresis. *Blood* **58**, 268–78.

Kunicki T.J., Russell N., Nurden A.T., Aster R.H. & Caen J.P. (1981c) Further studies of the human platelet receptor for quinine- and quinidine-dependent antibodies. *Journal of Immunology* **126**, 398–402.

Kurstjens R., Bolt C., Vossen M. & Haanen C. (1968) Familial thrombopathic thrombocytopenia. *British Journal of Haematology* **15**, 305–17.

Lackner H. (1973) Hemostatic abnormalities associated with dysproteinemias. *Seminars in Hematology* **10**, 125–33.

Lagarde M., Bryon P.A., Vargaftig B.B. & Dechavanne M. (1978) Impairment of platelet thromboxane A_2 generation and of the platelet release reaction in two patients with congenital deficiency of platelet cyclo-oxygenase. *British Journal of Haematology* **38**, 251–66.

Lages B., Malmsten C., Weiss H.J. & Samuelsson B. (1981) Impaired platelet response to thromboxane A_2 and defective calcium mobilization in a patient with a bleeding disorder. *Blood* **57**, 545–52.

Lages B., Scrutton M.C., Holmsen H., Day H.J. & Weiss H.J. (1975) Metal ion content of gel-filtered platelets from patients with storage pool disease. *Blood* **46**, 119–30.

Lee H., Nurden A.T., Thomaidis A. & Caen J.P. (1981) Relationship between fibrinogen binding and the platelet glycoprotein deficiencies in Glanzmann's thrombasthenia Type I and Type II. *British Journal of Haematology* **48**, 47–57.

Legrand C. & Caen J.P. (1976) Binding of ^{14}C-ADP by thrombasthenic platelet membranes. *Haemostasis* **5**, 231–8.

Legrand C. & Caen J.P. (1978) Binding of ^{14}C-ADP to normal human and thrombasthenic platelet membranes. Study of the dissociation of the nucleotide from its receptors. *Haemostasis* **7**, 339–51.

Levine P. (1973) A qualitative platelet defect in severe vitamin B_{12} deficiency: response, hyper-response and thrombosis after vitamin B_{12} therapy. *Annals of Internal Medicine* **78**, 533–9.

Levy-Toledano S., Tobelem G., Legrand C., Bredoux R., Degos L., Nurden A. & Caen J.P. (1978) An acquired IgG antibody occurring in a thrombasthenic patient; its effect on human platelet function. *Blood* **51**, 1065–71.

Libanska J., Falcão L., Gautier A., Ammon J., Spahr A., Vainer H. & Caen J. (1975) Thrombocytopénie thrombocytopathique hypogranulaire héréditaire. *Nouvelle Revue Française d'Hématologie* **15**, 165–82.

Lorez H.P., Richards J.G., Da Prada M., Picotti G.B., Pareti F.I., Capitano A. & Mannucci P.M. (1979) Storage pool disease: comparative fluorescence, microscopical cytochemical and biochemical studies on amine-storing organelles of human blood platelets. *British Journal of Haematology* **43**, 297–305.

McClure P.D., Casserly J., Monsier Ch. & Crozier D. (1970) Carbenicillin-induced bleeding disorders. *Lancet* **II**, 1307–8.

McClure P.D., Ingram G.I.C., Stacey R.S., Glass U.H. & Matchett M.O. (1966) Platelet function tests in thrombocythaemia and thrombocytosis. *British Journal of Haematology* **12**, 478–98.

McEver R.P., Baenziger N.L. & Majerus P.M. (1980) Isolation and quantitation of the platelet protein lacking in thrombasthenia using a monoclonal hybridoma antibody. *Clinical Research* (Abstract) **28**, 495A.

Malmsten C., Hamberg M., Svensson J. & Samuelsson B. (1975) Physiological role of an endoperoxide in human platelets: hemostatic defect due to platelet cyclo-oxygenase deficiency. *Proceedings of the National Academy of Sciences of the USA* **72**, 1446–50.

Malmsten C., Kindahl H., Samuelsson B., Levy-Toledano S., Tobelem G. & Caen J.P. (1977) Thromboxane synthesis and the platelet release reaction in Bernard-Soulier syndrome, thrombasthenia Glanzmann and Hermansky–Pudlak syndrome. *British Journal of Haematology* **35**, 511–20.

Matthias F.R. & Palinski W. (1977) Prostaglandin-endoperoxides and cyclic 3'-5'-AMP in platelets of patients with uremia. *Thrombosis and Haemostasis* (Abstract) **38**, 34.

Maurer H.M., McCue C.M., Caul J. & Still W.J.S. (1972) Impairment in platelet aggregation in congenital heart disease. *Blood* **40**, 207–16.

Mielke C.H. Jr, Levine P.H. & Zucker S. (1981) Preoperative prednisone therapy in platelet function disorders. *Thrombosis Research* **21**, 655–62.

Miletich J.P., Kane W.H., Hofmann S.L., Stanford N. & Majerus P.W. (1979) Deficiency of factor Xa-factor Va binding sites on the platelets of a patient with a bleeding disorder. *Blood* **54**, 1015–27.

Minkes M.S., Joist J.H. & Needleman P. (1979) Arachidonic acid-induced platelet aggregation independent of ADP-release in a patient with a bleeding disorder due to platelet storage pool disease. *Thrombosis Research* **15**, 169–79.

Mull M.M. & Hathaway W.E. (1970) Altered platelet function in newborns. *Pediatric Research* **4**, 229–37.

Mustard J.F., Kinlough-Rathbone R.L., Packham M.A., Perry D., Harfenist E.J. & Pai K.R.M. (1979) Comparison of fibrinogen association with normal and thrombasthenic platelets on exposure to ADP or chymotrypsin. *Blood* **54**, 987–93.

Nachman R.L., Jaffe A.E. & Weksler B.B. (1977) Immunoinhibition of ristocetin-induced platelet aggregation. *Journal of Clinical Investigation* **59**, 143–8.

Natelson E.A., Brown C.H. III, Bradshaw M.W., Alfrey C.P. & Williams T.W. Jr (1976) Influence of cephalosporin antibiotics on blood coagulation and platelet function. *Antimicrobial Agents and Chemotherapy* **9**, 91–3.

Neemeh J.A., Bowie E.J.W., Thompson J.H., Didisheim P. & Owen C.A. (1972) Quantitation of platelet aggregation in myeloproliferative disorders. *American Journal of Clinical Pathology* **57**, 336–47.

Nurden A.T. & Caen J.P. (1974) An abnormal platelet glycoprotein pattern in three cases of Glanzmann's thrombasthenia. *British Journal of Haematology* **28**, 253–60.

Nurden A.T. & Caen J.P. (1975) Specific roles for platelet surface glycoproteins in platelet function. *Nature* **255**, 720–2.

Okuma M., Takayama H. & Uchino H. (1982) Subnormal platelet response to thromboxane A_2 in a patient with chronic myeloid leukaemia. *British Journal of Haematology* **51**, 469–77.

Okuma M. & Uchino H. (1979) Altered arachidonate metabolism by platelets in patients with myeloproliferative disorders. *Blood* **54**, 1258–71.

Okumura T., Hasitz M. & Jamieson G.A. (1978) Platelet glycocalicin. Interaction with thrombin and role as thrombin receptor of the platelet surface. *Journal of Biological Chemistry* **253**, 3435–43.

Pareti F.I., Capitanio A. & Mannucci P.M. (1976) Acquired storage pool disease in platelets during disseminated intravascular coagulation. *Blood* **48**, 511–15.

Pareti F.I., Day H.J. & Mills D.C.B. (1974) Nucleotide and serotonin metabolism in platelets with defective secondary aggregation. *Blood* **44**, 789–800.

Peerschke E.I., Grant R.A. & Zucker M.B. (1979) Relationship between aggregation and binding of ^{125}I-fibrinogen and ^{45}calcium to human platelets. *Thrombosis and Haemostasis* (Abstract) **42**, 358.

Perkins H.A., McKenzie M.R. & Fudenberg H.H. (1970) Hemostatic defects in dysproteinemias. *Blood* **35**, 695–707.

Phillips D.R. (1978) Platelet membrane glycoproteins. In *Platelet Function Testing*. Day H.J., Holmsen H. & Zucker M.B. (eds). DHEW Publication No. (NIH) 78-1087, p. 240.

Phillips D.R. & Agin P.P. (1977) Platelet membrane defects in Glanzmann's thrombasthenia. Evidence for decreased amounts of two major glycoproteins. *Journal of Clinical Investigation* **60**, 535–45.

Phillips D.R., Jennings L.K. & Wiliams H.H. (1980) Identification of membrane proteins mediating the interaction of human platelets. *Journal of Cell Biology* **86**, 77–86.

Preston F.E., Emmanuel I.G., Winfield D.A. & Malia R.G. (1974) Essential thrombocythaemia and peripheral gangrene. *British Medical Journal* **III**, 548–52.

Rabiner S.F. & Hrodek O. (1968) Platelet factor-3 in normal subjects and patients with renal failure. *Journal of Clinical Investigation* **47**, 901–12.

Rabiner S.F. & Molinas F. (1970) The role of phenol and phenolic acids on the thrombocytopathy and defective platelet aggregation of patients with renal failure. *American Journal of Medicine* **49**, 346–51.

Raccuglia G. (1971) Gray platelet syndrome. A variety of qualitative platelet disorder. *American Journal of Medicine* **51**, 818–28.

Remuzzi G., Cavenaghi A.E., Mecca G., Donati M.B. & de Gaetano G. (1977) Prostacyclin-like activity and bleeding in renal failure. *Lancet* **II**, 1195–7.

Remuzzi G., Marchesi D., Livio M., Cavanaghi A.E., Mecca G., Donati M.B. & de Gaetano G. (1978) Altered platelet and vascular prostaglandin generation in patients with renal failure and prolonged bleeding times. *Thrombosis Research* **13**, 1007–15.

Remuzzi G., Mecca G. & de Gaetano G. (1980) *Hemostasis, Prostaglandins and Renal Disease.* Raven Press, New York.

Rendu F., Breton-Gorius J., Trugnan G., Castro-Malaspina H., Andrieu J.M., Bereziat G., Lebret M. & Caen J.P. (1978) Studies on a new variant of the Hermansky–Pudlak syndrome: qualitative ultrastructural and functional abnormalities of the platelet-dense bodies associated with a phospholipase A defect. *American Journal of Hematology* **4**, 387–99.

Rendu F., Lebret M., Nurden A. & Caen J.P. (1979a) Detection of an acquired platelet storage pool disease in three patients with a myeloproliferative disorder. *Thrombosis and Haemostasis* **42**, 794–6.

Rendu F., Nurden A.T., Lebret M. & Caen J.P. (1979b) Relationship between mepacrine-labelled dense body number, platelet capacity to accumulate ^{14}C-5-HT and platelet density in the Bernard–Soulier and Hermansky–Pudlak syndromes. *Thrombosis and Haemostasis* **42**, 694–704.

Roth G.J., Stanford N. & Majerus P.W. (1975) Acetylation of prostaglandin synthetase by aspirin. *Proceedings of the National Academy of Sciences of the USA* **72**, 3073–6.

Russell N.H., Keenan J.P. & Bellingham A.J. (1979) Thrombocytopathy in preleukaemia: association with a defect of thromboxane A_2 activity. *British Journal of Haematology* **41**, 417–25.

Russell N.H., Salmon J., Keenan J.P. & Bellingham A.J. (1981) Platelet adenine nucleotides and arachidonic acid metabolism in the myeloproliferative disorders. *Thrombosis Research* **22**, 389–97.

Salzman E.W. & Neri L.J. (1966) Adhesiveness of blood platelets in uremia. *Thrombosis et Diathesis Haemorrhagica* **15**, 84–92.

Salzman E.W., Rosenberg R.D., Smith M.H., Lindon J.N. & Favreali L. (1980) Effect of heparin and heparin fractions on platelet aggregation. *Journal of Clinical Investigation* **65**, 64–73.

Samama M., Lecrubier C., Conard J., Hotchen M., Breton-Gorius J., Vargaftig B., Chignard M., Lagarde M. & Dechavanne M. (1981) Constitutional thrombocytopathy with subnormal response to thromboxane A_2. *British Journal of Haematology* **48**, 293–303.

Smith J.B. & Willis A.L. (1971) Aspirin selectively inhibits prostaglandin production in human platelets. *Nature (New Biology)* **231**, 235–7.

Solum N.O., Hagen I. & Sletbakk T. (1980) Further evidence for glycocalicin being derived from a larger amphiphilic platelet membrane glycoprotein. *Thrombosis Research* **18**, 773–85.

Solum N.O., Rigoblot C., Budzyński A.Z. & Morder V.J. (1973) A quantitative evaluation of the inhibition of platelet aggregation by low molecular weight degradation products of fibrinogen. *British Journal of Haematology* **24**, 419–34.

Spaet T.H., Lejnieks I., Gaynor E. & Goldstein M.L. (1969) Defective platelets in essential thrombocythaemia. *Archives of Internal Medicine* **124**, 135–41.

Stewart J.H. & Castaldi P.A. (1967) Uraemic bleeding: a reversible platelet defect corrected by dialysis. *Quarterly Journal of Medicine* **36**, 409–23.

Stoff J.S., Stemerman M., Steer M., Salzman E. & Brown R.S. (1978) A unique defect in platelet aggregation in Bartter's syndrome: improvement by indomethacin. *Clinical Research* **26**, 508A.

Stoff J.S., MacIntyre D.E., Brown R.S. & Salzman E.W. (1979) Prostacyclin overproduction in Barrter's syndrome. *Lancet* **II**, 1196–7.

Stuart M.J. (1979) Platelet dysfunction in homozygous β-thalassemia. *Pediatric Research* **13**, 1345–9.

Stuart M.J., Stockman J.A. & Oski F.A. (1974) Abnormalities of platelet aggregation in the vaso-occlusive crisis of sickle-cell anemia. *Journal of Pediatrics* **85**, 629–32.

Thomas D.P. (1972) Abnormalities of platelet aggregation in patients with alcoholic cirrhosis. *Annals of the New York Academy of Sciences* **201**, 243–50.

Tobelem G., Levy-Toledano S., Bredoux R., Michel H., Nurden A. & Caen J.P. (1976) New approach to determination of specific functions of platelet membrane sites. *Nature* **263**, 427–9.

Tobelem G., Levy-Toledano S., Nurden A.T., Degos L., Caen J.P., Malmsten C. & Kindahl H. (1979) Further studies on a specific platelet antibody found in Bernard–Soulier syndrome and its effects on normal platelet function. *British Journal of Haematology* **41**, 427–36.

Tschopp T.B., Weiss H.J. & Baumgartner H.R. (1975) Interaction of thrombasthenic platelets with subendothelium: normal adhesion, absent aggregation. *Experientia (Basel)* **31**, 113–16.

Vainer H. & Bussel A. (1977) Altered platelet surface glycoproteins in chronic myeloid leukemia. *International Journal of Cancer* **19**, 143–9.

Vane J.R. (1971) Inhibition of prostaglandin synthesis as a mechanism of action for aspirin-like drugs. *Nature (New Biology)* **231**, 232–5.

Van Leeuwen E.F., Zonnefeld G.T.E., Von Reisz L.E., Jenkins C.S.P., van Mourik J.A. & Von dem Borne A.E.G.K. (1979) Absence of the complete platelet-specific alloantigens Zw (Pl[A]) on platelets in Glanzmann's thrombasthenia and the effect of anti-Zw[a] antibody on platelet function. *Thrombosis and Haemostasis* (Abstract) **42**, 422.

Walsh P.N. (1972) Platelet coagulant activities in thrombasthenia. *British Journal of Haematology* **23**, 553–69.

Walsh P.N., Mills D.C.B., Pareti F.I., Stewart G.I., Macfarlane D.E., Johnson M.M. & Egan J.J. (1975) Hereditary giant platelet syndrome: absence of collagen-induced coagulant activity and deficiency of factor XI binding to platelets. *British Journal of Haematology* **29**, 639–55.

Weiss H.J. (1967a) Platelet aggregation, adhesion and adenosine diphosphate release in thrombopathia (platelet factor 3 deficiency). A comparison with Glanzmann's thrombasthenia and von Willebrand's disease. *American Journal of Medicine* **43**, 570–8.

Weiss H.J. (1967b) The effect of clinical dextran on platelet aggregation, adhesion, and ADP release in man: *in vivo* and *in vitro* studies. *Journal of Laboratory and Clinical Medicine* **69**, 37–46.

Weiss H.J. & Ames R.P. (1973) Ultrastructural findings in storage pool disease and aspirin-like defects of platelets. *American Journal of Pathology* **71**, 447–66.

Weiss H.J. & Lages B. (1981) Platelet malondialdehyde production and aggregation responses induced by arachidonate, prostaglandin-G_2, collagen, and epinephrine in 12 patients with storage pool deficiency. *Blood* **58**, 27–33.

Weiss H.J. & Rogers J. (1972) Thrombocytopathia due to abnormalities in platelet release reaction—studies on six unrelated patients. *Blood* **39**, 187–96.

Weiss H.J., Tschopp T.B., Baumgartner H.R., Sussman I.I., Johnson M.M. & Egan J.J. (1974a) Decreased adhesion of giant (Bernard–Soulier) platelets to subendothelium. Further implications on the role of the von Willebrand factor in hemostasis. *American Journal of Medicine* **57**, 920–5.

Weiss H.J., Tschopp T., Brand H. & Rogers J. (1974b) Studies of platelet 5-hydroxytryptamine (serotonin) in patients with storage-pool disease and albinism. *Journal of Clinical Investigation* **54**, 421–32.

Weiss H.J., Vicic W.J., Lages B.A. & Rogers J (1979a) Isolated deficiency of platelet procoagulant activity. *American Journal of Medicine* **67**, 206–13.

Weiss H.J., Witte L.D., Kaplan K.L., Lages B.A., Chernoff A., Nossel H.L., Goodman D.S. & Baumgartner H.R. (1979b) Heterogeneity in storage pool deficiency: studies on granule-bound substances in 18 patients including variants deficient in α-granules, platelet factor 4, β-thromboglobulin, and platelet-derived growth factor. *Blood* **54**, 1296–319.

White G.C., Workman E.F. & Lundblad R.L. (1978) Thrombin binding to thrombasthenic platelets. *Journal of Laboratory and Clinical Medicine* **91**, 76–82.

White J.G. (1979) Ultrastructural studies of the gray platelet syndrome. *American Journal of Pathology* **95**, 445–62.

White J.G., Edson J.R., Desnick S.J. & Witkop C.J. (1971) Studies of platelets in a variant of the Hermansky–Pudlak syndrome. *American Journal of Pathology* **63**, 319–32.

Wilson P.A., McNicol G.P. & Douglas A.S. (1967) Platelet abnormality in human scurvy. *Lancet* **I**, 975–8.

Wu K.K. (1978) Platelet hyperaggregability and thrombosis in patients with thrombocythemia. *Annals of Internal Medicine* **88**, 7–11.

Wu K.K., LeBreton G.C., Tai H.-H. & Chen Y.-C. (1981) Abnormal platelet response to thromboxane A_2. *Journal of Clinical Investigation* **67**, 1801–4.

Zahavi J. & Marder V.J. (1974) Acquired 'storage pool disease' of platelets associated with circulating anti-platelet antibodies. *American Journal of Medicine* **56**, 883–90.

Zucker M.B. (1977) Heparin and platelet function. *Federation Proceedings* **36**, 47–9.

Zucker M.B., Pert J.H. & Hilgartner M.W. (1966) Platelet function in a patient with thrombasthenia. *Blood* **28**, 524–34.

Zucker S. & Mielke C.H. (1972) Classification of thrombocytosis based on platelet function tests. Correlation with hemorrhagic and thrombotic complications. *Journal of Laboratory and Clinical Medicine* **80**, 385–94.

Chapter 15
Platelets and Thrombosis

S. HEPTINSTALL *and* J. R. A. MITCHELL

Every year, in England and Wales, over 200 000 people die from conditions in which thrombosis plays a significant role, some 160 000 deaths being certified as due to coronary disease, 80 000 to stroke and 20 000 to venous thromboembolism. The way in which the liquid, flowing blood turns itself into a solid thrombotic mass is, however, unknown. Every junior student can confidently recite the 'causes' of thrombosis by quoting Virchow's triad, but closer scrutiny soon reveals that we do not know the nature of the postulated changes in vessel walls, in patterns of blood flow or in blood constituents which are thought to predispose to thrombosis.

We have acquired an extensive knowledge, extending down to the molecular level, of the sequence of events which leads to blood coagulation. Much of this detailed knowledge has arisen from studying those rare individuals who have defects of their clotting mechanism, but at the same time that nearly 300 000 people were dying in England and Wales from thrombosis, less than 200 died from primary bleeding disorders (haemophilia—10; purpura and other bleeding—133). We thus know a lot about what matters least, in terms of the general health of our community, and we know virtually nothing which is useful in a therapeutic or preventive sense about those conditions which are important in our community, because they lead to premature death and disability. The reasons for this paradox form the subject of this chapter, in which we try to identify the conditions in which thrombosis plays a crucial role, to define the contribution of platelets to thrombus formation, and to describe the patterns of platelet behaviour which may be relevant to their participation in thrombosis.

CLINICAL EVENTS RESULTING FROM THROMBUS FORMATION

One would not make much progress in developing a test for infection by studying patients with neoplasms, so before we start searching for a blood abnormality in thrombotic disease we need to be able to identify patients with the condition. This seems self-evident, but failure to apply this simple precept has contributed to our present confusion. If, for example, one cannot differentiate with confidence between patients who have sustained haemorrhagic and thrombotic strokes, then scrutinizing the blood behaviour of an undifferentiated group of strokes will be doomed to failure because they represent a mixture of two diametrically opposed processes (bleeding and thrombosis). Similarly, it would be of no value to assess the success of an antithrombotic agent by comparing the mortality rates in treated and untreated groups of myocardial infarct survivors unless one was certain that all the observed deaths were due to thrombotic events. If the main causes of death after infarction are the non-thrombotic consequences of the initial infarct, such as pump failure or arrhythmia, then we would have chosen the wrong model on which to assay our antithrombotic regimen.

As we shall see, none of the spontaneous diseases in man is ideal, but even with their various shortcomings they are still likely to prove more helpful than the injured-artery animal models (Honour and Mitchell 1964) since the gap between these models and disease in man is considerable. The four diseases that we must scrutinize are venous thromboembolism, heart attacks, strokes and peripheral arterial disease.

Venous thromboembolism

This should be an ideal model in that deep-vein thrombosis in the lower limbs is so common in certain situations (advanced age, immobility, operation, neoplasm, obesity) that one can study these high-risk groups and be confident that it will occur in a significant proportion of them (Sevitt and Gallagher 1959, Morris and Mitchell 1976a). It ought, therefore, to be possible to use these very high-risk patients to search for a 'thrombotic crasis' in the blood and to use their survival to validate effective antithrombotic treatment.

We need to recognize several ways in which the venous thromboembolic situation may provide incomplete answers:

1   *Venous versus arterial thrombosis.* A venous thrombus forms in a slow-flow system and the wall of the affected vein is usually normal. An arterial thrombus forms in a fast-flow system, in vessels whose walls are usually abnormal.

2   *Clotting versus thrombosis.* When a blood clot forms in a static system it has a very different structure from a well-developed arterial thrombus (Poole and French 1961). In the former, all the blood cells are trapped in a fine fibrin mesh in the proportions in which they occur in life, so that red cells dominate the scene, while platelets and white cells are relatively insignificant. In the latter, platelets dominate and the platelet masses are surrounded by polymorphs and by coarse fibrin strands. A typical venous thrombus has a relatively small

platelet-rich 'white head' and a long, clot-like 'red tail'. Although Paterson (1969) has emphasized that both elements may figure in the all-important, lethal pulmonary emboli, nevertheless the clot-like tail provides a greater contribution to the bulk of a venous thromboembolus than to an arterial thrombus which is dominated by platelet–leucocyte fibrin masses. Venous thromboembolism merits study in its own right, but the results obtained may not be relevant or directly transferable to arterial thrombosis.

3   *Occlusion versus embolism.* The major consequence of lower-limb venous thrombosis is death from pulmonary embolus. This is, of course, a function of thrombus movement or disintegration, whereas in arteries it is the non-movement and non-disintegration of a subtending arterial thrombus that leads to necrosis of the territory previously supplied. Thus one might prevent death from pulmonary embolus by persuading a venous thrombus to stay in the leg, whereas encouraging an arterial thrombus to remain stable and to stay *in situ* would not help the ischaemic heart, brain or limb.

4   *Diagnosis in life.* Clinical signs allow us to diagnose only a small proportion of leg-vein thrombi and pulmonary emboli (Browse 1978) and if we are to compare studies with each other we must be absolutely clear what end-point was taken to indicate venous thrombosis or embolism. We cannot compare two studies, one of which used ^{125}I labelled fibrinogen to detect calf-vein thrombosis, while the other used venography to detect thigh-vein thrombosis; nor can we compare a study on pulmonary embolism using an angiographic end-point with one which relied on the imperfect evidence provided by ventilation-perfusion isotope scanning of the lungs.

5   *Fact of death versus opinion about the cause of death.* If a condition is common and produces a fatal outcome then successful prevention should be reflected in the total death rate. If a regime does not reduce death rate then it is either ineffective or its beneficial effects on a particular cause of death are being swamped by deaths from other, unmodified conditions. We found (Morris and Mitchell 1976b) as had Salzman, Harris and De Sanctis (1966) that this was so in elderly women with fractured hips, where pulmonary embolism was eliminated by anticoagulation without the total death rate being significantly reduced.

Whereas total deaths form an objective end-point, deaths attributed by the pathologist to pulmonary embolism form an unacceptably subjective end-point. If a patient with advanced neoplastic disease, with massive myocardial infarction or with a major fracture, is found to have a pulmonary embolus at necropsy, how is blame to be apportioned between the alternative causes of death? Will the attribution be influenced by knowledge of the treatment that such a patient has had? These uncertainties are reflected in the inconclusive results of the multicentre trial on low-dose heparin after surgical operation (International Multicentre Trial 1975) where total deaths were not significantly different in the treated and untreated groups, whereas the deaths attributed to pulmonary emboli were different.

Heart attacks

These patient should pose no problems, since even in lay usage myocardial infarction has become equated with 'coronary thrombosis'. The reality is very different, and from the ill-assorted conditions lumped together as 'ischaemic heart disease', 'coronary heart/artery disease' and 'atherosclerotic heart disease', inevitable conflict has emerged about the role of thrombosis. Some workers argue that thrombosis is always present in patients dying after heart attacks (Harland and Holburn 1966), some argue that it is present but that it is a mere secondary consequence of the real events in the myocardium (Spain and Bradess 1960), while other workers deny that thrombi or wall disease are necessary accompaniments of the disease (Baroldi *et al.* 1974). As so often happens in such disagreements, all of them may be right, but they are talking about dissimilar processes. We must therefore break down the all-embracing 'ischaemic heart disease' into coherent subunits as follows:

1 *Myocardial infarction.* There is general agreement that patients who develop cardiac pain lasting for several hours, accompanied by *Q* waves and/or serial T and S-T segment changes in the ECG and by increased concentrations of cardiac enzymes, will be found at necropsy to have large areas of cardiac necrosis. Such patients will have severe coronary atheroma and will have at least one artery occluded by fresh thrombus (Mitchell and Schwartz 1965, Chandler *et al.* 1974). Thus an episode of transmural infarction serves as a valid indicator of thrombosis. Patients with transmural infarcts may die suddenly and can thus become confused with patients with unheralded sudden death. In such patients the findings at necropsy will depend on the interval between infarction and death, for within a few days an occluding recognizable thrombus can be transformed into a non-occluding or less characteristic mass (Mitchell and Schwartz 1965, Lichtlen and Engel 1978).

2 *Unheralded sudden death* differs from myocardial infarction at necropsy in that cardiac necrosis and coronary thrombi are not found (Schwartz and Gerrity 1975), although severe coronary atheroma is (Perper, Kuller and Cooper 1975). Although the role of microthrombi as a source of emboli is uncertain in these patients (Haerem 1972) unheralded sudden death has not been thought of as a thrombotic disease but new studies are now showing that plaque disruption often accompanied by thrombosis is commonly found in cardiac sudden death (Davies, Woolf and Robertson 1976).

3 *Heart failure and arrhythmias* can occur as a consequence of myocardial infarction, but can also have their origin in a wide variety of other cardiac diseases, some of which may have been unwisely included in 'ischaemic heart

disease' in the past. For example, focal areas of necrosis or scarring, which are often called 'small infarcts' by unwary pathologists and which may be responsible for arrhythmias such as Stokes–Adams attacks, are not directly related either to coronary atheroma or to thrombosis (Mitchell and Schwartz 1965). None of these manifestations (heart failure, arrhythmias or small areas of necrosis or scarring) should therefore be used as an indicator of thrombosis or of the failure of antithrombotic regimens.

In the field of 'ischaemic heart disease', only transmural cardiac infarction can therefore be used as a valid indicator of thrombosis in seeking patients to study for blood abnormalities in thrombotic disease or in collecting patients for clinical trials of potential antithrombotic drugs.

Strokes

If the study of heart disease perplexes the worker in the field of thrombosis, 'strokes' or 'cerebrovascular accidents' will confuse him even more. No great skill is required to perceive that a sudden neurological deficit, affecting limbs, speech or vision, has occurred. Attributing this episode to its true cause, however, calls for skills and for techniques which may not be available in those hospitals where the bulk of stroke episodes present.

As with 'heart attacks' we must progressively dissect 'strokes' until we find coherent subgroups which fulfil our criteria. We must discard two groups:

1 *Pseudo-strokes.* Cerebral tumours, abscesses, subdural haematomas, subarachnoid haemorrhages, epilepsy and hypoglycaemia may all present with focal neurological deficit of sudden onset which we must separate from true strokes.

2 *Primary intracerebral haemorrhage* arises from the rupture of minute, miliary aneurysms on arterioles in the brain substance. They were first described by Charcot and Bouchard (1868) and their significance and close relationship to age and to arterial hypertension have been re-emphasized (Russell 1963, Cole and Yates 1967). One would not wish to include patients with a vessel-rupturing, bleeding disorder in groups of patients thought to have thrombotic disease. At the present time, however, it is difficult to prevent this from happening, since it is not possible to separate cerebral haemorrhage from cerebral infarction on the basis of history and physical findings. The absence of neck stiffness and of blood from the cerebrospinal fluid (CSF) does not exclude intracerebral bleeding, since these signs indicate only that the haemorrhage has not been massive enough to break through into the ventricles. This is why the term 'athero-thrombotic brain infarction' (ABI) used in the Framingham surveys gives false precision to what should properly be called 'strokes with non-haemorrhagic CSF' (Kannel 1976). The advent of computerized axial tomography (CT scanning) represents a most important advance in stroke technology and it could be argued that access to CT scanning is mandatory for any study that attempts to link tests of thrombotic

behaviour with strokes or sets out to monitor the value of potential antithrombotic agents in the prevention of cerebral infarction.

Having identified patients with cerebral infarction, all should then be crystal clear. Unhappily, it is not, because two disparate events can produce infarction. First, a thrombus may form *in situ* in the cranial supply vessels, and, as in the coronary tree, this commonly occurs in association with severely diseased vessel walls, so the thrombi have the characteristic structure of arterial thrombi elsewhere. This group is thus the counterpart of transmural myocardial infarction in which there is subtending thrombotic occlusion of a diseased coronary artery. A second sort of occlusion occurs—namely an embolism. In many of the studies reported, emboli are thought to account for 60–70 per cent of cerebral infarcts (Adams and Vander Eecken 1953, Lhermitte, Gautier and Derouesné 1970). These emboli are of many and diverse kinds; some arise in the stagnant or slow-flow stream in the atria of patients with valvular disease and fibrillation, thus resembling venous thrombi and like them being influenced by anticoagulation. Some arise on the surface of transmural cardiac infarcts, while others form on the valves, as in bacterial or in non-bacterial endocarditis. Others form in the neck vessels themselves, especially the carotid sinus, and embolize. Finally, atheromatous material from neck artery plaques may embolize to the eye or brain, without any thrombotic element being involved. Thus cerebral infarction does not constitute a single coherent condition but is caused by thrombosis *in situ* and by a wide range of diseases where emboli of differing types come from different sources.

Short-lived episodes of functional deficit, which are labelled as transient ischaemic attacks (TIA), are even more complex. In some neurological centres the deficit must last for less than one hour to be classified as a TIA, whereas in the majority, attacks lasting up to 24 hours are put into the TIA category. In comparing results from different studies, the duration of the reported episodes must be carefully noted. The pattern of disease in the subtending neck vessels in TIAs differs markedly from that found in completed strokes, and thus the nature of the embolic masses that form could well differ (Harrison and Marshall 1976). Finally, it is not always easy to separate transient episodes that have an embolic or occlusive origin from other short-lived neurological problems, such as epilepsy, migraine, hypoglycaemia, and hypotension. If one wishes to use TIAs to study the nature of thrombotic disease or the effect of potential antithrombotic agents, the episodes must be defined very precisely by specifying the following:

1 The precise territory involved—the eye as in amaurosis fugax, the hemisphere or the brain-stem;
2 the precise duration of the deficit;
3 the state of neck arteries where this is known;
4 the nature of any cardiac lesions or arrhythmias.

Peripheral arterial disease

The accessibility of the limbs to clinical assessment or investigation and the ready availability of material derived from amputations and necropsies should have provided more information about peripheral arterial disease than we have succeeded in collecting about inaccessible organs such as the brain or heart. Perhaps the early development of surgical techniques (the centuries-old amputation, this century's sympathectomy and this generation's direct attack on vessels) has diverted attention away from basic pathology. If no effective treatment is available, as in stroke and heart attack, there is a strong incentive to collect basic information. In conditions for which treatment is thought to be available, basic research may, however, be neglected.

Like angina, intermittent claudication is a symptom and not a disease. Its natural history is variable (*British Medical Journal* 1976), it does not of itself kill, and the clinical methods available to assess peripheral pulses and flow are inaccurate and subject to observer error (Meade *et al.* 1968, Coffman 1972). Objective measurements of vascular patency, such as arteriography or plethysmography, can never be applied to large-scale field studies because they are either expensive in time and money or are not free from danger.

The limb can have its equivalent of TIAs, where digits can become temporarily malperfused. Like cerebral TIAs, such ischaemia is not necessarily thrombotic. Functional malperfusion caused by cold and by β-blocking agents, can give 'limb TIAs' while the major supply vessels remain patent. Local arteritis due to collagen disease can produce ischaemia even though the supply arteries are free from thrombi. Emboli of a variety of non-thrombotic types (atheromatous debris and bacterial vegetations from heart valves) can produce peripheral ischaemia and, finally, even if one is confident that a major vessel is occluded by a thrombotic embolus, it could be a slow-flow clot-like mass from a fibrillating atrium or a fast-flow, platelet–leucocyte–fibrin mass from the surface of a severely diseased aorta.

Once 'infarction' of the limb has occurred, the gangrenous extremity does not of itself lead to death. Removal of an infarcted limb, unlike the infarcted heart or brain, is compatible with survival, so the subsequent prognosis will depend on factors unrelated to the initial episode, for stroke and heart attack play a key role in determining the outcome in patients with claudication or gangrene (Singer and Rob 1960).

We cannot, therefore use the ischaemic limb as a direct guide to the presence of an arterial thrombus; claudication is a subjective symptom, temporary ischaemia can be confirmed objectively but has many causes, and gangrene can result from thrombosis *in situ* or from emboli of various kinds. Similarly, one cannot use survival after reconstructive surgery or amputation as an index of the natural history of limb artery thrombosis, since survival will largely be determined by subsequent heart attack and stroke. It has been assumed that the graft- or prosthesis-patency rate can be used as a measure of the tendency to re-thrombosis. However, artificial prostheses present an unnatural surface to the circulating blood and we cannot infer that when they become occluded the process is identical with spontaneous thrombosis in a diseased artery. Thus the patient who has had reconstructive surgery may be more akin to the injured-artery animal model (Honour and Mitchell 1964) than to the patient who develops spontaneous thrombotic occlusion in a diseased coronary or cerebral vessel and who then dies of a heart attack or stroke.

Conclusion

Thrombosis is a pathological process and can be identified with complete certainty only at necropsy or biopsy. Clinical and epidemiological labels are given by drawing inferences about the presence of thrombotic disease and, as we have seen, the confidence we can attach to these inferential labels varies widely from organ to organ. Unless we strive for precision, we will pay the price of perpetual uncertainty and confusion. If we cannot be precise, we should not shelter behind labels which give a false sense of accuracy. We should use clinical labels to describe clinical events, descriptive labels to characterize investigational results and reserve the pathological label of 'thrombosis' for situations in which we can prove without doubt or can infer with a high degree of certainty that a thrombus is present.

PATTERN OF PLATELET BEHAVIOUR IN THROMBOSIS

For centuries, it had been known that when blood was shed from blood vessels, either by injury or by the very common practice of blood-letting, it rapidly solidified. The mechanism that brought about this transformation was shown to reside in the blood plasma, so the concept of the evolution of a stringy material, fibrin, from a soluble precursor, fibrinogen, was readily established. The microscopes of the day also allowed the red and white cells to be characterized, but it was not until 1842 that a third type of blood cell, which we now know as the platelet, was first identified by Gulliver and by Addison (Robb-Smith 1967). Both these workers also noticed that fibrin strands developed around and between the platelets, so the seeds of the present controversy (do clotting and thrombotic mechanisms stimulate the platelets or do stimulated platelets activate the clotting–thrombotic system?) were sown at this very early stage. The relevance of these observations to *in vivo* events after injury was made clear by Wharton Jones in 1850, Bizzozero in 1882 and Schimmelbusch in 1885 (Robb-Smith 1967) who showed that when a vessel wall was breached or injured, the platelets adhered to the site and to each other, and the growing mass then became scaffolded by fibrin strands. It is curious that, despite the simultaneous recognition by Virchow in 1845 that the process of thrombosis or spontaneous blood solidification within the living blood vessels played an important part in human arterial and venous disease (Brinkhous 1969), interest in platelets rapidly waned after this initial creative era. In 1961 it was possible for Poole and French to remind readers that even 'in 1899 Welch had occasion to complain of the old and still common conception that a thrombus is essentially a blood coagulum'. They went on to comment that, 'so far, there is only a very little to add to the sum of knowledge available in the 1880s'.

The last 20 years have seen an explosive re-awakening of interest in platelets; attempts have been made to define the role of platelets in thrombus formation and to identify platelet abnormalities that might account for the fact that some individuals experience thrombotic events whereas others do not. However, studies of platelet reactivity in relation to thrombosis are not as simple as they might appear.

It is only possible to obtain detailed information about platelets after they have been removed from the body, exposed to foreign surfaces and anticoagulants, and separated from other blood cells. Once removed from the body they are studied in the absence of a vessel wall and thus of mechanisms in or on the vessel walls that might influence the way in which they behave. Thrombi contain fibrin as well as platelets, so studies of platelets in the absence of an intact coagulation pathway can only give us part of the information that is relevant to thrombus formation in that fibrin cannot be generated. In addition, anticoagulants can themselves influence the way in which platelets behave. Heparin induces aggregation (Eika 1972); citrate, by reducing the level of ionized calcium in the plasma, influences both the extent to which platelets aggregate and the extent to which they undergo release reactions (Macfarlane *et al.* 1975, Heptinstall and Mulley 1977, Heptinstall and Taylor 1979); EDTA completely inhibits those aspects of platelet behaviour that rely on some extracellular calcium being present (Born and Cross 1963). Because of these problems we should describe what we observe under such artificial conditions as platelet behaviour, and we must be aware that studies of platelet behaviour may only give a distorted reflection of true platelet functions.

Platelets are often studied in platelet-rich plasma (PRP), that is, in the absence of red cells and white cells, both of which can modify platelet behaviour. Platelet-rich plasma is prepared by differential centrifugation of the blood that has been collected. Imagine a situation in which a subpopulation of platelets that are hyperaggregable have clumped together (either before or after the blood was withdrawn) and are then removed from the remaining platelets along with the red and white cells during the preparation procedure.

In such a situation the platelets that were studied would not be representative of the platelets in the circulation.

Another problem relates to the timing of the platelet studies in relation to the thrombotic event. Most studies are carried out either during or after the thrombotic event, but at this stage one does not know whether any platelet abnormality is the cause of the event or a consequence of it. It would be better to study platelet behaviour before thrombosis occurred but such an approach is a formidable undertaking, expensive in both labour and time. A happy medium could involve a group of patients (e.g. those with diabetes or hyperlipidaemia) who are at high risk of developing vascular problems, but in this case any platelet abnormality might be a consequence of the existing disease and be unrelated to subsequent vascular complications.

It is possible to identify four aspects of platelet behaviour that may be relevant to their involvement in thrombosis: their ability to adhere to foreign surfaces, to aggregate, to undergo their various release reactions and to synthesize prostaglandins and thromboxanes. As we consider the progress that has been made through the study of each of these aspects of platelet behaviour, the reader will become aware of many other problems that make the study of platelets in relation to thrombosis a difficult task.

Adhesion of platelets to foreign surfaces

Platelets do not adhere to the normal endothelial lining of blood vessels but they do adhere to the subendothelial structures that are exposed when vascular tissue is damaged. The process is a complex one involving participation of platelet surface glycoproteins, plasma factors (including the von Willebrand factor), divalent cations and perhaps fibronectin, as well as collagen and other structures within the subendothelial layer. In itself this adhesive process may not be a disadvantage for a monolayer of platelets at a point of damage may help to protect the vasculature and secure haemostasis. Studies using injured rabbit arteries, however, have revealed that the formation of a platelet monolayer can be followed by the growth of larger masses so that thrombus formation results (Baumgartner 1974).

Platelets also have an affinity for artificial surfaces and this affinity may represent the initial stimulus to thrombus formation on artificial heart valves and prosthetic grafts. The factors that contribute to platelet–artificial surface interactions are less well understood than are the factors that lead to platelet deposition on subendothelium.

Measurements of the adhesiveness of platelets to artificial surfaces as a means of detecting a thrombotic crasis in the blood stem from the observation made by Wright (1941) that the number of platelets in anticoagulated blood fell progressively when the glass container holding the blood was rotated. This was believed to be due to the adhesion of platelets to the walls of the flask and Wright (1942) demonstrated that the platelet count fell at a greater rate in the post-partum and post-operative periods, a time when venous thrombosis is common. She thus provided suggestive evidence that measurements of platelet adhesiveness *in vitro* might reflect the tendency to thrombosis. Although we now know that in a rotating glass vessel it is the blood–air interface that causes platelet aggregation rather than the blood–glass interface (Page and Mitchell 1979), the observations of Wright were a stimulus for much work in this area. What has this work achieved?

Perhaps the acid test of success is the answer to the question, 'Would anyone now attempting to study the relation between platelets and thrombosis embark on studies of platelet adhesiveness?' We suspect that very few investigators would do so. Even if they were confident that they were using a procedure that was giving a measure of platelet adhesiveness (and most procedures fall far short of this ideal), and even though they applied the strictest control over experimental method, they would probably find that the range of values obtained for platelets from one healthy individual studied repeatedly would encompass the values obtained for most patients with thrombotic disease (Page and Mitchell 1979). Previous studies suggest that investigators may find that while mean platelet adhesiveness for a group of patients with thrombosis (acute myocardial infarction—Bygdeman and Wells 1969) or for a group of patients at risk of thrombosis (diabetes—Shaw *et al.* 1967) is higher than for a group without thrombosis, there would be a considerable overlap with the controls so they would not be able to relate increased adhesiveness to the thrombotic event in any individual. The uncertainty of the mechanisms involved in the adhesion of platelet to artificial surfaces, its variability and the failure of such measurements as a diagnostic tool have thus combined to discourage investigators.

Perhaps studies of platelet adhesiveness to damaged vasculature would prove of more value than studies of their interaction with artificial surfaces such as glass.

Platelet aggregation

Since it was found that adenosine diphosphate (ADP) and other agents induce platelets to aggregate together to form macroscopic clumps, interest has centred on the contribution of platelet aggregation to thrombosis. Certainly, it is known that aggregating agents such as ADP, adrenaline, noradrenaline, serotonin, prostaglandin G_2, prostaglandin H_2, thromboxane A_2, collagen and thrombin are present in circulating blood from time to time and platelet aggregates are seen in thrombi. However, what we do not know is whether the platelets are the prime movers in thrombus formation or whether they are merely attracted to a developing thrombus, like accident spectators who come to survey the scene. Does ADP or another aggregating agent produce platelet aggregation which in turn gives rise to procoagulant activity and fibrin formation? Or does platelet involvement occur after the coagulation cascade has been activated, since thrombin is a potent aggregating agent in its own right? The order of events is important because the way in which thrombus formation might be prevented will depend on it.

Platelet aggregation in PRP

Most studies of platelet aggregation involve the use of PRP because in this medium, platelet aggregation can be measured conveniently using aggregometers that record changes in light absorbance (Born 1962, Adams, Heptinstall and Mitchell 1975). Platelet aggregometry is a crude technique in that large clumps of platelets that are visible to the naked eye need to form before the amount of light transmitted through PRP changes. The 'aggregation traces' that are obtained thus reflect the size of the clumps and in no way represent the reaction-kinetics of the chemical processes accompanying aggregation. They have proved useful for assessing agents that induce aggregation and agents that inhibit it, but they have proved less useful as a means of identifying a thrombotic crasis in the blood.

I. SPONTANEOUS PLATELET AGGREGATION

Platelet aggregation can sometimes occur spontaneously when PRP is stirred. The aggregates are often very small and produce only slight changes in light absorbance, making spontaneous aggregation difficult to detect. The formation of the aggregates is presumably a consequence of some aspect of the preparation procedure. In most instances in which spontaneous aggregation has been observed, the PRP has contained citrate as the anticoagulant. Citrate encourages release reaction B (see below), and as both release reaction B and spontaneous aggregation can be inhibited by aspirin, perhaps spontaneous aggregation in stirred PRP relates to the anticoagulant that has been used.

Some investigators have claimed that spontaneous platelet aggregation is common after myocardial infarction (Zahavi and Dreyfuss 1969, Wu and Hoak 1976, Zahavi 1977), after ischaemic stroke and transient ischaemic attacks (Petrova, Pavlishchuk and Grigoriev 1975, Ten Cate *et al.* 1978) and that it occurs in PRP from some patients with venous thrombosis and peripheral vascular disease (Vreeken and van Aken 1971, Preston *et al.* 1974, Scrobohaci, Cunescu and Orha 1976, Wu and Hoak 1976). In contrast, it is only rarely seen in PRP from asymptomatic individuals (Kardinal, Wegener and Anderson 1975). Despite this, at the present time few publications that relate to spontaneous aggregation in stirred PRP are appearing in the literature. Perhaps this is because most investigators, including ourselves, have difficulty in demonstrating it except in occasional samples of PRP. This, in turn, may relate to its time-dependence; Wu and Hoak (1976) have indicated that it can only be observed for a short period after the blood has been taken and PRP has been prepared. Perhaps those investigators who would have continued to study it were diverted by the wave of enthusiasm that resulted from development in 1974 of a technique that purported to measure 'circulating' platelet aggregates rather than those that merely formed *in vitro* (see below).

2. AGENT-INDUCED PLATELET AGGREGATION

Although spontaneous aggregation in PRP is difficult to measure, the aggregation induced by agents such as ADP, adrenaline and collagen is not, since large clumps form in response to these agents and characteristic changes in light absorbance are obtained. When low (about 10^{-6}M) concentrations of ADP are added to PRP, the light absorbance of the sample falls, and then within two or three minutes begins to rise again to its starting value. The aggregation that is induced is thus reversible. When higher (about 10^{-5}M) concentrations of ADP are added to PRP, the light absorbance rapidly falls to a value that is close to that of platelet-free plasma. In this case the aggregation is irreversible. An intermediate concentration of ADP can sometimes be found at which aggregation occurs in two phases. An initial fall in light absorbance is followed by a period during which the light absorbance remains fairly steady before falling to a value close to that of platelet-free plasma. It is when the concentration of ADP is sufficient to induce this two-phase response or irreversible aggregation that a platelet release reaction occurs. The more extensive aggregation that occurs under these conditions is thought to result from the liberation of aggregating agents from intracellular storage granules during the release reaction and from the synthesis of proaggregatory prostaglandins and thromboxanes that occurs in association with the release reaction. Adrenaline produces aggregation traces that are similar to those produced by ADP. Collagen, however, differs in that it induces only a single, irreversible, phase of aggregation that is closely associated with the simul-taneous occurrence of a release reaction. Most of the attempts that have been made to detect abnormalities of aggregation in association with thrombosis have relied on analysis of the aggregation traces obtained using one or other of these three agents.

Unfortunately, although agent-induced aggregation is easy to observe, it suffers from several drawbacks as a tool for thrombosis research. As well as depending on the nature of the aggregating agent, its concentration, obvious factors such as the temperature at which the determinations are made and the number of platelets in the sample under investigation, the extent of aggregation also depends on the type and concentration of anticoagulant that is used and on the bench age of the PRP (Harrison, Emmons and Mitchell 1967, Warlow *et al.* 1974). Variable numbers of white cells in the preparation also influence the results that are obtained (Harrison, Emmons and Mitchell 1966). Thus, unless extreme care is taken in standardizing the technique, comparative studies of platelet aggregability are meaningless. The situation is made even worse by the inherent variability of aggregation in response to factors over which the investigator may have little control. It is influenced by physical exercise and mental stress (Harrison, Emmons and Mitchell 1967) and by commonly used drugs such as aspirin (O'Brien 1968, Weiss, Aledort and Kochwa 1968, Zucker and Peterson 1968). Perhaps it is not surprising, therefore, that studies of platelet aggregation in relation to thrombotic disease have not been definitive.

After a thrombotic event we might expect platelets to exhibit one of several types of behaviour. Firstly, they might be hyperactive and so aggregate more readily in response to a stimulus. This might reflect platelet hyperactivity as a contribution to the event or it might be a consequence of the event. Secondly, platelets might aggregate normally, or thirdly, they might be hypoactive and aggregate less readily in response to a stimulus. This might occur if a subpopulation of hyperactive platelets had been consumed in thrombus formation or had been lost during preparation of PRP, leaving less reactive platelets for examination. Platelets might also be hypoaggregable because they are 'exhausted', in that they have been utilized during thrombus formation and have subsequently returned to the circulation. Such a situation would parallel the well-known refractoriness of platelets to an aggregating agent after they have been activated by that agent *in vitro*. Finally, platelets might aggregate normally because platelet hyperactivity might not be a fundamental requirement for thrombus formation.

What has actually been observed? Unfortunately, and perhaps because of the difficulties inherent in measuring platelet aggregation, we are unable to supply a definitive answer. The consensus of opinion is that results obtained for groups of patients studied during or following events that have been designated thrombotic in origin (myocardial infarction, occlusive stroke, TIAs) indicate that platelets aggregate rather more extensively to ADP and to adrenaline than do platelets from groups of healthy volunteers (O'Brien, Heywood and Heady 1966, Zahavi and Dreyfuss 1969, Dreyfuss and Zahavi 1973, Petrova, Pavlischuk and Grigoriev 1975, Yamazaki, Takahashi and Sano 1975, Couch and Hassanein 1976, Dougherty, Levy and Weksler 1977) and tend to disaggregate less readily (Davis 1973). The concentration of ADP required to induce second phase aggregation in PRP tends to be lower than normal (Danta 1970, Anderson and Gormsen 1977, Lou *et al.* 1977) and platelets aggregate in response to lower concentrations of collagen than are normally required (Salky and Dugdale 1973). On the other hand, some investigators have been unable to demonstrate platelet hyperactivity in such circumstances and one group of workers believe that platelets are hypoactive rather than hyperactive immediately after myocardial infarction, platelet reactivity returning during the next few days (Knudsen *et al.* 1979). All measures of platelet reactivity after an acute painful episode should be interpreted with caution because pain-relieving drugs that the patient may have taken could have affected the results. The effect of aspirin on platelet reactivity, for instance, lasts for some ten days. In our own studies we have found that the extent of the ADP-induced release reaction (see below) is a more reliable indicator of recent aspirin ingestion than is the ability of the individual who donated the platelets to recall having taken it.

Some of the investigators who have observed platelet hyperaggregability shortly after an acute thrombotic episode believe it to be a transient phenomenon while others claim to have observed platelet hyperaggregability in some patients long after the acute event, so the question of cause or consequence remains unresolved. Platelet hyperaggregability would appear to be associated with hyperlipoproteinaemia (Colman 1977) and with diabetes (Colwell and Halushka 1980), conditions in which the risk of vascular disease in individual patients is high. But whether the platelet hyperaggregability is a cause of subsequent thrombotic events or is merely a reflection of the existing disease is not clear.

Circulating platelet aggregates

In 1974 Wu and Hoak developed a test that claimed to measure the number of platelet aggregates in circulating blood by collecting blood into two tubes, one containing EDTA and formaldehyde and another containing only EDTA. Platelet aggregates are readily dissociated by EDTA but it was thought that this would not occur when pre-formed aggregates are stabilized by a fixative such as formaldehyde. The tubes are then centrifuged to obtain PRP. Any aggregates in the tube that contains formaldehyde will be removed from the PRP during the centrifugation procedure, so the ratio of the number of individual platelets in the two samples has been taken to indicate the number of platelet aggregates in the blood as it was collected. Studies in a number of subjects revealed ratios in some patients with arterial insufficiency which differed from controls and it was concluded that these patients had 'circulating' platelet aggregates in their blood. Two questions arise. First, are such aggregates really circulating? Second, what is the relation between them and vascular disease?

Unfortunately there is no way of knowing whether such aggregates are circulating or not. Since blood comes into contact with foreign surfaces in the needle, the syringe and the tubes into which it is collected, and since foreign surfaces activate blood platelets, the very act of obtaining the blood might have caused the aggregates to form. Blood that flows directly from a peripheral vein, through a needle and then through a polythene tube and over a glass slide, contains large platelet aggregates that are readily visible through the microscope. We find it difficult to imagine that such clumps are pre-formed in the circulation.

The literature on the relation between 'circulating' platelet aggregates and vascular disease does not convince us that the technique has given a great deal of useful information. Contradictory reports abound. Some investigators have demonstrated platelet ratios to be abnormal after myocardial infarction, cerebral infarction and TIAs but others have not (compare the reports of Gjesdal 1976 and Mehta and Mehta 1979 with those of Prazitch *et al.* 1977 and Dalal *et al.* 1982). Kumpuris *et al.* (1980) found 'circulating' platelet aggregates in peripheral venous blood after exercise-induced angina but Dalal *et al.* (1982) could not confirm this. They concluded that methodological differences may be responsible for the different results in different laboratories. Although they could not find abnormal ratios in stable angina, Dalal *et al.* did find them in blood from those with unstable angina but, again, this contradicted the finding of Guyton and Willerson (1977).

The report of Lowe *et al.* (1979) suggests that abnormal platelet ratios are only a reflection of the high plasma fibrinogen levels that result from both vascular and non-vascular illness. On the one hand, this indicates that the measurements may not be telling us anything about vascular disease specifically, but on the other hand the finding is of interest because epidemiological investigations have linked high fibrinogen levels with coronary heart disease (Meade *et al.* 1980).

Platelet release reactions

Several materials that may contribute towards thrombosis are stored within intracellular granules in platelets and are liberated when platelets undergo their various release reactions. There are probably three types of intracellular granules: α granules, dense bodies and lysosomes (Fukami and Salganicoff 1977). The α granules contain β-thromboglobulin (βTG) and platelet factor 4 (PF4, a protein that has heparin-neutralizing activity) and it is likely that fibrinogen, together with a mitogenic factor for vascular cells and a factor that enhances vascular permeability, are also stored within them. The contents of the dense bodies include ADP, ATP, serotonin, calcium ions and probably adrenaline, noradrenaline and antiplasmin. The lysosomes contain hydrolases. Thus the materials that can be liberated from the cells include platelet aggregating agents, procoagulants, cofactors for aggregation and coagulation pathways, a mitogen, and factors that can influence vascular permeability both specifically and non-specifically.

Types of release reaction

Despite Holmsen's (1972, 1975) attempt to indicate that two types of release reaction exist, most publications refer to '*the* platelet release reaction' as though only one such event can occur. However, published evidence would now indicate that there are at least three types of release reaction which we will refer to as types A, B and C. In type A, only the contents of the α granules are liberated from the cells; in type B the contents of the dense bodies as well as the α granules are liberated; type C involves liberation of material from all three types of granule.

Release reaction A occurs whenever platelets are subjected to mild trauma. It occurs when blood is collected into an anticoagulant (Ludlam and Cash 1976) such as heparin, citrate, or EDTA (i.e. those anticoagulants that are routinely used for studies of platelet behaviour) and when blood is passed through a bubble oxygenator in patients undergoing cardio-pulmonary bypass surgery (Harker *et al.* 1980). Although only a small proportion of the platelets' store of granule contents is liberated during release reaction A, its occurrence has complicated attempts to estimate the extent to which platelets have been activated to undergo a release reaction *in vivo*. The amounts of βTG or of PF4 that are liberated during blood collection can be reduced by including an activator of adenylate cyclase (such as prostaglandin E_1) and an inhibitor of cyclic AMP phosphodiesterase (such as theophylline) in the anticoagulant (usually EDTA) and by rapidly cooling the sample of blood that has been collected (Ludlam and Cash 1976, Borsey *et al.* 1980, Franchi, Canciani and Mannucci 1980, Randi *et al.* 1981). Whether this procedure always prevents release reaction A, such that the level of βTG or PF4 in the plasma obtained from blood collected under such circumstances is a good reflection of the circulating level of the protein, is not clear. Another complicating factor is that a poor venepuncture can give rise to liberation of βTG and PF4 from the cells and Zahavi and Kakkar (1979) have warned against accepting high plasma levels of these proteins (even in blood collected into the anticoagulant mixture referred to above) as an indication of high circulating levels of these proteins unless the levels are consistently high in repeated determinations. Our own view is that even when consistently high values are obtained one cannot be sure that it is not the propensity of platelets to undergo release reaction A during venepuncture that is being measured rather than the true circulating level of the protein. Aspirin and other non-steroidal anti-inflammatory agents inhibit release reaction B, and partially inhibit release reaction C, but have no effect on release reaction A (see below). It is interesting, therefore, that neither aspirin nor sulphinpyrazone convincingly reduce plasma βTG or PF4 levels (Han *et al.* 1979, Kaplan *et al.* 1979, Ludlam *et al.* 1979a, Cortellaro *et al.* 1981, White and Marouf 1981).

Release reaction B can occur when platelets are induced to aggregate by agents such as ADP, adrenaline and low concentrations of collagen and thrombin and is equivalent to Holmsen's type I. When it occurs, the platelet aggregating agents that are stored in the dense bodies are liberated along with the constituents of the α granules (Kaplan *et al.* 1979) and can contribute to further aggregation. The second phase of the aggregation that can result when ADP or adrenaline is added to PRP is closely associated with the occurrence of release reaction B, and the extent of the aggregation that is induced by low concentrations of collagen is also closely related to the extent to which the release reaction occurs.

The extent to which release reaction B occurs in response to aggregating agents can be determined by measuring the amount of one of the dense body constituents that is liberated. Measurements of liberated ATP, serotonin and calcium ions have been used for this purpose, although measurements of the latter are only appropriate to platelet suspensions that contain less than about 50 μM calcium outside the cells because higher levels mask the relatively small amounts of calcium that are released. The most convenient means of determining the extent of release reaction B is to label platelets with ^{14}C- or ^{3}H-serotonin and to measure the amount of radiolabel that is ejected from the cells when the release reaction occurs. Platelets are effectively labelled by simply adding radiolabelled serotonin to blood or PRP when an active transport system rapidly transfers the serotonin to the inside of the cell. Provided that less than 1 μM serotonin is added to the platelet preparation all of the radiolabel is incorporated into the dense bodies (Costa and Murphy 1976).

Release reaction C (equivalent to Holmsen's type II) cannot be induced by ADP or adrenaline, but is induced by high concentrations of collagen or thrombin. As far as we are aware, measurements of the extent to which release reaction C occurs (by, for instance, measuring the amount of N-acetylglucos-aminidase that is liberated from lysosomes within the cells) have not yet been utilized in the search for platelet abnormalities in association with thrombosis.

Measurements of release in clinical practice

1.   BETA-TG AND PF4

The development of sensitive radioimmunoassays for the α granule consti-tuents βTG and PF4 led to several attempts to measure the levels of these proteins in blood plasma from different patient groups with a view to determining the extent to which platelets had been activated *in vivo*. It was thought that high levels might indicate significant platelet activation. Unfortunately, in nearly all the studies that have been carried out, a wide scatter of results has been obtained, and although mean values for groups of patients deemed to have thrombosis or to be at risk of thrombosis are usually higher than the mean values obtained for groups of individuals without vascular disease (Handin, McDonough and Lesch 1978, Zahavi and Kakkar 1979, Kutti *et al.* 1981, Levine *et al.* 1981, White and Marouf 1981, Zahavi *et al.* 1981), the tests have proved of little diagnostic or prognostic value. Thus we consider that measurements of βTG and PF4 have proved of no more value than those of platelet adhesion or of platelet aggregation.

2.   HEPARIN NEUTRALIZING ACTIVITY

Before radioimmunoassays for PF4 became available it could only be measured through its ability to neutralize heparin and thus alter the heparin-thrombin clotting time. Like PF4, the heparin neutralizing activity of plasma has been shown to be high in plasma taken from patients after myocardial infarction (O'Brien *et al.* 1975, Dana *et al.* 1976), from patients with peripheral vascular disease (Cella *et al.* 1979) and in association with deep venous thrombosis (O'Brien, Etherington and Shuttleworth 1977). Again, however, a wide scatter of results is always obtained. There is now some concern as to whether PF4 measured by radioimmunoassay and heparin neutralizing activity measurements are giving the same information since simultaneous measurements in plasmas derived from several individuals do not correlate with each other (Ludlam *et al.* 1979b).

3.   SEROTONIN

Measurements of the extent of the ADP-induced release reaction in PRP from a number of different individuals using ^{3}H- or ^{14}C-serotonin to adjudge its extent have revealed (Heptinstall and Mulley 1977) the following:
(i)   It is donor dependent. In PRP from some donors, ADP is much more effective in inducing a release reaction than in PRP from others.
(ii)   There is an inverse relation between the extent of the release reaction induced by a single high concentration of ADP and the amount of ADP that is required to induce irreversible aggregation, so the extent of the release reaction relates to the sensitivity of platelets to ADP.
(iii)   Two-phase aggregation in response to intermediate concentrations of ADP can only be observed when the release reaction is extensive. Thus the second phase of the aggregation induced by ADP is closely related to the occurrence of the release reaction.

(iv)   The extent of the release reaction depends on the type and concentration of anticoagulant in the platelet preparation (Heptinstall and Taylor 1979). In particular, the presence of citrate in the preparation increases the extent to which the release reaction occurs. On rare occasions, citrate can induce platelets to undergo a release reaction even in the absence of ADP. This effect of citrate is probably mediated via a reduced concentration of extracellular calcium ions in the plasma.

These observations prompted Heptinstall *et al.* (1980b) to measure the extent of the ADP-induced release reaction in PRP from patients who had just experienced a myocardial infarction. In view of the problems associated with the use of citrate they used heparin as an anticoagulant. The mean extent of the release reaction for the 26 patients was higher than that obtained for the group of healthy controls but the difference did not achieve statistical significance. Follow-up showed, however, that the results obtained for the patients who died within a year of infarction differed significantly from those who survived. The release reaction was extensive in PRP from six of the seven who died but only in four of the 18 who survived; thus an extensive release reaction was a marker of poor prognosis. The results gave no indication as to whether the extensive release reaction in these patients resulted from or pre-dated the myocardial infarction.

Prostaglandin and thromboxane synthesis

The most abundant precursor of prostaglandins and thromboxanes in platelets is arachidonic acid (Fig. 49). It can be released from membrane phospholipid directly via phospholipase A_2 (Bills, Smith and Silver 1976, 1977) or the phospholipid can be metabolized to either diglyceride (Bell *et al.* 1979), monoglyceride (Chan and Tai 1981) or phosphatidic acid (Billah, Lapetina and Cuatrecasas 1981) before the arachidonate is liberated. Part of the liberated fatty acid is then converted via the enzyme cyclooxygenase into prostaglandin G_2, and prostaglandin H_2 (Hamberg and Samuelsson 1974) which are then converted into thromboxane A_2 via the enzyme thromboxane synthetase (Hamberg, Svensson and Samuelsson 1975). Thromboxane A_2 is unstable and within a few minutes converts to thromboxane B_2. Malondialdehyde is produced at the same time as the thromboxanes and can be used as a marker of thomboxane production. The remainder of the arachidonic acid that has been liberated from phospholipid is converted via the enzyme lipoxygenase into non-prostanoids. The relevance of the non-prostanoids to platelet participation in thrombus formation is not known.

Prostaglandin G_2, prostaglandin H_2 and thromboxane A_2 may be of relevance to thrombus formation because they are aggregating agents

(Hamberg *et al.* 1974, Hamberg, Svensson and Samuelsson 1975), are vasoconstrictors and are involved in two of the three types of release reaction. Their contribution to the release reactions becomes clear when the effects of aspirin or of other non-steroidal anti-inflammatory agents are considered. These agents are inhibitors of the enzyme cyclooxygenase and prevent prostaglandin and thromboxane synthesis. They have little or no effect on release reaction A (Kaplan *et al.* 1979, Ryo, Proffitt and Deuel 1980), completely prevent release reaction B (Zucker and Peterson 1970, Cockbill, Heptinstall and Taylor 1979) and partially inhibit release reaction C (Evans *et al.* 1968, Smith and Willis 1971, MacIntyre 1977, Kaplan *et al.* 1979). Synthesized prostaglandins and thromboxanes are thus essential for the release reaction induced by agents such as ADP, and can contribute to the

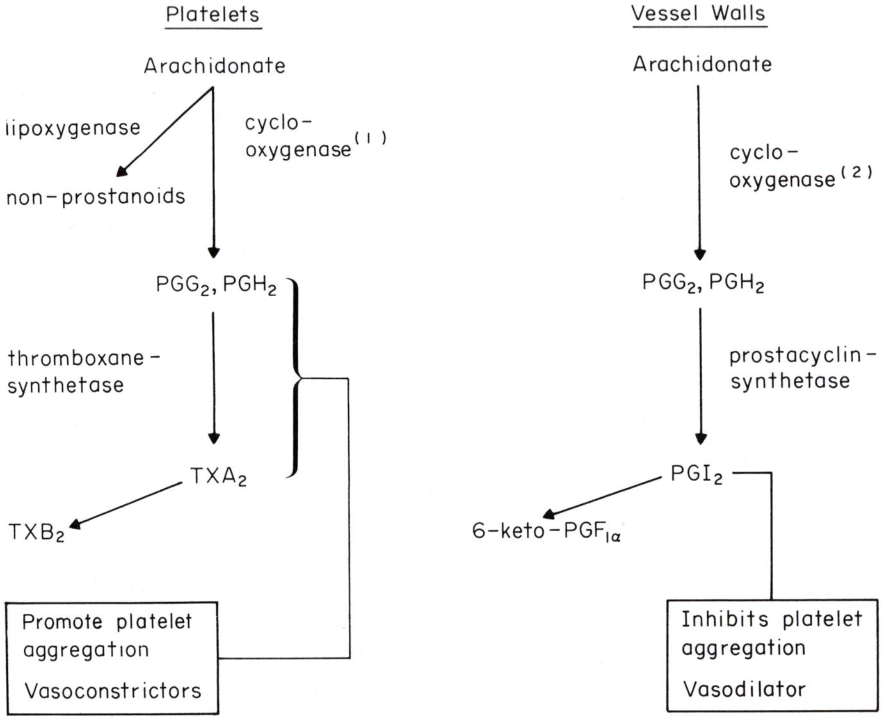

Fig. 49. Arachidonate metabolism in platelets and vessel walls.

release reaction induced by agents such as thrombin, but they are not necessary for the partial liberation of the contents of granules that occurs in response to mild trauma. The effectiveness of aspirin and similar agents as antithrombotic agents could, therefore, depend on which of the three release reactions contributes most to thrombus formation *in vivo*.

A cyclooxygenase that converts arachidonate into prostaglandin G_2 and prostaglandin H_2 is also present in vessel walls (Fig. 49). In this case, however, the prostaglandin endoperoxides are converted mainly into prostaglandin I_2 (prostacyclin; epoprostenol) via prostacyclin synthetase. Like thromboxane A_2, prostacyclin is unstable and converts to 6-keto-prostaglandin $F_{1\alpha}$. There is evidence that some thromboxane B_2 (and thus thromboxane A_2) is produced in vessel walls (Ally and Horrobin 1980) but the amount is believed to be small in relation to the amount of prostacyclin that is produced. Since prostacyclin is a potent inhibitor of nearly all aspects of platelet behaviour and is also a vasodilator its role may be to *prevent* thrombus formation. Thus the balance between platelet prostaglandin and thromboxane synthesis and vascular prostacyclin synthesis could be an important determinant in thrombosis. Perhaps clinical trials of aspirin as an antithrombotic agent have not proved successful because as well as inhibiting the cyclooxygenase in platelets it also inhibits the cyclooxygenase in blood vessel walls. It would seem that it is only when a dose of aspirin as low as 40 mg is administered to man that platelet cyclooxygenase is inhibited but that vascular cyclooxygenase is not (Hanley *et al.* 1981). Inhibitors of the platelet thromboxane synthetase may have more antithrombotic potential than inhibitors of cyclooxygenase since in theory any PGG_2 or PGH_2 produced by the platelets in the presence of the inhibitor might be redirected via prostaglandin synthetase in the vessel wall to produce PGI_2. Antagonists of TXA_2 may be another approach to the problem since they could block both the platelet and vasoconstrictor responses to TXA_2.

Most attempts to detect abnormalities in arachidonate metabolism in platelets and vessels have centred on diabetes. One approach has been to measure the capacity of platelets and vessels from patients with this condition to produce thromboxane and prostacyclin. The hypothesis that platelets from such patients might produce more thromboxane than normal and that vessels might produce less prostacyclin than normal seems to some extent to have been borne out. Increased thromboxane production has been claimed by Gensini *et al.* (1979), Stuart (1979), and Halushka *et al.* (1981); and decreased prostacyclin production by Johnson *et al.* (1979) and Silberbauer *et al.* (1979). Two groups of workers (Ziboh *et al.* 1979 and Butkus, Skrinska and Schumacher 1980) found that thromboxane production was highest in diabetics with vascular complications and Stuart *et al.* (1979) found that the platelets that produced most thromboxanes were the ones that aggregated most readily. All these experiments have, of course, been carried out *in vitro*.

Measurements of circulating levels of thromboxane B_2 or of 6-keto-prostaglandin $F_{1\alpha}$ are not worth reporting because there is continuing debate about what is actually being measured and, moreover, true circulating levels are probably too low for them to be measured accurately using the techniques available at present.

Selective inhibitors of the enzyme thromboxane synthetase have different effects on platelets from different individuals. In PRP from some donors they completely inhibit the irreversible aggregation and release reaction that stems from adding arachidonate to the PRP, but in other donors they do not prevent platelet aggregation or release (Heptinstall *et al.* 1980a). Fox *et al.* (1982) examined PRP from 21 diabetics and found that a thromboxane synthetase inhibitor did not prevent arachidonate-induced platelet behaviour in any of them. Halushka *et al.* (1981) had previously shown that imidazole, which also inhibits thromboxane synthetase, was a much less effective inhibitor of platelet behaviour in PRP from diabetics as compared with PRP from others.

Several interesting observations have also been made in conditions other than diabetes. Platelet thromboxane production has been shown to be increased in patients with prosthetic heart valves (Sullivan, Taylor and Samaha 1980). Perhaps this reflects increased turnover of platelets and the predominance of a younger population of platelets in the circulation. Platelets from hyperlipidaemics were shown to produce more thromboxane than platelets from controls (Tremoli *et al.* 1979, Zahavi *et al.* 1981) and so were platelets from patients with angina, irrespective of whether or not the patients were experiencing anginal pain at the time of blood sampling (Mehta, Mehta and Conti 1980). In the last study it was shown that the patients' platelets were also less sensitive to the anti-aggregatory effects of prostacyclin.

Szczeklik *et al.* (1978, 1979) carried out some experiments in which they determined the concentration of arachidonic acid that needed to be added to PRP to produce platelet aggregation. The determination of the threshold for arachidonate-induced aggregation is relatively unambiguous because, unlike other measures of platelet aggregation, it does not rely on graded responses. They found that platelets from some of a group of patients who had experienced a myocardial infarction were more sensitive to arachidonate in the days immediately after infarction. A more recent study (Sadurska *et al.* 1981) has shown that platelets from women who take oral contraceptives aggregate in response to lower concentrations of arachidonate, but the precise reason for differential sensitivity to arachidonate is unclear.

Such results are encouraging, if only because they represent fresh approaches to the problem of platelet involvement in thrombosis. However, it remains to be seen whether they will prove to be of any more value than have the other tests of platelet reactivity as diagnostic or prognostic indices.

Platelet survival

If platelets are being deposited in thrombotic or atherosclerotic masses, or are continually being activated *in vivo*, then the length of time that they survive in the circulation might be shortened. The most usual technique for measuring platelet survival is to isolate platelets, to label them with ^{51}Cr or ^{111}In, re-inject them and then follow the rate at which the radiolabel disappears from the circulation. The technique is not ideal because it is the survival of platelets that have come into contact with foreign surfaces, have been exposed to anticoagulants and have been handled to obtain PRP that is being measured, not that of the original population. Nevertheless, the technique has given some interesting information because the lifespan of the ^{51}Cr-labelled platelets has been shown to be considerably reduced in patients with prosthetic heart valves (Harker and Slichter 1970, Weily and Genton 1970, Weily *et al.* 1974, Steele *et al.* 1975, Steele, Rainwater and Vogel 1979) and in patients with rheumatic heart disease (Steele *et al.* 1974); in both groups of patients, shortened platelet survival appeared to correlate with thromboembolism. Platelet survival was also decreased in patients with recurrent deep vein thrombosis (Harker and Slichter 1972) and in patients with occluded coronary bypass grafts (Steele *et al.* 1976). Results obtained in established coronary artery disease and in patients studied within a few days or months of myocardial infarction have been less convincing. The mean platelet survival time in such platelets has usually proved to be shorter than that found in groups of individuals without vascular disease but there is always a considerable overlap of individual results (Steele *et al.* 1973, Steele, Battock and Genton 1975, Ritchie and Harker 1977, Kutti and Weinfeld 1979, Cortellaro *et al.* 1981). In contrast, there is a report that platelet survival is markedly reduced in patients with TIAs (Steele *et al.* 1977).

Mean platelet survival has been found to be short in diabetes. Some investigators have found it to be short only in groups of patients with vascular complications of the disease (Abrahamsen 1968, Jones, Paradise and Peterson 1981) whereas others have found it to be short in diabetics without vascular complications as well (Ferguson *et al.* 1975, Paton 1979, Tindall *et al.* 1981). It is interesting that the last three groups of investigators used different techniques to estimate platelet survival. Ferguson *et al.* labelled the platelets by injecting ^{75}Se selenomethionine into his volunteers, and Paton and Tindall used the irreversible inhibition of platelet cyclooxygenase by ingested aspirin (Stuart, Murphy and Oski 1975). So perhaps, *in vivo* labelling techniques are giving different information from techniques that rely on *in vitro* labelling. If so, these could prove more diagnostic or prognostic than studies of ^{51}Cr-labelled platelet survival in arterial disease.

Conclusion

Studies of platelets *in vitro* have indicated ways in which platelets may participate in thrombus formation but have so far given few clues as to why thrombosis occurs in some individuals but not in others. Abnormalities of platelet adhesiveness, platelet aggregation or in the abilities of platelets to undergo their various release reactions and to synthesize prostaglandins and thromboxanes have only been described for groups of patients who have thrombosis or are at risk of thrombosis rather than in individual subjects. At the present time we cannot confidently ascribe the cause of thrombosis in any one individual to platelet dysfunction, nor could we recommend a single test for detecting or monitoring a thrombotic tendency.

THE PAST AND THE FUTURE

The swing of the pendulum in the first half of this century away from platelets and towards disordered coagulation as the prime mover in thrombosis (the concept that thrombosis is just clotting in the wrong place) was related to the discovery of heparin and the coumarin anticoagulants, for in respect of venous thrombosis their ability to prevent thromboembolism was soon apparent (Sevitt and Gallagher 1959, Mitchell 1979b). It was assumed that the presence of platelets in a thrombus was merely a secondary phenomenon brought about by thrombin generated from the clotting cascade. The next swing of the pendulum, which was away from this concept, was triggered by the apparent inability of anticoagulants to modify the natural history of arterial thrombosis (Mitchell 1981). This period of disillusionment coincided with the rediscovery of the platelet as a major thrombus constituent and with the discovery that materials unrelated to the clotting chain, such as ADP (Gaarder *et al.* 1961), serotonin and the catecholamines (Mitchell and Sharp 1964) and collagen (Zucker and Borrelli 1962) could aggregate platelets. This produced a loss of interest in the relationship between clotting and thrombosis which was as complete as the swing away from platelets had been between 1900 and 1950. It led to the belief that thrombosis was merely platelet aggregation in the wrong place. The extremity of this swing may now have been reached by the further extrapolation that thrombosis represents inappropriate aggregation, brought about by an excess of 'bad' material generated by stimulated platelets (thromboxane A_2) and a deficiency of 'good' material generated by vessel walls (prostacyclin). Concentration on the prostaglandin balance to the exclusion of all other mechanisms is unlikely to be rewarding because many platelet activities are independent of the arachidonate–thromboxane pathway and because thrombi do actually contain fibrin. The necessity to swing the pendulum away from a consideration of platelets in isolation is coinciding with our inability to produce convincing evidence that platelet abnormalities are responsible for thrombosis, that anti-aggregants are antithrombotic and with the reaffirmation that anti-coagulants may, after all, modify arterial thromboembolism (Sixty-Plus Reinfarction Group 1980, Mitchell 1981).

As in many previously irreconcilable conflicts (was rickets, for example, due to lack of sunlight or to dietary deficiencies?), it seems probable that extreme views are likely to be wrong so that both clotting and platelet activities will be found to contribute to thrombosis. It is foolish to ignore the structure of thrombi and to concentrate on one mechanism to the exclusion of the other.

REFERENCES

Abrahamsen A.F. (1968) Platelet survival in man with special reference to haemostasis and thrombosis. *Scandinavian Journal of Haematology* Suppl. 3, 1–53.

Adams J., Heptinstall S. & Mitchell J.R.A. (1975) A six-channel automated platelet aggregometer. *Thrombosis et Diathesis Haemorrhagica* **34**, 821–4.

Adams R.D. & Vander Eecken H.M. (1953) Vascular diseases of the brain. *Annual Reviews of Medicine* **4**, 213–52.

Ally A.I. & Horrobin D.F. (1980) Thromboxane A_2 in blood vessel walls and its physiological significance: relevance to thrombosis and hypertension. *Prostaglandins and Medicine* **4**, 431–8.

Anderson L.A. & Gormsen J. (1977) Platelet aggregation and fibrinolytic activity in transient cerebral ischema. *Acta Neurologica Scandinavica* **55**, 76–82.

Baroldi G., Radice F., Schmid G. & Leone A. (1974) Morphology of acute myocardial infarction in relation to coronary thrombosis. *American Heart Journal* **87**, 65–75.

Baumgartner H.R. (1974) The subendothelial surface and thrombosis. *Thrombosis et Diathesis Haemorrhagica* Suppl. 59, 91–105.

Bell R.L., Kennerly D.A., Stanford N. & Majerus P.W. (1979) Diglyceride lipase: a pathway for arachidonate release from human platelets. *Proceedings of the National Academy of Sciences of the USA* **76**, 3238–41.

Billah M.M., Lapetina E.G. & Cuatrecasas P. (1981) Phospholipase A_2 activity specific for phosphatidic acid. A possible mechanism for the production or arachidonic acid in platelets. *Journal of Biological Chemistry* **256**, 5399–404.

Bills T.K., Smith J.B. & Silver M.J. (1976) Metabolism of ^{14}C-arachidonic acid by human platelets. *Biochemica et Biophysica Acta* **424**, 303–14.

Bills T.K., Smith J.B. & Silver M.J. (1977) Selective release of arachidonic acid from the phospholipids of human platelets in response to thrombin. *Journal of Clinical Investigation* **60**, 1–6.

Born G.V.R. (1962) Aggregation of blood platelets by adenosine diphosphate and its reversal. *Nature* **194**, 927–9.

Born G.V.R. & Cross M.J. (1963) The aggregation of blood platelets. *Journal of Physiology* **168**, 178–95.

Borsey D.Q., Dawes J., Fraser D.M., Prowse C.V., Elton R.A. & Clarke B.F. (1980) Plasma beta-thromboglobulin in diabetes mellitus. *Diabetologia* **18**, 353–7.

Brinkhous K.M. (1969) The problem in perspective. In *Thrombosis.* Sherry S.,

Brinkhous K.M., Genton E. & Stengle J.M. (eds). pp. 335–8. National Academy of Sciences, Washington.

British Medical Journal (1976) Intermittent claudication. **I**, 1165–6.

Browse N. (1978) Diagnosis of deep vein thrombosis. *British Medical Bulletin* **34**, 163–7.

Butkus A., Skrinska V.A. & Schumacher P. (1980) Thromboxane production and platelet aggregation in diabetic subjects with clinical complications. *Thrombosis Research* **19**, 211–23.

Bygdeman S. & Wells R. (1969) Studies of platelet adhesiveness, blood viscosity and the microcirculation in patients with thrombotic disease. *Journal of Atherosclerosis Research* **10**, 33–9.

Cella G., Zahavi J., de Haas H.A. & Kakkar V.V. (1979) B-thromboglobulin, platelet production time and platelet function in vascular disease. *British Journal of Haematology* **43**, 127–36.

Chan L.Y. & Tai H.H. (1981) Release of arachidonate from diglyceride in human platelet requires the sequential action of a diglyceride lipase and a monoglyceride lipase. *Biochemical and Biophysical Research Communications* **100**, 1688–95.

Chandler A.B., Chapman I., Erhardt L.R., Roberts W.C., Schwartz C.J., Sinapius D., Spain D.M., Sherry S., Ness P.M. & Simon T.L. (1974) Coronary thrombosis in myocardial infarction. *American Journal of Cardiology* **34**, 823–33.

Charcot J.M. & Bouchard C. (1868) Nouvelles recherches sur la pathogenie de l'hemorrhagie cérébrale. *Archives de Physiologie, Normale et Pathologique* **I**, 110–27, 643–65, 725–34.

Cockbill S.R., Heptinstall S. & Taylor P.M. (1979) A comparison of the abilities of acetylsalicylic acid, flurbiprofen and indomethacin to inhibit the release reaction and prostaglandin synthesis in human blood platelets. *British Journal of Pharmacology* **67**, 73–8.

Coffman J.D. (1972) Detection of obstructive arterial disease. *New England Journal of Medicine* **287**, 612–13.

Cole F.M. & Yates P.O. (1967) The occurrence and significance of intra-cerebral micro-aneurysms. *Journal of Pathology and Bacteriology* **93**, 393–411.

Colman R.W. (1977) Platelet function in hyperbetalipoproteinaemia. *Thrombosis and Haemostasis* **39**, 284–93.

Colwell J.A. & Halushka P.V. (1980) Platelet function in diabetes mellitus. *British Journal of Haematology* **44**, 521–6.

Cortellaro M., Boschetti C., Beggi P. & Polli E.E.(1981) *In vivo* platelet hyperactivity and factor VIII related antigen increase long after myocardial infarction. *Scandinavian Journal of Haematology* **26**, 106–14.

Costa J.L. & Murphy D.L. (1976) Changes in human platelet storage packet size following incubation with labelled serotonin. *Life Science* **18**, 1413–17.

Couch J.R. & Hassanein R.S. (1976) Platelet aggregation, stroke and transient ischemic attack in middle-aged and elderly patients. *Neurology* **26**, 888–95.

Dalal J.J., Penny W.J., Saunders K.C., Sheridan D.J., Bloom A.L. & Henderson A.H. (1982) Platelet counts and aggregates in coronary artery disease. *European Heart Journal* **3**, 107–13.

Dana B., Ellman L., Carvalho A., Daggett W.M. & Hutter A.M. (1976) Plasma heparin neutralizing activity in coronary artery disease. *American Journal of Cardiology* **38**, 9–11.

Danta G. (1970) Second phase aggregation induced by adenosine diphosphate in patients with cerebral vascular disease and in control subjects. *Thrombosis et Diathesis Haemorrhagica* **23**, 159–69.

Davies M.J., Woolf N. & Robertson W.B. (1976) Pathology of acute myocardial infarction with particular reference to occlusive coronary thrombi. *British Heart Journal* **38**, 659–64.

Davis J.W. (1973) Defective platelet aggregation associated with occlusive arterial disease. *Angiology* **24**, 391–7.

Dougherty J.H., Levy D.E. & Weksler B.B. (1977) Platelet activation in acute cerebral ischaemia. Serial measurements of platelet function in cerebrovascular disease. *Lancet* **I**, 821–4.

Dreyfuss F. & Zahavi J. (1973) Adenosine diphosphate induced platelet aggregation in myocardial infarction and ischaemic heart disease. *Atherosclerosis* **17**, 107–20.

Eika C. (1972) The platelet aggregating effect of eight commercial heparins. *Scandinavian Journal of Haematology* **9**, 480–2.

Evans G., Packham M.A., Nishizawa E.E., Mustard J.F. & Murphy E.A. (1968) The effect of acetylsalicylic acid on platelet function. *Journal of Experimental Medicine* **128**, 877–94.

Ferguson J.C., Mackay N., Philip J.A.D. & Sumner D.J. (1975) Determination of platelet and fibrinogen half-life with (^{75}Se) selenomethionine: studies in normal and diabetic subjects. *Clinical Science and Molecular Medicine* **49**, 115–20.

Finlayson R. (1965) Spontaneous arterial disease in exotic animals. *Journal of Zoology* **147**, 239–343.

Fox S.C., Hanley S.P., Heptinstall S. & Peacock I. (1982) Inhibition of prostaglandin and thromboxane synthesis in blood platelets from healthy individuals and from diabetics. *Transactions of the Biochemical Society* **10**, 254–5.

Franchi F., Canciani M.T. & Mannucci P.M. (1980) The B-thromboglobulin test. *Thrombosis and Haemostasis* **44**, 107.

Fukami M.H. & Salganicoff L. (1977) Human platelet storage organelles. A review. *Thrombosis and Haemostasis* **38**, 963–70.

Gaarder A., Jonsen J., Laland S., Hellem A.J. & Owren P.A. (1961) Adenosine diphosphate in red cells as a factor in the adhesiveness of human blood platelets. *Nature* **192**, 531–2.

Gensini G.F., Abbate R., Favilla S. & Neri-Serneri G.G. (1979) Changes of platelet function and blood clotting in diabetes mellitus. *Thrombosis and Haemostasis* **42**, 983–93.

Gjesdal K. (1976) Platelet function and free fatty acids during acute myocardial infarction and severe angina pectoris. *Scandinavian Journal of Haematology* **17**, 205–12.

Guyton J.R. & Willerson J.T. (1977) Peripheral venous platelet aggregates in patients with unstable angina pectoris and acute myocardial infarction. *Angiology* **28**, 695–701.

Haerem J.W. (1972) Platelet aggregates in intra-myocardial vessels of patients dying suddenly and unexpectedly of coronary artery disease. *Atherosclerosis* **15**, 199–213.

Halushka P.V., Rogers R.C., Loadholt C.B. & Colwell J.A. (1981) Increased platelet thromboxane synthesis in diabetes mellitus. *Journal of Laboratory and Clinical Medicine* **97**, 87–96.

Hamberg M. & Samuelsson B. (1974) Prostaglandin endoperoxides. Novel transformations of arachidonic acid in human platelets. *Proceedings of the National Academy of Sciences of the USA* **71**, 3400–4.

Hamberg M., Svensson J. & Samuelsson B. (1975) Thromboxanes: A new group of biologically active compounds derived from prostaglandin endoperoxides. *Proceedings of the National Academy of Sciences of the USA* **72**, 2944–8.

Hamberg M., Svensson J., Wakabayashi T. & Samuelsson B. (1974) Isolation and structure of two prostaglandin endoperoxides that cause platelet aggregation. *Proceedings of the National Academy of Sciences of the USA* **71**, 345–9.

Han P., Turpie A.G.G., Genton E. & Gent M. (1979) The effect of antiplatelet drugs on plasma betathromboglobulin in coronary artery disease. *Thrombosis and Haemostasis* **42**, 59.

Handin R.I., McDonough M. & Lesch M. (1978) Elevation of platelet factor four in acute myocardial infarction: measurement by radioimmunoassay. *Journal of Laboratory and Clinical Medicine* **91**, 340–9.

Hanley S.P., Bevan J., Cockbill S.R. & Heptinstall S. (1981) Differential inhibition by low dose aspirin of human venous prostacyclin synthesis and platelet thromboxane synthesis. *Lancet* **I**, 969–71.

Harker L.A., Malpass T.W., Branson H.E., Hessell H.E.A., & Slichter S.J. (1980) Mechanisms of abnormal bleeding in patients undergoing cardiopulmonary bypass: acquired transient platelet dysfunction associated with selective-granule release. *Blood* **56**, 824–34.

Harker L.A. & Slichter S.J. (1970) Studies of platelet and fibrinogen kinetics in patients with prosthetic heart valves. *New England Journal of Medicine* **283**, 1302–5.

Harker L.A. & Slichter S.J. (1972) Platelet and fibrinogen consumption in man. *New England Journal of Medicine* **287**, 999–1005.

Harland W.A. & Holburn A.M. (1966) Coronary thrombosis and myocardial infarction. *Lancet* **II**, 1158–60.

Harris W.H., Salzman E.W., Athanasoulis C.A., Waltman A.C. & De Sanctis R.W. (1977) Aspirin prophylaxis of venous thromboembolism after total hip replacement. *New England Journal of Medicine* **297**, 1246–9.

Harrison M.J.G., Emmons P.R. & Mitchell J.R.A. (1966) The effect of white cells on platelet aggregation. *Thrombosis et Diathesis Haemorrhagica* **16**, 105–21.

Harrison M.J.G., Emmons P.R. & Mitchell J.R.A. (1967) The variability of human platelet aggregation. *Journal of Atherosclerosis Research* **7**, 197–205.

Harrison M.J.G. & Marshall J. (1976) Angiographic appearance of carotid bifurcation in patients with completed stroke, transient ischaemic attacks and cerebral tumour. *British Medical Journal* **I**, 205–7.

Heptinstall S., Bevan J., Cockbill S.R., Hanley S.P. & Parry M.J. (1980a) Effects of a selective inhibitor of thromboxane synthetase on human blood platelet behaviour. *Thrombosis Research* **20**, 219–30.

Heptinstall S. & Mulley G.P. (1977) Adenosine diphosphate induced platelet aggregation and release reaction in heparinized platelet rich plasma and the influence of added citrate. *British Journal of Haematology* **36**, 565–71.

Heptinstall S., Mulley G.P., Taylor P.M. & Mitchell J.R.A. (1980b) Platelet release reaction in myocardial infarction. *British Medical Journal* **I**, 80–1.

Heptinstall S. & Taylor P.M. (1979) The effects of citrate and extracellular calcium ions on the platelet release reaction induced by adenosine diphosphate and collagen. *Thrombosis and Haemostasis* **42**, 778–93.

Holmsen H. (1972) The platelet: Its membrane, physiology and its biochemistry. In *Clinics in Haematology*. Vol. 1:2. pp. 235–66. O'Brien J.R. (ed.). W.B. Saunders, London.

Holmsen H. (1975) Biochemistry of the platelet release reaction. In *Biochemistry and Pharmacology of Platelets* (Ciba Foundation Symposium 35). pp. 175–205. Elsevier Science Publishing Co., New York.

Honour A.J. & Mitchell J.R.A. (1964) Platelet clumping in injured vessels. *British Journal of Experimental Pathology* **45**, 75–87.

International Multicentre Trial (1975) Prevention of fatal post-operative pulmonary embolism by low doses of heparin. *Lancet* **II**, 45–51.

Johnson M., Harrison H.E., Raftery A.T. & Elder J.B. (1979) Vascular prostacyclin may be reduced in diabetes in man. *Lancet* **I**, 325–6.

Jones R.L., Paradise C. & Peterson C.M. (1981) Platelet survival in patients with diabetes mellitus. *Diabetes* **30**, 486–9.

Kaegi A., Pineo G.F., Shimizu A., Trivedi H., Hirsch J. & Gent M. (1975) The role of sulfinpyrazone in the prevention of arteriovenous shunt thrombosis. *Circulation* **52**, 497–500.

Kannel W.B. (1976) Epidemiology of cerebrovascular disease. In *Cerebral Arterial Disease*. Ross Russell R.W. (ed.). Churchill Livingstone, Edinburgh.

Kaplan K.L., Broekman J., Chernoff A., Lesznik G.R. & Drillings M. (1979) Platelet α-granule proteins: studies on release and subcellular localization. *Blood* **53**, 604–18.

Kardinal C.G., Wegener L.T. & Anderson L.K. (1975) Spontaneous platelet aggregation. Occurrence in an asymptomatic individual. *American Journal of Clinical Pathology* **63**, 559–63.

Knudsen J.G., Gormsen J., Skagen K. & Amtorp O. (1979) Changes in platelet functions, coagulation and fibrinolysis in uncomplicated cases of acute myocardial infarction. *Thrombosis and Haemostasis* **42**, 1513–22.

Kumpuris A.G., Luchi R.J., Waddell C.C. & Miller R.R. (1980) Production of circulating platelet aggregates by exercise in coronary patients. *Circulation* **61**, 62–5.

Kutti J., Safai-Kutti S., Svärdsudd K., Swedberg K. & Wadenvik H. (1981) Plasma levels of platelet factor 4 in patients admitted to a coronary care unit. *Scandinavian Journal of Haematology* **26**, 235–40.

Kutti J. & Weinfeld A. (1979) Platelet survival and platelet production in acute myocardial infarction. *Acta Medica Scandinavica* **205**, 501–4.

Levine P.H., Fisher M., Fullerton A.L., Duffy C.P. & Hoogasian J.J. (1981) Human platelet factor 4: preparation from outdated platelet concentrates and application in cerebral vascular disease. *American Journal of Hematology* **10**, 375–85.

Lhermitte F., Gautier J.C. & Derouesné C. (1970) Nature of occlusions of the middle cerebral artery. *Neurology* **20**, 82–8.

Lichtlen P.R. & Engel H.-J. (1978) Angiographic aspects of CHD in young women. In *Coronary Disease in Young Women*. Oliver M.F. (ed.) Churchill Livingstone, Edinburgh.

Lou H.C., Nielsen J.D., Bomholt A. & Gormsen J. (1977) Platelet hyperaggregability in young patients with completed stroke. *Acta Neurologica Scandinavica* **56**, 326–34.

Lowe G.D.O., Reavey M.M., Johnston R.V., Forbes C.D. & Prentice C.R.M. (1979)

Increased platelet aggregates in vascular and non-vascular illness: correlation with plasma fibrinogen and effect of Ancrod. *Thrombosis Research* **14**, 377–86.

Ludlam C.A., Allen M., Blandford R.B., Dowdle R., Bentley N. & Bloom A.L. (1979a) β-Thromboglobulin and platelet survival in patients with rheumatic heart disease and prosthetic cardiac valves and their treatment with sulphinpyrazone. *Thrombosis and Haemostasis* **42**, 329.

Ludlam C.A. & Cash J.D. (1976) Studies on the liberation of β-thromboglobulin from human platelets *in vitro*. *British Journal of Haematology* **33**, 239–47.

Ludlam C.A., O'Brien J.R., Bolton A.E. & Etherington M. (1979b) A comparison between the plasma concentration of immunologically assayed platelet factor 4 and β-thromboglobulin and the heparin thrombin clotting time. *Thrombosis Research* **15**, 523–30.

Macfarlane D.E., Walsh P.N., Mills D.C.B., Holmsen H. & Day H.G. (1975) The role of thrombin in ADP-induced platelet aggregation and release: a critical evaluation. *British Journal of Haematology* **30**, 457–63.

MacIntyre D.E. (1977) Platelet aggregation: prostaglandin synthase dependent and independent mechanisms. *Drugs in Experimental Clinical Research* **2**, 99–104.

Meade T.W., Gardner M.J., Cannon P., Richardson P.C. (1968) Observer variability in recording the peripheral pulses. *British Heart Journal* **30**, 661–5.

Meade T.W., North W.R.S., Chakrabarti R., Stirling Y., Haines A.P., Thompson S.G. & Brozović M. (1980) Haemostatic function and cardiovascular death; early results of a prospective study. *Lancet* **I**, 1050–4.

Medical Research Council Steering Committee (1972) Effect of aspirin on post-operative venous thrombosis. *Lancet* **II**, 441–5.

Mehta J., Mehta P. & Conti C.R. (1980) Platelet function studies in coronary heart disease. IX. Increased platelet prostaglandin generation and abnormal platelet sensitivity to prostacyclin and endoperoxide analog in angina pectoris. *American Journal of Cardiology* **46**, 943–7.

Mehta P. & Mehta J. (1979) Platelet function studies in coronary artery disease. V. Evidence for enhanced platelet microthrombus formation activity in acute myocardial infarction. *American Journal of Cardiology* **43**, 757–60.

Mitchell J.R.A. (1969) Anticoagulant therapy in ischaemic heart disease. *Abstracts of World Medicine* **43**, 249–58.

Mitchell J.R.A. (1976) Has our basic knowledge of cerebrovascular disease led to effective and rational treatment? In *Stroke*. Gillingham F.J., Mawdsley C. & Williams A.E. (eds). Churchill Livingstone, Edinburgh.

Mitchell J.R.A. (1979a) *Strokes in Perspective*. British Medicine, 23–28 Interface, London.

Mitchell J.R.A. (1979b) Can we really prevent post-operative pulmonary emboli? *British Medical Journal* **I**, 1523–4.

Mitchell J.R.A. (1981) Anticoagulants in coronary heart disease retrospect and prospect. *Lancet* **I**, 257–62.

Mitchell J.R.A. & Schwartz C.J. (1965) *Arterial Disease*. Blackwell Scientific Publications, Oxford.

Mitchell J.R.A. & Sharp A.A. (1964) Platelet clumping *in vitro*. *British Journal of Haematology* **10**, 78–93.

Morris G.K. & Mitchell J.R.A. (1976a) Prevention and diagnosis of venous thrombosis in patients with hip fractures. *Lancet* **II**, 867–9.

Morris G.K. & Mitchell J.R.A. (1976b) Warfarin sodium in prevention of deep venous thrombosis and pulmonary embolism in patients with fractured neck of femur. *Lancet* **II**, 869–72.

Morris G.K. & Mitchell J.R.A. (1977) Preventing thromboembolism in elderly patients with hip fractures: studies of low-dose heparin, dipyridamole, aspirin and flurbiprofen. *British Medical Journal* **I**, 535–7.

O'Brien J.R. (1968) Effects of salicylates on human platelets. *Lancet* **I**, 779–83.

O'Brien J.R., Etherington M., Jamieson S., Lawford P., Sussex J. & Lincoln S.V. (1975) Heparin neutralizing activity test in the diagnosis of acute myocardial infarction. *Journal of Clinical Pathology* **28**, 975–9.

O'Brien J.R., Etherington M.D. & Shuttleworth R. (1977) β-Thromboglobulin and heparin-neutralizing activity test in clinical conditions. *Lancet* **I**, 1153–4.

O'Brien J.R., Heywood J.B. & Heady J.A. (1966) The quantitation of platelet aggregation induced by four compounds: a study in relation to myocardial infarction. *Thrombosis et Diathesis Haemorrhagica* **16**, 752–67.

Page R.L. & Mitchell J.R.A. (1979) Platelet adhesiveness to glass. *Thrombosis and Haemostasis* **42**, 705–25.

Paterson J.C. (1969) The pathology of venous thrombi. In *Thrombosis*. Sherry S., Brinkhous K.M., Genton E. & Stengle J.M. (eds). National Academy of Sciences, Washington.

Paton R.C. (1979) Platelet survival in diabetes mellitus using an aspirin-labelling technique. *Thrombosis Research* **15**, 793–802.

Perper J.A., Kuller L.H. & Cooper M (1975) Arteriosclerosis of coronary arteries in sudden unexpected death. *Circulation* **51–52** (Suppl. III), 27–33.

Petrova T.R., Pavlishchuk S.A. & Grigoriev G.I. (1975) Phase analysis of platelet aggregation in acute disturbances of cerebral circulation. *Cor Vasa* **17**, 102–11.

Poole J.C.F. & French J.E. (1961) Thrombosis. *Journal of Atherosclerosis Research* **1**, 251–73.

Prazitch J.A., Rapaport S.I., Samples J.R. & Englen R. (1977) Platelet aggregate ratios—standardization of technique and test results in patients with myocardial ischaemia and patients with cerebrovascular disease. *Thrombosis and Haemostasis* **38**, 597–605.

Preston F.E., Emmanuel I.G., Winfield D.A. & Malia R.G. (1974) Essential thrombocythaemia and peripheral gangrene. *British Medical Journal* **III**, 548–52.

Randi M.L., Fabris F., Casonato A. & Girolami A. (1981) The effect of anticoagulant mixtures on BTG and PF4 levels. *Thrombosis and Haemostasis* **46**, 569.

Ritchie J.L. & Harker L.A. (1977) Platelet and fibrinogen survival in coronary atherosclerosis. Response to medical and surgical therapy. *American Journal of Cardiology* **39**, 595–8.

Robb-Smith A.H.T. (1967) Why the platelets were discovered. *British Journal of Haematology* **13**, 618–37.

Russell R.W.R. (1963) Observations on intracerebral aneurysms. *Brain* **86**, 425–42.

Ryo R., Proffitt R.T. & Deuel T.F. (1980) Human platelet factor 4, subcellular localization and characteristics of release from intact platelets. *Thrombosis Research* **17**, 629–44.

Sadurska B., Tacconi M.T., di Minno G., Roncaglioni M.C., Pangrazzi J., Donati M.B., Bizzi A. & Silver M.J. (1981) Plasma and platelet lipid composition and platelet aggregation by arachidonic acid in women on the pill. *Thrombosis and Haemostasis* **45**, 150–3.

Salky N. & Dugdale M. (1973) Platelet abnormalities in ischaemic heart disease. *American Journal of Cardiology* **32**, 612–17.

Salzman E.W., Harris W.H. & De Sanctis R.W. (1966) Anticoagulation for prevention of thromboembolism following fractures of the hip. *New England Journal of Medicine* **275**, 122–30.

Schwartz C.J. & Gerrity R.G. (1975) Anatomical pathology of sudden unexpected cardiac death. *Circulation* **51–52** (Suppl. III), 18–26.

Scrobohaci M.L., Cunescu V. & Orha I. (1976) Recurrent thromboembolism with spontaneous platelet aggregation. *Thrombosis and Haemostasis* **36**, 645–6.

Sevitt S. & Gallagher N.G. (1959) Prevention of venous thrombosis and pulmonary embolism in injured patients. *Lancet* **II**, 981–9.

Shaw S., Pegrum G.D., Wolff S. & Ashton W.L. (1967) Platelet adhesiveness in diabetes mellitus. *Journal of Clinical Pathology* **20**, 845–7.

Silberbauer K., Schernthaner G., Siuzinger H., Piza-Katzer H. & Winter M. (1979) Decreased vascular prostacyclin in juvenile-onset diabetes. *New England Journal of Medicine* **300**, 366.

Singer A. & Rob C. (1960) The fate of the claudicator. *British Medical Journal* **II**, 633–6.

Sixty-Plus Reinfarction Group (1980) A double blind trial to assess long-term anticoagulant therapy in elderly patients after myocardial infarction. *Lancet* **II**, 989–94.

Smith J.B. & Willis A.L. (1971) Aspirin selectively inhibits prostaglandin production in human platelets. *Nature (New Biology)* **231**, 235–8.

Spain D.M. & Bradess V.A. (1960) The relationship of coronary thrombosis to coronary atherosclerosis and ischemic heart disease. *American Journal of Medical Sciences* **240**, 701–10.

Steele P., Battock D. & Genton E. (1975) Effects of clofibrate and sulphinpyrazone on platelet survival time in coronary artery disease. *Circulation* **52**, 473–6.

Steele P., Battock D., Pappas G. & Genton E. (1976) Correlation of platelet survival time with occlusion of saphenous vein aorto-coronary bypass grafts. *Circulation* **53**, 685–7.

Steele P., Carroll J., Overfield D. & Genton E. (1977) Effect of sulfinpyrazone on platelet survival time in patients with transient cerebral ischaemic attacks. *Stroke* **8**, 396–9.

Steele P., Rainwater J. & Vogel R. (1979) Platelet suppressant therapy in patients with prosthetic cardiac valves. Relation of clinical effectiveness to alteration of platelet survival time. *Circulation* **60**, 910–13.

Steele P.P., Weily H.S., Davies H. & Genton E. (1973) Platelet function studies in coronary artery disease. *Circulation* **48**, 1194–200.

Steele P.P., Weily H.S., Davies H. & Genton E. (1974) Platelet survival in patients with rheumatic heart disease. *New England Journal of Medicine* **290**, 537–9.

Steele P., Weily H., Davies H., Pappas G. & Genton E. (1975) Platelet survival time following aortic valve replacement. *Circulation* **51**, 358–62.

Stuart M.J. (1979) Platelet malondialdehyde formation: an indicator of platelet hyperfunction. *Thrombosis and Haemostasis* **42**, 649–54.

Stuart M.J., Elrad H., Graeber J.E., Hakanson D.O., Sunderji S.G. & Barvinchak M.K. (1979) Increased synthesis of prostaglandin endoperoxides and platelet hyperfunction in infants of mothers with diabetes mellitus. *Journal of Laboratory and Clinical Medicine* **94**, 12–17.

Stuart M.J., Murphy S. & Oski F.A. (1975) A simple non-radioisotope technic for the determination of platelet life-span. *New England Journal of Medicine* **292**, 1310–13.

Sullivan J.M., Taylor J.C. & Samaha J.L. (1980) Platelet malondialdehyde in cardiovascular disease: effect of prosthetic heart valves and cardioactive drugs on production. *Thrombosis and Haemostasis* **44**, 76–80.

Szczeklik A., Gryglewski R.J., Musial J., Grudzinska L., Serwońska M. & Marcinkiewicz E. (1978) Thromboxane generation and platelet aggregation in survivals of myocardial infarction. *Thrombosis and Haemostasis (Stuttgart)* **40**, 66–74.

Szczeklik A., Serwońska M., Lukasiewicz W., Mruk J. & Musial J. (1979) Arachidonate versus ADP-induced platelet aggregation in acute myocardial infarction. *Thrombosis and Haemostasis* **42**, 822–3.

Ten Cate J.W., Vos J., Oosterhuis H., Prenger D. & Jenkins C.S.P. (1978) Spontaneous platelet aggregation in cerebrovascular disease. *Thrombosis and Haemostasis* **39**, 223–9.

Tindall H., Paton R.C., Zuzel M. & McNicol G.P. (1981) Platelet life-span in diabetics with and without retinopathy. *Thrombosis Research* **21**, 641–8.

Tremoli E., Maderna P., Sirtori M. & Sirtori C.R. (1979) Platelet aggregation and malondialdehyde formation in type IIA hypercholesteralaemic patients. *Haemostasis* **8**, 47–53.

Virchow R. (1858) *Die cellular Pathologie in ihrer Begründung auf physiologische und Pathologische Gewebelehre.* Hirschwald, Berlin.

Vreeken J. & van Aken W.G. (1971) Spontaneous aggregation of blood platelets as a cause of idiopathic thrombosis and recurrent painful toes and fingers. *Lancet* **II**, 1394–7.

Warlow C., Corina A., Ogston D. & Douglas A.S. (1974) The relationship between platelet aggregation and time interval after venepuncture. *Thrombosis et Diathesis Haemorrhagica* **31**, 133–41.

Weily H.S. & Genton E. (1970) Altered platelet function in patients with prosthetic mitral valves. Effect of sulphinpyrazone therapy. *Circulation* **42**, 967–72.

Weily H.S., Steele P.P., Davies H., Pappas G. & Genton E. (1974) Platelet survival in patients with substitute heart valves. *New England Journal of Medicine* **290**, 534–7.

Weiss H.J., Aledort L.M. & Kochwa S. (1968) The effect of salicylates on the hemostatic properties of platelets in man. *Journal of Clinical Investigation* **47**, 2169–80.

Weksler B.B. & Goldstein T.M. (1980) Prostaglandins: Interactions with platelets and polymorphonuclear leucocytes in hemostasis and inflammation. *American Journal of Medicine* **68**, 419–28.

White G.C. & Marouf A.A. (1981) Platelet factor 4 levels in patients with coronary artery disease. *Journal of Laboratory and Clinical Medicine* **97**, 369–78.

Wright H.P. (1941) The adhesiveness of blood platelets in normal subjects with varying concentrations of anticoagulants. *Journal of Pathology and Bacteriology* **53**, 255–62.

Wright H.P. (1942) Changes in the adhesiveness of blood platelets following parturition and surgical operations. *Journal of Pathology and Bacteriology* **54**, 461–8.

Wu K.K. & Hoak J.C. (1974) A new method for the quantitative detection of platelet aggregates in patients with arterial insufficiency. *Lancet* **II**, 924–7.

Wu K.K. & Hoak J.C. (1976) Spontaneous platelet aggregation in arterial insufficiency: mechanisms and complications. *Thrombosis and Haemostasis* **35**, 702–11.

Yamazaki H., Takahashi T. & Sano T. (1975) Hyperaggregability of platelets in thromboembolic disorders. *Thrombosis et Diathesis Haemorrhagica* **34**, 94–105.

Zahavi J. (1977) The role of platelet in myocardial infarction, ischemic heart disease, cerebrovascular disease, thromboembolic disorders and acute idiopathic pericarditis. *Thrombosis and Haemostasis* **38**, 1073–84.

Zahavi J., Betteridge J.D., Jones N.A.G., Galton D.J. & Kakkar V.V. (1981) Enhanced *in vivo* platelet release reaction and malondialdehyde formation in patients with hyperlipidemia. *American Journal of Medicine* **70**, 59–64.

Zahavi J. & Dreyfuss F. (1969) An abnormal pattern of adenosine diphospate-induced platelet aggregation in acute myocardial infarction. *Thrombosis et Diathesis Haemorrhagica* **21**, 76–88.

Zahavi J. & Kakkar V.V. (1979) B-thromboglobulin—a specific marker of *in vivo* platelet release reaction. *Thrombosis and Haemostasis* **42**, 23–9.

Ziboh V.A., Maruta H., Lord J. & Cagle W.D. (1979) Increased biosynthesis of thromboxane A_2 by diabetic platelets. *European Journal of Clinical Investigation* **9**, 223–8.

Zucker M.B. & Borrelli J. (1962) Platelet clumping produced by connective tissue suspensions and by collagen. *Proceedings of the Society for Experimental Biology and Medicine* **109**, 779–87.

Zucker M.B. & Peterson J. (1968) Inhibition of adenosine diphosphate-induced secondary aggregation and other platelet functions by acetylsalicylic acid ingestion. *Proceedings of the Society for Experimental Biology and Medicine* **127**, 547–51.

Zucker M.B. & Peterson J. (1970) Effect of acetylsalicylic acid, other non-steroidal anti-inflammatory agents, and dipyridamole on human blood platelets. *Journal of Laboratory and Clinical Medicine* **76**, 66–75.

Chapter 16
The Fibrinolytic Enzyme System*

B. BENNETT, D. OGSTON *and* A. S. DOUGLAS

Fibrinolysis is the term applied to the process of dissolution of fibrin clots or deposits within the body. The principal interest in the process has arisen from its potential role in the limitation or removal of intravascular thrombi and the possibility of altering the system in order to achieve this therapeutically. The process may also clearly play a major role in the healing and repair of injured tissues in which fibrin is frequently deposited in a diffuse manner and there is evidence too that its modification by tumour cells may be important in tumour growth or dissemination.

The process of fibrinolysis results from the action of an enzyme system, the fibrinolytic enzyme system, which bears certain superficial similarities to the coagulation system with which it interacts at certain points. Whereas, however, the sequence of events in the enzyme cascade of the coagulation pathways is understood in considerable detail, largely due to studies on the plasmas of individuals with single factor deficiencies, the sequence of events in reactions leading to fibrinolysis is less clearly defined, partly perhaps because individuals deficient in specific enzymes have been less commonly discovered.

It is clear, however, that the system operates finally via the protease plasmin, which is generated from the circulating proenzyme plasminogen, the two proteins occupying positions analogous to prothrombin and thrombin in the clotting mechanism. Plasmin is very rarely detectable in free form in circulating plasma due to the action of the principal antiplasmin of the blood, known as α_2-antiplasmin, which combines with and neutralizes formed plasmin very rapidly and thus performs a function analogous to that of antithrombin III in clotting. The molecular nature and action of these agents is understood in detail, but the agents responsible for conversion of plasminogen to plasmin in the body are less clearly understood as yet. It is known that activators of plasminogen may occur in circulating blood, in vascular endothelium and in many tissues but their interrelationships and relative importance are only beginning to be understood. Activators arising from the blood itself are sometimes termed 'intrinsic activators' while those arising exterior to the flowing blood are termed 'extrinsic activators'. While a

* This chapter contains references to material published or in press before January 1982.

comparison of fibrinolytic pathways with those of coagulation is interesting and instructive, analogies between the two should not be pursued too far. Fig. 50 presents an outline diagram of the fibrinolytic enzyme system as currently perceived. The following section outlines the known properties of individual components of the fibrinolytic system and is followed by a description of the agents known to inhibit fibrinolysis in the blood. Thereafter the possible interaction of the individual agents to produce *in vivo* fibrinolysis will be discussed, and an indication given of the mechanisms underlying physiological and pathological fibrinolysis in man.

Plasminogen

Plasminogen, a β-globulin of molecular weight 80–90 000 (Sjöholm, Wiman and Wallen 1973, Robbins 1977) exhibits electrophoretic heterogeneity. It exists in plasma as a single polypeptide chain the sequence of which is known (Wiman and Wallen 1975, Sottrup-Jensen *et al.* 1978). It occupies a position in the fibrinolytic pathways analogous to that of prothrombin in coagulation. Like prothrombin it has a large number of internal disulphide bridges, forming several triple loop ('kringle') structures (Sottrup-Jensen *et al.* 1978). NH_2-terminal glutamic acid characterizes the circulating form of the protein, 'glu-plasminogen' (Wallen and Wiman 1972), but other forms, mainly with NH_2-terminal lysine, 'Lys-plasminogen' (Robbins *et al.* 1967), are produced by the action of plasmin which hydrolyses Arg 67-Met 68, Lys 76-Lys 77 or Lys 77-Val 78 bonds with resultant removal of a small peptide. Lys-plasminogen is readily cleaved by plasminogen activators at a single site, Arg 560-Val 561 (Robbins *et al.* 1967, Sottrup-Jensen *et al.* 1978), to form plasmin, a two-chain molecule. Glu-plasminogen is converted to plasmin less readily than is Lys-plasminogen; in the presence of plasmin inhibitors, the conversion is achieved by cleavage at the same Arg 560-Val 561 bond (Summaria *et al.* 1975, Violand and Castellino 1976). In the absence of plasmin inhibitors further cleavage at Arg 67-Met 68, Lys 76-Lys 77, etc. occurs (Wiman and Wallen 1973). The *in vivo* sequence of events is unclear but it has been proposed that conversion of Glu- to Lys-plasminogen may occur by the action of traces of plasmin and that this form, more susceptible to plasminogen activators, is rapidly converted to plasmin (Violand and Castellino 1976).

Plasmin

Plasmin, formed as above, is a serine protease with His 602, Asp 645 and Ser 740 in its active site. As indicated, it comprises two chains bound by two disulphide bonds (Summaria *et al.* 1975, Sottrup-Jensen *et al.* 1978, Wiman 1978). The active centre is situated in the light (B) chain (Robbins *et al.* 1973,

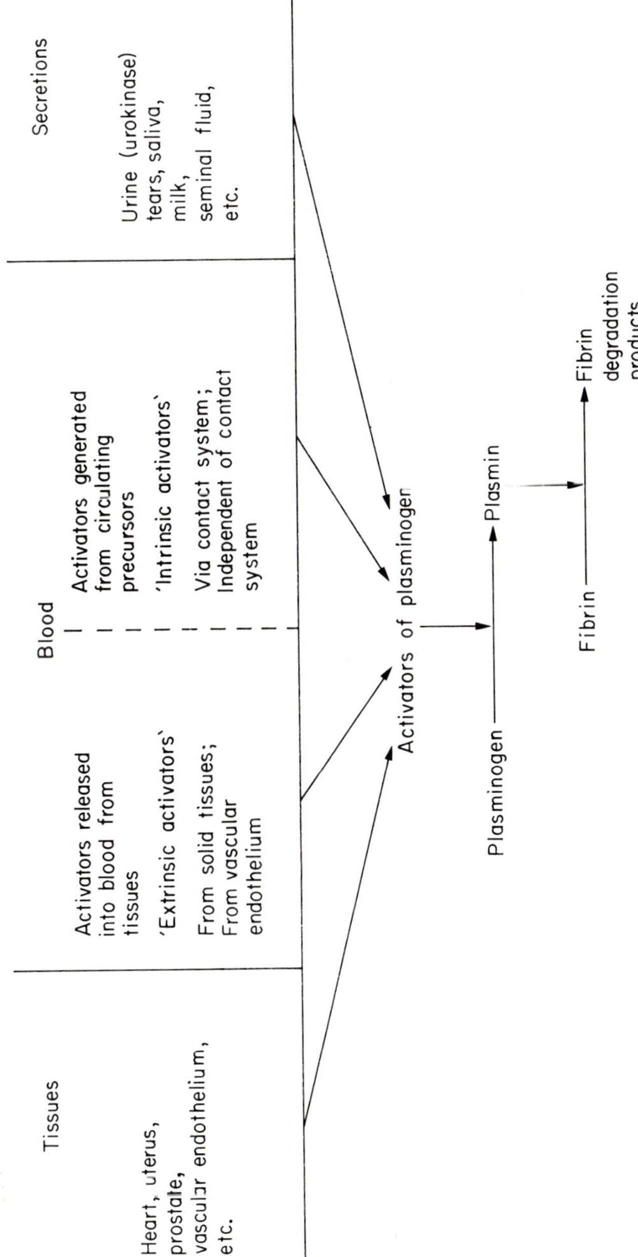

Fig. 50. The fibrinolytic enzyme system, indicating the source from which activators of plasminogen may be derived. The interrelationships of these activators are not yet fully defined.

Sottrup-Jensen *et al.* 1978). The heavy (A) chain contains the triple loops and the so-called lysin-binding sites (Rickli and Otavsky 1975) which are blocked by various fibrinolytic inhibitors (lysine, EACA, tranexamic acid, etc.) and participate in the absorption of plasmin on to fibrin.

Plasmin, like trypsin, is a serine protease (Groskopf *et al.* 1969) capable of digestion of a number of proteins in pure systems including fibrin, fibrinogen, factors V and VIII and casein, various peptides, amino acid esters and amides (Robbins 1977). Thus its unmodified release in the circulating blood would have disastrous effects. Its rapid interaction with α_2-antiplasmin, resulting in its neutralization (at a rate even faster than the interaction of trypsin with its inhibitors), usually protects the plasma proteins from its action. As the adsorption on to formed fibrin involves the lysine-binding sites which modify the rate of its interaction with α_2-antiplasmin, once such adsorption has occurred it is relatively protected from the effect of the inhibitors. This phenomenon probably accounts for limitation of its action to formed fibrin *in vivo*.

Plasminogen activators

While the molecular nature of plasminogen and plasmin together with that of the antiplasmins is understood in great detail, less information on the agents converting plasminogen to plasmin is available. It is known that plasminogen activators are present in many tissues, urine and other secretions, and in the blood itself, but their precise nature, interrelationships, relative importance and function remain to be established. Figure 50 outlines the possible sources of plasminogen activator in the body. It should be emphasized that, while clinicians probably conceive of fibrinolysis primarily as an intravascular event as their preoccupations often concern either haemorrhage or thrombosis, fibrin deposition and fibrinolysis also occur in the extravascular compartment. Thus, while investigation tends naturally to concern itself with fibrinolysis in circulating blood, extravascular fibrinolysis may be important though inaccessible to direct investigation in patients.

Tissue plasminogen activators

Most human tissues produce plasminogen activators from which they can be extracted for study. Plasminogen activators have been prepared from human uterine tissues (Kok 1979a, Rijken *et al.* 1979). The molecular weight of one was 64 000–69 000 and the agent existed as a two-chain molecule, the smaller chain (31 000 mol.wt) containing the active site as deduced by incorporation of radiolabelled DFP (Rikjen *et al.* 1979). It seems possible that the two-chain form represents proteolytic degradation of a single chain molecule (Wallen *et al.* 1981).

Activator has also been isolated from porcine and human myocardial tissue (Rickli and Zaugg 1970, Cole and Bachmann 1977, Booth and Bennett 1981). The porcine preparation had a molecular size of 51 500 on gel filtration. Activator from human myocardium has been found to have a molecular size of 65 000 as judged by polyacrylamide gel electrophoresis (Booth and Bennett 1981).

Endothelial plasminogen activators

Using a histochemical technique, Todd demonstrated in 1959 that plasminogen activator was present in the endothelium of blood vessels, and is particularly rich in venous endothelium. Activator may be washed from the vascular tree of human cadavers and is presumed to derive from the vascular endothelium; on gel filtration the material has been judged to have a molecular weight of 65 000 (Aoki and von Kaulla 1971a). A more highly purified preparation was assigned a molecular weight of 70–75 000 by gel filtration and ultracentrifugation and, unlike the tissue preparation mentioned above, appears to exist as a single chain (Binder, Spragg and Austen 1979). Our own studies on endothelial plasminogen activator indicate a molecular weight identical to that of human heart activator on polyacrylamide gel electrophoresis; with progressive purification, both forms of activator became contaminated with active fragments of smaller molecular size in spite of inclusion of protease inhibitors throughout the purification (Booth and Bennett 1981). Other workers have also isolated active material of similar molecular size from cadaveric vessel washouts (Aasted 1980, Allen and Pepper 1981); in one case reduction suggested that a two-chain molecule had been identified.

Plasminogen activator in circulating blood

Small quantities of plasminogen activator are detectable in plasma obtained from resting subjects. Levels are markedly enhanced by a number of stimuli such as exercise, adrenalin, stress, and venous occlusion (Biggs, Macfarlane and Pilling 1947, Sherry *et al.* 1959, Bennett, Ogston and Ogston 1968). Characterization of plasma plasminogen activator(s) has been impeded by its (their) lability and the fact that only tiny quantities are present. It seems probable that activators in blood may be of two basic types: those released into the blood from tissues and vascular endothelium, activators of extrinsic origin, and those arising from the blood itself, activators of intrinsic origin.

'EXTRINSIC' PLASMINOGEN ACTIVATORS

The activator which appears in human blood after prolonged venous occlusion has been partially purified (Ogston, Bennett and Mackie 1976, Mackie, Booth and Bennett 1981). It behaves as a serine protease and chromatographs with proteins of large molecular size in buffers of low ionic strength; in buffers containing high salt concentrations it chromatographs with albumin as if disassociation of a large complex had occurred. This material is immunologically distinct from urokinase and similar in its physical properties to purified activator from tissue and from cadaveric endothelium (Mackie, Booth and Bennett 1981). Other workers have purified what are probably similar activators from human blood and have also found molecular weights of 60 000 and other properties similar to those of endothelial activator (Radcliffe and Heinze 1978, Kok 1979b). Similarity between post-occlusion activator and endothelial or tissue activator has been demonstrated immunologically (Rijken, Wijngaards and Welbergen 1980, 1981).

It appears, therefore, that one type of plasminogen activator in blood is chemically and immunologically related to that in vascular endothelium and other tissues; it is presumed that it is released into the blood by various stimuli and is thus designated 'extrinsic' activator.

'INTRINSIC' PLASMINOGEN ACTIVATORS

Plasma from resting subjects contains only traces of plasminogen activator and this activator may differ from that present after the stimuli mentioned above. It is clear that, in addition to an activator present and directly demonstrable in plasma, activator may be *generated* from plasma by stimuli known to activate the contact system such as exposure to kaolin, dextran or ellagic acid (Niewiarowski and Prou-Wartelle 1959, Iatridis, Iatridis and Ferguson 1966, Astrup and Rosa 1974). Generation of such activator is defective in plasmas deficient in factor XII (Hageman factor), prekallikrein (Fletcher factor) and high molecular weight kininogen (Fitzgerald factor) (Ogston *et al.* 1969, Wuepper 1973, Saito *et al.* 1975). Thus each of these agents, necessary for the generation of activity in one of the coagulation pathways, is necessary for generation of activity in a fibrinolytic pathway. It may be that incompletely defined agents other than the above are also involved (Ogston *et al.* 1969). The nature of the agent finally responsible for activation of plasminogen in this pathway is not certain; though kallikrein itself and factor XII fragments have been reported as having this property (Colman 1969, Laake and Vennerod 1974, Goldsmith, Saito and Ratnoff 1978), they may not represent the final activator of the pathway (Binder, Beckman and Jorg 1981). This activator may be generated from plasma depleted of activator and plasminogen by lysine sepharose which thus presumably does not absorb the proenzymes necessary for maintenance of the path to activator formation. Although this 'contact-generated' activator has not been completely defined, some of its physical properties in partially purified form are similar to those of circulating, vascular endothelial and tissue activators (Mackie, Booth and Bennett 1981). Using a different approach, it has been shown that a proportion of the total plasminogen activator activity in the plasma euglobulin fraction is inhibited by C1 inactivator (C1 Ina) while the remainder resisted this agent (Kluft 1978). Fluctuations in level of the resistant fraction seemed to parallel fluctuations induced by exercise, whereas the C1 Ina-sensitive fraction was optimally recovered by the use of dextran; it was suggested that C1 Ina-sensitive fraction represented activator intrinsic to the blood while the resistant fraction represented activator released from vascular endothelium or tissues. Activators of intrinsic origin have been further divided into factor XII-dependent and factor XII-independent moieties, the latter possibly being immunologically related to urokinase (Kluft, Wijngaards and Jie 1981, Wijngaards and Kluft 1981).

Plasminogen activators in secreted fluids

Urokinase is the human activator of plasminogen which has received most detailed study. Fibrinolytic activity was observed in human urine over 30 years ago (Macfarlane and Pilling 1947, Williams 1951) and the responsible agent, urokinase, isolated in pure crystalline form in 1965 (Lesuk, Terminiello and Traver 1965, Lesuk *et al.* 1967). The molecular weight was found to be 50 000 though two molecular forms are now generally recognized with weights of 54 000 and 31 000 (White, Barlow and Mozen 1966). An agent identical to urokinase has been observed in renal tissue cultures (Bernik and Kwaan 1967). The relationship of urokinase to plasma and tissue activators is conflicting (Kucinski, Fletcher and Sherry 1968, Aoki and von Kaulla 1971b, Bernik *et al.* 1974) but, as indicated above, a proportion of plasma activator may be related to urokinase and this may explain in part the discrepant observations of different groups.

Plasminogen activators have been identified and described in a large number of secretions other than urine, including tears, saliva, milk and semen (Astrup and Sterndorff 1953, von Kaulla and Shettles 1953, Albrechtsen and Thaysen 1955, Storm 1955). The activity in tears and saliva is immunologically similar to tissue activator, while semen contains activators similar to tissue activator and to urokinase (Rijken, Wijngaards and Welbergen 1981).

Activators in cultured tissues

Plasminogen activators are produced by a number of cell types in tissue culture, notably vascular endothelial cells, cells from various tumours and cells having undergone oncogenic transformation by a number of stimuli. Culture of endothelial cells and examination of the activator produced (Levin and Loskutoff 1981, Loskutoff and Edgington 1977, 1981, Loskutoff 1981) will be a useful tool in examining endothelial activator which cannot be readily sampled *in vivo* while the production of activator by cultured human tumour cells is already being exploited (Korninger *et al.* 1981, Rijken and Collen 1981) to produce large quantities of activator not obtainable by other means.

Streptokinase

This material, produced by β-haemolytic streptococci Lancefield group C, has received detailed study concerning its ability to activate plasminogen. It interacts with plasminogen or with plasmin to produce a $1:1$ molecular complex which behaves as a plasminogen activator. It is not a physiological activator and so is discussed in detail in the next chapter.

Inhibitors of fibrinolysis

Alpha$_2$-antiplasmin

Free plasmin is rarely demonstrable by functional assays in circulating blood. This is due to the activity of the major plasma antiplasmin known as α_2-plasmin inhibitor, α_2-antiplasmin, fast-acting antiplasmin or simply antiplasmin (Mullertz 1974, Collen, De Cock and Verstraete 1975, Moroi and Aoki 1976, Wiman and Collen 1977, Hedner and Abildgaard 1978). This recently described protein has a molecular weight of between 60 000 and 70 000 (Moroi and Aoki 1976, Wiman and Collen 1977), migrates as an α_2-globulin on electrophoresis, is a single chain glycoprotein in its native form and has been partially sequenced (Lijnen *et al.* 1981). Levels are reduced in severe liver disease (Aoki and Yamanaka 1978) suggesting that it may be synthesized in the liver though other interpretations of the observation exist.

Alpha$_2$-antiplasmin binds to and inhibits plasmin very rapidly, and irreversibly (Moroi and Aoki 1976, Wiman and Collen 1977). The stable complex is formed by reaction with the light chain of plasmin which contains the active site. Blocking of the active site by substrate or of the lysine-binding sites on plasmin slows complex formation markedly (Christensen and Clemmensen 1977, Wiman and Collen 1978a) indicating that both the lysine-binding and active enzyme sites participate in complex formation. Alpha$_2$-antiplasmin also impedes absorption of plasminogen by fibrin (Moroi and Aoki 1977a). Plasmin-α_2-antiplasmin complexes may be demonstrated in plasma by two-dimensional immunoelectrophoresis *in vitro*, after activation of plasminogen by urokinase (Aoki *et al.* 1977), in plasma of patients undergoing therapy with streptokinase (Verstraete, Vermylen and Schetz 1978) and have also been observed in the plasma of patients with spontaneous fibrinolytic bleeding (Booth and Bennett 1982).

Alpha$_2$-macroglobulin

This protein was believed to be the major plasma antiplasmin until the recent description of α_2-antiplasmin as a separate entity. Alpha$_2$-macroglobulin has a molecular weight of approximately 725 000, exists as a tetramer of four apparently identical subunits and the molecular characteristics have been described in detail. It is capable of binding a number of plasma enzymes including plasmin. Its reaction with plasmin is slower than that of α_2-antiplasmin and it is now suggested that its role is the neutralization of plasmin formed in excess of the inhibitory capacity of α_2-antiplasmin (Collen 1976, Mullertz and Clemmensen 1976). Alpha$_2$-macroglobulin–plasmin complexes have been demonstrated to appear in plasma to which plasmin or urokinase had been added (Harpel 1981). Greater quantities of the complexes were noted when plasminogen was activated endogenously by urokinase than when plasmin was added directly. Small amounts of the complexes have been demonstrated *in vivo* during urokinase infusions but were not detected in patients with DIC.

In addition to its ability to inhibit plasmin, α_2-macroglobulin is also *in vitro* an inhibitor of thrombin, urokinase and kallikrein (Harpel 1970b, Ogston *et al.* 1973, Abildgaard 1979).

Alpha$_1$-antitrypsin

Norman and Hill, who described two different antiplasmin activities in 1958, identified one such agent with α_1-mobility. This was noted by others (Shamash and Rimon 1966) who confirmed that it was heat and acid labile and had a molecular size similar to that of α_1-antitrypsin. Plasmin inhibition by α_1-antitrypsin, a single-chain glycoprotein of molecular weight approximately 54 000, is a time-dependent reaction (Bundy and Mehl 1959, Crawford 1973) the mechanism remaining incompletely defined; one suggestion has been that α_1-antitrypsin has enzymic activity which degrades the plasmin molecule (Rimon, Shamash and Shapiro 1966). The quantitative importance of α_1-antitrypsin as an inhibitor of plasmin is probably minor; no haemorrhagic disorder is associated with α_1-antitrypsin deficiency (Kahn 1978).

C1s̄-Inactivator (C1 Ina)

This protein, a neuramino-glycoprotein of molecular weight 104 000 and α_2-mobility inhibits C1 esterase (C1s̄) activity (Ratnoff and Lepow 1957,

Pensky, Levy and Lepow 1961, Pensky and Schwick 1969). In purified systems it inhibits the fibrinolytic and esterolytic activities of plasmin (Ratnoff *et al.* 1969, Schreiber, Kaplan and Austen 1973). It has been suggested that C1 Ina is a substrate for plasmin as it has been shown that the two form an equimolar complex (Harpel 1970a), after which C1 Ina is degraded, one of the derivatives retaining the ability to complex with plasmin (Harpel and Cooper 1975).

C1 Ina, in addition to inhibiting plasmin, also inhibits factor XIIa, factor XIa and kallikrein (Harpel 1976, Schapira, Scott and Colman 1981). It appears to be the principal plasma inhibitor of factor XIIa and shares with α_2-macroglobulin the plasma inhibitory activity against kallikrein. Thus it may influence fibrinolysis at stages earlier than that of formed plasmin, as by inhibiting these two agents it may impede the factor XII-dependent generation of plasminogen activator.

Patients with hereditary C1 Ina deficiency and hereditary angio-oedema show some decrease in plasma inhibition of plasmin. However, the significance of this agent as a plasmin inhibitor is minor and deficient patients do not show haemorrhagic features as do those with α_2-antiplasmin deficiency.

Antithrombin III (AT III)

AT III, in addition to possessing heparin cofactor and progressive antithrombin activities, (see Chapter 6), also inhibits plasmin in a progressive time-dependent manner forming an undissociable equimolar complex with the enzyme; this reaction is accelerated by heparin (Highsmith and Rosenberg 1974, Crawford and Ogston 1975). This property is probably of minor importance *in vivo*. Patients with AT III deficiency do not show any evidence of enhanced fibrinolysis.

Inter-α-trypsin inhibitor

This labile glycoprotein, which inhibits a number of enzymes, also interacts with plasmin (Heide, Heimburger and Haupt 1965, Schwick, Heimburger and Haupt 1967, Steinbuch 1971) but is unlikely to contribute major antiplasmin activity *in vivo*.

In summary, plasma inhibition of plasmin is principally due to α_2-antiplasmin. Alpha$_2$-macroglobulin may be called into play if the capacity of α_2-antiplasmin is overwhelmed. The other inhibitors mentioned probably play an insignificant role in the inhibition of plasmin in the blood if normal quantities of α_2-antiplasmin and α_2-macroglobulin are present (Mullertz 1974, Collen 1976).

Inhibition of plasminogen activator

Many groups have sought to establish the presence of inhibitors of plasminogen activator (Paraskevas, Nilsson and Martinsson 1962, Bennett 1967, 1970, Lauritsen 1968). Methodological problems, principally the absence of a specific substrate for activator, other than plasminogen itself, have impeded progress since the use of plasminogen as substrate has meant that assay systems have always been influenced by antiplasmin properties of any molecules examined. Additionally, until recently, preparations of blood and tissue activators have not been available for such studies so investigation has centred on the detection of inhibitors of urokinase- or streptokinase-induced lysis. Alpha$_2$-antiplasmin and α_1-antitrypsin will inhibit urokinase slowly (Clemmensen and Christensen 1976, Moroi and Aoki 1977b) and α_2-macroglobulin will produce some immediate inhibition of urokinase activity (Ogston *et al.* 1973). A further protein has been described which will inhibit some of the enzymic properties of urokinase but not that of lysing clots (Gallimore 1980). Urokinase inhibitors have also been noted in the placenta (Kawano, Morimoto and Uemura 1968), and in amniotic fluid (Walker, Campbell and Ogston 1980). Thus there are several agents capable of inhibiting urokinase-induced clot lysis but, as activators discrete from urokinase abound in the body, these inhibitors will play a restricted role in physiological fibrinolysis, though they will clearly influence therapeutic lysis with urokinase. One well-characterized protein, detected originally by its ability to inhibit urokinase-induced clot lysis has been shown to inhibit clot lysis induced by activated factor XII, and so may have a role in controlling fibrin lysis *in vivo* (Hedner 1980).

Agents which appear to inhibit tissue or circulating activator have less commonly been described. Several agents inhibiting fibrinolysis by activator from pig heart have recently been noted in human plasma, one of which did not inhibit urokinase (Walker and Ogston 1981), and inhibitor of plasminogen activator has been noted in cultured endothelial cells (Loskutoff and Edgington 1981). These agents are not fully characterized, their role is as yet unknown and some workers doubt the physiological significance of specific inhibitors of tissue activator, suggesting that control of activator activity in the circulation is via clearance mechanisms rather than by neutralization (Collen 1980, Korninger and Collen 1981).

Histidine-rich glycoprotein

This protein has recently been identified as being capable of interacting with the high-affinity lysine-binding sites of plasmin and thus reducing the rate at which plasmin–α_2-antiplasmin complexing occurs (Lijnen, Hoylaerts and

Collen 1980). It might thus be expected to modify fibrinolysis considerably. In *in vitro* studies it caused a limited increase in the rate of activation of plasminogen by urokinase but retarded the lysis of ^{125}I-labelled fibrin clots by tissue activator and plasminogen; the latter finding was thought to indicate that it impeded binding of plasminogen to fibrin due to its interaction with the binding sites. The molecular weight of this protein is 60 000. Its physiological role is unknown but by interaction with lysine-binding sites on plasminogen or plasmin it may significantly influence fibrinolytic processes.

Mechanism of fibrinolysis

It will be evident that, under normal circumstances, any plasmin formed in the circulation will be very rapidly neutralized by the action of α_2-antiplasmin. Free plasmin is thus almost never detectable in the blood. If thrombi or other fibrin deposits are removed it clearly must therefore be by the action of plasmin preferentially in these fibrin-containing areas, that is, by local fibrinolysis with the neutralization in the blood of any plasmin diffusing away from the area of activity. Any concept of the mechanism of fibrinolysis must explain why plasmin can act locally and escape the influence of α_2-antiplasmin while plasmin diffusing into the blood is usually neutralized immediately.

Role of fibrin

The preferential adsorption of individual agents on to formed fibrin has long been proposed as the means whereby local fibrinolysis is promoted. Early theories suggested that preferential adsorption of plasminogen (Alkjaersig, Fletcher and Sherry 1959), or of plasmin from postulated circulating plasmin-antiplasmin complexes (Ambrus and Marcus 1962), on to formed fibrin were crucial. Evidence illuminating these possibilities has been conflicting. This may partly reflect the fact that early studies probably examined principally the adsorption of native Glu-plasminogen, as it has recently been shown that while Glu-plasminogen is absorbed rather reluctantly by fibrin, Lys-plasminogen is absorbed more powerfully (Thorsen 1975, Cederholm-Williams 1977). It appears, too, that the lysine-binding sites of plasminogen, recently demonstrated, play a major role in the adsorption or otherwise of plasminogen on to fibrin, as their blockade by 6-aminohexanoic acid prevents adsorption in both pure and plasma-containing systems (Moroi and Aoki 1972, Thorsen 1975, Rakoczi, Wiman and Collen 1978).

Fibrin is also capable of adsorbing plasminogen activators and such binding varies according to the activator preparation used. Urokinase, for example, binds poorly to fibrin but the SK-plasminogen activator complex is adsorbed (Chesterman, Allington and Sharp 1972). In contrast, the more recently purified human activators which have been studied are adsorbed avidly on to formed or forming fibrin. Plasma activator (Ogston, Bennett and Mackie 1976), tissue activator (Thorsen, Glas-Greenwalt and Astrup 1972) and endothelial activator (Mackie and Bennett 1978), are adsorbed in this way. Additionally, the ability of several forms of these activators to activate plasminogen is enhanced in purified systems by the presence of fibrin or fibrin monomer (Allen and Pepper 1981, Binder, Beckman and Jorg 1981). Whether this enhancement depends on adsorption is not established but seems probable (Hoylaerts *et al.* 1981, Libeskind, Lipinski and Gurewich 1981, Lloyd, Cederholm-Williams and Sharp 1981).

Many of the adsorption studies mentioned have been carried out in purified systems, and, where repeated in plasma-containing systems, adsorption has been modified quantitatively by plasma protease inhibitors, though qualitatively similar adsorptions occurred (Rakoczi, Wiman and Collen 1978). It is thus clear that formed or forming fibrin will adsorb both plasminogen and some of the plasminogen activators found in the body. Adsorption of plasminogen involves its lysine-binding sites, involvement of which will markedly reduce the susceptibility of plasmin, formed from such molecules, to inhibition by α_2-antiplasmin which also acts via these sites. The preferential adsorption of activators and plasminogen sets the scene for plasmin generation on the surface of its substrate fibrin, in a form which renders it unlikely to be rapidly inhibited by α_2-antiplasmin. Any plasmin formed which diffuses off the fibrin strands will presumably free its lysine-binding sites and thus render itself susceptible to rapid inhibition by α_2-antiplasmin in the circulation; in this way, fibrinolysis is limited to the solid fibrin deposit and release of plasmin in an active form into the circulation or its generation there is prevented.

Many questions remain unanswered which may influence this concept which is based largely on that of Wiman and Collen (1978b). The relative importance of activator or plasminogen adsorbed on to fibrin during its formation, or diffusing into fibrin deposits thereafter, is uncertain. The nature and relative importance of the different types of plasminogen activator need to be established, as does the relationship and function of one- and two-chain forms of activator, which appear to show similar activity (Rijken, Hoylaerts and Collen 1981), and the existence and role of inhibitors of plasminogen activator need to be confirmed and defined.

Identification of fibrinolysis in the body

Episodes of fibrinolysis in the body may be sustained or transient, generalized or local events. If they are sustained and generalized, their identification is easy. Thus patients with haemorrhage due to systemic fibrinolysis will have evidence in their circulating blood of grossly increased amounts of plasmin or of plasminogen activator. These may be identified by such simple techniques as:

(a) the whole blood clot-lysis time

(b) the euglobulin clot-lysis time

which do not differentiate plasmin from plasminogen activator, or

(c) lysis of preformed fibrin plates which, by the use of plasminogen-containing and plasminogen-free fibrin, can be made to differentiate plasmin from activator.

These tests are all that are necessary to establish that fibrinolytic activity sufficient to cause bleeding is or is not present. They are, however, useful only in detecting *systemic* hyperfibrinolysis. If an episode of fibrinolysis has been transient or localized, demonstration that it has occurred is more difficult.

Past attempts at showing that fibrinolysis has occurred recently or is occurring locally within the body have depended upon efforts to demonstrate the presence of products of fibrin digestion in the serum. As yet, methods widely available to clinical laboratories do not distinguish fibrin from fibrinogen breakdown products nor will they distinguish them from soluble fibrin monomer with complete certainty and so may not invariably separate intravascular clotting from fibrinolysis. An alternative method, more recently developed, for demonstration that *in vivo* fibrinolysis has undoubtedly occurred depends on the demonstration that plasmin has been formed (even though it may not be measured in functional assays) by means of identifying plasmin–α_2-antiplasmin complexes in circulating blood.

Products of plasmin degradation of fibrinogen or fibrin

Agents resulting from the degradation of fibrin or fibrinogen by plasmin were recognized first by Stormorken (1957), Triantaphyllopoulos (1958) and Niewiarowski and Kowalski (1958). Five molecular entities, designated A, B, C, D and E were identified as products of fibrinogen digestion by plasmin *in vitro* by Nussenzweig and Seligmann (1960) and Nussenzweig *et al.* (1961). Other labile intermediate derivatives have also been noted and are known as the X and Y fragments and by other terms (Fletcher *et al.* 1966, Larrieu, Marder and Inceman 1966, Mossesson *et al.* 1967). These agents have been studied in detail and schemes from their sequential production from the fibrinogen molecule proposed and reviewed (Marder, Shulman and Carroll 1969, Mossesson 1973, Gaffney 1977). These fragments possess properties which may influence haemostasis. Some may themselves be coagulable by thrombin, albeit at a slower rate than fibrinogen, if they retain the fibrinopeptide-containing portions of the molecule and those containing the binding sites responsible for fibrin monomer polymerization (Fisher *et al.* 1967); others are incoagulable. Some such products, by competing for the action of thrombin, may delay its action in clotting fibrinogen (Wallen and Bergstrom 1958) while fibrin clots formed in presence of significant amounts of these agents may be structurally defective (Bang *et al.* 1962). Early products of fibrinogen digestion, if injected into dogs thus impede the thrombin–fibrinogen reaction and produce bleeding while late products impair fibrin polymerization (Kowalski *et al.* 1964). Early products alter platelet release reactions in response to thrombin, kaolin and other agents (Hirsch, Fletcher and Sherry 1965, Jerushalmy and Zucker 1966, Kopec *et al.* 1966). In clinical situations these agents may be detected free in serum by immunological techniques such as immunodiffusion, immunoelectrophoresis and tanned red cell haemagglutination inhibition (Ferreira and Murat 1963, Nilehn and Nilsson 1964, Merskey, Kleiner and Johnson 1966, Merskey, Lalezari and Johnson 1969).

It is not surprising that the products released from polymerized fibrin differ structurally from those released from soluble fibrinogen though they have shown considerable immunological similarity with these. It is to be expected, and has been found to be the case, that the products of plasmin-induced lysis of non-cross-linked fibrin are somewhat similar to those resulting from lysis of fibrinogen itself (Gaffney 1973, Pizzo *et al.* 1973), whereas those released from lysis of fibrin, which has been cross-linked by the action of factor XIII, are of different structure. The fibrin fragment which has received most attention is the dimer of the D fragment, with the γ-γ glutamyl lysine cross-link formed by thrombin-activated factor XIII (Gaffney and Brasher 1973, Pizzo *et al.* 1973), known as the D-dimer. It has since become apparent that this fragment may exist complexed to an E fragment (Fedderson and Gormsen 1971, Olexa and Budzynski 1979) and this may represent the form in which it is found *in vivo* as it appears to be the end-stage product of lysis in plasma systems (Gaffney 1979).

The distinction between the products of fibrinogen and fibrin digestion in the serum of patients is conceptually important as the former should indicate a systemic hyperfibrinolytic state with digestion of plasma fibrinogen while the latter may represent the lysis of local deposits of formed fibrin within the body. Such distinction cannot be made by the generally available latex agglutination assays which, as they employ antibodies to fibrinogen's D and E fragments will not differentiate between fibrinogen and fibrin fragments in serum. Further, though it was initially believed that the detection of antigens related to fibrinogen/fibrin in the serum might reasonably be expected to reflect *lysis* of fibrinogen or fibrin at least, Shainoff and Page (1962) and Sasaki *et al.* (1966) have demonstrated that fibrin monomer may form soluble complexes with fibrinogen or with some of its larger degradation products, and that these may or may not be clottable. This finding indicates that agents produced by the action of thrombin, without necessarily the participation of plasmin, may appear in the serum and so be detected by assays dependent upon antisera to fibrinogen or some of its fragments, due to cross-reactions between these antisera. Thus assays originally believed to detect fibrinogen or fibrin-degradation products (FDP) and to reflect fibrinolytic activity may actually detect antigens which could reflect either fibrinolytic activity *or* coagulant activity in the serum and may not distinguish between them. The assays, therefore, do not specifically detect FDP, but detect FDP or soluble fibrin monomer–fibrinogen complexes, and have been correctly reassessed as measuring fibrin/fibrinogen-related antigens (FRA), a term which encompasses both entities. Various neoantigens have been identified on the formation of certain of the degradation products of fibrinogen. Antisera raised to these have not, however, yet proved of value in clinical situations. Other methods of approaching the distinction between *in vivo* coagulation and fibrinolysis depended upon the demonstration of abnormally precipitable fibrinogen derivatives in the plasma of patients; so the demonstration of fibrin monomer, precipitable by cooling (Shainoff and Page 1962), by addition of protamine sulphate (Lipinski and Worowski 1968) or ethanol (Godal and Abildgaard 1966), has been advocated as evidence of intravascular clotting as opposed to fibrinolysis. Whether these methods distinguish clearly between the coagulant and fibrinolytic components of bleeding syndromes remains uncertain. An alternative but more complex approach to the problem lies in an attempt to establish the relative size of molecules reacting with antisera to fibrinogen in plasma. The detection of such molecules larger in size than fibrinogen itself might be regarded as a demonstration of polymerization products reflecting hypercoagulable and thrombotic states (Fletcher *et al.* 1977), while agents smaller than fibrinogen might be expected to reflect fibrinolysis *in vivo*. This approach, while conceptually attractive, remains too complex for routine use in clinical laboratories.

Plasmin–α_2-antiplasmin complex formation

It is, therefore, clear that detection of fibrin/fibrinogen-related antigens by the present generally available techniques may not always distinguish intravascular clotting from fibrinolysis or quantitate the relative contribution of each to a bleeding episode, and will not do so until techniques are available for clinical use which make meaningful and accurate distinctions between fibrin monomer–fibrinogen complexes, and fragments of fibrin or fibrinogen. Another approach to this distinction of intravascular clotting from fibrinolysis recommends itself as promising in this area. Recent observation on the protease inhibitors in plasma have clearly identified AT III and α_2-antiplasmin as the principal inhibitors of thrombin and of plasmin respectively. It is also established that these inhibitors form complexes with the enzymes they inhibit. Such complexes can be detected distinct from the uncomplexed inhibitors by the simple technique of two-dimensional immunoelectrophoresis. The presence of complexes of AT III with activated procoagulants has been demonstrated in cases of intravascular clotting (Collen 1977). Fig. 51 illustrates the findings in a patient with acute severe DIC in respect of such complexes and also in respect of plasmin–α_2-antiplasmin complexes and compares them with the findings in normal plasma. It is clear that both complexed AT III and complexed α_2-antiplasmin are present in the patient's plasma. These findings persisted for some time after the acute event when the coagulation derangement was returning to normal and detectable hyperfibrinolysis had disappeared. It was, therefore, evident that both intravascular clotting and plasmin generation had contributed to the haemostatic derangement clinically manifest by gross depletion of clotting factors. This approach can also be used to define the rarer situation in which hyperfibrinolysis alone is responsible for haemorrhage; this is shown by the presence of plasmin–α_2-antiplasmin complexes without thrombin–AT III complexes and such cases have been described (Booth and Bennett 1982, Booth *et al.* 1983). The technique of two-dimensional immunoelectrophoresis is relatively insensitive and demonstrates complexes only when formed in large quantities. A useful refinement of this approach may come if the suggestion is verified that the AT III complexed to activated procoagulants and α_2-antiplasmin complexed with plasmin exhibit antigenic sites different from those of the uncomplexed molecules (Collen 1977). There is already some evidence that this may be the case and attempts at devising immunological methods specific for the complexes are underway (Collen 1977, Plow, De Cock and Collen 1979, Harpel 1981). If these methods can be shown to be completely specific for the inhibitor-enzyme complexes, and are uninfluenced by the uncomplexed proteins, these methods can be made quantitative and sensitive and will greatly assist in the assessment of the relative contributions of intravascular coagulation and fibrinolysis to haemostatic disorders.

Physiological variation in fibrinolysis

Fibrinolytic activity is associated with the endothelium of blood vessels (Todd 1959), particularly that of veins, and activity is significantly higher in peripheral venous than in arterial blood (Ogston, Ogston and Bennett 1966), due primarily to increased activator levels since no difference in plasminogen, fibrinogen or inhibitors of fibrinolysis was noted.

The most striking physiological variation in fibrinolytic activity is the increase seen after exercise, first noted by Biggs and her colleagues (1947). This is due to a rise in activator level (Sawyer *et al.* 1960) and, in spite of very striking rises in activator after sustained physical exercise, detectable change in plasminogen or fibrinogen levels does not occur (Bennett, Ogston and

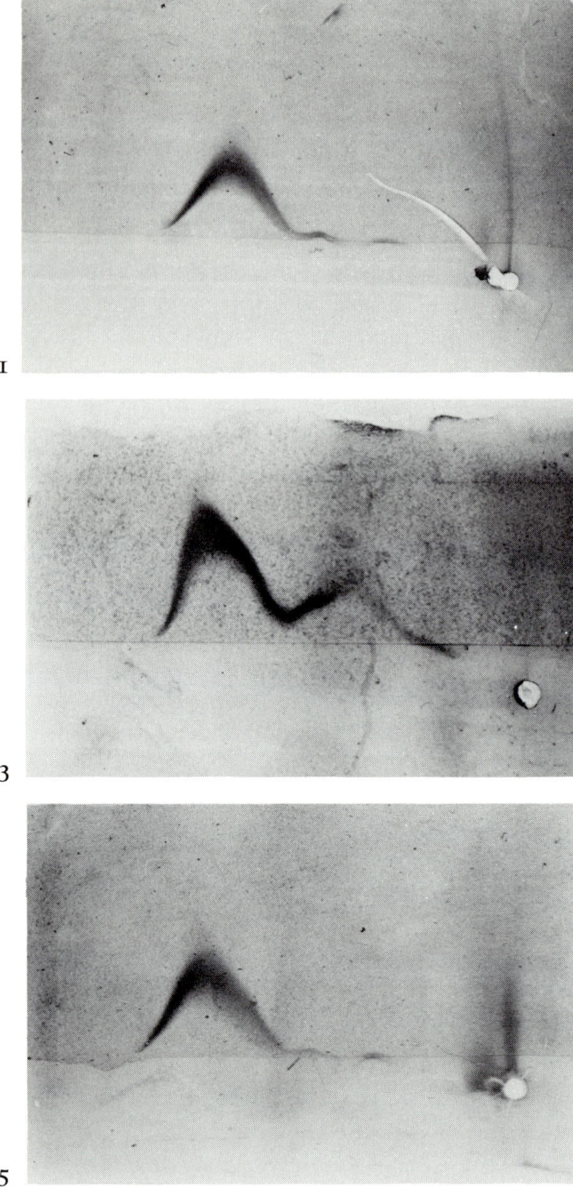

Fig. 51. Two-dimensional immunoelectrophoresis (2-DIEP) of plasma against antiserum to antithrombin III (AT III)—panels 1, 3 and 5, and against antiserum to α_2-antiplasmin (α_2AP)—panels 2, 4 and 6. Panels 1 and 2 are from normal human plasma; panels 3 and 4 are from a patient (A) with severe acute DIC and panels 5 and 6 are from a patient (B) with primary fibrinolytic haemorrhage. Patient A shows a large slow-moving second peak in the run against antiserum to AT III and a very large slow-moving peak in that against antiserum to α_2AP; these are due to thrombin–AT III complex and plasmin–α_2AP complexes respectively, and indicate

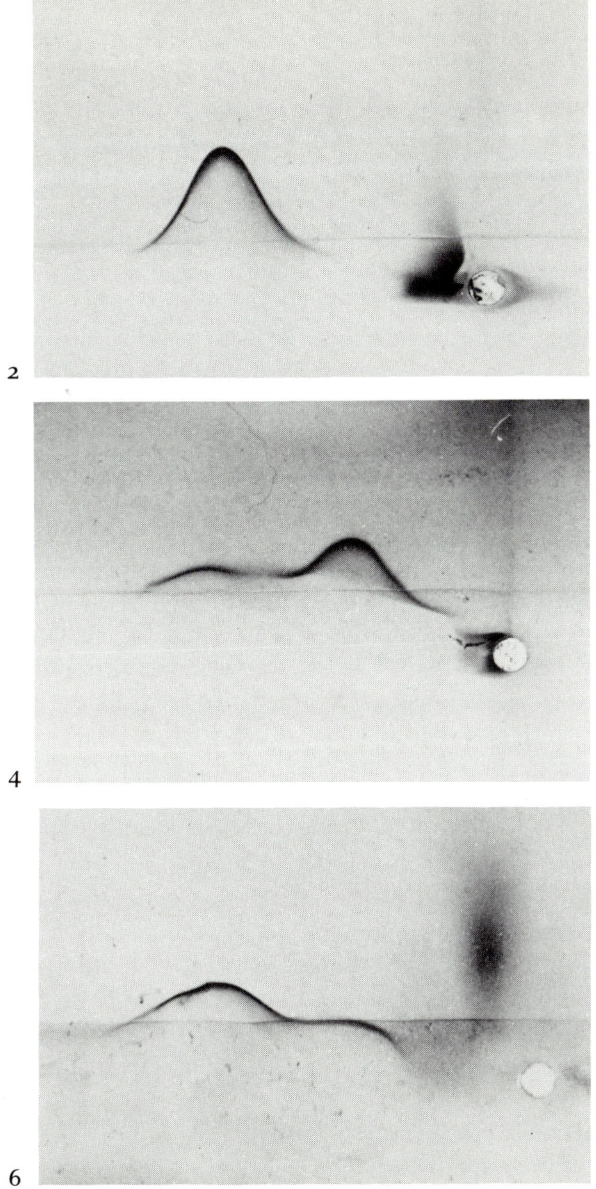

that both coagulation and fibrinolysis has occurred *in vivo*. Patient B shows no thrombin–AT III complex but has plasmin–α_2AP complex in his plasma confirming that fibrinolysis alone was responsible for his bleeding disorder (Booth *et al.* 1981, 1983).

(Reproduced from Booth N.A. & Bennett B. (1984) Plasmin–α_2–antiplasmin complexes in bleeding disorders characterized by primary or secondary fibrinolysis. *British Journal of Haematology* **56**, 545–56.)

Ogston 1968). Adrenalin injection increases fibrinolytic activity (Biggs, Macfarlane and Pilling 1947, Fearnley and Lackner 1955) and the exercise-induced increase might therefore reflect catecholamine activity, though this is not clearly supported by studies using α- and β- adrenergic blockers (Cash, Woodfield and Allen 1970, Britton *et al.* 1974). Possibly some of the changes observed directly reflect altered blood flow over the endothelium of capillaries and venules (Rennie, Bennett and Ogston 1977).

Acute mental stress increases fibrinolytic activity measured by techniques primarily reflecting activator levels (Macfarlane and Biggs 1946, Truelove 1951); catecholamines may play a part in this response. The effect of prolonged stress is not established. Evidence for a diurnal variation in fibrinolytic activity is available with levels lowest in the early morning and rising during the course of the day. Though such change may reflect exercise levels or stress, they apparently occur in bedfast patients and independent of work patterns (Fearnley, Balmforth and Fearnley 1957, Fearnley 1960).

Normal pregnancy results in profound changes in fibrinolysis which have been recently summarized (Bennett and Ogston 1977). Fibrinogen and plasminogen levels rise, activator levels fall and antiplasmin rises. By term, activator levels in circulating blood are very low, but rise within a few hours of delivery to the non-pregnant range. The newborn child has low plasma plasminogen and high activator levels, the latter falling in the first few days of life. No major change in overall fibrinolytic activity occurs with age though plasminogen levels rise slightly.

Striking ethnic differences have been recorded. In several studies, Africans have been noted to have higher fibrinolytic activity than is observed in white subjects, reflecting higher activator and plasminogen levels and possibly lower overall antiplasmin activity (Bennett and Ogston 1977). Whether this is environmentally mediated is not clear, though a study of black and white individuals matched for age, height, weight and activity levels, but not for socio-economic class, in the USA indicated increased fibrinolytic activity in the black group; it was noted, however, that this tended to decrease with rising social class (Szczeklik *et al.* 1980).

Obesity is associated with reduced fibrinolytic activity (Goldrick 1961) due primarily to low activator levels (Bennett *et al.* 1966). Activity rises during dietary restriction in both obese and non-obese (Ogston and McAndrew 1964). Studies on the influence of dietary fats and alimentary lipaemia on fibrinolysis have produced numerous and conflicting reports (Bennett and Ogston 1977).

Hereditary haemorrhage and fibrinolysis

Alpha$_2$-antiplasmin deficiency

Hereditary deficiency of plasma α_2-antiplasmin is associated with a severe haemorrhagic disorder characterized typically by prolonged bleeding after even trivial injuries, less frequent 'spontaneous' bleeding into joints or other body cavities (Aoki *et al.* 1979, 1980, Kluft, Vellenga and Brommer 1979). An individual so affected has been described in detail. His α_2-antiplasmin level was 3 per cent that of normal plasma and overall fibrinolysis *in vitro*, as judged by the whole blood clot lysis time, was grossly increased. Fibrinogen, plasminogen and serum FRA levels were, however, normal as were levels of the other plasma inhibitors of plasmin and all the other procoagulants. Thus it appeared that *in vivo* fibrinolysis did not occur continuously. *In vitro*, the abnormality was totally corrected by the addition of purified α_2-antiplasmin, and plasma transfusion and tranexamic acid produced clinical benefit. The patient was the product of a consanguineous marriage between two individuals, themselves sprung from marriages of cousins from two branches of a single large family. Many of the patient's siblings and other relatives thus had α_2-antiplasmin levels of approximately 50 per cent of normal; none of these individuals, however, showed any haemorrhagic symptoms and assessment of their coagulation and fibrinolytic status in the laboratory was normal, indicating that α_2-antiplasmin levels of 50 per cent are compatible with totally normal haemostasis. The disorder thus appears autosomal recessive and clinically abnormality is expressed only in homozygotes. These very rare abnormalities illustrate the major role played by fibrinolysis and its control in normal haemostasis.

Plasminogen activator excess

A second lifelong and presumably hereditary disorder of fibrinolysis resulting in a severe haemorrhagic state has been described (Booth *et al.* 1981, 1983). The individual affected also showed prolonged bleeding after minor trauma, particularly dental extractions, had occasionally spontaneous bleeding into joints and finally a spontaneous cerebral haemorrhage. The disorder was characterized by normal coagulation and platelet function but grossly increased overall fibrinolysis as measured by the whole blood clot lysis time. This individual had, however, totally normal levels of all known inhibitors of fibrinolysis, and his disorder was the result of a grossly increased circulating level of a plasminogen activator chemically and immunologically similar to tissue activator. Unlike the patient with α_2-antiplasmin deficiency, however, this individual showed mildly reduced fibrinogen levels, markedly raised levels of serum FRA and, though plasmin activity was not demonstrable in his plasma, plasmin–α_2-antiplasmin complexes were demonstrable immunologically (Booth *et al.* 1983); these abnormalities were reversed by treatment with tranexamic acid. This disorder, therefore, appeared to be due to increased levels of activator with no demonstrable deficiency of any inhibitor. The individual had a gross hyperlipidaemia in addition to his bleeding disorder and very extensive arterial atheroma. He had a marked family history of myocardial infarction, but no family history of haemorrhage and so the two disorders appeared unrelated.

Acquired disorders of fibrinolysis

Haemorrhage due to excessive fibrinolysis occurs when plasminogen conversion to plasmin takes place to a degree and at a rate sufficient to overwhelm the ability of plasmin inhibitors, principally α_2-antiplasmin, to neutralize the active enzyme.

Thrombolytic therapy

Fibrinolytic bleeding may most simply be seen to occur during thrombolytic therapy, discussed in the following chapter, during which large quantities of urokinase or streptokinase are infused in the attempt to produce lysis of thrombi. In this situation plasmin is rapidly generated in the circulating blood and plasmin–α_2-antiplasmin complexes are formed (Collen and Wiman 1979) but under some circumstances free plasmin activity is demonstrable. When this occurs marked depletion of plasma fibrinogen, factor VIII and V procoagulant activity occurs as the enzyme digests the proteins in the circulation. This represents a clear-cut and well-defined hyperplasminaemic state and is one in which FRA are generated in large quantity which further interfere with haemostasis as described above. Such FRA may be expected to be generated both from circulating fibrinogen and from the thrombus under attack and would thus be expected to comprise both fibrinogen- and fibrin-degradation products which are not at present distinguishable by currently widely available tests for FRA. Such hyperplasminaemia is an undesirable consequence of treatment, the aim of which is the dissolution of a local thrombus without, if possible, the production of systemic hyperplasminaemia, and reflects the fact that urokinase and streptokinase are not avidly absorbed on to formed fibrin. It is possible that, in the future, thrombolytic regimes may be developed which achieve local thrombolysis successfully and avoid systemic hyperplasminaemia if sufficient quantities of *tissue* activator can be produced to be used in such programmes, as this activator *is* absorbed specifically on to formed fibrin. Tissue activator produced by cultured human melanoma cells has been used in this way in dog experiments and in man (Weimar *et al.* 1981) and has achieved significant lysis of thrombi without producing detectable activation of plasminogen in the circulation, consumption of α_2-antiplasmin, fibrinogen breakdown or bleeding. This is in contrast to the use of urokinase which, in doses producing lesser degrees of thrombolysis, resulted in systemic activation of the fibrinolytic system and a significant degree of bleeding (Matsuo, Rijken and Collen 1981).

Activator release from tumours or injured tissue

Hyperfibrinolysis due to urokinase or streptokinase therapy represents a highly defined state due specifically to the intravenous injection of plasminogen activators. Similar situations occasionally arise spontaneously. Proteolytic states, probably reflecting activator release, have been described in metastatic carcinoma of the prostate (Tagnon, Whitmore and Schulman 1952) or pancreas (Ratnoff 1952), cirrhosis of the liver (Grossi, Moreno and Rousselot 1961, Fletcher *et al.* 1964), leukaemia (Mikata *et al.* 1959) and disseminated lupus (Zywicka *et al.* 1961). In this department we have recently demonstrated primary fibrinolytic bleeding due to excessive amounts of plasminogen activator with plasmin–α_2-antiplasmin complex formation, depletion of total antiplasmin activity and severe haemorrhage in the absence of any coagulation disorder in two patients, one with disseminated breast carcinoma and the other with metastatic carcinoma of the prostate (Booth and Bennett 1984). Fibrinolytic bleeding may occasionally occur after damage to tissue containing plasminogen activator during surgery, particularly involving extracorporeal circulation (von Kaulla and Swan 1958, Gans and Krivit 1962, Douglas *et al.* 1966). Such rare episodes are due to primary fibrinolysis, that is fibrinolysis due to release of activator alone, in which DIC does not exist and any depletion of clotting factors is due only to the digestion by plasmin.

Fibrinolysis secondary to disseminated intravascular clotting (DIC)

A commoner event is fibrinolysis secondary to DIC as the primary or initiating event. DIC is discussed elsewhere in this volume and will not be described in detail here, but may occur in a variety of clinical situations such as a number of complications of pregnancy, in widespread malignant disease, after major trauma, after incompatible blood transfusion and during septicaemic states. In some forms of DIC, excessive fibrinolytic activity contributes to the global haemostatic disturbances but its quantitative contribution is often difficult to assess and varies in different situations. The time course with which DIC evolves and the nature of the initiating event vary and further complicate assessment of the contribution of fibrinolysis to the overall disorder. The acute disorders which complicate pregnancy such as abruptio placentae or amniotic fluid embolism provide good examples of the evolution of such disorders from a single acute event. Some workers (Bonnar *et al.* 1969) have noted reduced plasminogen activator and plasminogen with elevated FRA levels in such disorders while others report increased fibrinolytic activity (Weiner, Reid and

Table 35. Sequence of changes in fibrinolytic system after amniotic fluid embolism.

Time after initiating event	Plasma plasminogen activator	Plasma plasmin-α_2AP complex	Serum FRA	Plasma fibrinogen
1 hour	+ + + +	+ + + +	+ + + +	<50 mg/100 ml
2 hours	+ + + +	+ + + +	+ + + +	70 mg/100 ml
3 hours	+	+ + +	+ + + +	100 mg/100 ml
24 hours	−	+ +	+ + + +	150 mg/100 ml

Raby 1953, Beller *et al.* 1963, Skøjdt 1965, Philips, Montgomery and Taylor 1967). It seems most probable that variation in these findings reflects the time at which blood samples are studied, relative to the initiating event. Table 35, which summarizes findings in a patient studied over a period of hours after amniotic fluid embolism and placental abruption, indicates a burst of fibrinolytic activity reflected by high activator levels and the presence of plasmin–α_2-antiplasmin complexes at the onset of the disorder followed by disappearance of activator within a few hours; by this time the only evidence that a fibrinolytic phase has occurred is the persistence of plasmin–α_2-antiplasmin complexes and raised FRA levels, and interpretation of the latter, as indicating the fibrinolytic as opposed to the coagulant aspect of the disorder, may be difficult as already discussed. It seems likely in these situations that intravascular clotting is initiated immediately by the release into the circulation of thromboplastic agents from the uterus and that fibrinolysis occurs simultaneously either, (a) by concurrent release of uterine plasminogen activator, or (b) in response to acute deposition of fibrin within the microcirculation itself. Fibrinolysis thus probably contributes to the initial haemostatic disaster but plasmin is rapidly neutralized in the circulation by complex formation with α_2-antiplasmin, by which time peripheral blood sampling can detect that it has happened only by demonstration of such complexes and not by demonstration of high activator or plasmin levels in functional assays.

Fibrinolysis in liver disease

The overall haemostatic defect in liver disease is extremely complex and varies with:

1   the type of liver disease;

2   the degree to which impaired synthesis of clotting and fibrinolytic factors occurs;

3   the degree to which increased consumption of these factors in the circulation (by intravascular clotting or fibrinolysis) occurs;

4   the degree to which hepatic clearance of clotting or fibrinolytic factors occurs.

Thus the discussion of fibrinolysis in relation to liver disease requires that liver disease be defined, and many publications on the subject do not do this precisely. Goodpasture in 1914 knew that clots made from blood of patients with cirrhosis lysed rapidly, an observation confirmed repeatedly since (Ratnoff 1977). Similarly, rapid fibrinolysis is not observed in obstructive jaundice, primary biliary cirrhosis (Jedrychowski *et al.* 1973), carcinoma of the liver (Ratnoff 1949) or metastatic liver disease (Ogston, Bennett and Ogston 1971). The mechanisms underlying such observations are not completely defined but clearly those listed under 2–4 above may all contribute. Plasminogen levels, for instance, are regularly found to be reduced in uncomplicated cirrhosis and may reflect either decreased synthesis or increased consumption or both (Collen, Rouvier and Verstraete 1972). Plasminogen activator levels are elevated in cirrhosis; the activator measured is probably not synthesized in the liver but may be released from vascular endothelium and raised levels presumably reflect either decreased inhibition of activator in the blood or its delayed clearance from the circulation (Fletcher *et al.* 1964); additionally, cirrhotic liver does contain activator which might possibly be released under some circumstances (Astrup *et al.* 1960) though information on this is lacking. Reduced levels of inhibitors of fibrinolysis in cirrhosis may occur (Ogston, Bennett and Ogston 1971, Aoki and Yamanaka 1978), reflecting either impaired synthesis or increased consumption or both.

In forms of liver disease, other than compensated cirrhosis, rapid fibrinolysis is not the rule. Presumably in these disorders, in addition to the factors listed above, must be added the possibility that proteins may be released from damaged tissues into the circulation and may directly then influence fibrinolysis. This clearly may occur in acute hepatitis and hepatic necrosis and may conceivably occur in various forms of malignant disease of the liver. The striking change from high to low fibrinolytic activity noted in connection with development of hepatoma in cirrhotic patients certainly suggests that some tumours may release inhibitory agents (Kwaan and McFadzean 1959).

The dissection out of the very complex haemostatic disorders, which may complicate liver disease of that portion attributable specifically to abnormal fibrinolysis, and the definition of the mechanisms involved is clearly difficult. Detection of high activator levels or plasmin–α_2-antiplasmin complexes may tell us that fibrinolysis is occurring in various forms of liver disease but, until discrimination between FRA is precise enough to identify separately such antigens as soluble fibrin monomer–fibrinogen complexes, fibrin- or fibrinogen-breakdown products, the quantitative contribution of the fibrinolytic system will remain undefined. Even if this is possible it will not be clear whether it represents a primary event or is secondary to other factors.

In practical terms, at present, the fibrinolytic contribution to haemorrhage is probably not major in most patients with liver disease. Fibrinolytic inhibitors may be helpful in some cases but has not had a beneficial effect in studies on variceal bleeding (Lewis and Doyle 1964, Tytgat, Collen and Verstraete 1971). As DIC complicates several forms of liver disease to varying degrees, the use of such inhibitors in undefined bleeding disorders arising in liver disorders cannot be recommended.

Fibrinolysis and thrombosis

Many thrombi disappear or shrink relatively rapidly in the body presumably as a result of spontaneous fibrinolysis and it is established that the body's fibrinolytic system may be harnessed to achieve therapeutic dissolution of formed thrombi. It may be postulated that thrombi which persist and produce symptoms represent a failure of the body's fibrinolytic mechanism. This is a plausible concept and an enormous literature seeks to examine the possibility. Broadly speaking, three types of study have been carried out:

1. Assessment of fibrinolytic activity in patients with an established thrombus

Innumerable such studies have been performed but cannot establish whether depressed fibrinolysis thus demonstrated is a response to, rather than a cause of, the thrombosis.

2. Assessment of fibrinolytic activity in disorders or clinical situations predisposing to thrombosis

It is thus established that reduced blood fibrinolytic activity occurs in association with obesity, bed rest, cardiac failure, the post-operative period, pregnancy and the post-partum period, after myocardial infarction and after femoral fracture. All these situations are associated with deep venous thrombosis, but the depressed fibrinolysis demonstrated cannot be held to be the only cause of such thrombosis as many other factors operate, and, where sequential changes in fibrinolysis have been recorded, maximum depression of activity appears to occur later than the period during which thrombus development is commonest.

3. Assessment of disordered fibrinolysis and its use in the prediction of future thrombotic disease.

Here, evidence is available that points to a causal relationship between depressed fibrinolysis and thrombosis. Several patients have now been described who possess variant forms of the plasminogen molecule (Aoki *et al.* 1978, Sakata and Aoki 1980, Wohl, Summaria and Robbins 1979, Wohl *et al.* 1981). The abnormalities have been summarized (Robbins 1981) and concern variously the function of the molecules, their active sites, ability to form activator complexes, the binding of activator to the zymogens, cleavage characteristics and isoelectric forms in which they appear in plasma. Essentially, the ease with which they were converted to plasmin was reduced and the affected individuals had a history of recurrent thrombosis. In one case the disorder appeared hereditarily based (Aoki *et al.* 1978). In these patients a clear association was established between a pre-existing fibrinolytic disorder and venous thrombosis. Secondly, a number of individuals have been described in whom 'recurrent idiopathic venous thrombosis' was associated with defective production of plasminogen activator by samples of venous endothelium examined after vein biopsy (Isacson and Nilsson 1972); here it is not totally clear whether the abnormality antedated the thrombotic event but it seems possible. Finally, depressed fibrinolytic activity has been found of value (in association with a number of other factors) in predicting the occurrence of venous thrombosis after surgery (Clayton, Anderson and McNicol 1976, Crandon *et al.* 1980). These observations, particularly the first, do now provide a link between depressed fibrinolytic activity and subsequent development of venous thrombosis. Many other factors clearly play a role in thrombus generation, however, and the quantitative importance of normal fibrinolysis in preventing thrombosis or in limiting small thrombi before they reach clinical significance, remains uncertain.

Fibrinolysis and neoplasia

A link between fibrin formation and tumour growth or dissemination has been proposed for many years and it has been suggested that fibrinolytic factors may be implicated (Donati and Poggi 1980, Marcus *et al.* 1980). Production of fibrinolytically active agents has been associated with malignant transformation of cells in culture (Reich 1973). These agents are principally plasminogen activators (Roblin *et al.* 1981); they differ according to the cell line from which they originate, some being related and others unrelated to urokinase (Vetterlein *et al.* 1979). Inhibition of growth of experimental tumours by tranexamic acid has been reported (Peterson 1968, 1977) and such agents have been employed in protocols for the treatment of cancer in humans (Astedt, Mattsson and Trope 1977). Whether production of plasminogen activators is a marker of neoplasia is not established since not all malignant cells produce them (Kucinski, Fletcher and Sherry 1968). An alternative possibility concerns a role for activator in the ability of a tumour to metastasize (Mott *et al.* 1974, Wang *et al.* 1980). It is evident that, while the fibrinolytic system may play a part in the behaviour of malignant cells, its role is not yet defined.

Concluding remarks

It will be evident that fibrin, during or after its formation, may adsorb plasminogen and some of its activators, and thus concentrates on its surface the agents which are capable of generating plasmin. In this way, from the complex series of enzymes and inhibitors of the fibrinolytic system, fibrin abstracts the elements necessary for its own ultimate destruction; activity of this system is held in check, remote from fibrin deposits, by the powerful inhibitors described in this chapter. Uncontrolled over-activity of the system is rare, easy to detect and causes a severe haemorrhagic disorder. Under-activity of the system is difficult to quantify but may contribute to the persistence of intravascular thrombi or fibrin deposited in tissues injured by any pathological process. The problem of quantifying under-activity of the system and relating this clearly to the persistence of fibrin deposits has, in general, not been solved. The system may, however, be harnessed for the removal of thrombi in a number of ways discussed in the next chapter. It is possible, but not established, that it may play a role in the behaviour of certain malignant cells.

Acknowledgment

Previously unpublished studies reported in this chapter were supported by project grant G/978/718-S from the Medical Research Council of Great Britain and were carried out by Dr N.A. Booth.

REFERENCES

Aasted B. (1980) Purification and characterisation of human vascular plasminogen activator. *Biochemica et Biophysica Acta* **621**, 241–54.

Abildgaard U. (1979) A review of antithrombin III. In *The Physiological Inhibitors of Blood Coagulation and Fibrinolysis*. Collen D., Wiman B. & Verstraete M. (eds). pp. 19–29, 31–3, 239–41. Elsevier, Amsterdam.

Albrechtsen O.K. & Thaysen J.H. (1955) Fibrinolytic activity in human saliva. *Acta Physiologica Scandinavica* **35**, 138.

Alkjaersig N., Fletcher A.P. & Sherry S. (1959) The mechanism of clot dissolution by plasmin. *Journal of Clinical Investigation* **38**, 1086–95.

Allen R.A. & Pepper D.S. (1981) Isolation and properties of human vascular plasminogen activator. *Thrombosis and Haemostasis* **45**, 43–50.

Ambrus C.M. & Markus G. (1962) Plasmin-antiplasmin complex as a reservoir of fibrinolytic enzyme. *American Journal of Physiology* **199**, 491.

Aoki N., Moroi M., Matsuda M. & Tachiya K. (1977) The behaviour of α_2-plasmin inhibitor of fibrinolytic states. *Journal of Clinical Investigation* **60**, 361–9.

Aoki N., Moroi M., Sakata Y., Yoshida N. & Matsuda M. (1978) Abnormal plasminogen. A hereditary molecular abnormality found in a patient with recurrent thrombosis. *Journal of Clinical Investigation* **61**, 1186–95.

Aoki N., Saito H., Kamiya T., Koie K., Sakata Y. & Kabakura M. (1979) Congenital deficiency of α_2-plasmin inhibitor associated with severe hemorrhagic tendency. *Journal of Clinical Investigation* **63**, 877–84.

Aoki N., Sakata Y., Matsuda M. & Tateno K. (1980) Fibrinolytic states in a patient with congenital deficiency of α_2-plasmin inhibitor. *Blood* **55**, 483–8.

Aoki N. & von Kaulla K.N. (1971a) The extraction of vascular plasminogen activator from human cadavers and a description of its properties. *American Journal of Clinical Pathology* **55**, 171–9.

Aoki N. & von Kaulla K.N. (1971b) Dissimilarity of human vascular plasminogen activator and human urokinase. *Journal of Laboratory and Clinical Medicine* **78**, 354–62.

Aoki N. & Yamanaka T. (1978) The α_2-plasmin inhibitor levels in liver disease. *Clinica Chimica Acta* **84**, 99–105.

Astedt B., Mattsson W. & Trope C. (1977) Treatment of advanced breast cancer with chemotherapeutics and inhibitor of coagulation and fibrinolysis. *Acta Medica Scandinavica* **201**, 491–5.

Astrup T., Rasmussen J., Amery A. & Poulsen H.E. (1960) Fibrinolytic activity of cirrhotic liver. *Nature* **185**, 619–20.

Astrup T. & Rosa A.T. (1974) A plasminogen proactivator-activator system in human blood effective in absence of Hageman factor. *Thrombosis Research* **4**, 609–13.

Astrup T. & Sterndorff I. (1953) A fibrinolytic system in human milk. *Proceedings of the Society for Experimental Biology and Medicine* **84**, 605–8.

Bang N.U., Fletcher A.P., Alkjaersig N. & Sherry S. (1962) Pathogenesis of the coagulation defect developing during pathological plasma proteolytic (fibrinolytic) states III. Demonstration of abnormal clot structure by electron microscopy. *Journal of Clinical Investigation* **41**, 935–48.

Beller F.K., Douglas G.W., Debrovner C.H. & Robinson R. (1963) The fibrinolytic enzyme system in amniotic fluid embolism. *American Journal of Obstetrics and Gynecology* **87**, 48–55.

Bennett B. (1967) A method for the quantitative assay of inhibitors of plasminogen activation in human serum. *Thrombosis et Diathesis Haemorrhagica* **17**, 12–22.

Bennett B. (1970) Further studies on an inhibitor of plasminogen activation in human serum: release of the inhibitor during coagulation and thrombus formation. *Thrombosis et Diathesis Haemorrhagica* **23**, 553–61.

Bennett B., Ogston C.M., McAndrew G.M. & Ogston D. (1966) Studies on the fibrinolytic enzyme system in obesity. *Journal of Clinical Pathology* **19**, 241–3.

Bennett B., Ogston C.M. & Ogston D. (1968) The effect of prolonged exercise on the components of the blood fibrinolytic enzyme system. *Journal of Physiology* **198**, 479–85.

Bennett B. & Ogston D. (1977) Physiological variations in coagulation, fibrinolysis and platelet behaviour. In *Haemostasis: Biochemistry, Physiology and Pathology*. Ogston D. & Bennett B. (eds). John Wiley & Sons, New York.

Bernik M.B. & Kwaan H.C. (1967) Origin of fibrinolytic activity in cultures of human kidney. *Journal of Laboratory and Clinical Medicine* **70**, 650–61.

Bernik M.B., White W.F., Oller E.P. & Kwaan H.C. (1974) Immunologic identity of plasminogen activator in human urine blood vessels and tissue culture. *Journal of Laboratory and Clinical Medicine* **84**, 546–58.

Biggs R., Macfarlane R.G. & Pilling F. (1947) Observations on fibrinolysis: Experimental production by exercise and adrenaline. *Lancet* I, 402–5.

Binder B.R., Beckman R. & Jorg M. (1981) Plasminogen activator activity of urokinase, the vascular plasminogen activator, plasma kallikrein and Hageman factor in the presence and absence of fibrin. *Thrombosis and Haemostasis* **46**, 12.

Binder B.R., Spragg J. & Austen K.F. (1979) Purification and characterisation of human vascular plasminogen activator derived from blood vessel perfusate. *Journal of Biological Chemistry* **254**, 1998–2003.

Bonnar J., Davidson J.F., Pidgeon C.F., McNicol G.P. & Douglas A.S. (1969) Fibrin degradation products in normal and abnormal pregnancy and parturition. *British Medical Journal* III, 137–40.

Booth N.A. & Bennett B. (1980, 1981) Unpublished observations.

Booth N.A. & Bennett B. (1982) Plasmin-α_2-antiplasmin complexes as an indicator of *in vivo* fibrinolysis. *British Journal of Haematology* **50**, 537–41.

Booth N.A. & Bennett B. (1984) Plasmin-α_2-antiplasmin complexes in bleeding disorders characterized by primary or secondary fibrinolysis. *British Journal of Haematology* **56**, 545–56.

Booth N.A., Bennett B., Wijngaards G. & Grieve J.H.K. (1983) A new life-long haemorrhagic disorder due to excess of plasminogen activator. *Blood* **61**, 267–75.

Booth N.A., Cumming A.M., Cook I.A., Knox J., Dawson A.A. & Bennett B. (1981) Hyperactive fibrinolysis in a patient with gross hyperlipidaemia. In *Progress in Chemical Fibrinolysis & Thrombolysis*, Vol. 5. Davidson J.F., Nilsson I.M. & Astedt B. (eds). pp. 342–4. Churchill Livingstone, Edinburgh.

Britton B.J., Hawkey C., Wood W.G. & Peele M. (1974) Stress—a significant factor in venous thrombosis? *British Journal of Surgery* **61**, 814–20.

Bundy H.F. & Mehl J.W. (1959) Trypsin inhibitors of human serum. II. Isolation of the α_2-inhibitor and its partial characterisation. *Journal of Biological Chemistry* **234**, 1124–8.

Cash J.D., Woodfield D.G. & Allen A.G.E. (1970) Adrenergic mechanisms in the systemic plasminogen activator response to adrenaline in man. *British Journal of Haematology* **18**, 487–94.

Cederholm-Williams S. (1977) The binding of plasminogen (mol. wt. 84,000) and plasmin to fibrin. *Thrombosis Research* II, 421–3.

Chesterman C.N., Allington M.J. & Sharp A.A. (1972) Relationship of plasminogen activator to fibrin. *Nature (New Biology)* **288**, 15–17.

Christensen U. & Clemmensen I. (1977) Kinetic properties of the primary inhibitor of plasmin from human plasma. *Biochemical Journal* **163**, 389–91.

Clayton J.K., Anderson J.A. & McNicol G.P. (1976) Preoperative prediction of postoperative deep vein thrombosis. *British Medical Journal* II, 910–12.

Clemmensen I. & Christensen F. (1976) Inhibition of urokinase by complex formation with human α_1-antitrypsin. *Biochemical et Biophysica Acta* **429**, 591–9.

Cole E.R. & Bachmann F.W. (1977) Purification and properties of a plasminogen activator from pig heart. *Journal of Biological Chemistry* **252**, 3729–37.

Collen D. (1976) Identification and some properties of a new fast reacting plasmin inhibitor in human plasma. *European Journal of Biochemistry* **69**, 209–16.

Collen D. (1977) Thrombin-antithrombin III and plasmin–antiplasmin complex as indicators of *in vivo* activation of the coagulation and/or fibrinolytic systems. *Acta Clinica Belgica* **32**, 398–402.

Collen D. (1980) Biochemical background of fibrinolytic therapy. In *Fibrinolysis and Urokinase*. Tilsner V. & Lenau H. (eds). pp. 9–17. Proceedings of the Serono Symposia, Vol. 31. Academic Press, London.

Collen D., De Cock F. & Verstraete M. (1975) Immunochemical distinction between antiplasmin and α_1-antitrypsin. *Thrombosis Research* **7**, 245–9.

Collen D., Rouvier J. & Verstraete M. (1972) Metabolism of iodine-labelled plasminogen and prothrombin in cirrhosis of the liver. *Clinical Research* **20**, 483.

Collen D. & Wiman B. (1979) Turnover of antiplasmin, the fast-acting plasmin inhibitor of plasma. *Blood* **53**, 313–24.

Colman R.W. (1969) Activation of plasminogen by human plasma kallikrein. *Biochemical and Biophysical Research Communications* **35**, 273–9.

Crandon A.J., Peel K.R., Anderson J.A., Thompson V. & McNicol G. (1980) Postoperative deep vein thrombosis: identifying high risk patients. *British Medical Journal* **281**, 343–4.

Crawford G.P.M. & Ogston D. (1975) The action of antithrombin III on plasmin and activators of plasminogen. *Biochimica et Biophysica Acta* **391**, 189–92.

Crawford I.P. (1973) Purification and properties of normal human α_1-antitrypsin. *Archives of Biochemistry and Biophysics* **156**, 215–22.

Donati M.B. & Poggi A. (1980) Malignancy and haemostasis. *British Journal of Haematology* **44**, 173–82.

Douglas A.S., McNicol G.P., Bain W.H. & Mackay W.A. (1966) The haemostatic defect following extracorporeal circulation. *British Journal of Surgery* **53**, 455–67.

Fearnley G.R. (1960) Spontaneous fibrinolysis. *American Journal of Cardiology* **6**, 371–7.

Fearnley G.R., Balmforth G. & Fearnley E. (1957) Evidence of diurnal fibrinolytic rhythm with a simple method for measuring natural fibrinolysis. *Clinical Science* **16**, 645–50.

Fearnley G.R. & Lackner R (1955) The fibrinolytic activity of normal blood. *British Journal of Haematology* **1**, 189–98.

Fedderson C. & Gormsen J. (1971) Plasmin digestion of stabilized and non-stabilized fibrin. *Scandinavian Journal of Haematology* **8**, 461–9.

Ferriera H.C. & Murat L.G. (1963) An immunological method for demonstrating fibrin degradation products in serum and its use in the diagnosis of fibrinolytic states. *British Journal of Haematology* **9**, 299–310.

Fisher S., Fletcher A.P., Alkjaersig N. & Sherry S. (1967) Immunoelectrophoretic characterization of plasma fibrinogen derivatives in patients with pathological plasma proteolysis. *Journal of Laboratory and Clinical Medicine* **70**, 903–22.

Fletcher A.P., Alkjaersig N., Fisher S. & Sherry S. (1966) The proteolysis of fibrin by plasmin. The identification of thrombin-clottable fibrinogen derivatives which polymerize abnormally. *Journal of Laboratory and Clinical Medicine* **68**, 780–802.

Fletcher A.P., Alkjaersig N., O'Brien J.R. & Tulevski V. (1977) Fibrinogen catabolism in the surgically operated patient and in those with postoperative venous thrombosis. Correlation of plasma fibrinogen chromatographic findings with ^{125}I-labelled fibrinogen scan findings. *Journal of Laboratory and Clinical Medicine* **89**, 1349–64.

Fletcher A.P., Biederman O., Moore D., Alkjaersig N. & Sherry D. (1964) Abnormal plasminogen—plasmin system activity (fibrinolysis) in patients with hepatic cirrhosis; its cause and consequences. *Journal of Clinical Investigation* **43**, 681–95.

Gaffney P.J. (1973) Subunit relationships between fibrinogen and fibrin degradation products. *Thrombosis Research* **2**, 201–18.

Gaffney P.J. (1977) The biochemistry of fibrinogen and fibrin degradation products. In *Haemostasis: Biochemistry, Physiology and Pathology.* Ogston D. & Bennett B. (eds). pp. 105–68. J. Wiley & Sons, New York.

Gaffney P.J. (1979) The relevance of D dimer-E-complex to the lysis of cross-linked fibrin. In *Progress in Chemical Fibrinolysis and Thrombolysis.* Davidson J.F., Cepelak V.N., Samama M.M. & Desnoyers P.C. (eds). Vol. 4. pp. 424–32. Churchill Livingstone, Edinburgh.

Gaffney P.F. & Brasher M. (1973) Subunit structure of the plasmin-induced degradation products of cross-linked fibrin. *Biochimica et Biophysica Acta* **295**, 308–13.

Gallimore M.J. (1980) Studies on plasma inhibitors of urokinase using a chromogenic peptide substrate for urokinase. In *Fibrinolysis and Urokinase.* Tilsner V. & Lenau H. (eds). pp. 27–34. Proceedings of the Serono Symposia, Vol. 31. Academic Press, London.

Gans H. & Krivit W. (1962) Problems in haemostasis during and after open heart surgery VI. Overall changes in blood coagulation mechanism. *Journal of the American Medical Association* **179**, 145–8.

Godal H.C. & Abildgaard U. (1966) Gelation of soluble fibrin by ethanol. *Scandinavian Journal of Haematology* **3**, 342–50.

Goldrick R.B. (1961) Fibrinolysis, blood clotting, serum lipids and body build in natives of New Guinea and Australians. *Australasian Annals of Medicine* **10**, 20–8.

Goldsmith G.H. Jr, Saito H. & Ratnoff O.D. (1978) The activation of plasminogen by Hageman factor (factor XII) and Hageman factor fragments. *Journal of Clinical Investigation* **62**, 54–60.

Goodpasture E.W. (1914) Fibrinolysis in chronic hepatic insufficiency. *Bulletin of the Johns Hopkins Hospital* **25**, 330–6.

Groskopf W.R., Hsieh B., Summaria L. & Robbins K.C. (1969) Studies on the active centre of human plasmin. The serine and histidine residues. *Journal of Biological Chemistry* **244**, 359–65.

Grossi C.E., Moreno A.H. & Rousselot L.M. (1961) Studies on spontaneous fibrinolytic activity in patients with cirrhosis of the liver and its inhibition by epsilon amino caproic acid. *Annals of Surgery* **153**, 383–93.

Harpel P.C. (1970a) Cl Inactivator inhibition by plasmin. *Journal of Clinical Investigation* **49**, 568–75.

Harpel P.C. (1970b) Human plasma alpha$_2$-macroglobulin: an inhibitor of plasma kallikrein. *Journal of Experimental Medicine* **132**, 329–52.

Harpel P.C. (1976) Cl Inactivator. *Methods in Enzymology* **45**, 751–60.

Harpel P.C. (1981) α_2-Plasmin inhibitor and α_2-macroglobulin–plasmin complexes in plasma. Quantitation by an enzyme-linked differential antibody immuno absorbent assay. *Journal of Clinical Investigation* **68**, 46–55.

Harpel P.C. & Cooper N.R. (1975) Studies on human plasma Cl inactivator–enzyme interactions 1. Mechanisms of interaction with Cls, plasmin and trypsin. *Journal of Clinical Investigation* **55**, 593–604.

Hedner U. (1980) Inhibitors of plasminogen activation distinct from the other plasma protein inhibitors. In *Fibrinolysis and Urokinase.* Tilsner V. & Lenau H. (eds). pp. 19–25. Proceedings of Serono Symposia, Vol. 31. Academic Press, London.

Hedner U. & Abildgaard U. (1978) Report on the joint meeting of the task forces on

Nomenclature and Standards of Inhibitors of Coagulation and Fibrinolysis. *Thrombosis and Haemostasis* **38**, 524–5.

Heide K., Heimburger N. & Haupt H. (1965) An inter-alpha-trypsin inhibitor of human serum. *Clinica Chimica Acta* **11**, 82–5.

Highsmith R.F. & Rosenberg R.D. (1974) The inhibition of human plasmin by human antithrombin—heparin cofactor. *Journal of Biological Chemistry* **249**, 4335–8.

Hirsch J., Fletcher A.P. & Sherry S. (1965) The effect of fibrin and fibrinogen proteolysis products on clot physical properties. *American Journal of Physiology* **209**, 415–24.

Hoylaerts M., Rijken D.C., Lijnen H.R. & Collen D. (1981) Kinetics of plasminogen activation by tissue plasminogen activator. *Thrombosis and Haemostasis* **46**, 162.

Iatridis S.G., Iatridis P.G. & Ferguson J.H. (1966) Effects of ellagic acid upon human fibrinolytic enzyme system. *Thrombosis et Diathesis Haemorrhagica* **16**, 657–67.

Isacson S. & Nilsson I.M. (1972) Defective fibrinolysis in blood and vein walls in recurrent 'idiopathic' venous thrombosis. *Acta Chirurgica Scandinavica* **138**, 313–19.

Jacobsen R.J., Wagner S., Weinberg R. & Björnsson S. (1971) Bleeding complications in fulminant hepatitis. *Lancet* **II**, 1426.

Jedrychowski A., Hillenbrand P., Ajdukiewicz A.B., Parbhoo S.P. & Sherlock S. (1973) Fibrinolysis in cholestatic jaundice. *British Medical Journal* **I**, 640–2.

Jerushalmy Z. & Zucker M.B. (1966) Some effects of fibrinogen degradation products (FDP) on blood platelets. *Thrombosis et Diathesis Haemorrhagica* **15**, 413–19.

Kawano T., Morimoto K. & Uemura Y. (1968) Urokinase inhibitor in human placenta. *Nature* **217**, 253.

Khan M.J.P. (1978) Blood clotting activity by individuals without α_1-antitrypsin activity. *Proceedings of the International Society of Haematology XVIII Congress* p. 520.

Kluft C. (1978) Cl-Inactivator resistant fibrinolytic activity in plasma euglobulin fractions. Its relationship to vascular activator in the blood and its role in euglobulin fibrinolysis. *Thrombosis Research* **13**, 135–51.

Kluft C., Vellenga E. & Brommer E.J.P. (1979) Homozygous α_2-antiplasmin deficiency. *Lancet* **II**, 209.

Kluft C., Wijngaards G. & Jie A.F.H. (1981) The factor XII–independent plasminogen proactivator system of plasma includes urokinase-related material. *Thrombosis and Haemostasis* **46**, 343.

Kok P. (1979a) Separation of plasminogen activators from human uterine tissue and comparison with activators from human urine and porcine tissue. *Thrombosis and Haemostasis* **41**, 718–33.

Kok P. (1979b) Separation of plasminogen activators from human plasma and a comparison with activators from human uterine tissue and urine. *Thrombosis and Haemostasis* **41**, 734–44.

Kopec M., Budzynski A., Stachurska J., Wegrzynowicz Z. & Kowalski E. (1966) Studies on the mechanism of interference by fibrinogen degradation products (FDP) with the platelet function. *Thrombosis et Diathesis Haemorrhagica* **15**, 476–90.

Korninger C. & Collen D. (1981) Inhibition of human tissue plasminogen activator by human plasma: no evidence for a specific antiactivator. *Thrombosis and Haemostasis* **46**, 280.

Korninger C., Matsuo O., Suy R., Stassen J.M. & Collen D. (1981) Thrombolytic properties of purified human tissue plasminogen activator in a dog femoral vein thrombosis model. *Thrombosis and Haemostasis* **46**, 209.

Kowalski E., Budzynski A.Z., Kopec M., Latallo Z.S., Lipinski B. & Wegrzynowicz Z.

(1964) Studies on the molecular pathology and pathogenesis of bleeding in severe fibrinolytic states in dogs. *Thrombosis et Diathesis Haemorrhagica* **12**, 69–74.

Kucinski C.S., Fletcher A.P. & Sherry S. (1968) Effect of urokinase antiserum on plasminogen activators: demonstration of immunologic dissimilarity between plasma plasminogen activators and urokinase. *Journal of Clinical Investigation* **47**, 1238–53.

Kwaan H.C., Lo R. & McFadzean A.J.S. (1959) Antifibrinolytic activity in primary carcinoma of the liver. *Clinical Science* **18**, 251–61.

Laake K. & Vennerod A.M. (1974) Factor XII-induced fibrinolysis: studies on the separation of pre-kallikrein, plasminogen proactivator and factor XI in human plasma. *Thrombosis Research* **4**, 285–302.

Larrieu M.-J., Marder V.J. & Inceman S. (1966) *Diffuse Intravascular Clotting.* Transactions of the Conference of International Committee on Haemostasis and Thrombosis, p. 215. Schattauer-Verlag, Stuttgart.

Lauritsen O.S. (1968) Urokinase inhibitor in human plasma. *Scandinavian Journal of Clinical and Laboratory Investigation* **22**, 314–21.

Lesuk A., Terminiello L. & Traver J.H. (1965) Crystalline human urokinase, some properties. *Science* **147**, 880–1.

Lesuk A., Terminiello L., Traver J.H. & Groff J.L. (1967) Biochemical and biophysical studies of human urokinase. *Thrombosis et Diathesis Haemorrhagica* **18**, 293–4.

Levin E.G. & Loskutoff D.J. (1981) Multiple molecular forms of plasminogen activator produced by cultured bovine endothelial cells. *Thrombosis and Haemostasis* **46**, 83.

Lewis J.H. & Doyle A.P. (1964) Effect of epsilon aminocaproic acid on coagulation and fibrinolytic mechanisms. *Journal of the American Medical Association* **188**, 56–63.

Libeskind I.C., Lipinski B. & Gurewich V. (1981) Binding of blood plasminogen activator to fibrinogen, fibrin monomer and fibrin. *Thrombosis and Haemostasis* **46**, 163.

Lijnen H.R., Hoylaerts M. & Collen D. (1980) Isolation and characterisation of a human plasma protein with affinity for lysine-binding sites in plasminogen. Role in regulation of fibrinolysis and identification as histidine-rich glycoprotein. *Journal of Biological Chemistry* **255**, 10214–22.

Lijnen H.R., Wiman B., Van Hoef B. & Collen D. (1981) Partial primary structure of human α_2 antiplasmin. *Thrombosis and Haemostasis* **46**, 282.

Lipinski B. & Worowski K. (1968) Detection of soluble fibrin complexes in blood by means of protamine sulphate test. *Thrombosis et Diathesis Haemorrhagica* **20**, 44.

Lloyd D.A., Cederholm-Williams S.A. & Sharp A.A. (1981) Binding of plasminogen and vascular plasminogen activator to fibrin and the fibrin alpha-chain. *Thrombosis and Haemostasis* **46**, 163.

Loskutoff D.J. (1981) Effect of thrombin on the production of plasminogen activator by endothelial cells. *Thrombosis and Haemostasis* **46**, 82.

Loskutoff D.J. & Edgington T.S. (1977) Synthesis of a fibrinolytic activator and inhibitor by endothelial cells. *Proceedings of the National Academy of Sciences of the USA* **74**, 3903–7.

Loskutoff D.J. & Edgington T.S. (1981) An inhibitor of plasminogen activator in rabbit endothelial cells. *Thrombosis and Haemostasis* **46**, 82.

Macfarlane R.G. & Biggs R. (1946) Observations on fibrinolysis, spontaneous activity associated with surgical operations, trauma, etc. *Lancet* **II**, 862–4.

Macfarlane R.G. & Pilling J. (1947) Fibrinolytic activity of normal urine. *Nature* **159**, 779.

Mackie M. & Bennett B. (1978) Unpublished observations.

Mackie M., Booth N.A. & Bennett B. (1981) Comparative studies on human activators of plasminogen. *British Journal of Haematology* **47**, 77–90.

Marder V.J., Shulman N.R. & Carroll W.R. (1969) High molecular weight derivatives of human fibrinogen produced by plasmin. *Journal of Biological Chemistry* **244**, 2111–19.

Markus G., Takita H., Camiolo S.M., Corasanti J.G., Evers J.L. & Hobika G.H. (1980) Content and characterization of plasminogen activators in human lung tumours and normal lung tissue. *Cancer Research* **40**, 841–8.

Matsuo O., Rijken D.C. & Collen D. (1981) Thrombolysis by human tissue plasminogen activator and urokinase in rabbits with experimental pulmonary embolus. *Nature* **291**, 590–1.

Merskey C., Kleiner G.J. & Johnson A.J. (1966) Quantitative estimation of split products of fibrinogen in human serum, relation to diagnosis and treatment. *Blood* **28**, 1–18.

Merskey C., Lalezari P. & Johnson A.J. (1969) A rapid, simple, sensitive method of measuring fibrinolytic split products in human serum. *Proceedings of the Society for Experimental Biology and Medicine* **131**, 871–5.

Mikata I., Hasegawa M., Igarashi T., Shirakura N. & Hohida M. (1959) Plasmin in haemorrhagic blood disease. *Keio Journal of Medicine* **8**, 278–83.

Moroi M. & Aoki N. (1972) Inhibition of plasminogen binding to fibrin by α_2 plasmin inhibitor. *Thrombosis Research* **10**, 851–6.

Moroi M. & Aoki N. (1976) Isolation and characterisation of α_2 plasmin inhibitor from human plasma. *Journal of Biological Chemistry* **251**, 5956–65.

Moroi M. & Aoki N. (1977a) Inhibition of plasminogen binding to fibrin by α_2 plasmin inhibitor. *Thrombosis Research* **10**, 851–6.

Moroi M. & Aoki N. (1977b) Inhibition of proteases in coagulation, kinin-forming and complement systems by α_2-plasmin inhibitor. *Journal of Biochemistry* **82**, 969–72.

Mossesson M.W. (1973) The fibrinogenolytic pathway of fibrinogen catabolism. *Thrombosis Research* **2**, 185–200.

Mossesson M.W., Alkjaersig N., Sweet B. & Sherry S. (1967) Human fibrinogen of relatively high solubility. Comparative biophysical, biochemical and biological studies with fibrinogen of lower solubility. *Biochemistry* **6**, 3279–87.

Mott D.M., Fabisch P.H., Sani B.P. & Sorof S. (1974) Lack of correlation between fibrinolysis and the transformed state of cultured mammalian cells. *Biochemical and Biophysical Research Communications* **61**, 621–7.

Mullertz S. (1974) Different molecular forms of plasminogen and plasmin produced by urokinase in human plasma and their relation to protease inhibitors and lysis of fibrinogen and fibrin. *Biochemical Journal* **143**, 273–83.

Mullertz S. & Clemmensen I. (1976) The primary inhibitor of plasmin in human plasma. *Biochemical Journal* **159**, 545–53.

Niewierowski S. & Kowalski E. (1958) Un nouvel anticoagulant dérivé du fibrinogène. *Revue d'Hématologie* **13**, 320.

Niewierowski S. & Prou-Wartelle O. (1959) Rôle du facteur contact (Facteur Hageman) dans la fibrinolyse. *Thrombosis et Diathesis Haemorrhagica* **3**, 593–603.

Nilehn J.-E. & Nilsson I.M. (1964) Demonstration of fibrinolytic split products in human serum by an immunological method in spontaneous and induced fibrinolytic states. *Scandinavian Journal of Haematology* **1**, 313–30.

Norman P.S. & Hill B.M. (1958) Studies of the plasmin system III. Physical properties of the two plasmin inhibitors of plasma. *Journal of Experimental Medicine* **108**, 639–49.

Nussenzweig V. & Seligmann M. (1960) Analyse par les methodes immunochimiques de la dégradation par la plasmine du fibrinogène humain et de la fibrine à différents stades. *Revue d'Hématologie* **15**, 451.

Nussenzweig V., Seligmann M., Pelmont J. & Grabar P. (1961) Les produits de dégradation du fibrinogène humain par la plasmine. *Annales de l'Institut Pasteur* **100**, 377–87.

Ogston D., Bennett B., Herbert R.D. & Douglas A.S. (1973) The inhibition of urokinase by alpha$_2$-macroglobulin. *Clinical Science* **44**, 73–9.

Ogston D., Bennett B. & Mackie M. (1976) Properties of a partially purified preparation of a circulating plasminogen activator. *Thrombosis Research* **8**, 276–84.

Ogston D., Bennett B. & Ogston C.M. (1971) The fibrinolytic enzyme system in hepatic cirrhosis and malignant metastases. *Journal of Clinical Pathology* **24**, 822–6.

Ogston D. & McAndrew G.M. (1964) Fibrinolysis in obesity. *Lancet* **II**, 1205–7.

Ogston D., Ogston C.M. & Bennett B. (1966) Arterio-venous differences in components of the fibrinolytic enzyme system. *Thrombosis et Diathesis Haemorrhagica* **16**, 32–7.

Ogston D., Ogston C.M., Ratnoff O.D. & Forbes C.D. (1969) Studies on a complex mechanism for the activation of plasminogen by kaolin and by chloroform. The participation of Hageman factor and additional co-factors. *Journal of Clinical Investigation* **48**, 1786–801.

Olexa S.A. & Budzynski A.Z. (1979) Primary soluble plasmic degradation products of crosslinked human fibrin. Isolation and stoichiometry of the (DD)E complex. *Biochemistry* **18**, 991–5.

Paraskevas M., Nilsson I.M. & Martinsson G. (1962) A method for determining serum inhibitor of plasminogen activation. *Scandinavian Journal of Clinical and Laboratory Investigation* **14**, 138–44.

Pensky J., Levy L.R. & Lepow I.H. (1961) Partial purification of a serum inhibitor of Cl-esterase. *Journal of Biological Chemistry* **236**, 1674–9.

Pensky J. & Schwick H.G. (1969) Human inhibitor of Cl esterase: identity with α_2 neuraminoglycoprotein. *Science* **163**, 698.

Peterson H.-I. (1968) Experimental studies on fibrinolysis in growth and spread of tumour. *Acta Chirurgica Scandinavica*, Suppl. 394, 1–42.

Peterson H.-I. (1977) Fibrinolysis and antifibrinolytic drugs in the growth and spread of tumours. *Cancer Treatment Reviews* **4**, 213–17.

Philips L.L., Montgomery G. Jr & Taylor H.C. (1957) The role of the fibrinolytic enzyme system in obstetrical afibrinogenaemia. *American Journal of Obstetrics and Gynecology* **73**, 43–56.

Pizzo S.V., Taylor L.M., Schwartz M.L., Hill R.L. & McKee P.A. (1973) Subunit structure of fragment D from fibrinogen and cross-linked fibrin. *Journal of Biological Chemistry* **248**, 4584–90.

Plow E.F., De Cock F. & Collen D. (1979) Immunochemical characterisation of the plasmin–antiplasmin system. Basis for the specific detection of plasmin antiplasmin complex by latex agglutination assays. *Journal of Laboratory and Clinical Medicine* **93**, 199–209.

Radcliffe R. & Heinze T. (1978) Isolation of plasminogen activator from human plasma by chromatography on lysine-sepharose. *Archives of Biochemistry and Biophysics* **189**, 185–94.

Rakoczi I., Wiman B. & Collen D. (1978) On the biological significance of the specific interaction between fibrin and plasminogen and anti-plasmin. *Biochimica et Biophysica Acta* **540**, 295–300.

Ratnoff O.D. (1949) Studies on a proteolytic enzyme in human plasma: IV. The role of lysis of plasma clots in normal and diseased individuals, with particular reference to hepatic disease. *Bulletin of the Johns Hopkins Hospital* **84**, 29–42.

Ratnoff O.D. (1952) Studies on a proteolytic enzyme in human plasma VII. A fatal haemorrhagic state associated with excessive plasma proteolytic activity in a patient undergoing surgery for carcinoma of the head of the pancreas. *Journal of Clinical Investigation* **31**, 521–8.

Ratnoff O.D. (1977) The haemostatic effects of liver disease. In *Haemostasis: Biochemistry, Physiology and Pathology*. Ogston D. & Bennett B. (eds). John Wiley & Sons, New York.

Ratnoff O.D. & Lepow I.H. (1957) Some properties of an esterase derived from preparations of the first component of complement. *Journal of Experimental Medicine* **106**, 327–43.

Ratnoff O.D., Pensky J., Ogston D. & Naff G.B. (1969) The inhibition of plasmin, plasma kallikrein, plasma permeability factor and the Clr subcomponent of the first component of complement by serum Cl esterase inhibitor. *Journal of Experimental Medicine* **129**, 315–31.

Reiche E. (1973) Tumour associated fibrinolysis. *Federation Proceedings* **32**, 2174–5.

Rennie J.A.R., Bennett B. & Ogston D. (1977) Effect of local exercise and venous occlusion on fibrinolytic activity. *Journal of Clinical Pathology* **30**, 350–2.

Rickli E.E. & Otavsky W.I. (1975) A new method of isolation and some properties of the heavy chain of human plasmin. *European Journal of Biochemistry* **59**, 441–7.

Rickli E.E. & Zaugg H. (1970) Isolation and purification of highly enriched tissue plasminogen activator from pig heart. *Thrombosis et Diathesis Haemorrhagica* **23**, 64–76.

Rijken D.C. & Collen D. (1981) Purification and characterisation of the plasminogen activator secreted by human melanoma cells in culture. *Journal of Biological Chemistry* **256**, 7035–41.

Rijken D.C., Hoylaerts M. & Collen D. (1981) On the fibrinolytic properties of single chain and two chain human tissue plasminogen activator. *Thrombosis and Haemostasis* **46**, 12.

Rijken D.C., Wijngaards G. & Welbergen J. (1980) Relationships between tissue plasminogen activator and the activators in blood and vascular wall. *Thrombosis Research* **18**, 815–30.

Rijken D.C., Wijngaards G. & Welbergen J. (1981) Immunological characterisation of plasminogen activator activities in human tissues and body fluids. *Journal of Laboratory and Clinical Medicine* **97**, 477–86.

Rijken D.C., Wijngaards G., Zaal de Jong M. & Welbergen J. (1979) Purification and partial characterisation of plasminogen activator from human uterine tissue. *Biochemica et Biophysica Acta* **580**, 140–53.

Rimon A., Shamash Y. & Shapiro B. (1966) The plasmin inhibitor of human plasma IV. Its action on plasmin, trypsin, chyrotrypsin and thrombin. *Journal of Biological Chemistry* **241**, 5102–7.

Robbins K.C. (1977) The biochemistry of plasminogen and plasmin. In *Haemostasis: Biochemistry, Physiology and Pathology*. Ogston D. & Bennett B. (eds). pp 208–20. John Wiley & Sons, New York.

Robbins K.C. (1981) The regulation and control of the blood fibrinolytic system. In *Progress in Chemical Fibrinolysis and Thrombolysis*, Vol. 5. Davidson J.F., Nilsson I.M. & Astedt B. (eds). pp. 3–13. Churchill Livingstone, Edinburgh.

Robbins K.C., Bernabe P., Arzedon L. & Summaria L. (1973) The primary structure of human plasminogen II. The histidine loop of human plasmin; light (B) chain active centre histidine sequence. *Journal of Biological Chemistry* **248**, 1631–3.

Robbins K.C., Summaria L., Hsieh B. & Shah R.J. (1967) The peptide chains of human plasmin. Mechanism of activation of human plasminogen to plasmin. *Journal of Biological Chemistry* **242**, 2333–42.

Roblin R., Vetterlein D.A., McLellan W.L., Young P.L., Bell T.E. & Eichorg B. (1981) Regulation of plasminogen activator activity in embryonic and tumour derived human cell cultures. In *Progress in Chemical Fibrinolysis and Thrombolysis*, Vol. 5. Davidson J.F., Nilsson I.M. & Astedt B. (eds). pp. 90–5. Churchill Livingstone, Edinburgh.

Saito H., Ratnoff O.D., Waldmann R. & Abraham J.P. (1975) Fitzgerald trait: deficiency of a hitherto unrecognised agent, Fitzgerald factor, participating in surface mediated reactions of clotting, fibrinolysis, generation of kinins and the property of diluted plasma enhancing vascular permeability (PF/Dil). *Journal of Clinical Investigation* **55**, 1082–9.

Sakata Y. & Aoki N. (1980) Molecular abnormality of plasminogen. *Journal of Biological Chemistry* **255**, 5442–7.

Sasaki T., Page I.H. & Shainoff J.R. (1966) Stable complex of fibrinogen and fibrin. *Science* **152**, 1069–71.

Sawyer W.D., Fletcher A.P., Alkjaersig N. & Sherry S. (1960) Studies on the thrombolytic activity of normal plasma. *Journal of Clinical Investigation* **39**, 426–34.

Schapira M., Scott C.F. & Colman R.W. (1981) Relative importance of plasma protease inhibitors in the inactivation of kallikrein in human plasma. *Thrombosis and Haemostasis* **46**, 259.

Schreiber A.D., Kaplan A.P. & Austen K.F. (1973) Plasma inhibitors of the components of the fibrinolytic pathway in man. *Journal of Clinical Investigation* **52**, 1394–401.

Schwick H.G., Heimburger N. & Haupt H. (1967) Purification and chemical-physical properties of some proteinase inhibitors of plasma. *Thrombosis et Diathesis Haemorrhagica* **18**, 302.

Shainoff J.R. & Page I.H. (1962) Significance of cryoprofibrin in fibrinogen-fibrin conversion. *Journal of Experimental Medicine* **116**, 687–707.

Shamash Y. & Rimon A. (1966) The plasmin inhibitors of human plasma III. Purification and partial characterization. *Biochimica et Biophysica Acta* **121**, 35–41.

Sherry S., Lindemeyer R.I., Fletcher A.P. & Alkjaersig N. (1959) Studies on enhanced fibrinolytic activity in man. *Journal of Clinical Investigation* **38**, 810–22.

Sjöholm I., Wiman B. & Wallen P. (1973) Studies on the conformational changes of plasminogen induced during activation to plasmin and by 6-aminohexanoic acid. *European Journal of Biochemistry* **39**, 471–9.

Skøjdt P. (1965) Amnotic fluid embolism. *Acta Obstetrica Gynaecologica Scandinavica* **44**, 437–57.

Sottrup-Jensen L., Claeys H., Zajdel M., Petersen T.E. & Magnussen S. (1978) The primary structure of human plasminogen. In *Progress in Chemical Fibrinolysis and Thrombolysis*, Vol. 3. Davidson J.F., Rowan R.M., Samama M.M. & Desnoyers P.C. (eds). pp. 191–209. Raven Press, New York.

Steinbuch M. (1971) Les antiproteases du plasma. *Revue Française de Transfusion* **14**, 61–82.

Storm O. (1955) Fibrinolytic activity in human tears. *Scandinavian Journal of Clinical and Laboratory Investigation* **7**, 239–43.

Stormorken H. (1957) Reactivity of stored plasma to thrombin with reference to the fibrinogen conversion accelerator and heparinoid activity. *British Journal of Haematology* **3**, 299–310.

Summaria L., Arzadon L., Bernabe P. & Robbins K.C. (1975) The activation of plasminogen to plasmin by urokinase in the presence of the plasmin inhibitor Trasylol. *Journal of Biological Chemistry* **250**, 3988–95.

Szczeklik A., Dischinger P., Kueppers F., Tyroler H.A., Hames C.G., Cassel J. & Creagan S. (1980) Blood fibrinolytic activity, social class and habitual physical activity II. A study of black and white men in Southern Georgia. *Journal of Chronic Diseases* **33**, 291–9.

Tagnon H.J., Whitmore W.F. & Schulman N.R. (1952) Fibrinolysis in metastatic carcinoma of the prostate. *Cancer* **5**, 9–12.

Thorsen S. (1975) Differences in the binding to fibrin of native plasminogen and plasminogen modified by proteolytic degradation. Influence of omega-amino carboxylic acids. *Biochimica et Biophysica Acta* **393**, 55–65.

Thorsen S., Glas-Greenwalt P. & Astrup T. (1972) Differences in the binding to fibrin of urokinase and tissue plasminogen activator. *Thrombosis et Diathesis Haemorrhagica* **28**, 65–74.

Todd A.S. (1959) The histological localisation of fibrinolysin activator. *Journal of Pathology and Bacteriology* **78**, 281–3.

Triantaphyllopoulos D.C. (1958) Anticoagulant effect of incubated fibrinogen. *Canadian Journal of Biochemistry and Physiology* **36**, 249–59.

Truelove S.C. (1951) Fibrinolysis and the eosinophil count. *Clinical Science* **10**, 229–40.

Tytgat G.N., Collen D. & Verstraete M. (1971) Metabolism of fibrinogen in cirrhosis of the liver. *Journal of Clinical Investigation* **50**, 1690–701.

Verstraete M., Vermylen J. & Schetz J. (1978) Biochemical changes noted during intermittent administration of streptokinase. *Thrombosis and Haemostasis* **39**, 61–8.

Vetterlein D., Young P.L., Bell T.E. & Roblin R. (1979) Immunological characterisation of multiple molecular weight forms of human cell plasminogen activator. *Journal of Biological Chemistry* **254**, 575–8.

Violand B.N. & Castellino F.J. (1976) Mechanism of urokinase activation of human plasminogen. *Journal of Biological Chemistry* **251**, 3906–12.

von Kaula K.N. & Shettles B. (1953) The relationship between human seminal fluid and the fibrinolytic system. *Proceedings of the Society for Experimental Biology and Medicine* **83**, 692–4.

von Kaulla K.N. & Swan H. (1958) Clotting deviations in man during cardiac bypass: fibrinolysis and circulating anticoagulant. *Journal of Thoracic Surgery* **36**, 519–30.

Walker J.E., Campbell D.M. & Ogston D. (1980) Inhibitors of fibrinolysis in amniotic fluid. *Thrombosis and Haemostasis* **44**, 32–4.

Walker J.E. & Ogston D. (1981) The inhibition of tissue activators and urokinase by human plasma. *Thrombosis and Haemostasis* **46**, 280.

Wallen P. & Bergstrom K. (1958) Action of thrombin in plasmin digested fibrinogen. *Acta Chemica Scandinavica* **12**, 572 8.

Wallen P., Ranby M., Bergsdorf N. & Kok P. (1981) Purification and characterization of tissue plasminogen activator: on the occurrence of two different forms and their enzymatic properties. In *Progress in Chemical Fibrinolysis and Thrombolysis*, Vol. 5. Davidson J.F., Nilsson I.M. & Astedt B. (eds). pp. 16–23. Churchill Livingstone, Edinburgh.

Wallen P. & Wiman B. (1972) Characterisation of human plasminogen II. Separation and partial characterisation of different molecular forms of human plasminogen. *Biochimica et Biophysica Acta* **257**, 122–34.

Wang B.A., McLouchlin G.A., Richie J.P. & Mannick J.A. (1980) Correlation of the production of plasminogen activator with tumour metastasis in B16 mouse melanoma cell lines. *Cancer Research* **40**, 288–92.

Weimar W., Stibbe J., van Seyen A.J., Billiau A., De Somer P. & Collen D. (1981) Specific lysis of an iliofemoral thrombus by administration of extrinsic (tissue type) plasminogen activator. *Lancet* **II**, 1018–20.

Weiner A.E., Reid D.E. & Raby C.C. (1953) Incoagulable blood in severe premature separation of the placenta: a method of management. *American Journal of Obstetrics and Gynecology* **66**, 475–99.

White W.F., Barlow G.H. & Mozen M.M. (1966) The isolation and characterisation of plasminogen activators (urokinase) from human urine. *Biochemistry* **5**, 2160–9.

Wijngaards G. & Kluft C. (1981) Urokinase-related fibrinolytic activity in human plasma. *Thrombosis and Haemostasis* **46**, 385.

Williams J.R.B. (1951) The fibrinolytic activity of urine. *British Journal of Experimental Pathology* **32**, 530–7.

Wiman B. (1978) Biochemistry of the plasminogen to plasmin conversion. In *Fibrinolysis: Current Fundamental and Clinical Concepts.* Gaffney P.J. & Balkuv-Ulutin S.M. (eds). pp. 47–60. Academic Press, London.

Wiman B. & Collen D. (1977) Purification and characterisation of human antiplasmin, the fast acting plasmin inhibitor of plasma. *European Journal of Biochemistry* **78**, 19–26.

Wiman B. & Collen D. (1978a) On the kinetics of the reaction between human antiplasmin and plasmin. *European Journal of Biochemistry* **84**, 573–8.

Wiman B. & Collen D. (1978b) Molecular mechanism of physiological fibrinolysis. *Nature* **272**, 549–50.

Wiman B. & Wallen P. (1973) Activation of human plasminogen by an insoluble derivative of urokinase. *European Journal of Biochemistry* **36**, 25–31.

Wiman B. & Wallen P. (1975) Structural relationships between 'glutamic acid' and 'lysine' forms of human plasminogen and their interaction with the amino terminal activator peptide as studied by affinity chromatography. *European Journal of Biochemistry* **50**, 489–94.

Wohl R.C., Summaria L., Chediak J., Rosenfeld S. & Robbins K.C. (1982) Human plasminogen variant Chicago III. *Thrombosis and Haemostasis* **48**, 146–52.

Wohl R.C., Summaria L. & Robbins K.C. (1979) Physiological activation of the human fibrinolytic system. Isolation and characterisation of human plasminogen variants Chicago I and Chicago II. *Journal of Biological Chemistry* **254**, 9063–9.

Wuepper K.D. (1973) Prekallikrein deficiency in man. *Journal of Experimental Medicine* **138**, 1345–55.

Zywicka H., Kopec M., Latallo Z. & Kowalski E. (1961) Anticoagulant circulant ressemblant à l'antithrombin IV au cours d'un lupus erythémateux disseminé. *Thrombosis et Diathesis Haemorrhagica* **6**, 63–72.

Chapter 17
Thrombolytic Therapy and Fibrinolytic Inhibitors

D. OGSTON, B. BENNETT *and* A. S. DOUGLAS

Thrombolytic therapy

Thromboembolic occlusive vascular disease remains a major cause of morbidity and mortality. While the dominant role of platelets in arterial thrombosis is recognized, fibrin both contributes to the structure and cohesion of arterial thrombi and constitutes the major component of venous thrombi.

The harnessing of the potential activity of the fibrinolytic enzyme system to remove unwanted fibrin deposits has been a goal of investigators for many years. Thrombolytic therapy offers the theoretical advantage over anticoagulant therapy in affording the possibility of removing intravascular thrombi before the production of irreversible tissue damage. Anticoagulant therapy can merely prevent extension of the thrombus and with its use the restoration of the obstructed circulation depends on the natural physiological thrombolytic mechanism or on recanalization.

The potential therapeutic value of thrombolytic therapy in man was demonstrated by Johnson and McCarthy (1959) who used a systemic infusion of streptokinase to lyse artificial thrombi in the arm veins of volunteers. Over the succeeding years a variety of thrombolytic agents administered in various schedules has been used in a number of conditions associated with fibrin deposition. Unfortunately, trials of such agents of a size and design which could provide definitive conclusions on advantages over other forms of therapy have been scanty. Enthusiasm for the use of thrombolytic therapy in the management of thromboembolic disease has waxed and waned and there is considerable variation in the extent of its use between different countries. At the present time thrombolytic therapy with presently available agents is not universally accepted as the treatment of choice for any condition.

Thrombolytic agents

Agents with the property of contributing to the removal of intravascular fibrin deposits may be classified into three main groups. Firstly, drugs may be introduced into the circulation which directly degrade fibrin by proteolysis: examples of such materials are plasmin and proteases from species of *Aspergillus*. Secondly, agents which activate endogenous plasminogen directly, for example, urokinase, or indirectly (streptokinase) may be used. Thirdly, drugs may be administered which enhance the synthesis or release of the vascular wall activator within the body: examples of this group of drugs are nicotinic acid and the anabolic steroids. Use of these latter drugs is at present aimed at prevention of the build-up of intravascular fibrin rather than at removal of existing thrombi.

The mechanism of thrombolysis

The mechanism of thrombolysis is considered in detail in the chapter on the fibrinolytic enzyme system (Chapter 16), but it is pertinent to briefly consider here the principal hypotheses of the thrombolytic mechanism since the rational use of thrombolytic agents demands this background knowledge. One hypothesis, now largely discounted, is that plasmin generated in the circulation is bound to plasma inhibitors: the plasmin–antiplasmin complex dissociates in the presence of fibrin due to the higher affinity of plasmin for fibrin than for inhibitor (Ambrus and Markus 1960). If such a hypothesis was correct it would be logical to employ thrombolytic regimes aimed at inducing high levels of circulating plasmin.

A second hypothesis gives to plasminogen activator the key role in the lysis of thrombi. Alkjaersig and her colleagues (1959) postulated that considerable quantities of plasminogen are adsorbed on to fibrin during clotting. Diffusion of circulating plasminogen activator into the thrombus activates the intrinsic adsorbed plasminogen: the plasmin formed at this site is free to hydrolyse fibrin, unimpeded by the circulating antiplasmins. In this hypothesis high activator levels would be desirable while plasma plasminogen depletion should not impair thrombolysis and, indeed, would prevent sustained hyperplasminaemia and consequent plasma protein proteolysis.

In the theory proposed by Chesterman, Allington and Sharp (1972) activators bind selectively to fibrin while plasminogen diffuses into the thrombus and is converted to plasmin in this site. Under this hypothesis optimal thrombolysis would require high activator levels with the presence of plasminogen in the circulation to replenish the thrombus plasminogen.

The discovery of the fast-acting α_2-antiplasmin with new knowledge of the biochemistry of plasminogen has led to a further proposal to explain the mechanism of thrombolysis (Wiman and Collen 1978) in which the lysine-binding sites of plasminogen play a central role. Plasminogen is bound to fibrin through its lysine-binding sites. Plasminogen activator is also absorbed on to the fibrin surface and its activating properties are enhanced leading to the localized formation of plasmin with consequent cleavage of fibrin. When associated with fibrin the lysine-binding sites of plasmin are occupied; as a result its inactivation by α_2-antiplasmin is very slow. Any free plasmin released into the plasma is rapidly bound and inactivated by the inhibitor. At the present time a vascular/tissue activator with high affinity for fibrin is not generally available for therapeutic use. It is probable, however, that it is from this direction that improved thrombolytic agents will emerge. Indeed, at the time of writing, a tissue activator purified from the culture fluid of human melanoma cells has been shown to produce greater thrombolysis than urokinase of experimental thrombi in isolated segments of femoral veins in dogs without significant activation of circulating plasminogen, breakdown of fibrinogen or consumption of α_2-antiplasmin and freedom from bleeding complications (Korninger *et al.* 1981). The efficacy of the same activator has been compared to urokinase in experimental pulmonary emboli in rabbits and found to induce thrombolysis at lower dosage than urokinase without impairment of haemostatic function (Matsuo, Rijken and Collen 1981), while the resolution of venous thrombosis in two patients without systemic fibrinolytic activation after the use of this tissue-type plasminogen activator has been reported (Weimar *et al.* 1981).

Streptokinase

It was observed by Tillett and Garner (1933) that a filtrate of some β-haemolytic streptococci could cause the rapid dissolution of human plasma clots. Christensen and MacLeod (1945) showed later that the agent produced by streptococci acted on plasminogen to form a protease. The activator was termed streptokinase and its therapeutic possibilities were stimulated by the demonstration of Johnson and Tillett (1952) that infusions of streptokinase lysed thrombi induced by sodium morrhuate in the ear veins of rabbits.

Streptokinase, a protein of molecular weight 47000, is a catabolic by-product of the Group C β-haemolytic streptococcus. It does not activate plasminogen directly, but binds in a 1:1 stoichiometric reaction to human plasminogen. This reaction results in the formation of an active proteolytic site on the plasminogen moiety of the complex which becomes a plasminogen activator. This complex is rapidly altered to a streptokinase–plasmin complex which is also a potent plasminogen activator (Robbins and Markus 1978, Castellino 1979). The light chain of plasminogen can also form an active activator complex with streptokinase (Summaria and Robbins 1976). The streptokinase of the complex undergoes proteolysis into a number of inactive components (Siefring and Castellino 1976). The highest activator activity is found in complexes which contain intact streptokinase or its high molecular weight fragments (Wohl *et al.* 1978).

Free streptokinase is rapidly removed from the circulation and there does not appear to be any natural inhibitor of the activator complex (Summaria *et al.* 1977).

STREPTOKINASE ANTIBODIES

Streptococcal infections or therapy with streptokinase stimulates the production of antibodies against streptokinase. These precipitating antibodies are of the IgG class (Spöttl and Kaiser 1974) and neutralize administered streptokinase with the formation of inactive complexes which are rapidly eliminated from the circulation.

Urokinase

The presence of fibrinolytic activity in normal urine was first described by Macfarlane and Pilling (1947). The evidence that this activity was due to a plasminogen activator was provided by the experiments of Williams (1951), and the name urokinase was given to the urinary activator by Sobel and colleagues (1952).

Urokinase is a direct activator of plasminogen, cleaving the specific arginyl–valine bond in the carboxyl-terminal position of plasminogen to form the two-chain plasmin molecule. Urokinase consists of a single polypeptide chain and can exist in two molecular forms, one of molecular weight 54 700 and the other of 31 300. The latter can be derived from the former by the action of plasmin. The relative therapeutic efficacy of the two forms is not established.

There are two sources of urokinase for use in thrombolytic therapy, that prepared from human urine and the other produced by human fetal cells in tissue culture. These preparations appear to be identical.

Urokinase is non-antigenic in man (Genton and Claman 1970) and is not pyrogenic. A major disadvantage lies in its relative lack of adsorption on to fibrin; tissue activator possesses this property, but is not yet generally available for thrombolytic therapy.

Different units for urokinase activity are used. The Ploug unit is equivalent to 1.35 CTA (Committee on Thrombolytic Agents) units while the international unit (iu) is equivalent to the CTA unit.

Plasmin

Commercial preparations of plasmin have been widely used in the past for thrombolysis. Plasmin introduced into the circulation is rapidly neutralized by the excess of antiplasmins, in particular, α_2-antiplasmin and α_2-macroglobulin, and early studies demonstrated that no plasma proteolytic activity was present after plasmin infusions (Sawyer *et al.* 1961). More recently it has been confirmed that plasminaemia and systemic fibrinolysis only occur after depletion of α_2-antiplasmin (Collen and Vestraete 1979). Any thrombolytic activity found in early preparations of plasmin was attributed to its streptokinase content. Others have used activator-free porcine plasmin (Amris and Amris 1963), but controlled trials to establish its clinical value are lacking. A possible use for plasmin or other direct proteolytic enzyme would be to dissolve local fibrin deposits of low plasminogen content, for example, clotted arterio-venous shunts. Intra-arterial regional perfusion of a plasmin preparation containing streptokinase has been used successfully in patients with thrombosis of the palmar arch or digital arteries not amenable to surgical removal, but no control group was included (Kartchner and Wilcox 1976). The same mixture infused into a coronary artery close to the site of an occlusion was claimed to achieve patency of the artery in the majority of patients with evolving myocardial infarction treated (Ganz *et al.* 1981).

ACYL-ACTIVATOR AND ACYL-PLASMIN

Acylated derivatives of plasmin and streptokinase-plasmin (ogen) complexes have been proposed as thrombolytic agents (Smith *et al.* 1981). Such derivatives are enzymatically inert and unable to degrade proteins or to react with plasma inhibitors, but may still bind to fibrin through the lysine binding sites which are separate from the catalytic centre. After binding, deacylation may take place to provide fibrin-bound plasmin, and thrombolysis consequently takes place. The theoretical advantages of acyl-plasmins and acyl-activators are reduced systemic hyperplasminaemia with reduction in the consequent bleeding risk and less wasteful inhibition by α_2-antiplasmin. In preliminary observations both acyl-plasmin and acyl-activator produced significant thrombolysis of venous clots in rabbits and dogs whereas free plasmin or non-acylated streptokinase-plasmin activator were much less effective.

Dosage schedules for thrombolytic therapy

STREPTOKINASE

Circulating streptokinase antibodies must be neutralized before a therapeutic thrombolytic effect can be achieved. The antibody combines with and inactivates administered streptokinase and the complexes formed are rapidly cleared from the blood stream. The concentration of antibody, however, varies over a wide range from patient to patient.

Before starting treatment the quantity of streptokinase which must be infused to overcome the antibodies and other inhibitors can be estimated by an *in vitro* assay (titrated initial dose: streptokinase resistance test). These assays require, however, both time and laboratory facilities. The dose calculated from such a test is then infused over a period of 30 minutes. Therapy is continued with a maintenance dose of some 100 000 units/hour.

An alternate approach is to use a standard dosage schedule which is likely to neutralize the antibodies in a large proportion of the community. An initial dose of 1 250 000 units was found by Verstraete and colleagues (1966) to neutralize circulating antibody in 97 per cent of the population studied. In fact, a smaller initial dose can produce a thrombolytic action, probably because of the relatively slow reaction between streptokinase and antibody, thus allowing complex formation between streptokinase and plasminogen to proceed. An initial loading dose of 250 000 units given over 30 minutes followed by 100 000 units/hour has been found to produce acceptable activation of plasminogen in 95 per cent of patients (Urokinase-Streptokinase Embolism Trial 1974). Most now use a standard initial dose of between 250 000 and 600 000 units given over a period of 30 minutes which is followed by a maintenance dose of 100 000 units/hour.

UROKINASE

The usual regime for urokinase therapy is a loading dose of 4000 CTA units/kg body weight given intravenously over 10 to 30 minutes. This is followed by a maintenance dose of 4000 CTA units/kg body weight/hour for 12 to 72 hours.

Anticoagulant therapy following thrombolytic therapy

The use of thrombolytic therapy for vascular occlusion should be followed by anticoagulant therapy. In its absence the incidence of re-thrombosis is unacceptably high with the possible added hazard that any thrombus which does form may be unlysable if a plasminogen-depleting dose of streptokinase has been used. It is usual practice to give intravenous heparin (1500 units/hour) for at least 24 hours after the completion of the streptokinase or urokinase infusion and, at the same time, to start oral anticoagulant therapy. An alternative strategy is the use of a defibrinating agent after streptokinase therapy (Tibbutt *et al.* 1977).

Alternative strategies for administration of thrombolytic agents

A number of modifications to the basic streptokinase administration schedules have been proposed with the aim of increasing its efficacy and reducing the incidence of haemorrhagic complications.

It would be theoretically advantageous to increase the adsorption of plasminogen to fibrin in order to enhance the potential quality of plasmin which could be formed locally. Lys-plasminogen has a higher affinity for fibrin than native glu-plasminogen and its use in thrombolytic therapy could, therefore, be beneficial: in a small trial Kakkar, Sagar and Lewis (1975) obtained increased thrombolysis in venous thrombosis using a regime of intermittent plasminogen, mainly in the lys-form, and streptokinase infusion.

A further potentially helpful manoeuvre would be reduction of the plasma fibrinogen level prior to the start of thrombolytic therapy which would decrease the quantity of the anticoagulant fibrinogen degradation products formed. With this aim the defibrinating agent ancrod has been used in sequence with streptokinase and reported to be therapeutically effective without producing haemorrhagic side-effects (Forbes, Barbenell and Prentice 1976). In another study, however, the combination was associated with bleeding at venepuncture (Latallo and Lopaciuk 1973).

The infusion of thrombolytic agent at comparatively low dosage directly to the site of a thrombus would have the advantages of reduced cost and the avoidance of systemic hyperplasminaemia and potential bleeding. Streptokinase has been used successfully in this way in the management of arterial thrombosis (Chesterman, Nash and Biggs 1971, Dotter, Rösch and Seaman 1974) and pulmonary embolism (Gallus *et al.* 1975). In one trial of locally infused urokinase, venographic evidence of lysis of iliofemoral thrombosis was obtained in some patients (Mavor *et al.* 1969), although the overall results were unsatisfactory due to rethrombosis.

Complications of thrombolytic therapy

HAEMORRHAGIC COMPLICATIONS

Free circulating plasmin causes the proteolysis of fibrinogen and certain coagulation factors, in particular, factors V and VIII. The degradation products resulting from the breakdown of fibrinogen interfere with fibrin polymerization, inhibit thrombin, and affect platelet function. In addition, cross-links cannot be formed even in the presence of normal concentrations of factor XIII due to the loss of the carboxyl-terminal ends of the α-chains in the X fragments: any fibrin formed from these is therefore more sensitive to plasmin digestion. As a consequence of these effects on the haemostatic mechanism, bleeding is a common and important complication of thrombolytic therapy and occurs particularly at sites of previous trauma. The risks of bleeding in such situations as recent surgical wounds is greater with thrombolytic therapy than anticoagulant therapy, but there appears to be little difference between urokinase and streptokinase in the incidence of haemorrhagic complications. If significant bleeding does occur, cessation of the infusion is usually all that is required since both urokinase and streptokinase are rapidly cleared from the circulation. In occasional instances blood transfusion and epsilon-aminocaproic acid, tranexamic acid or aprotinin may be required to control severe bleeding or to allow emergency surgery to be performed.

ALLERGIC COMPLICATIONS

Allergic reactions are due to the antigenic nature of streptokinase and are not seen with urokinase. Mild allergic reactions are common and include urticaria, flushing, headache and muscle and skeletal pain. Rarely bronchospasm, hypotension or angioedema develops. Mild fever is common and marked pyrexial reactions can occur. Hydrocortisone cover of the infusion does not reduce the incidence of febrile reactions.

Contraindications to systemic thrombolytic therapy

It is mandatory that thrombolytic agents should be avoided in situations where severe haemorrhagic complications are likely to be produced. Absolute contraindications are, therefore, the presence of an active or potential bleeding site such as a duodenal ulcer or ulcerative colitis, or the existence of an intracranial neoplasm or a recent cerebrovascular accident.

In the absence of a pressing indication thrombolytic therapy should be avoided in patients who have had a major surgical procedure within the past ten days, and this stricture includes organ biopsy and arterial puncture. Patients who have had recent gastrointestinal bleeding or trauma with possible internal injuries should only receive thrombolytic therapy where the strongest indication for its use exists. It is usually recommended that thrombolytic agents should be withheld from those with severe hyper-tension.

Other contraindications include severe acute or chronic hepatic or renal disease; conditions where there is a risk of central nervous system embolism, for example, mitral valve disease with atrial fibrillation or subacute bacterial endocarditis; the presence of haemostatic defects such as thrombocytopenia; pregnancy; age in excess of 75; and diabetic haemorrhagic retinopathy. In general, patients receiving anticoagulant therapy or who have had platelet aggregation inhibitors during the previous ten days should not be started on thrombolytic therapy, while those who have had a recent streptococcal infection with consequent high anti-streptokinase levels, or who have recently received a course of streptokinase are not usually suitable for therapy with streptokinase.

These relative contraindications must be carefully evaluated and the additional risks of thrombolytic agents in these situations weighed against the possible therapeutic benefits.

Laboratory control of thrombolytic therapy

Thrombolytic therapy has now been administered to many patients without prior laboratory estimation of the required initial dosage or control of subsequent dosage by utilizing standardized dose schedules, and the need for strict laboratory control is arguable. There is no single test which will reliably identify those patients who will develop haemorrhagic complications and, therefore, the emphasis must be on the careful selection of patients and close clinical observation during therapy so that rapid action can be instituted if bleeding occurs.

Laboratory monitoring of therapy can be useful in establishing that a lytic state has been achieved by the given dosage level. The thrombin clotting time is valuable in reflecting the degree of hyperplasminaemia induced through its effect on fibrinogen level and fibrinogen degradation product production. After the first six hours of continuous infusion of streptokinase a prolongation of the thrombin time up to four times the control value is usual and acceptable. Markedly prolonged times suggest excessive plasmin formation and an increased risk of haemorrhage: if it occurs consideration must be given to either stopping the infusion for a period of hours or increasing the dosage to achieve rapid plasminogen depletion. Lack of prolongation of the thrombin time suggests that the circulating streptokinase antibodies were not adequately neutralized by the initial dose.

Further information on the current thrombolytic state may be obtained from assays of plasma fibrinogen and the circulating thrombolytic activity. Plasma fibrinogen is best measured by a thrombin-clottable technique, but precipitation methods are more rapid and may be adequate. The euglobulin clot lysis time, fibrin plate or a labelled fibrin substrate may be used to assess plasma thrombolytic activity. The fibrin plate and labelled fibrin substrate assays have the advantage of being independent of the circulating fibrinogen and plasminogen levels, but take a number of hours to obtain a result.

Aspergillus **proteases**

Stefanini and Marin (1958) noted that a number of strains of *Aspergillus oryzae* produced a proteolytic enzyme capable of lysing fibrin. Purification of the protease was achieved with the aim of providing a thrombolytic agent. *Aspergillus ochraceus* contains very similar proteases.

The protease from *Aspergillus oryzae* (brinase) has a molecular weight of about 21 000: it degrades fibrinogen some six times as fast as it lyses fibrin, but has no plasminogen activator activity. Plasma inhibitors neutralize brinase and its dosage must be calculated on the basis of the quantity required to prevent too great a reduction in inhibitor level. If this occurs, the free plasma proteolysis results in hydrolysis of a number of plasma proteins with consequent haemorrhage and hypotension.

While thrombolysis has been achieved in experimental animals with brinase (Roschlaw and Tosoni 1965, Ele, Amundsen and Rø 1972), the therapeutic value of this agent has not been established.

Therapeutic uses of thrombolytic therapy

The use of thrombolytic therapy for a variety of thromboembolic conditions has been widely investigated. Many of the studies, however, have been anecdotal or have lacked appropriate control groups, and the number of acceptably randomized and controlled studies available to assess the precise value of thrombolytic therapy in particular situations is small. Conditions in which thrombolytic therapy has been used are listed in Table 36.

DEEP VEIN THROMBOSIS

Deep vein thrombosis is a potentially hazardous disorder recognized to be common after operations or immobility of the lower limbs. The development of isotopic techniques has led to the recognition that it also occurs frequently following medical disorders such as myocardial infarction and cerebrovascular accidents (Warlow, Ogston and Douglas 1972, Warlow *et al.* 1973). Its principal complication is pulmonary embolization, but valvular damage leading to the postphlebitic syndrome may be responsible for considerable long-term morbidity. The site of thrombosis influences the frequency of

Table 36. Disorders in which thrombolytic therapy has been employed.

Deep vein thrombosis
Pulmonary embolism
Myocardial infarction
Peripheral arterial occlusion
Cerebrovascular occlusion
Retinal vessel occlusion
Vitreous haemorrhage
Arterio-venous shunt occlusion
Thrombotic thrombocytopenia purpura
Removal of fibrin deposits in meningitis
Hyphaema
Haemothorax and empyema
Renal cortical necrosis
Heart valve prosthesis obstruction

complications: emboli usually originate from non-occlusive thrombi in the iliofemoral segment while impaired valve function and the postphlebitic syndrome follows occlusive thrombosis in this site. Calf vein thrombosis is of less significance, but extension upwards to the iliofemoral segment may take place.

The treatment of deep vein thrombosis is by anticoagulants, surgical thrombectomy or thrombolytic therapy. Anticoagulant therapy markedly decreases the mortality from pulmonary embolism (Barritt and Jordan 1960), and is the standard against which other methods of treatment are judged. Such therapy is probably adequate for thrombosis confined to the calf veins. Thrombectomy has lost favour, partly because of the high incidence of re-thrombosis. To assess the therapeutic value of thrombolytic therapy, objective evaluation using pre- and post-treatment venography is essential. Approaches have been made to quantify the venographic changes in the mass of thrombus (Marder *et al.* 1977).

It is clear from a number of studies comparing patients with deep venous thrombosis treated with an anticoagulant with those receiving thrombolytic agents that thrombolytic therapy, usually streptokinase, induces partial or complete clearance of thrombus in the majority of cases, whereas heparin-treated patients show little or no clearance (Kakkar *et al.* 1969a, Tsapogas *et al.* 1973, Tibbutt *et al.* 1974, Duckert *et al.* 1975, Arnesen *et al.* 1978). Indeed, extension of thrombus has been seen in spite of adequate heparin treatment (Marder 1979).

Venous thrombi become less susceptible to lysis as they age and patients with symptoms of thrombosis for more than a week usually show little lysis. However, in one trial about half of the deep venous occlusions of 10–15 days duration were abolished after streptokinase treatment (Duckert *et al.* 1975). It is clear that the risk of re-thrombosis after thrombolytic therapy is much less than after thrombectomy.

The efficiency of thrombolytic therapy in preserving valve function and preventing the post-phlebetic syndrome is not finally decided, but the few trials in which this has been specifically studied point to a distinct advantage in favour of thrombolytic agents. Kakkar and colleagues (1969b) used ascending functional cinephlebography to assess venous valve function and found that this was normal 6–12 months after streptokinase therapy in those in whom the diagnosis was made within 36 hours and the thrombus rapidly and completely dissolved. Essentially identical findings were reported by Johansson, Ericson and Zetterquist (1976) and by Elliot *et al.* (1979). The benefit from thrombolytic therapy contrasts with the valvular destruction seen after venous thrombectomy.

There is the theoretical possibility of detachment of a portion of the thrombus during thrombolytic therapy with resultant pulmonary embolism.

Small fragments of the thrombus may well embolize, but are rapidly broken up in the lung by the induced systemic fibrinolytic state. The incidence of pulmonary embolism during thrombolytic therapy for deep vein thrombosis has varied: Hess (1969) reported an incidence of 1.1 per cent fatal and 2.9 per cent non-fatal emboli and Robertson, Nilsson and Nylander (1970) had evidence of embolization in one of nine treated patients. Duckert and colleagues (1975) found that the incidence of non-fatal pulmonary embolism was greater in the heparin than in the streptokinase groups.

It is concluded that thrombolytic therapy in leg vein thrombosis should be reserved for patients with extensive iliofemoral thrombus of recent onset.

PULMONARY EMBOLISM

The management of pulmonary embolism by thrombolytic therapy has a number of theoretical attractions: the emboli will be predominantly composed of fibrin, the pulmonary vessels will themselves be healthy, and the therapy should concurrently remove the source of further possible emboli. There is, however, the problem that a high proportion of patients with a large pulmonary embolus die very rapidly (Gorham 1961a, b), certainly before thrombolytic therapy can be instituted and become effective. Its use, therefore, is restricted to those with an embolus of a size which is causing right heart failure, but which will allow survival for at least 12 hours. Numbers of suitable patients are necessarily small and this has hampered the completion of adequately sized trials to compare the efficacy of heparin and thrombolytic therapy.

There is very substantial evidence that thrombolytic therapy with either streptokinase or urokinase dissolves recent pulmonary emboli much more readily than heparin. One large-scale trial (Urokinase Pulmonary Embolism Trial Study Group (1970) compared heparin with urokinase followed by heparin: the mortality between the two groups was similar, but at 24 hours the urokinase group showed greater resolution of emboli. No difference, however, was seen in lung scan appearances between the two groups after six months. In a more recent study (Sharma, Burleson and Sasahara 1980) pulmonary-capillary blood volume and diffusing capacity measurements were used to assess the long-term resolution of pulmonary emboli after different forms of therapy: those treated with urokinase or streptokinase had greater resolution both at two weeks and one year.

Other studies have shown that streptokinase produces more rapid clearance of pulmonary emboli as assessed by angiography than heparin (Miller 1972) and a greater fall in pulmonary artery resistance (Hirsch, MacDonald and O'Sullivan 1971, Miller *et al.* 1971). In a controlled randomized trial of 30 patients with life-threatening pulmonary embolism,

Tibbutt and colleagues (1974) found that the streptokinase-treated patients had greater lysis and greater reduction in systolic and mean pulmonary arterial pressures than the heparin-treated group. Similar findings were reported by Ly and associates (1978).

It is concluded from the data available that thrombolytic therapy is the treatment of choice for the comparatively few patients with massive pulmonary embolism and acute right heart failure, but who are not deteriorating so rapidly that death is likely to ensue before thrombolysis can take place. Whether its wide use is justified in smaller emboli to prevent subsequent persistent pulmonary hypertension is uncertain.

MYOCARDIAL INFARCTION

Formidable difficulties attend both the use of thrombolytic therapy in myocardial infarction and the assessment of its benefit. In spite of these, the mortality and morbidity attending this common disorder have encouraged physicians to attempt to improve its prognosis by the use of thrombolytic agents. Its aim in this situation is to improve the circulation in the infarcted area of the myocardium, either by removing the fibrin component of any coronary artery thrombus present or by the removal or prevention of microthrombi. The benefits from this, however, may be only marginal since delayed removal of a thrombus may not prevent death from electrical instability of the myocardium or from cardiogenic shock and, in any event, infarction may result from causes of coronary occlusion not amenable to thrombolysis, for example, a ruptured atheromatous plaque or a subendothelial haemorrhage.

A number of early studies, while not fulfilling the criteria of controlled trials, demonstrated that thrombolytic therapy for myocardial infarction was feasible, safe and did not increase the risk of cardiac rupture or aneurysm formation (Fletcher *et al.* 1959, Dewar, Horler and Cassells-Smith 1961, Lippschutz *et al.* 1965). Any decision or recommendation for widespread use must depend, however, on the results obtained from well-designed trials.

A considerable number of trials on the use of streptokinase or urokinase in myocardial infarction have now been carried out. They have, however, differed in a number of ways including the diagnostic criteria employed for entry to the trial, the method of randomization into control and treatment groups, the time interval between the onset of symptoms and the start of treatment, and in the dosage of thrombolytic agent and the duration of its administration. Details of many of the trials are provided in the review by Duckert (1979).

The variability in design makes valid comparison between the results of the different trials very difficult. The results of some of the earlier clinical trials, largely conducted outwith coronary care units, suggested that mortality could be reduced by the early administration of streptokinase (Schmutzler *et al.* 1966, European Working Party 1971, Heikinheimo *et al.* 1971). In contrast, later controlled trials carried out in coronary care units have shown no significant benefit from either streptokinase or urokinase in terms of mortality (Dioguardi *et al.* 1971, Bett *et al.* 1973, European Collaborative Study 1975, Aber *et al.* 1976). A further trial was organized by the European Cooperative Study Group (1979). Three hundred and fifteen of the 2338 patients admitted to the coronary care units of the 11 participating centres were entered into a randomized trial. All received coumarin anticoagulants and a streptokinase infusion was commenced in the treatment group within 12 hours of the onset of symptoms in a dosage of 250 000 iu over 20 minutes followed by 100 000 iu/hour for 24 hours. The difference in mortality within a six-month period between the streptokinase-treated group (15.6 per cent) and the control group (30.6 per cent) was significant at the 1 per cent level. The reduction in mortality in the treatment group was particularly marked in the three-week to six-month post-infarction period: the reason for this reduction in late deaths is obscure, but could reflect the differences between the control and treatment groups in the frequency of risk factors.

It must be concluded that the information presently available on the treatment of myocardial infarction with thrombolytic agents does not justify a recommendation for its widespread adoption.

Peripheral arterial occlusion

The use of thrombolytic therapy in the management of recent occlusions of peripheral arteries has been reported from a number of centres and shown by angiography to produce partial or complete removal of thrombi in a high proportion of patients (McNicol *et al.* 1963, Amery, Vermylen and Verstraete 1969, Persson, Thompson and Patman 1973, Reichle *et al.* 1977). Success in achieving clearance of occluded arteries is increased by early treatment (Amery, Vermylen and Verstraete 1969). A small randomized study comparing heparin and streptokinase has been reported in favour of thrombolytic therapy (Reichle *et al.* 1977), but results of controlled trials comparing surgical and thrombolytic therapy are not available.

In addition to systemic thrombolytic therapy for arterial occlusion, low dose intra-arterial infusions of streptokinase have been used following partial clearing by endarterectomy or the Fogarty balloon catheter (Chesterman, Nash and Biggs 1971, Dotter, Rösch and Seaman 1974).

Acute arterial occlusions may threaten the limb, and sufficient time to achieve thrombolysis with streptokinase may not be available. The use of streptokinase in this situation is, therefore, limited, but it may have a place in the management of acute arterial occlusions too distally placed to allow other techniques of treatment.

Streptokinase has also been used in chronic arterial occlusions with generally indifferent results. A review of a number of the reported studies is available (Martin 1979). The arteriographically demonstrated lysis in a proportion of the chronic obstructions of the lower limbs treated with streptokinase suggests that the organization of thrombi in larger arteries may be delayed for some months. Lysis appears to be more frequent in large vessels such as the iliac arteries than in more distal ones such as the popliteal, while chronic arterial obstructions in the upper part of the body have shown no benefit from streptokinase therapy. In contrast to the encouraging results reported from some centres, other studies have shown little or no benefit, clinically or arteriographically, in patients with chronic arterial obstruction treated with streptokinase (Verstraete, Vermylen and Donati 1971, Persson, Thompson and Patman 1973).

RETINAL VESSEL OCCLUSION

Occlusion of a retinal vessel is an important cause of visual loss in the elderly and is without effective treatment. The retinal vasculature has the advantage for the evaluation of thrombolytic therapy in that the retinal vessels can be directly visualized while changes in visual acuity can be readily measured. Some uncontrolled studies have suggested that fibrinolytic agents might be of benefit in retinal vein occlusion (Hawkey and Howell 1964, Den Ottolander and Craandijk 1968). The results of one controlled clinical trial in which 40 patients with retinal vein occlusion were randomly allocated to a streptokin- ase-treated group and a control group have been made available (Kohner *et al.* 1976): the return of vision was slightly but significantly better in the treated group, but three of the treated patients developed a vitreous haemorrhage with permanent loss of vision while receiving streptokinase. It seems, therefore, that the value of thrombolytic therapy in retinal vein occlusion is limited.

MISCELLANEOUS CONDITIONS

Thrombolytic therapy has been claimed to produce beneficial effects in a variety of conditions associated with the deposition of fibrin. These include the haemolytic-uraemic syndrome (Powell and Ekert 1974, Stuart *et al.* 1974), acute obstruction of heart valve prostheses (Luluaga *et al.* 1971), and renal artery thrombosis with impending renal cortical necrosis (Jones *et al.* 1975). The numbers treated and results obtained do not permit definite conclusions or recommendations.

Pharmacological enhancement of natural fibrinolytic activity

A rise in the potential thrombolytic activity of the blood might be achieved by increasing the synthesis or release of plasminogen activator from stores, in particular, the vessel wall. A detailed review of synthetic fibrinolytic agents is available (Davidson and Walker 1979). Early studies suggested that both the diguanide phenformin and the anabolic steroid ethylestrenol could induce increased fibrinolytic activity, but given singly resistance developed in a few months. A combination of anabolic steroid and phenformin, however, was claimed to produce a persistent increase in plasma fibrinolytic activity (Fearnley, Chakrabarti and Hocking 1967) and it was later demonstrated that such a combination increases the activator content of the vessel wall, presumably by stimulating synthesis. A disadvantage of phenformin lies in its liability to cause lactic acidosis.

It was found later that the 17-α-alkyl anabolic steroid stanozolol given alone induced a sustained enhancement of fibrinolytic activity in man (Davidson *et al.* 1972), particularly in those with impaired fibrinolytic activity. It was believed that fibrinolytic enhancement by anabolic steroids required some weeks, but a recent study has shown increased fibrinolytic activity as early as two days after starting stanozolol (Preston *et al.* 1981). The 17-α-alkyl steroids have been found to produce changes in other components of the haemostatic mechanism: plasma levels of fibrinogen and α_2-macroglobulin are reduced and plasminogen increased (Walker *et al.* 1975, Preston *et al.* 1981). Antithrombin III levels also may be increased (Walker *et al.* 1975).

The usual dose of stanozolol is 5–10 mg/day. Masculinizing effects make the drug unsuitable for women while recorded complications of anabolic steroids include cholestatic jaundice and hypersensitivity jaundice.

Evidence for a pharmacological influence of anabolic steroids on fibrinolysis is convincing, but it is far from established that the increase in fibrinolytic activity produced has a therapeutic action in the prevention or treatment of thrombotic disease. Nilsson (1975) has claimed that a combination of phenformin and ethylestrenol reduces the frequency of thrombotic episodes in patients with idiopathic recurrent venous thrombosis. In contrast, a similar drug combination given for three weeks before and one week after gynaecological surgery did not reduce the incidence of radioisotopically detected deep venous thrombosis (Fossard *et al.* 1974).

Fibrinolytic inhibitors

A number of agents, synthetic and natural, have the ability to inhibit the fibrinolytic enzyme system, and some of these have been used therapeutically in haemostatic and other disorders. The three inhibitors available for use in man are epsilon-aminocaproic acid, aminomethyl cyclohexane carboxylic acid, and the polypeptide aprotinin.

Epsilon-aminocaproic acid (EACA: 6-aminohexanoic acid)

EACA was first described as an antiplasmin agent by Okamoto and colleagues (1959), but was later shown to be capable of competitively inhibiting the activation of plasminogen at concentrations of 10^{-4} M and higher, whereas it acted as a non-competitive inhibitor of plasmin and other proteases at concentrations above 5×10^{-2} M (Ablondi *et al.* 1959, Alkjaersig, Fletcher and Sherry 1959).

The omega-aminocarboxylic acids including EACA and aminomethyl cyclohexane carboxylic acid (Fig. 52) bind in a 1:1 stoichiometric complex with plasminogen (Abiko, Iwamoto and Tomikawa 1969) through its lysine-binding site (Wiman and Wallén 1977). The binding results in a conformational change in the plasminogen molecule (Sjöholm, Wiman and Wallén 1973), which probably explains the more ready activation of the complex than of native plasminogen by urokinase in purified systems. The *in vivo* inhibitory action of these amino acids is probably the result of dissociation of plasminogen from the fibrin surface with consequent prevention of its activation (Thorsen 1975, Wiman and Wallén 1977).

In addition to its effects on the fibrinolytic system, EACA is capable of inhibiting the activation of the first component of complement (Soter, Austen and Gigli 1975) and, at high concentration, has been reported to decrease the amount of thymidine incorporation into lymphocytes (Hirscholm *et al.* 1971).

PHARMACOKINETICS OF EACA

EACA is rapidly and almost completely absorbed from the gastrointestinal tract: after a single oral dose the plasma EACA concentration reaches its

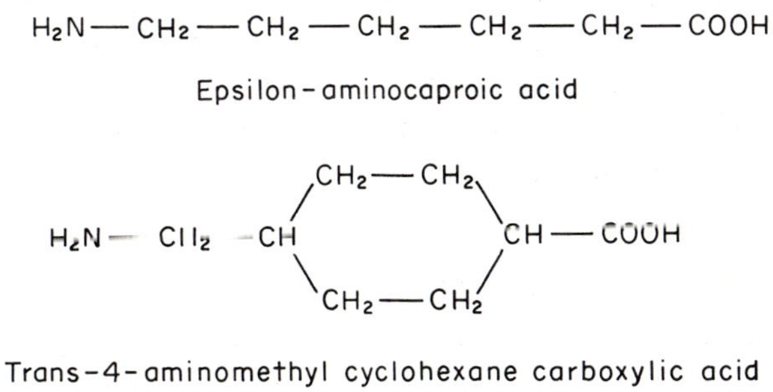

$$H_2N - CH_2 - CH_2 - CH_2 - CH_2 - CH_2 - COOH$$

Epsilon-aminocaproic acid

Trans-4-aminomethyl cyclohexane carboxylic acid

Fig. 52. Structure of omega-aminocarboxylic acid fibrinolytic inhibitors.

maximum in about two hours (McNicol *et al.* 1962). Most is excreted in the urine within 12 hours, primarily by glomerular filtration, but also by tubular secretion. Intravenous EACA in a dose of 10 g produces a high initial plasma concentration of some 150 mg/100 ml which falls to a level of around 3.5 mg/100 ml within 3–4 hours (Andersson *et al.* 1968). Over 80 per cent is found in the urine within 4–6 hours (McNicol *et al.* 1962): concentration during excretion results in high urinary levels.

The major portion of administered EACA is not metabolized in the body. It is able to enter and leave cells down concentration gradients and is therefore widely distributed throughout the extracellular and intracellular compartments.

Inhibition of circulating activator activity requires a plasma EACA concentration of 1 mmol (13 mg/100 ml) which can be achieved by an oral or intravenous loading dose of 4–6 g followed by a maintenance dose of 1 g hourly given orally or by continuous infusion. Inhibition of urinary fibrinolytic activity can be obtained by smaller doses, 3 g three times daily being adequate (Nilsson, Andersson and Björkman 1966).

Trans-4-aminomethyl cyclohexane carboxylic acid (AMCA: tranexamic acid)

Tranexamic acid is a water-soluble synthetic amino acid. Its properties are similar to those of EACA. but it is some ten times more potent. Control of systemic fibrinolytic activity requires a plasma concentration of around 10–15 μg/ml.

PHARMACOKINETICS OF TRANEXAMIC ACID

Studies on the absorption, distribution and excretion of tranexamic acid after oral or intravenous administration have been reported (Andersson *et al.* 1965, 1968, Eriksson *et al.* 1974). After intravenous administration of tranexamic acid at a dose of 10 mg/kg body weight some 30 per cent of the dose was recovered in the urine during the first hour and the plasma concentration at one hour was 18 μg/ml. Tranexamic acid is not so readily absorbed from the gut as EACA: after oral administration the maximum plasma concentration was 2 μg/ml after three hours with some 40 per cent of the dose being recoverable from the urine within 24 hours. Urinary excretion is by glomerular filtration (Eriksson *et al.* 1974). The biological half-life was calculated to be 80 minutes (Kaller 1967); a longer time was found in two subjects by Eriksson *et al.* (1974).

Tranexamic acid is widely distributed throughout the extracellular and intracellular compartments. After repeated intravenous or oral administration

(10–20 mg/kg) an antifibrinolytic concentration (10 μg/ml) was maintained in the tissues for up to 17 hours (Andersson *et al.* 1968). Tranexamic acid is able to enter the cerebro-spinal fluid (Tovi, Nilsson and Thulin 1972) and joint fluid (Ahlberg, Eriksson and Kjellman 1976) and can cross the placenta into the fetal plasma (Kullander and Nilsson 1970).

The dose of tranexamic acid used therapeutically has varied widely. Nilsson (1980) has recommended 10 mg/kg intravenously or 30–50 mg/kg orally 3–4 hourly for the management of systemic fibrinolysis. Control of local tissue bleeding 10–20 mg/kg orally 3–4 times daily was deemed adequate, while for urinary tract bleeding 10 mg/kg intravenously or 20 mg/kg orally 2–3 times daily was suggested.

Side-effects of EACA and AMCA

The incidence of side-effects of EACA used in therapeutic dosage is relatively low and any which occur are usually mild. Gastrointestinal upset including pain, diarrhoea, nausea and vomiting, hypotension, dizziness, nasal stuffiness, and allergic reactions have all been reported (Andersson 1962, McNicol *et al.* 1962, Andersson *et al.* 1965). Myopathy occurs rarely and only after some weeks of a dosage of 18–30 g daily (Bennett 1972, Lane *et al.* 1979). An acute delirious state has also been described (Wysenbeek *et al.* 1978). The incidence of side-effects in patients receiving AMCA appears to be less than for EACA.

A potential hazard of antifibrinolytic therapy is intravascular thrombosis and occasional patients have developed thrombosis while on therapy (Naeye 1962, Rydin and Lundberg 1976, Hoffman and Koo 1979). Many of the patients, however, had diseases which predispose to thrombosis. In one large series the mortality from myocardial infarction and pulmonary embolism was similar in the untreated and EACA-treated patients (Vinnicombe and Shuttleworth 1966), while the incidence of ^{125}I-fibrinogen uptake-detected venous thrombosis was not significantly different between an AMCA-treated and a placebo group of post-prostatectomy patients (Hedlund 1975). It is concluded that the danger of inducing thrombosis in EACA- or AMCA-treated patients is small, particularly during short-term therapy.

A further possible hazard of antifibrinolytic therapy lies in the formation of extravascular blood clots which are resistant to natural fibrinolytic removal. Urinary tract obstruction in patients with haematuria treated with EACA has been reported (McNicol 1961, Stark *et al.* 1965, Gobbi 1967). Because of the risk of hydronephrosis, antifibrinolytic drugs are best avoided in patients with bleeding in the kidney or upper urinary tract. Intrathoracic clots resistant to lysis have also been reported (McNicol 1962).

Aprotinin (Kunitz bovine trypsin inhibitor: Trasylol)

Aprotinin, commercially prepared from bovine lung, is a polypeptide of molecular weight 6000 which can inhibit many serine proteases including trypsin, chymotrypsin, kallikrein and plasmin (Feeney, Means and Bigler 1969).

The reaction between plasmin and aprotinin proceeds in two steps, a rapid phase followed by a slower phase: it can also inhibit the plasmin–streptokinase complex, but much more slowly than plasmin (Wiman 1980). In addition to its inhibitory effect on plasmin, aprotinin has been shown to be a competitive inhibitor of plasminogen activation and to have an anticoagulant action (Dubber *et al.* 1968). The latter was found to be due principally to inhibition of activated factors XII and XI (Prentice, McNicol and Douglas 1970). In therapeutic dosage, however, aprotinin is a relatively weak anticoagulant.

Aprotinin has been recommended for use in the defibrination syndrome, particularly in pregnancy, but results from controlled clinical trials are not available to provide a basis for firm conclusions on its efficacy. None of the physiological protease inhibitors react readily with the plasmin–streptokinase complex: aprotinin's property of inhibiting this complex may theoretically be of value in the control of bleeding complications resulting from streptokinase therapy.

Clinical uses of fibrinolytic inhibitors

On theoretical grounds antifibrinolytic therapy would be beneficial in situations where haemorrhage results from excessive fibrinolytic activity, either generalized or localized, or where a defective coagulation mechanism produces inadequate fibrin which is easily disrupted by normal physiological fibrinolytic activity. The situations in which therapy with fibrinolytic inhibitors has been used are listed in Table 37.

Table 37. Situations in which use of fibrinolytic inhibitors has been suggested.

Systemic hyperplasminaemic states
Urinary tract bleeding
Primary menorrhagia
Haemophilia
Gastrointestinal bleeding
Subarachnoid haemorrhage
Epistaxis
Tonsillectomy
Traumatic hyphaema
Hereditary angioedema

PRIMARY HYPERPLASMINAEMIA

Primary hyperplasminaemia (primary fibrinolysis) is a rare condition in which plasminogen is converted to plasmin in sufficient quantity and speed to temporarily overwhelm the neutralizing capacity of the plasma protease inhibitors. The effect of the presence of free circulating plasmin is the proteolysis and depletion of fibrinogen and coagulation factors, in particular V and VIII, and the formation of fibrinogen degradation products with an anticoagulant action. In contrast to the much commoner disseminated intravascular coagulation (DIC) with a secondary fibrinolytic response, thrombocytopenia will not necessarily be present. If the diagnosis of primary fibrinolysis is made on the basis of the presence of a predisposing clinical condition, markedly accelerated clot lysis, defective clotting and defibrination, and DIC can be excluded, treatment with EACA or tranexamic acid is merited. Secondary fibrinolysis in disseminated intravascular coagulation is a protective mechanism and antifibrinolytic drugs are contraindicated in this situation.

HAEMOPHILIA

A number of uncontrolled studies have suggested that EACA might reduce the frequency of bleeding events in patients with haemophilia (Abe *et al.* 1962, Mainwaring and Keidan 1962, Reid, Hodge and Cerutti 1967). The results of four controlled trials, two with EACA and two with tranexamic acid, are available. In a double-blind controlled trial of EACA in ten patients with severe haemophilia, Gordon and associates (1965) obtained a reduction in the number of spontaneous bleeds while on the drug, but the results did not reach the 5 per cent level of significance. A further double-blind cross-over study of tranexamic acid or placebo showed a significant reduction in the incidence of haemorrhagic events (Rainsford, Jouhar and Hall 1973). In contrast, others have found no benefit from the prophylactic use of EACA (Strauss, Kevy and Diamond 1965) or tranexamic acid (Bennett, Ingram and Inglish 1973) in haemophilia.

Fibrinolytic inhibitors have also been used to reduce bleeding from tooth sockets after extraction in haemophilic patients. Some early reports pointed to a reduction in blood loss after dental extraction in patients given EACA (Reid *et al.* 1964, Cooksey, Perry and Raper 1966, Tavenner 1968) or AMCA (Björlin and Nilsson 1973). This impression has received support from the results of double-blind studies comparing EACA and placebo (Walsh *et al.* 1971) or tranexamic acid and placebo (Forbes *et al.* 1972). Antifibrinolytic drugs have also been reported to help in the control of bleeding after synovectomy (Storti *et al.* 1972).

Haematuria in haemophilic patients can also be controlled by EACA or tranexamic acid (McNicol *et al.* 1961, Barkhan 1964, Tsevrenis and Mandalaki 1965), but the incidence of clot retention with renal obstruction is unacceptably high (Stark *et al.* 1965, Hilgartner 1966, van Itterbeek, Vermylen and Verstraete 1968).

MENORRHAGIA

A suggestion that increased local fibrinolytic activity contributes to excessive menstrual blood loss (Astrup 1958) was supported by the finding of higher levels of plasminogen activator in the endometrium of women with excessive menstrual bleeding than in those with normal menstrual loss (Rybo 1966). Double-blind trials have provided conclusive evidence that menstrual bleeding can be reduced by treatment with EACA (Nilsson and Rybo 1965) or tranexamic acid (Nilsson and Rybo 1967, Vermylen *et al.* 1968, Callender, Warner and Cope 1970).

Excessive and irregular menstrual bleeding complicating the use of intra-uterine devices has also been shown by controlled trials to be decreased by therapy with EACA (Kasonde and Bonnar 1975) or tranexamic acid (Weström and Bengtsson 1970).

PROSTATECTOMY

Bleeding is a common problem after prostatectomy. This complication is related to the high content of plasminogen activator in the prostatic capsule and the urinary urokinase bathing the prostatic cavity, the local fibrinolytic activity contributing to premature dissolution of haemostatic fibrin clots. The initial report on the use of antifibrinolytic drugs to reduce post-prostatectomy bleeding came from McNicol and colleagues (1961): blood loss was reduced after both suprapubic prostatectomy and transurethral resection in patients given EACA. This effect has been confirmed in a number of controlled trials (Lawrence, Ward-McQuaid and Holdom 1966, Madsen and Strauch 1966, Vinnicombe and Shuttleworth 1966, Smart, Turnbull and Jenkins 1974). Tranexamic acid has a similar beneficial effect in reducing post-prostatectomy blood loss (Hedlund 1969).

GASTROINTESTINAL BLEEDING

Evidence for the presence of plasminogen activator in blood vessels of the gastric and intestinal submucosa and mucosa and in mucosal cells has been reviewed by Poller (1980). The local fibrinolytic activity may impair haemostasis in ulcer craters; consequently, antifibrinolytic drugs have been employed in the management of upper gastrointestinal bleeding. Three double-blind trials of tranexamic acid have provided some evidence of therapeutic benefit. In one trial, in which the drug was only given orally, there was a significant difference in favour of tranexamic acid in terms of cessation of bleeding and lack of requirement for further transfusion or surgery, but only when patients with hiatus hernia or bleeding varices were excluded from analysis (Cormack *et al.* 1973). In the trial of Biggs, Hugh and Dodds (1976) the tranexamic acid-treated group, who received intravenous and oral therapy at the start with continuation orally, had a significantly lower requirement for surgical intervention to manage continuous or recurrent bleeding. In a further double-blind study, patients receiving tranexamic acid had significantly lower transfusion requirements (Engqvist *et al.* 1979).

The use of antifibrinolytic therapy in the management of bleeding in ulcerative colitis has been reported with apparent benefit (Nilsson, Andersson and Björkman 1966, Salter and Read 1970), but results from a double-blind cross-over study failed to show a significant reduction in blood loss while on EACA (Mowat *et al.* 1973).

SUBARACHNOID HAEMORRHAGE

The risk of rebleeding following rupture of an intracranial aneurysm and subarachnoid haemorrhage is high. Many studies on the use of antifibrinolytic therapy to reduce the incidence of rebleeding in the first two or three weeks after initial rupture have been reported, the rationale being to prevent premature dissolution of haemostatic fibrin around the aneurysmal site. Two controlled clinical trials carried out have shown a significantly lower rebleeding rate in the patients treated with tranexamic acid (Fodstad *et al.* 1978, Maurice-Williams 1978). In contrast, two other trials have failed to demonstrate any benefit from therapy (Van Rossum *et al.* 1977, Kaste and Ramsay 1979). In addition, there has been a suggestion that tranexamic acid-treated patients have an increased incidence of cerebral vasospasm with consequent reduction in blood flow (Fodstad 1980). At the present time no firm recommendation can be given for the use of antifibrinolytic drugs to prevent rebleeding following rupture of an intracranial aneurysm.

OTHER SITES OF LOCAL BLEEDING

Antifibrinolytic drugs have been used in a variety of other forms of localized bleeding, but results from double-blind controlled trials are available only for bleeding after adenotonsillectomy and for recurrent epistaxis. Both EACA and tranexamic acid have been shown to reduce blood loss following adenotonsillectomy (Verstraete, Vermylen and Tyberghein 1968, Verstraete *et al.* 1977).

Suggestive evidence for a favourable influence on epistaxis was obtained by Petruson (1974): recurrent epistaxes were less frequent and less severe in the tranexamic-treated group than in the placebo group. Recurrent abruptio placentae (Astedt and Nilsson 1978) and traumatic hyphaema (Bramsen 1977, Mortensen and Sjolie 1978) have also been managed by tranexamic acid with apparent benefit.

HEREDITARY ANGIOEDEMA

An inherited deficiency of $C\bar{1}$ inactivator allowing uninhibited $C1$-esterase to cleave a kinin-like permeability factor from $C2$ appears to be the basic abnormality in hereditary angioedema. Activation of $C1$ may be achieved by plasmin, providing a rationale for the use of antifibrinolytic drugs in this condition. A number of uncontrolled trials have suggested that long-term EACA therapy is of benefit in this condition (Nilsson, Andersson and Björkman 1966, Lundh *et al.* 1968, Champion and Lachmann 1969). Double-blind trials of both EACA (Frank *et al.* 1972) and tranexamic acid (Blohmé 1972, Sheffer, Austen and Rosen 1972) have provided further evidence for the efficacy of antifibrinolytic therapy in reducing the frequency and severity of attacks of angioedema.

REFERENCES

Abe T., Sato A., Kazama M. & Matsumura T. (1962) Effect of ε-aminocaproic acid in haemophilia. *Lancet* II, 405.

Aber C.P., Bass N.M., Berry C.L., Carson P.H.M., Dobbs R.J., Fox K.M., Hamblin J.J., Haydu S.P., Howitt G., MacIver J.E., Portal R.W., Raftery E.B., Rousell R.H. & Stock J.P.P. (1976) Streptokinase in acute myocardial infarction: a controlled multicentre study in the United Kingdom. *British Medical Journal* II, 1100–4.

Abiko Y., Iwamoto M. & Tomikawa M. (1969) Plasminogen-plasmin system V. A stoichiometric equilibrium complex of plasminogen and a synthetic inhibitor. *Biochimica et Biophysica Acta* 185, 424–31.

Ablondi F.B., Hagan J.J., Philips M. & De Renzo E.C. (1959) Inhibition of plasmin, trypsin and the streptokinase-activated fibrinolytic system by ε-aminocaproic acid. *Archives of Biochemistry and Biophysics* 82, 153–60.

Ahlberg A., Eriksson O. & Kjellman H. (1976) Diffusion of tranexamic acid to the joint *Acta Orthopaedica Scandinavica* 47, 486–8.

Alkjaersig N., Fletcher A.P. & Sherry S. (1959) The mechanism of clot dissolution by plasmin. *Journal of Clinical Investigation* 38, 1086–95.

Ambrus C.M. & Markus G. (1960) Plasmin–antiplasmin complex as a reservoir of fibrinolytic enzyme. *American Journal of Physiology* 199, 491–4.

Amery A., Vermylen J. & Verstraete M. (1969) Recent progress in thrombolytic therapy. *Journal of Clinical Pathology* 22, 371.

Amris C.J. & Amris A. (1963) Investigations concerning activator-free porcine plasminogen. *Scandinavian Journal of Clinical and Laboratory Investigation* 15, 189–97.

Andersson L. (1962) Studies on fibrinolysis in urinary tract disease and its treatment with epsilon-amino-caproic acid. *Acta Chirurgica Scandinavica* Suppl. 301, 1–29.

Andersson L., Nilsson I.M., Colleen S., Granstrand B. & Melander A. (1968) Role of urokinase and tissue activator in sustaining bleeding and the management thereof with EACA and AMCA. *Annals of the New York Academy of Sciences* 146, 642–56.

Andersson L., Nilsson I.M., Niléhn J.-E., Hedner U., Granstrand B. & Melander B. (1965) Experimental and clinical studies on AMCA, the antifibrinolytically active isomer of p-aminomethyl cyclohexane carboxylic acid. *Scandinavian Journal of Haematology* 2, 230–47.

Arnesen H., Heilo A., Jakobsen E., Ly B. & Skaga E. (1978) A prospective study of streptokinase and heparin in the treatment of deep vein thrombosis. *Acta Medica Scandinavica* 203, 457–63.

Astedt B. & Nilsson I.M. (1978) Recurrent abruptio placentae treated with the fibrinolytic inhibitor tranexamic acid. *British Medical Journal* I, 756–7.

Astrup T. (1958) The haemostatic balance. *Thrombosis et Diathesis Haemorrhagica* 2, 347–57.

Barkhan P. (1964) Haematuria in a haemophiliac treated with ε-aminocaproic acid. *Lancet* II, 1061.

Barritt D.W. & Jordan S.C. (1960) Anticoagulant drugs in the treatment of pulmonary embolism. A controlled trial. *Lancet* I, 1309–12.

Bennett A.E., Ingram G.I.C. & Inglish P.J. (1973) Antifibrinolytic treatment in haemophilia: a controlled trial of prophylaxis with tranexamic acid. *British Journal of Haematology* 24, 83–8.

Bennett J.R. (1972) Myopathy from ε-aminocaproic acid: a second case. *Postgraduate Medical Journal* 48, 440–2.

Bett J.H.N., Biggs J.C., Castaldi P.A., Chesterman C.N., Hale G.S., Hirsch J., Isbister J.A., McDonald I.G., McLean K.H., Morgan J.J., O'Sullivan E.F. & Rosenbaum M. (1973) Australian multicentre trial of streptokinase in acute myocardial infarction. *Lancet* I, 57–60.

Biggs J.C., Hugh T.B. & Dodds A.J. (1976) Tranexamic acid and upper gastrointestinal haemorrhage—a double-blind trial. *Gut* 17, 729–34.

Björlin G. & Nilsson I.M. (1973) Tooth extractions in haemophiliacs after administration of a single dose of factor VIII or factor IX concentrate supplemented with AMCA. *Oral Surgery, Oral Medicine, Oral Pathology* 36, 482–9.

Blohmé G. (1972) Treatment of hereditary angioneurotic oedema with tranexamic acid. *Acta Medica Scandinavica* 192, 293–8.

Bramsen T. (1977) Traumatic hyphaema treated with the antifibrinolytic drug tranexamic acid II. *Acta Ophthalmologica* 55, 616–20.

Callender S.T., Warner G.T. & Cope E. (1970) Treatment of menorrhagia with tranexamic acid. A double-blind trial. *British Medical Journal* IV, 214–16.

Castellino F.J. (1979) Aspects of the structure and activation of human plasminogen. In *The Chemistry and Physiology of the Human Plasma Proteins*. Bing D.H. (ed.) pp. 299–313. Pergamon Press, New York.

Champion R.H. & Lachmann P.J. (1969) Hereditary angio-oedema treated with ε-aminocaproic acid. *British Journal of Dermatology* 81, 763–5.

Chesterman C.N., Allington M.J. & Sharp A.A. (1972) Relationship of plasminogen activator to fibrin. *Nature (New Biology)* **238**, 15–17.

Chesterman C.N., Nash T. & Biggs J.C. (1971) Small-vessel thrombosis following vascular injury. Successful treatment with a low-dose intra-arterial infusion of streptokinase. *British Journal of Surgery* **58**, 582–5.

Christensen L.R. & McLeod C.M. (1945) A proteolytic enzyme of serum: chracterization, activation, and reaction with inhibitors. *Journal of General Physiology* **28**, 559–83.

Collen D. & Verstraete M. (1979) Alpha$_2$-antiplasmin consumption and fibrinogen breakdown during thrombolytic therapy. *Thrombosis Research* **14**, 631–9.

Cooksey M.W., Perry C.B. & Raper A.B. (1966) Epsilon-aminocaproic acid therapy for dental extractions in haemophiliacs. *British Medical Journal* **II**, 1633–4.

Cormack F., Chakrabarti R.R., Jouhar A.J. & Fearnley G.R. (1973) Tranexamic acid in upper gastrointestinal haemorrhage. *Lancet* **I**, 1207–8.

Davidson J.F., Lochhead M., McDonald G.A. & McNicol G.P. (1972) Fibrinolytic enhancement by stanozolol: a double-blind trial. *British Journal of Haematology* **22**, 543–59.

Davidson J.F. & Walker I.D. (1979) Synthetic fibrinolytic agents. *Progress in Cardiovascular Diseases* **21**, 375–96.

Den Ottolander G.J.H. & Craandijk A. (1968) Treatment of thrombosis of the central retinal vein with streptokinase. *Thrombosis et Diathesis Haemorrhagica* **20**, 415–19.

Dewar H.A., Horler A.R. & Cassells-Smith A.J. (1961) Fibrinolytic treatment of coronary thrombosis. A pilot study. *British Medical Journal* **II**, 671–5.

Dioguardi N., Mannucci P.M., Lotto A., Rossi P., Levi G.F., Lomanto B., Rota M., Mattei G., Proto C., Fiorelli G. & Agostoni A. (1971) Controlled trial of streptokinase and heparin in acute myocardial infarction. *Lancet* **II**, 891–5.

Dotter C.T., Rösch J. & Seaman A.J. (1974) Selective clot lysis with low-dose streptokinase. *Radiology* **111**, 31–7.

Dubber A.H.C., McNicol G.P., Uttley D. & Douglas A.S. (1968) *In vitro* and *in vivo* studies with Trasylol, an anticoagulant and a fibrinolytic inhibitor. *British Journal of Haematology* **14**, 31–49.

Duckert F. (1979) Thrombolytic therapy in myocardial infarction. *Progress in Cardiovascular Diseases* **21**, 342–50.

Duckert F., Müller G., Nyman D., Benz A., Prisender S., Madar G., Da Silva M.A., Widner L.K. & Schmitt H.E. (1975) Treatment of deep vein thrombosis with streptokinase. *British Medical Journal* **II**, 479–81.

Ele H., Amundsen E. & Rø J.S. (1972) Thrombolytic treatment with brinase of dogs with experimental pulmonary embolism. *Scandinavian Journal of Thoracic and Cardiovascular Surgery* **6**, 164–71.

Elliot M.S., Immelman E.J., Jeffery P., Benatar S.R., Funston M.R., Smith J.A., Shepstone B.J., Ferguson A.D., Jacobs P., Walker W. & Louw J.H. (1979) A comparative randomized trial of heparin versus streptokinase in the treatment of acute proximal venous thrombosis: an interim report of a prospective trial. *British Journal of Surgery* **66**, 838–43.

Engqvist A., Broström O., von Feilitzen F., Halldin M., Nyström B., Ost A., Reichard H., Sandqvist S., Törngren S. & Wedlund J.E. (1979) Tranexamic acid in massive haemorrhage from the upper gastrointestinal tract: a double-blind study. *Scandinavian Journal of Gastroenterology* **14**, 839–44.

Eriksson O., Kjellman H., Pilbrant Å. & Schannong M. (1974) Pharmacokinetics of tranexamic acid after intravenous administration to normal volunteers. *European Journal of Clinical Pharmacology* 7, 375–80.

European Collaborative Study (1975) Controlled trial of urokinase in myocardial infarction. *Lancet* II, 624–6.

European Cooperative Study Group for Streptokinase Treatment in Acute Myocardial Infarction (1979) Streptokinase in acute myocardial infarction. *New England Journal of Medicine* 301, 797–802.

European Working Party (1971) Streptokinase in recent myocardial infarction. A controlled multicentre trial. *British Medical Journal* III, 325–31.

Fearnley G.R., Chakrabarti R. & Hocking E.D. (1967) Fibrinolytic effects of diguanides plus ethyloestrenol in occlusive vascular disease. *Lancet* II, 1008–11.

Feeney R.E., Means G.E. & Bigler J.C. (1969) Inhibition of human trypsin, plasmin and thrombin by naturally occurring inhibitors of proteolytic enzymes. *Journal of Biological Chemistry* 244, 1957–60.

Fletcher A.P., Sherry S., Alkjaersig N., Smyrniotis F.E. & Jick S. (1959) The maintenance of a sustained thrombolytic state in man. II Clinical observations on patients with myocardial infarction and other thrombo-embolic disorders. *Journal of Clinical Investigation* 38, 1111–19.

Fodstad H. (1980) Tranexamic acid (AMCA) in aneurysmal subarachnoid haemorrhage. *Journal of Clinical Pathology* 33, Suppl. 14, 68–73.

Fodstad H., Liliequist B., Schannong M. & Thulin C.A. (1978) Tranexamic acid in the preoperative management of ruptured intracranial aneurysms. *Surgical Neurology* (*Boston*) 10, 9–15.

Forbes C.D., Barbenell J. & Prentice C.R.M. (1976) Treatment of thrombosis by sequential therapy with ancrod followed by streptokinase: clinical pharmacology and rheology. *Haemostasis* 5, 348–54.

Forbes C.D., Barr R.D., Reid G., Thomson C., Prentice C.R.M., McNicol G.P. & Douglas A.S. (1972) Tranexamic in control of haemorrhage after dental extraction in haemophilia and Christmas disease. *British Medical Journal* II, 311–13.

Fossard D.P., Friend J.R., Field E.S., Corrigan T.P., Kakkar V.V. & Flute P.T. (1974) Fibrinolytic activity and postoperative deep-vein thrombosis. *Lancet* I, 9–11.

Frank M.M., Sergent J.S., Kane M.A. & Alling D.W. (1972) Epsilon aminocaproic acid therapy of hereditary angioneurotic oedema. *New England Journal of Medicine* 286, 808–12.

Gallus A.S., Hirsch J., Cade J.F., Turpie A.G.G., Walker J.R. & Gent M. (1975) Thrombolysis with a combination of small doses of streptokinase and full doses of heparin. *Seminars in Thrombosis and Hemostasis* 2, 14–32.

Ganz W., Buchbinder N., Marcus H., Mondkar A., Maddahi J., Charuzi Y., O'Connor L., Shell W., Fishbein M.C., Kass R., Miyamoto A. & Swan H.J.C. (1981) Intracoronary thrombolysis in evolving myocardial infarction. *American Heart Journal* 101, 4–13.

Genton E. & Claman H.N. (1970) Urokinase: antigenic studies in patients following thrombolytic therapy. *Journal of Laboratory and Clinical Medicine* 75, 619–21.

Gobbi F. (1967) Use and misuse of aminocaproic acid. *Lancet* II, 472–3.

Gordon A.M., McNicol G.P., Dubber A.H.C., McDonald G.A. & Douglas A.S. (1965) Clinical trial of epsilon-aminocaproic acid in severe haemophilia. *British Medical Journal* I, 1632–5.

Gorham L.W. (1961a) A study of pulmonary embolism. Part I. A clinicopathological investigation of 100 cases of massive embolism of the pulmonary artery; diagnosis by physical signs and differentiation from acute myocardial infarction. *Archives of Internal Medicine* **108**, 8–22.

Gorham L.W. (1961b) A study of pulmonary embolism. Part II. The mechanism of death; based on a clinicopathological investigation of 100 cases of massive and 285 cases of minor embolism of the pulmonary artery. *Archives of Internal Medicine* **108**, 189–207.

Hawkey C. & Howell M. (1964) Intravenous streptokinase in the treatment of retinal vascular occlusion. *Journal of Clinical Pathology* **17**, 363–4.

Hedlund P.O. (1969) Antifibrinolytic therapy with cyklokapron in connection with prostatectomy. *Scandinavian Journal of Urology and Nephrology* **3**, 177–82.

Hedlund P.O. (1975) Postoperative venous thrombosis in benign prostatic disease. A study of 316 patients, using the ^{125}I-fibrinogen uptake test. *Scandinavian Journal of Urology and Nephrology* (Suppl.) **27**.

Heikinheimo R., Ahrenberg P., Honkapohja H., Iisalo E., Kallio V., Konttinen Y., Leskinen O., Mustaniemi H., Reinikainen M. & Siitonen L. (1971) Fibrinolytic treatment in acute myocardial infarction. *Acta Medica Scandinavica* **189**, 7–13.

Hess H. (1969) Zur Streptokinase-Therapie akuter Verschlüsse von Gliedmassen gefässen. *Thrombosis et Diathesis Haemorrhagica* **32** (Suppl.), 275–7.

Hilgartner M.W. (1966) Intrarenal obstruction in haemophilia. *Lancet* **I**, 486.

Hirsch J.L., McDonald I. & O'Sullivan E. (1971) Comparison of the effects of streptokinase and heparin in the early rate of resolution of major pulmonary emboli. *Journal of the Canadian Medical Association* **104**, 488–91.

Hirschhorn R., Grossman J., Troll W. & Weissmann G. (1971) The effect of epsilon aminocaproic acid and other inhibitors of proteolysis upon the response of human peripheral blood lymphocytes to phytohemagglutinin. *Journal of Clinical Investigation* **50**, 1206–17.

Hoffman E. P. & Koo A.H. (1979) Cerebral thrombosis associated with amicar therapy. *Radiology* **131**, 687–9.

Johansson E., Ericson K. & Zetterquist S. (1976) Streptokinase treatment of deep venous thrombosis of the lower extremity. Clinical, phlebographic and plethysmographic evaluation of early and late results. *Acta Medica Scandinavica* **199**, 89–94.

Johnson A.J. & McCarthy W.R. (1959) The lysis of artificially induced intravascular clots in man by intravenous infusions of streptokinase. *Journal of Clinical Investigation* **38**, 1627–43.

Johnson A.J. & Tillett W.S. (1952) Lysis in rabbits of intravascular blood clots by the streptococcal fibrinolytic system (streptokinase). *Journal of Experimental Medicine* **95**, 449–63.

Jones F.E., Black P.J., Cameron J.S., Chantler C., Gill D., Maisey M.N., Ogg C.S. & Saxton H. (1975) Local infusion of urokinase and heparin into renal arteries in impending renal cortical necrosis. *British Medical Journal* **IV**, 547–9.

Kakkar V.V., Flanc C., Howe C.T., O'Shea M. & Flute P.T. (1969a) Treatment of deep vein thrombosis. A trial of heparin, streptokinase, and arvin. *British Medical Journal* **I**, 806–10.

Kakkar V.V., Howe C.T., Laws J.W. & Flanc C. (1969b) Late results of treatment of deep vein thrombosis. *British Medical Journal* **I**, 810–11.

Kakkar V.V., Sagar S. & Lewis M. (1975) Treatment of deep-vein thrombosis with intermittent streptokinase and plasminogen infusion. *Lancet* **II**, 674–6.

Kaller H. (1967) Enterale Resorption, Verteilung und Elimination von 4-Aminomethylcyclohexancarbonsäure (AMCHA) und ε-Aminocapronsäure (ACS) beim Menschen. *Naunyn-Schmiederberg's Archives of Pharmacology* **256**, 160–8.

Kartchner M.M. & Wilcox W.C. (1976) Thrombolysis of palmar and digital arterial thrombosis by intra-arterial thrombolysin. *Journal of Hand Surgery* **1**, 67–74.

Kasonde J. M. & Bonnar J. (1975) Effect of ethamsylate and aminocaproic acid on menstrual blood loss in women using intrauterine devices. *British Medical Journal* **IV**, 21–2.

Kaste M. & Ramsay M. (1979) Tranexamic acid in subarachnoid haemorrhage: a double-blind study. *Stroke* **10**, 519–22.

Kohner E.M., Pettit J.E., Hamilton A.M., Bulpitt C.J. & Dollery C.T. (1976) Streptokinase in central retinal vein occlusion: a controlled clinical trial. *British Medical Journal* **I**, 550–3.

Korninger C., Matsuo O., Suy R., Stassen J.M. & Collen D. (1981) Thrombolytic properties of purified human tissue plasminogen activator in a dog femoral vein thrombosis model. *Thrombosis and Haemostasis* **46**, 209.

Kullander S. & Nilsson I.M. (1970) Human placental transfer of an antifibrinolytic agent (AMCA). *Acta Obstetricia et Gynecologica Scandinavica* **49**, 241–2.

Lane R.J.M., McLelland N.J., Martin A.M. & Mastaglia F.L. (1979) Epsilon aminocaproic acid (EACA) myopathy. *Postgraduate Medical Journal* **55**, 282–5.

Latallo Z.S. & Lopaciuk S. (1973) New approach to thrombolytic therapy. The use of defibrase in connection with streptokinase. *Thrombosis and Haemostasis* **56** (Suppl.), 253–64.

Lawrence A.C.K., Ward-McQuaid J.N. & Holdom G.L. (1966) The effect of epsilon aminocaproic acid on the blood loss after retropubic prostatectomy. *British Journal of Urology* **38**, 308–10.

Lippschutz E.J., Ambrus J.L., Ambrus C.M., Constant J., Rekate A.C., Collins G.L. & Sokal J.E. (1965) Controlled study of the treatment of coronary occlusion with urokinase-activated human plasmin. *American Journal of Cardiology* **16**, 93–8.

Luluaga I.T., Carrera D., D'Oliveira J., Cantaluppi C.G., Santin H., Molteni L., Ferreira R., Zwolinski E. & de Luluaga I.I. (1971) Successful thrombolytic therapy after acute tricuspid-valve obstruction. *Lancet* **I**, 1067–8.

Lundh B., Laurell A.B., Wetterqvist H., White T. & Granerus G. (1968) A case of hereditary angioneurotic oedema, successfully treated with ε-aminocaproic acid: studies on C′1 esterase inhibitor, C′1 activation, plasminogen level and histamine metabolism. *Clinical and Experimental Immunology* **3**, 733–45.

Ly B., Arnesen H., Eie H. & Hol R. (1978) A controlled clinical trial of streptokinase and heparin in the treatment of major pulmonary embolism. *Acta Medica Scandinavica* **203**, 465–70.

Macfarlane R.G. & Pilling J. (1947) Fibrinolytic activity of normal urine. *Nature* **159**, 779.

McNicol G.P., Fletcher A.P., Alkjaersig N. & Sherry S. (1961) The use of epsilon-aminocaproic acid, a potent inhibitor of fibrinolytic activity, in the management of post-operative haematuria. *Journal of Urology* **86**, 829–37.

McNicol G.P., Fletcher A.P., Alkjaersig N. & Sherry S. (1962) The absorption, distribution, and excretion of ε-aminocaproic acid in man. *Journal of Laboratory and Clinical Medicine* **59**, 15–24.

McNicol G.P., Reid W., Bain W.H. & Douglas A.S. (1963) Treatment of peripheral arterial occlusion by streptokinase perfusion. *British Medical Journal* **I**, 1508–12.

Madsen P.O. & Strauch A.E. (1966) The effect of aminocaproic acid on bleeding following transurethral prostatectomy. *Journal of Urology (Baltimore)* **96**, 255–6.

Mainwaring K. & Keidan S.E. (1965) Fibrinolysis in haemophilia: the effect of ε-aminocaproic acid. *British Journal of Haematology* **11**, 682–8.

Marder V.J. (1979) Guidelines for thrombolytic therapy of deep-vein thrombosis. *Progress in Cardiovascular Diseases* **21**, 327–32.

Marder V.J., Soulen R.L., Atichartakarn V., Budzynski A.Z., Parulekar S., Kim J.R., Edward N., Zahavi J. & Algazy K.M. (1977) Quantitative venographic assessment of deep vein thrombosis in the evaluation of streptokinase and heparin therapy. *Journal of Laboratory and Clinical Medicine* **89**, 1018–29.

Martin M. (1979) Thrombolytic therapy in arterial thromboembolism. *Progress in Cardiovascular Diseases* **21**, 351–74.

Matsuo O., Rijken D.C. & Collen D. (1981) Thrombolysis by human tissue plasminogen activator and urokinase in rabbits with experimental pulmonary embolus. *Nature* **291**, 590–1.

Maurice-Williams R.S. (1978) Prolonged antifibrinolysis: an effective non-surgical treatment for ruptured intracranial aneurysms? *British Medical Journal* **I**, 945–7.

Mavor G.E., Ogston D., Galloway J.M.D. & Karmody A.M. (1969) Urokinase in iliofemoral venous thrombosis. *British Journal of Surgery* **56**, 571–4.

Miller G.A.H. (1972) The diagnosis and management of massive pulmonary embolism. *British Journal of Surgery* **59**, 837–9.

Miller G.A.H., Sutton G.C., Kerr I.H., Gibson R.V. & Honey M. (1971) Comparison of streptokinase and heparin in treatment of isolated acute massive pulmonary embolism. *British Medical Journal* **II**, 681–4.

Mortensen K. & Sjolie A.K. (1978) Secondary haemorrhage following traumatic hyphaema. A comparative study of conservative and tranexamic acid treatment. *Acta Ophthalmologica* **56**, 763–8.

Mowat N.A.G., Douglas A.S., Brunt P.W., McIntosh J.A.R., King P.C. & Boddy K. (1973) Epsilon-aminocaproic acid therapy in ulcerative colitis. *American Journal of Digestive Diseases* **18**, 959–65.

Naeye R.L. (1962) Thrombotic state after a haemorrhagic diathesis, a possible complication of therapy with epsilon-aminocaproic acid. *Blood* **19**, 694–701.

Nilsson I.M. (1975) Phenformin and ethyloestrenol in recurrent venous thrombosis. In *Progress in Chemical Fibrinolysis and Thrombolysis*. Vol. 1. Davidson J.F., Samama M.M. & Desnoyers P.C. (eds). pp. 1–12, Raven Press, New York.

Nilsson I.M. (1980) Clinical pharmacology of aminocaproic and tranexamic acids. *Journal of Clinical Pathology* **33** Suppl. 14, 41–7.

Nilsson I.M., Andersson L. & Björkman S.E. (1966) Epsilon-aminocaproic acid (E-ACA) as a therapeutic agent. Based on 5 years clinical experience. *Acta Medica Scandinavica* Suppl. 448, 1–46.

Nilsson L. & Rybo G. (1965) Treatment of menorrhagia with epsilon-aminocaproic acid. *Acta Obstetricia et Gynecologica Scandinavica* **44**, 467–73.

Nilsson L. & Rybo G. (1967) Treatment of menorrhagia with an antifibrinolytic agent, tranexamic acid (AMCA). A double-blind investigation. *Acta Obstetricia et Gynecologica Scandinavica* **46**, 572–80.

Okamoto S., Nakajima T., Okamoto U., Watanabe J., Iguchi Y., Igawa T., Chien Ching-Chun & Hayashi T. (1959) A suppressing effect of ε-amino-N-caproic acid on the bleeding of dogs, produced with the activation of plasmin in the circulatory blood. *Keio Journal of Medicine* **8**, 247–66.

Persson A.V., Thompson J.E. & Patman R.D. (1973) Streptokinase as an adjunct to arterial surgery. *Archives of Surgery* **107**, 779–90.

Petruson B. (1974) Epistaxis: A clinical study with special reference to fibrinolysisk. *Acta Otolaryngica* Suppl. 317, 1–73.

Pierse D. & LeGrice H. (1963) Urokinase in ophthalmology. *Lancet* **II**, 1143–4.

Poller L. (1980) Fibrinolysis and gastrointestinal haemorrhage. *Journal of Clinical Pathology* **33** (Suppl. 14), 63–7.

Powell R.H. & Ekert H. (1974) Streptokinase and antithrombic therapy in the hemolytic-uremic syndrome. *Journal of Pediatrics* **84**, 345–9.

Prentice C.R.M., McNicol G.P. & Douglas A.S. (1970) Studies on the anticoagulant action of aprotinin (Trasylol). *Thrombosis et Diathesis Haemorrhagica* **24**, 265–72.

Preston F.E., Burakowski B.K., Porter N.R. & Malia R.G. (1981) The fibrinolytic response to stanozolol in normal subjects. *Thrombosis Research* **22**, 543–51.

Rainsford S.G., Jouhar A.J. & Hall A. (1973) Tranexamic acid in the control of spontaneous bleeding in severe haemophilia. *Thrombosis et Diathesis Haemorrhagica* **30**, 272–9.

Reichle F.A., Rao N.S., Chang K.H.Y., Marder V. & Algazy K. (1977) Thrombolysis of acute or subacute non-embolic arterial thrombosis. *Journal of Surgical Research* **22**, 202–8.

Reid W.O., Hodge S.M. & Cerutti E.R. (1967) The use of EACA in preventing or reducing haemorrhage in the hemophiliac. *Thrombosis et Diathesis Haemorrhagica* **18**, 179–89.

Reid W.O., Lucas O.N., Francisco J., Geisler P.J. & Erslev A.J. (1964) The use of epsilon-aminocaproic acid in the management of dental extractions in the haemophiliac. *American Journal of Medical Sciences* **248**, 184–8.

Robbins K.C. & Markus G. (1978) The interaction of human plasminogen with streptokinase. In *Fibrinolysis: Current Fundamental and Clinical Concepts.* Gaffney P.J. & Balkuv-Ulutin S. (eds). pp. 61–75. Academic Press, London.

Robertson B.R., Nilsson I.M. & Nylander G. (1970) Thrombolytic effect of streptokinase as evaluated by phlebography of deep venous thrombi of the leg. *Acta Chirurgica Scandinavica* **136**, 173–80.

Roschlaw W.H.E. & Tosoni A.L. (1965) Thrombolytic therapy with CA-7 (fibrinolytic enzyme from *Aspergillus oryzae*) in the dog. *Canadian Journal of Physiology and Pharmacology* **43**, 731–40.

Rybo G. (1966) Plasminogen activators in the endometrium. II. Clinical aspects. *Acta Obstetricia et Gynecologica Scandinavica* **45**, 429–50.

Rydin E. & Lundberg P.O. (1976) Tranexamic acid and intracranial thrombosis. *Lancet* **II**, 49.

Salter R.H. & Read A.E. (1970) Epsilon aminocaproic acid therapy in ulcerative colitis. *Gut* **11**, 585–7.

Sawyer W.D., Fletcher A.P., Alkjaersig N. & Sherry S. (1961) Thrombolytic therapy: basic and therapeutic considerations. *Archives of Internal Medicine* **107**, 274–89.

Schmutzler R., Heckner F., Kortge P., van de Loo J., Pezold F.A., Poliwoda H., Praetorius F. & Zekorn D. (1966) Zur thrombolytischen therapie des frischen lieozinfarktes. I. Einfuhrung, behandleinapplane, klinische ergebnisse. *Deutsche Medizinische Wochenschrift* **91**, 581–7.

Sharma G.V.R.K., Burleson V.A. & Sasahara A.A. (1980) Effect of thrombolytic therapy on pulmonary-capillar blood volume in patients with pulmonary embolism. *New England Journal of Medicine* **303**, 842–5.

Sheffer A.L., Austen K.F. & Rosen F.S. (1972) Tranexamic acid therapy in hereditary angioneurotic oedema. *New England Journal of Medicine* **287**, 452–4.

Siefring G.E. & Castellino F.J. (1976) Interaction of streptokinase with plasminogen. Isolation and characterization of a streptokinase degradation product. *Journal of Biological Chemistry* **251**, 3913–20.

Sjöholm I., Wiman B. & Wallén P. (1973) Studies on the conformational changes of plasminogen induced during activation to plasmin and by 6-aminohexanoic acid. *European Journal of Biochemistry* **39**, 471–9.

Smart C.J., Turnbull A.R. & Jenkins J.D. (1974) The use of furosemide and epsilon-aminocaproic acid in transurethral prostatectomy. *British Journal of Urology* **46**, 521–5.

Smith R.A.G., Dupe J.R., English P.D. & Green J. (1981) Fibrinolysis with acyl-enzymes: a new approach to thrombolytic therapy. *Nature* **290**, 505–8.

Sobel G.W., Mohler S.R., Jones N.W., Dowdy A.B.C. & Guest M.M. (1952) Urokinase: an activator of plasma profibrinolysin extracted from urine. *American Journal of Physiology* **171**, 768–9.

Soter N.A., Austen K.F. & Gigli I. (1975) Inhibition by ε-aminocaproic acid of the activation of the first component of the complement system. *Journal of Immunology* **114**, 928–32.

Spöttl F. & Kaiser R. (1974) Rapid detection and quantitation of precipitating streptokinase-antibodies. *Thrombosis et Diathesis Haemorrhagica* **32**, 608–16.

Stark S.N., White J.G., Langer L. & Krivit W. (1965) Epsilon-aminocaproic acid therapy as a cause of intrarenal obstruction in haematuria of haemophiliacs. *Scandinavian Journal of Haematology* **2**, 99–107.

Stefanini M. & Marin H. (1958) Fibrinolytic activity of extracts from non-pathogenic fungi. *Proceedings of the Society for Experimental Biology and Medicine* **99**, 504–7.

Storti E., Ascari E., Turpini R., Molinari E., Gamba G. & Pettene A. (1972) Epsilon-aminocaproic acid for synovectomy in haemophilic patients. *Acta Haematologica* **47**, 146–56.

Strauss H.S., Kevy S.V. & Diamond L.K. (1965) Ineffectiveness of prophylactic epsilon-aminocaproic acid in severe hemophilia. *New England Journal of Medicine* **273**, 301–4.

Stuart J., Winterborn M.H., White R.H.R. & Flinn R.M. (1974) Thrombolytic therapy in haemolytic-uraemic syndrome. *British Medical Journal* **III**, 217–21.

Summaria L., Boreisha I.G., Arzadon L. & Robbins K.C. (1977) The dissolution of human cross-linked plasma fibrin clots by the equimolar human plasmin-derived light (B) chain-streptokinase complex. The acceleration of clot lysis by pretreatment of fibrin clots with the light (B) chain. *Thrombosis Research* **11**, 377–89.

Summaria L.E. & Robbins K.C. (1976) Isolation of a human plasmin-derived, functionally active, light (B) chain capable of forming with streptokinase an equivalent light (B) chain-streptokinase complex with plasminogen activator activity. *Journal of Biological Chemistry* **251**, 5810–13.

Tavenner R.W.H. (1968) Epsilon-aminocaproic acid in the treatment of haemophilia and Christmas disease with special reference to the extraction of teeth. *British Dental Journal* **124**, 19–22.

Thorsen S. (1975) Differences in the binding to fibrin of native plasminogen and plasminogen modified by proteolytic degradation. Influence of ω-aminocarboxylic acids. *Biochimica et Biophysica Acta* **393**, 55–65.

Tibbutt D.A., Chesterman C.N., Williams E.W., Faulkner T. & Sharp A.A. (1977) Controlled trial of the sequential use of streptokinase and ancrod in the treatment of deep vein thrombosis of lower limb. *Thrombosis and Haemostasis* **37**, 222–32.

Tibbutt D.A., Williams E.A., Walker M.W., Chesterman C.N., Holt J.M. & Sharp A.A. (1974) Controlled trial of ancrod and streptokinase in the treatment of deep vein thrombosis of lower limb. *British Journal of Haematology* **27**, 407–14.

Tillett W.S. & Garner R.L. (1933) The fibrinolytic activity of haemolytic streptococci. *Journal of Experimental Medicine* **58**, 485–502.

Tovi D., Nilsson I.M. & Thulin C.-A. (1972) Fibrinolysis and subarachnoid haemorrhage. Inhibitory effect of tranexamic acid. *Acta Neurologica Scandinavica* **48**, 393–402.

Tsapogas M.J., Peabody R.A., Wu.K.T., Karmody A.M., Devaraj K.T. & Eckert C. (1973) Controlled study of thrombolytic therapy in deep vein thrombosis. *Surgery* **74**, 973–84.

Tsevrenis H. & Mandalaki T. (1965) Haematuria in a haemophiliac treated with ε-aminocaproic acid. *Lancet* **I**, 610.

Urokinase Pulmonary Embolism Trial Study Group (1970) Phase 1 results. A cooperative study. *Journal of the American Medical Association* **214**, 2163–72.

Urokinase-Streptokinase Embolism Trial (1974) Phase 2 results. A cooperative study. *Journal of the American Medical Association* **229**, 1606–13.

van Itterbeek H., Vermylen J. & Verstraete M. (1968) High obstruction of urine flow as a complication of the treatment with fibrinolysis inhibitors of haematuria in haemophiliacs. *Acta Haematologica* **39**, 237–42.

van Rossum J., Wintzen A.R., Endtz L.J., Schoen J.H.R. & de Jonge H. (1977) Effect of tranexamic acid on rebleeding after subarachnoid hemorrhage: a double-blind controlled clinical trial. *Annals of Neurology* **2**, 238–42.

Vermylen J., Verhaegen-Declercq M.L., Verstraete M. & Fierens F. (1968) A double-blind study of the effect of tranexamic acid in essential menorrhagia. *Thrombosis et Diathesis Haemorrhagica* **20**, 583–7.

Verstraete M., Tyberghein J., Degreef Y., Daems L. & Van Hoof A. (1977) Double-blind trials with ethamsylate, batroxobin or tranexamic acid on blood loss after adenotonsillectomy. *Acta Clinica Belgica* **32**, 136–41.

Verstraete M., Vermylen J., Amery A. & Vermylen C. (1966) Thrombolytic therapy with streptokinase using a standard dosage scheme. *British Medical Journal* **I**, 454–6.

Verstraete M., Vermylen J. & Donati M.B. (1971) The effect of streptokinase infusion on chronic arterial occlusions and stenoses. *Annals of Internal Medicine* **74**, 377–82.

Verstraete M., Vermylen J. & Tyberghein J. (1968) Double-blind evaluation of the haemostatic effect of adrenochrome monosemicarbazone, conjugated oestrogens and epsilonaminocaproic acid after adenotonsillectomy. *Acta Haematologica* **40**, 154–61.

Vinnicombe J. & Shuttleworth K.E.D. (1966) Aminocaproic acid in the control of haemorrhage after prostatectomy. A controlled trial. *Lancet* **I**, 230–2.

Walker I.D., Davidson J.F., Young P. & Conkie J.A. (1975) Effect of anabolic steroids on plasma antithrombin III, α_2-macroglobulin and α_1-antithrypsin levels. *Thrombosis et Diathesis Haemorrhagica* **34**, 106–14.

Walsh P.N., Rizza C.R., Matthews J.M., Eipe J., Kernoff P.B.A., Coles M.D., Bloom A.L., Kaufman B.M., Beck P., Hanan C.M. & Biggs R. (1971) Epsilon-aminocaproic acid therapy for dental extractions in haemophilia and Christmas disease: a double-blind controlled trial. *British Journal of Haematology* **20**, 463–75.

Warlow C., Beattie A.G., Terry G., Ogston D., Kenmure A.C.F. & Douglas A.S. (1973) A double-blind trial of low doses of subcutaneous heparin in the prevention of deep-vein thrombosis after acute myocardial infarction. *Lancet* **II**, 934–6.

Warlow C., Ogston D. & Douglas A.S. (1972) Venous thrombosis following strokes. *Lancet* **I**, 1305–6.

Weimar W., Stibbe J., van Seyen A.J., Billiau A., De Somer P. & Collen D. (1981) Specific lysis of an iliofemoral thrombus by administration of extrinsic (tissue-type) plasminogen activator. *Lancet* **II**, 1018–20.

Weström L. & Bengtsson L.P. (1970) Effect of tranexamic acid (AMCA) in menorrhagia with intrauterine contraceptive devices. A double-blind study. *Journal of Reproductive Medicine* **5**, 154–61.

Williams J.R.B. (1951) The fibrinolytic activity of urine. *British Journal of Experimental Pathology* **32**, 530–7.

Wiman B. (1980) On the reaction of plasmin or plasmin–streptokinase complex with aprotinin or α_2-antiplasmin. *Thrombosis Research* **17**, 143–52.

Wiman B. & Collen D. (1978) Molecular mechanism of physiological fibrinolysis. *Nature* **272**, 549–50.

Wiman B. & Wallén P. (1977) The specific interaction between plasminogen and fibrin. A physiological role of the lysine-binding site in plasminogen. *Thrombosis Research* **10**, 213–22.

Wohl R.C., Summaria L., Arzadon L. & Robbins K.C. (1978) Steady state kinetics of activation of human and bovine plasminogens by streptokinase and its equimolar complexes with various activated forms of human plasminogen. *Journal of Biological Chemistry* **253**, 1402–7.

Wysenbeek A.J., Sella A., Vardi M. & Yeshurun D. (1978) Acute delirious state after ε-aminocaproic acid. *Lancet* **I**, 221.

Chapter 18
Antithrombotic Therapy

A. S. DOUGLAS, B. BENNETT *and* D. OGSTON

This chapter describes the drugs administered with the aim of preventing or limiting thrombosis and the problems encountered in their use. The therapeutic intention of those using these drugs varies from the prevention of extension of any established thrombus to the prevention of thrombosis itself, whether it be *new thrombosis*—in patients entering high-risk situations such as surgery, or *recurrent thrombosis*—in patients who have already sustained an arterial or venous vascular occlusion.

The literature on antithrombotic therapy is extensive and selection of particular aspects is necessary. This account will be confined to drugs which are used as follows:

1   to prevent fibrin formation (heparin, coumarin drugs, ancrod);
2   to prevent platelet adhesion and aggregation (aspirin, dipyridamole—'Persantin', sulphinpyrazone—Anturan, dextrans and hydroxychloroquine). Thrombolytic enzymes and pharmacological fibrinolytic activators are considered in Chapter 17.

In vascular disease, antithrombotic drugs may not be the most important aspect of patient management. Venous thromboembolic disease is often a disorder consequent on hospitalization; early mobilization, active leg exercise, graded pressure stockings and a variety of other physical methods may be of more importance than heparin and warfarin therapy in the prophylaxis of deep venous thrombosis. Similarly, the treatment of hypertension and the cessation of cigarette smoking are likely to make a much more important contribution to the prevention of arterial occlusions than any drug which limits fibrin formation or platelet function.

The object of antithrombotic therapy is to interfere with fibrin formation or platelet function. Neither of these two processes can be divorced one from the other. Warfarin therapy interferes with the production of fibrin by diminishing the generation of thrombin; thrombin aggregates platelets. Anti-platelet drugs interfere with aggregation and release of a range of substances from platelets; some of these released materials play a role in blood coagulation. Once fibrin is formed it attracts platelets to its surface; this is particularly obvious in venous thrombi as indicated by the lines of Zahn. Thus intervention in the process of fibrin formation alters platelet function and vice versa.

There are two comparisons, which need to be made to provide the rationale for antithrombotic therapy:

1   *between blood clotting and thrombosis;*
2   *between arterial and venous thrombosis.*

1.   Blood clotting and thrombosis

Over a century ago, it was known that there was a major difference between a thrombus and a blood clot, but the distinction was ignored for many years thereafter, until Poole drew renewed attention to this (Poole 1959, 1960). A blood clot is a structure formed in static blood in a container outside the body and consists of red cells, white cells and platelets randomly dispersed in a fibrin network. On the other hand, a thrombus is formed in moving blood within the body and is not homogeneous. The part of the thrombus which is attached to the vessel wall consists of platelet aggregates with numerous white cells, but very few red cells and a limited amount of fibrin. As the head first forms, the platelets are adherent one to another, and only later does fibrin appear between individual platelets. The fibrin may form strands traversing this platelet 'head' of the thrombus; electron microscopy also demonstrates fibrin between individual platelets. The red 'tail' which flows from the platelet head consists largely of fibrin with entrapped red cells rather than platelets.

2.   Arterial and venous thrombosis

In normal haemostasis, when a small blood vessel is severed a platelet 'plug' forms. The first step is adhesion of platelets to the damaged vessel wall. Further platelets are added to form a loosely constructed platelet plug. This, however, is unstable and abnormal haemorrhage will occur unless reinforcement with fibrin follows rapidly, so platelet reactions and fibrin formation participate in normal haemostasis. These two phenomena contribute to intravascular thrombus generation, though the trigger is not severance of a blood vessel but damage to the blood vessel endothelium; in arteries this may occur at the site of a complicated atheromatous plaque and in veins it may perhaps follow mechanical injury or a combination of this with reduced blood flow for a variety of reasons. Venous and arterial thrombi differ, however, in the quantitative contribution of platelets and fibrin to the thrombus mass. In the venous system the platelet head of a thrombus may be small, attaching the thrombus to the vessel often in the region of a valve cusp while a relatively large red tail streams away in the direction of blood flow. The structure of this tail is the closest approach *in vivo* to that of a blood clot formed in static blood in the test-tube. An arterial thrombus has a much larger platelet head which may be sufficient to occlude a blood vessel without a major mass of fibrin. If such a thrombus does not occlude the lumen, or if platelet-induced retraction allows renewed flow in the vessel, a fibrin-containing tail to the thrombus may be formed in the streaming blood.

Thrombi, arterial or venous, therefore consist of mixtures of fibrin and platelets. Because venous thrombi have a relatively large fibrin component it is reasonable to expect anticoagulant drugs to be more effective than the anti-platelet agents, while drugs modifying platelet function might be expected to be more effective in the prevention of arterial thrombosis. The use of both types of drug, while they may prevent thrombus formation in their respective ways, will similarly impair normal haemostatic mechanisms, and the degree to which this occurs has a major bearing on their value and acceptability.

Embolism

In arteries or veins, occlusive thrombi will often declare themselves by local symptoms and may have major immediate and long-term local effects ranging from organ infarction to chronic venous or arterial insufficiency. In contrast, non-occlusive thrombi may be locally silent or produce relatively minor local symptoms but declare themselves only when they become detached and embolize causing acute infarction or transient ischaemia of distant organs such as brain or lungs. Additionally, the long-term local sequelae to non-occlusive thrombi are often undefined. Thus agents may be used in management of thrombotic disorders with two separate clinical aims: firstly, the prevention or mitigation of the local effects of blood vessel occlusion, such as acute myocardial infarction or chronic arterial or venous insufficiency of a limb, or secondly, the prevention of embolization and its sequelae, such as pulmonary infarction or transient ischaemic attacks. These aims may not be identical, though clearly total prevention of local thrombosis will prevent both local and embolic problems completely.

Clinical trials of antithrombotic therapy

In certain thrombotic disorders, the value of antithrombotic therapy is clear. In many, the best clinical trials have usually demonstrated trends in favour of antithrombotic agents but these have failed to reach the chosen levels of statistical significance. There are, furthermore, numerous studies which are inadequate in design and do not allow firm conclusions; in others, where the design has been satisfactory, the numbers of patients entered have been too small to encourage acceptance of the results without reservation.

The natural history of 'thrombotic' disease; the numbers of patients required to enter a study

Coronary artery disease is used to illustrate the issues. Despite the debate to the contrary, let us assume for the present that myocardial infarction is a 'thrombotic' disease. Death rates after myocardial infarction can be used to illustrate the problem. Of 100 deaths from this disorder, the following represents an approximation of their distribution in time:

100 deaths

Fail to reach hospital alive	45
Further deaths in the first 24 hours	15
Further deaths in the first month	10
Further deaths in the next six months	8
Further deaths up to one year	6
Thereafter annual death rate of 4 per cent	
—up to 5 years	say 16
	———
	100

Once past the first six months the death rate is of the order of 4–5 per cent per year. The difficulty then is to show that in a treated group with a death rate of 3 per cent there is a real difference when compared with a placebo group with a mortality of 5 per cent per annum. Where the death rate in the placebo group is so small, then the numbers of patients required to enter the study is so enormous that the study becomes laborious and expensive. Additionally, even if a small percentage benefit is shown to be significant by such effort, the regime examined is unlikely to be widely valued unless it is simple to administer and manage and acceptably free from troublesome side-effects.

The historical lessons from past studies of antithrombotic therapy

In the conduct of further trials the lessons learnt from the history of previous endeavours to test the anticoagulant and antiplatelet drugs must not be forgotten.

For the 15–20 years after the introduction of anticoagulant drugs of coumarin type, nearly all the studies were of inadequate design. Over the last 20 years a number of well-designed and well-conducted studies of anti-coagulants have been published, but the results have sometimes failed to provide the clear answers which were expected. There has been 'therapeutic greed' (Mitchell 1981a); clinical investigators have been disappointed because the trend of the results toward benefit in some disorders has been small. Because a difference has been too small to be of statistical significance, the conclusion has been that the trial result was negative. The difference in death rate in a trial may be below the technical level of significance adopted by statisticians, but 'not significant' is not equivalent to 'there is no difference'. It corresponds merely to 'not proven' and indicates that there are insufficient numbers to allow one to dismiss chance as an alternative explanation.

This problem has extended even into recent large clinical trials in the field of antiplatelet agents. This has led to the suggestion by some that there should be no more multi-centre trials of antithrombotic agents and that a return to the 'best clinical judgment' should be made without further studies on the despairing argument that digitalis derivatives have been used for generations without controlled trials. The control of atrial fibrillation, however, is an event which may be directly related to the institution of digoxin; the prevention of an episode of thrombosis cannot be related to a therapeutic regimen in an individual patient, and thus the term 'clinical judgment' is simply an euphemism for guesswork or uncritical faith. Despite the disappointments encountered in the past, there is clearly a crucial role for properly conducted trials of antithrombotic therapy in the future. The problems and shortcomings in the design of early trials are quite understandable as the principles of sound trial design were only coming into recognition when they were conducted. Today it is simpler to plan a trial of sound design once clear objectives have been identified and appropriate pilot studies performed to isolate unforeseen problems. Their execution is more difficult.

While we cannot abandon the critical application of properly designed therapeutic trials of agents for the prevention of thrombotic disorders, a philosophical rather than a scientific problem requires to be confronted when considering trials in which statistically significant but small benefits can be shown to result from the use of any prophylactic regimen. This is, perhaps, particularly relevant to recent trials concerned with the secondary prevention of myocardial infarction. If it is shown that a particular drug reduces the death rate in the years after a primary episode of myocardial infarction from, say, 4 to 2 per cent and that this is statistically significant, to whom is the regime valuable? Is it to the individual patient or to society as a whole? It will be apparent that both the individual patient and the society in which he exists may assess the value of such a benefit by widely differing criteria, unrelated to statistical factors and influenced crucially by the convenience and acceptibility of the regime, the nature and frequency of side-effects, the complexity or otherwise of measures necessary to control its safety and its cost in monetary terms or in the time necessarily spent in its supervision. The medical profession has certainly ignored statistical significance in the past in face of some of these factors, and doubtless, along with individual patients and society as a whole, will do so again in the future.

The multi-centre trial

It is usually difficult to obtain adequate numbers of patients at a single centre for trials of the prevention of thrombosis with currently available agents; it usually requires many participants at many centres, each possessed with much tenacity of purpose to carry it to its completion. The doctors at the participating centres must be capable of sinking their own personalities sufficiently to allow them to participate in a cooperative study, from which no individual credit will accrue; they must admit into the trial only patients approved by an independent team, conform to an agreed plan of patient care and submit their patient records for scrutiny and, if required, criticism by a central organization. This may need national or international endeavour.

These trials will involve many clinicians who have little or no training in statistical methods; to ensure continued cooperation, the design must be simple and easily understood. It is a mistake to try to answer too many questions and the temptation to collect non-essential additional information must be resisted. Where these rules are not adhered to, the antithrombotic trial may answer no simple question clearly or completely. The responsible statistician must be concerned with the design of the trial from the time of its original planning. No statistician can accept the responsibility of assessing the results of a trial when he has not been consulted about the initial design.

A multi-centre trial should be coordinated by a centre with experience of this type of scientific effort. These studies are sometimes funded by the pharmaceutical industry; when this is so, the coordinating centre should not be 'in house'; and should be entirely independent of the pharmaceutical company.

Criteria of selection

Those planning the study must insist that the criteria of selection are precise. A consequence may be that many patients have to be excluded from the trial. For example, in a study of aspirin in secondary prevention of myocardial infarction, many patients may have to be excluded because of longstanding dyspepsia, or because of other available evidence of intolerance of aspirin. On completion of the study, the investigators should be able to report the number of potential patients who were ineligible and be able to give the reasons why they were not recruited into the study.

Random allocation

The method of allocation to treatment and placebo group must be strictly random. Of the many aspects of trial design this is probably the single most important feature to ensure that the groups compared differ only in the preparation assigned to them. Cards indicating allocation to one or other treatment group are made out; each is sealed in an individual envelope and the envelopes are arranged in a strictly random order. The physician in charge must first decide whether each patient is suitable for inclusion in the trial. Only after a firm decision that a patient can be entered in the trial may the next envelope in the series be opened. The content of the envelope alone decides to which group the patient is allocated. Unless this procedure is adhered to rigidly, bias is introduced and the value of the trial negated.

The method of provision of random allocation and the immediacy of its availability may vary according to the clinical situation under study. For example, if the value of a drug is to be tested in patients in whom the first dose is administered immediately upon suspicion of vascular occlusion, such as pulmonary embolism or myocardial infarction, allocation envelopes must be available on site or allocations be immediately obtainable from a continuously manned telephone in the coordinating office of the trial centre. In contrast, if the trial concerns the effect of a drug on a less acutely presenting disorder such as transient ischaemic attacks or stable coronary artery disease, allocations may be obtained less urgently from the coordinating centre, which will also be able to screen the individual patient's criteria for suitability for admission to the trial.

Random allocation by this method may, of course, by chance not succeed in providing strictly comparable groups. In the recent AMIS (see p. 522) study testing the effect of aspirin in survivors of myocardial infarction, such an allocation procedure did not provide equal distribution of risk factors in spite of including 4000 patients. In general, however, if the sample size is large enough, strictly random allocation should ensure that the groups studied are comparable in spite of variation between individuals; the method supersedes the unacceptable practices of the past in which comparisons between units and hospitals using different regimes or between current practices and historical controls within units were made.

Once allocation has been made, follow-up and management of the different study groups must be identical. Follow-up must include collection of data on patients who discontinue medication in any group for any reason, such as the development of side-effects, personal inclination, change of address, etc. Patients lost to follow-up present a major problem which may threaten the validity of a trial's interpretation. This will be discussed again below, but it must be emphasized that total follow-up is necessary. That is to say it should be possible to determine what has happened to all patients randomized whether or not they have withdrawn from a study group.

Patients will require various treatments, separate from that under trial, as events related or unrelated to thrombotic disease occur. Individual physicians must be at liberty to institute therapy appropriate to these. Though some of these may be foreseen and guidelines agreed upon by participants for the management of anticipated new events, it is clearly impossible to obtain identical management in a multi-centre trial, though within individual centres standard management may be possible. Random allocation should be arranged so that each participating centre has equal number of patients allocated to each study group to maintain comparability of management of groups throughout the study.

The numbers of patients initially randomized may be decided in advance using an estimate of the total needed to show a benefit of therapy thought to be worthwhile in the context of the disorder under study. It may, however, be a mistake to stop the trial too early as the required numbers may actually only become evident as a result of observations made as the study progresses.

Ethical issues

From the ethical viewpoint the design of trials needs careful consideration, and, as such, may be scientifically far from ideal. If a physician believes that a particular treatment cannot be withheld from patients he clearly cannot participate in such trials. Similarly, if early trials indicate that a specific treatment confers significant benefit, is it possible for later trials to contain a control group receiving placebo, or should all trials compare new treatments with those already shown to be of value? If a patient in a placebo group develops a further thrombotic episode, should he continue to receive placebo or be commenced upon alternative therapy and, if so, how should further events in such patients be analysed? These and other questions make the design of control groups and the analysis of results exceedingly difficult. The design of a trial must permit treatment changes under specified circumstances. In the study of the value of, for example, coumarin therapy, if a patient develops serious haemorrhage the clinician concerned must be free to reverse the anticoagulant effect if he so decides. Similarly, if a patient in a trial of an agent believed to influence coronary artery disease develops deep venous thrombosis his physician must be able to treat the patient with oral anticoagulants. Such treatment changes or withdrawals from initial treatment allocation have created problems in the interpretation of results as such changes may not be randomly assigned. One important method of dealing with this problem is to count the eventual outcome against the initial treatment allocation regardless of intervening events.

'Explicative' or 'pragmatic intention to treat' designs

This topic is reviewed by Sackett and Gent (1979) and Hampton (1981). In his paper, Hampton makes an excellent case for a standard method of data presentation that clarifies what was done, makes trial comparison easier and allows readers to make their own judgment of the results. Fig. 53 is reproduced from Hampton's paper.

The box in the top line (1) represents the total number of patients from which those entering the trial were chosen. In recent large multi-centre trials of anti-platelet therapy no information is given on this. Without this, the applicability of the results to the broad spectrum of patients suffering from the clinical problems cannot be appreciated. The trials are, of course, testing a therapy in a group of patients with well-defined criteria of inclusion or exclusion. However, for the general physician, the patient population studied

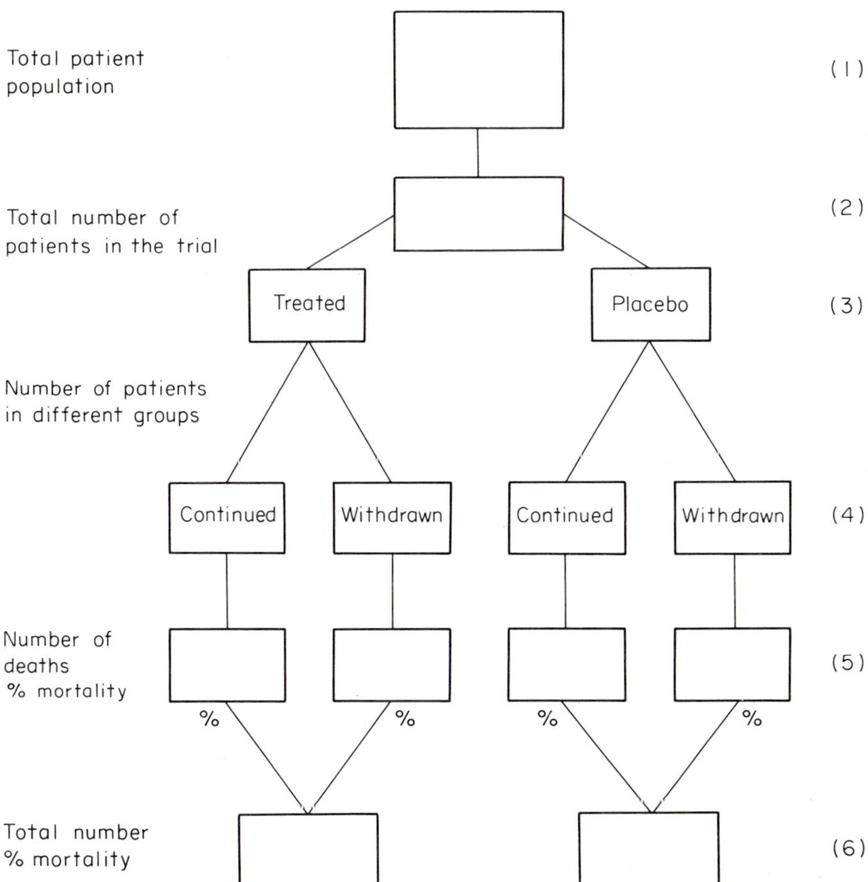

Fig. 53. Plan for uniformity of trial reporting proposed by Professor J.R. Hampton (see text).

needs to be set in the overall context of the disorder in a general hospital population. The second box gives the total number of patients included in the trial. If the number in box 2 is small as compared with box 1 then this should be explained by the authors describing the study. The reasons for exclusion should be recorded. The number of patients randomly allocated is shown in line 3. If the numbers are large, then good matching is usual. However, as noted earlier in one of the largest of the well-conducted clinical trials, randomization of 4000 patients failed to provide a good match of important risk factors.

The boxes on line 4 show the numbers allocated who continued in the study or were withdrawn. If the numbers of patients withdrawn are substantially greater in the treated as compared with the placebo group, then the active treatment is unlikely to find widespread clinical acceptance.

The boxes on the fifth line show the number (and, below the number, the percentages) of patients who died in each of the subgroups, i.e. both the groups who continued treatment or were withdrawn from treatment (active or placebo).

The boxes on line 6 give the number of deaths among the patients allocated to the original treatment intention.

Those favouring the 'explicative' approach will look at line 5 and will compare the percentage mortality in those continued on active therapy compared with those continued on placebo. This form of analysis appeals to those who take the viewpoint of the pharmacologist that once a patient is off therapy then it is not fair to count his death against the treated group. The alternative approach is to conduct the trial analysis based on 'all patients randomized—intention to treat basis'. Here, fatality rate is counted against initial treatment intention, whether the patient was continued on therapy or not. This method of assessment is the one which is most trusted by the scientific community. However, as Sackett and Gent (1979) emphasize, real differences in the efficacy of the therapy may well be obscured by this approach as any benefit in those continuing may be diluted by those who stop therapy. For the present, those who use the explicative approach with its analysable and non-analysable deaths should provide sufficient data in their reports to allow readers to apply the pragmatic approach if they so wish.

Avoidance of 'data dredging'

Once a trial has been completed, particularly if its result is inconclusive, there is a temptation to try to identify subgroups in which differences may be apparent. This is risky 'data dredging', and the figures must be viewed with extreme caution. The problem is that with a large study it is likely that some subgroup will show a much larger difference than is found in the analysis of all patients randomized. Any such differences must not be accepted as proven. It is, however, proper to note these differences as areas for further study.

Double-blinding

It is desirable that physicians as well as patients should be unaware of the nature of the preparation the patient receives. This has been possible in recent large trials of the use of sulphinpyrazone, aspirin, and aspirin with dipyridamole. It is much more difficult to run a study double-blind when agents such as oral anticoagulants are employed because of the necessity to adjust dosage according to the variable anticoagulant effect in individuals. It has been achieved using two observers—one responsible for control of therapy and the other clinically responsible for all other aspects of management. In double-blind studies there will be a small number of circumstances in which unblinding is needed and haemorrhage during trials of coumarin-related agents typifies these. In some other situations it may be possible to discontinue therapy without unblinding.

Precision of diagnosis—criteria for entry and end-points

In some trials there may be time for a fairly leisurely appraisal of a patient's suitability for entry. In studies which allowed entry weeks or months after a myocardial infarction, for example, precision of diagnosis before entry could be demanded. With the realization that mortality is highest immediately after infarction and that greatest benefits of any treatment are likely to be achieved during this period, patients may have to be entered on the basis of a working clinical diagnosis on available evidence, sometimes refuted later by sequential electrocardiographic and enzyme changes. This is not an insuperable problem. It is quite possible and proper to design and execute a satisfactory trial in which patients are entered on the basis of a working clinical diagnosis. In a proportion the diagnosis will not be substantiated. Effective randomization should ensure that equal numbers of such individuals are distributed in each study group. The analysis must be a pragmatic one as the question asked is that which faces the clinician on first seeing the patient with chest pain—should treatment be given before proof of diagnosis is available in the knowledge that the diagnosis, if substantiated, carries a high risk? It will be permissible later to look at the results of the treatment in those patients proven to have myocardial infarction, but this approach will answer a question different from that answered by the pragmatic one.

In addition to the problem of precision of diagnosis before entry, precision in identifying end-points must be considered. If mortality is the parameter studied, this is simple. Standard identification of the *cause* of mortality in a multi-centre trial is much less easy to achieve, as is standard identification of various thrombotic events. Methods for identification of venous thrombosis, for example, may differ at different centres, as may standards of assessment of the same method at different centres; central 'blind' reading of cardiographs, venograms or the various methods of scanning is desirable, and evidence on end points should be considered by a mortality and morbidity committee. Even when trials are not double-blind such a group codes the nature and cause of end point episodes, fatal or non-fatal, without knowledge of treatment groups. Where they disagree with the responsible clinician their decision must be final to ensure uniformity in a multi-centre trial. A hallmark of a well-designed trial is the selection of end-points simple to identify, with causes which may also be objectively determined.

Multiple looks at the data

In a multi-centre study the coordinating centre must be responsible for monitoring progress to ensure that the trial can be stopped should difference between the groups reach the agreed level of significance. On the other hand, the level of significance should be set relatively high, say at the 1 per cent level to avoid premature cessation of entry or follow-up.

Some leading world authorities on clinical trials insist that a price has to be paid for interim looks at the data, i.e. the more looks there are at the data the more strictly set should be the level of significance required.

Assessment of results/end-points

In assessment of results, death from all causes is the most important end-point. It is permissible, of course, to look at the deaths by cause (e.g. cancer or fatal cardiovascular events). These results are of less consequence than deaths from all causes. Non-fatal events should be simple to identify clinically and must be amenable to investigation by widely available and comparable methods as indicated above.

Conclusion

In antithrombotic drug trials the design must be such that the conclusion can be correlated with the treatment given; scrutiny of many published trials reveals that clinicians studying patients record accurately what was observed, but fail to appreciate that what was observed was not necessarily related to the antithrombotic therapy given, because trial design was inadequate to allow that conclusion.

The intention now is to proceed to review the best of the evidence regarding the current therapeutic role of the conventional anticoagulants (heparin and coumarins), ancrod and the antiplatelet drugs. Elsewhere in this book or in recent reviews (Winter and Douglas 1981, Mackie and Douglas 1982) will be found the following relevant topics.

ANTICOAGULANT DRUGS

Oral anticoagulants
> Mechanism of action (p. 38), Control of oral anticoagulant therapy (p. 176), Methods for comparison of results, between different laboratories (p. 177). Sites of haemorrhage (p. 153), Management of excessive anticoagulation and bleeding in patients on oral anticoagulants (p. 303).

(Pharmacology of drug interaction is dealt with below.)

Heparin
> Mode of action (p. 83), Laboratory control (p. 177), Haemorrhage on heparin therapy (p. 153), Management of haemorrhage due to heparin therapy (p. 303).

ANTIPLATELET DRUGS

Dipyridamole
Sulphinpyrazone
Hydroxychloroquine

PHARMACOLOGY OF WARFARIN AND DRUG INTERACTIONS

Warfarin reduces the synthesis of normally functioning vitamin K-dependent clotting factors but has no effect on their subsequent metabolism. Therefore, the level of the various vitamin K-dependent clotting factors in the blood, following institution of oral anticoagulant treatment is related to the half-life of the appropriate factor. This varies, ranging from about seven hours for factor VII to approximately 60 hours for factor II. It can thus be estimated that some 4–5 days of therapy is needed before all the vitamin K-dependent factors reach their lowest levels. From this, important practical implications emerge for the safe and effective use of oral anticoagulants. The effect of warfarin on the coagulation system is conventionally measured by the one-stage prothrombin time which reflects reductions in factor VII and X and to a lesser extent II, but which is insensitive to changes in the concentration of factor IX. Factor VII falls most rapidly because it has the shortest half-life, and in the first place the prolongation of the prothrombin time reflects this. The patient may appear well anticoagulated on the basis of the test result from the laboratory, but the full antithrombotic effect has still not been reached, because the other vitamin K-dependent factors have not reached their nadir. It has thus become customary to overlap the warfarin effect by a period of continuous intravenous heparin.

Until recently it was common clinical practice to give a large loading dose of warfarin. However it is now realized that this does not lead to a more rapid reduction in factors II, VII, IX and X when compared to the start of therapy with much smaller repeated dosages. Some investigators believe that the large loading dose of warfarin causes a precipitous and dangerous fall in factor VII, exposing the patient to the risk of haemorrhage because of the overshoot (Mackie and Douglas 1982). Most physicians now agree that it is safer and not less effective to start warfarin therapy with 10 mg daily on each of the first two days stopping the heparin on the third day and checking the prothrombin time 3–4 hours after stopping the heparin.

Warfarin is well absorbed orally and is highly bound to plasma albumin; commercial warfarin is a racemic mixture of two isomers R(+) and S(−). The latter is four times more potent than R(+), but is more rapidly eliminated. Metabolism of warfarin is achieved by hepatic microsomal enzymes and the rate of metabolism of each isomer can be established, an issue of particular use when studying mechanisms of drug interaction.

A more detailed review of the above aspects is provided by Mackie and Douglas (1982).

Drug interactions with oral anticoagulants

Patients may receive anticoagulants for a few weeks or for their entire life-time. There is ample time for exposure to other drugs. Much of the literature is confusing and anecdotal. The patients are often on many drugs, making identification of the offender difficult. In hospitals and primary care situations in the UK about one-third of the patients on anticoagulants are at risk of having a drug interaction.

Drugs are thought to have the potential for interference with the action of oral anticoagulants and/or increase the risk of haemorrhage by altering the following:

1   Drug absorption.
2   Protein binding.
3   Receptor site affinity.
4   Metabolism and excretion.
5   Additional parameters of the haemostatic mechanism.

In practical terms, any change in drug therapy in a patient on anticoagulants should be made with the recognition of a potential drug interaction in mind.

Interactions can reduce the therapeutic efficacy of the anticoagulant. Barbiturates act in this way by enzyme induction. If a patient is stabilized on long-term anticoagulant therapy together with a barbiturate, and the latter is stopped, then there is a serious risk of haemorrhage unless the dose of the anticoagulant is reduced. While some of the more commonly used drugs causing interaction may be memorized, this will not be possible with many of the others. Those to be memorized are included in Table 38.

A more detailed review of drug interaction with anticoagulants is provided by Mackie and Douglas (1982).

The following section consists of a review of some of the well-conducted clinical trials of antithrombotic drugs. These studies have investigated the efficacy of such drugs in preventing thrombus or arresting the propagation of an existing thrombus. They do not dissolve thrombi, but the vessel lumen may become patent as the channel enlarges by thrombus retraction or the natural fibrinolytic mechanism.

Table 38. Warfarin—drug interaction.

Warfarin effect enhanced	Proposed mechanism
Phenylbutazone	Inhibition of S($-$) isomer
Cimetidine	Inhibition of S($-$) isomer
Cotrimoxazole	Inhibition of S($-$) isomer
Metronidazole	Inhibition of S($-$) isomer
Anabolic steroids	Unknown mechanism
Aspirin	Additive effect of platelet defect to coagulation abnormality
Allopurinol	? Inhibition of metabolism
Ethacrynic acid	? Displacement of protein binding
Quinidine	? Decreased synthesis of vitamin K-dependent factors
Thyroxine	? Increased catabolism of vitamin-dependent factors
Dextropropoxyphene	Action unknown

Warfarin effect reduced	Proposed mechanism
Barbiturates	Induction of hepatic enzymes
Rifampicin	Induction of hepatic enzymes
Cholestyramine	Inhibition of absorption

VENOUS THROMBOSIS

The conventional anticoagulants are used in the prophylaxis and treatment of deep venous thrombosis and pulmonary embolism. Much of the evidence in favour of *prophylaxis* is convincing; despite widespread use in the management of *established* venous thromboembolic disease, the evidence for efficacy is scanty; much is opinion and not fact. This opinion, however, has been translated into established clinical practice.

In the study of prophylaxis it is possible to rank patients in groups at high risk. Frequently these are patients who enter hospital for the management of other specified disorders. Table 39 lists recognized positive risk factors in venous thrombosis.

Cigarette smoking may be a negative risk factor.

It is clearly desirable to identify patients at high risk of developing venous thrombosis. Clayton, Anderson and McNicol (1976) studied the frequency of isotopically diagnosed venous thrombosis in general surgical patients. Using an equation constructed by them, it was possible to identify 95 per cent of patients who developed evidence of venous thrombosis with misallocation of only 28 per cent of those who did not develop venous thrombosis. The equation is based on three clinical variables—age, varicose veins and percentage overweight, and two tests of coagulation—the euglobulin lysis time and fibrin-related antigen.

Table 39. Recognized positive risk factors in venous thrombosis.

Increasing age
Immobility
Obesity
Pregnancy
Surgery
Malignant disease
Previous venous thrombotic disease
Myocardial infarction
Varicose veins
Oral contraceptives, especially in older women
Heart failure
Post-operative infection
Intravenous infusions and cannulae
Trauma
Polycythaemia

An exercise separate from the prediction of venous thrombosis by such methods is the detection of established thrombosis. Clinical diagnosis is difficult and uncertain. Venography is the method which may be regarded as the yardstick against which all other methods are measured. It is not, however, necessarily freely available in all hospitals and has disadvantages in that it is sometimes painful and some contrast media themselves can irritate veins and lead to thrombosis. Less uncomfortable and possibly safer methods for establishing the presence of venous thrombus use isotope labelling techniques but here a result is less immediately available. [125]Iodine-labelled fibrinogen injection with serial scanning of the legs is reliable as a detector of thrombus in the calf veins but less reliable as a guide to its presence in the iliofemoral veins where its presence is of more clinical importance because of the greater risk of pulmonary embolism; as an approximation, possibly a quarter of calf vein thromboses have a dangerous proximal extension. From the time of injection of fibrinogen, serial counting may detect the subsequent development of thrombus over a period of up to a week. This method has a major advantage in that it does not require that the patient move to the scanner and can thus be used in the detection of calf vein thrombi in patients entering high-risk situations associated with immobility such as surgery or pinning of femoral neck fractures. Its major disadvantage is the uncertainty with which it detects the clinically important proximally placed thrombi. A newer, less widely studied technique of some promise involves the use of radio-labelled platelets. These autologous platelets labelled with indium-111 are reinjected and the patient scanned by gamma camera 24 hours later. Concentrations of the label detected in this way correlate well with venous thrombi detected by venography as if the labelled platelets adhered to the thrombus (Fenech *et al.* 1981). This method requires movement of the patient, but is superior to the labelled fibrinogen technique in that it detects thrombi in the iliofemoral segments and inferior vena cava. Methods involving other isotopes have been employed and the use of Doppler ultrasound and impedence plethysmography also give a reasonable correlation with venography but may miss the presence of certain thrombi.

Pulmonary embolism is the complication of deep venous thrombosis most trials seek to prevent. The Registrar General's statistics probably underestimate its contribution to fatality. Clinical diagnosis, like that of some forms of venous thrombosis, is difficult and uncertain. Even combination of ventilation and perfusion scanning with radiography of the chest leaves some uncertainties, and pulmonary angiography remains the most certain method available to establish the diagnosis without doubt. Even when it is available patients may be too unwell to allow the use of the technique. The unexpected finding of pulmonary embolism at post mortem is frequent though some occur as terminal events in other irremediable disorders. Trials of antithrombotic therapy should, of course, be directed at the prevention of venous thrombosis and pulmonary embolism in patients at risk but with remediable problems. However, even in major hospitals autopsy rates may not be high with the result that trials aimed at influencing the incidence of pulmonary embolism are sometimes faced with the difficulty of establishing whether it has, in fact, occurred. Although the autopsy evidence on incidence of pulmonary embolism is incomplete, it suggests that possibly in half of those in whom it was detected it was the cause of death. If this supposition is correct then preventable deaths from pulmonary embolism could equal those due to road traffic accidents (Morris and Mitchell 1978).

The post-phlebitic limb syndrome has received less attention than pulmonary embolism as a complication of deep venous thrombosis and is probably underestimated because of the time lapse, which may be many years, between the acute event and the development of the itching, swollen eczematous and ulcerated leg which is its hallmark. It is, however, a complication causing considerable morbidity and should not be overlooked.

In spite of the many reservations expressed above on the identification of venous thrombosis, the approximate incidence of venous thrombi after various events and detected by objective criteria (usually the labelled fibrinogen technique) is as shown in Table 40.

Table 40. Incidence of venous thrombosis.

	Approximate %	Reference
Fractured femur in the elderly	70	Morris & Mitchell (1976a)
Total hip replacement	50	Morris, Henry & Preston (1974)
Knee replacement	50	McKenna *et al.* (1976)
Suprapubic prostatectomy	50	Nicolaides *et al.* (1972)
Cerebral infarction	50	Warlow (1981)
General surgery in patients over 40 years	35	Nicolaides *et al.* (1972)
Hysterectomy for non-malignant disease	15	Bonnar & Walsh (1972)
Myocardial infarction	10–30	Warlow *et al.* (1973)
		Miller *et al.* (1976)

Prophylaxis of deep venous thrombosis
(see Morris and Mitchell 1978)

A. Clinical situations where the evidence on prevention of leg vein thrombosis and pulmonary embolism is convincing

I. ORAL ANTICOAGULANTS IN FRACTURED NECK OF FEMUR

There is strong evidence indicating that oral anticoagulants prevent deep venous thrombosis and pulmonary embolism. Twenty years ago Sevitt and Gallagher (1959) conducted a trial of phenindione in 300 patients with hip fractures; these patients were divided into anticoagulant and non-anticoagulant groups. Using human brain thromboplastin, those on phenindione had their prothrombin time test prolonged to 2–3 times the control value. It was reported that patients with these fractures could be operated upon without troublesome haemorrhage while therapy was maintained. There were 42 deaths (in 150 patients) in the control patients and 25 deaths (in 150 patients) in the anticoagulated patients. No pulmonary embolism was detected in the phenindione-treated patients, whereas in the control series this developed in 18 per cent of the patients and was fatal in 10 per cent. The clinical evidence of reduced thrombosis was supported by very careful autopsy studies. Significant venous thrombus was observed at autopsy in 83 per cent of the control patients who died but in only 14 per cent of the treatment group. Salzman, Harris and De Sanctis (1966) reported a further study of oral anticoagulants in elderly patients with hip fractures. Almost all the patients had received a loading dose of warfarin before surgery and many were fully anticoagulated because of delays in operation due to complicating medical illness. Thromboembolic complications occurred in 22 of 83 control patients, but in only 7 of 83 treated patients.

This prophylactic role of oral anticoagulants in fractured hips has been confirmed by several other groups of investigators (Borgstrom *et al.* 1965, Neu, Waterfield and Ash 1965, Eskeland, Solheim and Skjorten 1966, Salzman, Harris and De Sanctis 1966, Morris and Mitchell 1976a). Despite this evidence, most orthopaedic surgeons fail to implement the policy of routine use of oral anticoagulants. The fear of increased haematoma formation and therefore greater risk of sepsis prevent widespread use (Simon and Stengle 1974, Morris and Mitchell 1976b). There is also reluctance to accept that there is a high incidence of deep vein thrombosis and pulmonary embolism principally because it is clinically silent so often.

Despite the low level of clinical application, all the trials mentioned above provide strong evidence in favour of the use of coumarins as soon as possible after the fracture of the hip and before surgery. The risk of haemorrhage was small and acceptable given good laboratory control. The first took place over 20 years ago but the orthopaedic community chooses to ignore the evidence.

2. ORAL ANTICOAGULANTS IN OTHER SURGICAL SITUATIONS

Table 41 lists sources of reasonable evidence in support of prophylactic anticoagulant therapy.

Table 41. Evidence in support of prophylactic use of oral anticoagulants.

Type of patient or procedure	Reference
Injured and burned patients	Sevitt & Gallagher (1961)
General and gynaecological surgery	Kistner & Smith (1954)
General surgery	{ Matis (1961) { Dick, Matis & Mayer (1959)
Gynaecological surgery	{ Turnbull (1960) { Bottomley, Lloyd & Chalmers (1964)
Thoracic including cardiac surgery	Storm (1958)
Elective hip surgery and high-risk general surgical patients	Clagett & Salzman (1974)

The evidence suggests that the oral anticoagulant effect should be established before the operation.

B. Clinical situations where the evidence of prophylaxis of venous thromboembolic disease is reasonably strong but not permitting of final judgment

1. LOW-DOSE HEPARIN IN GENERAL SURGERY

In this second category there is good evidence that low-dose heparin (5000 units subcutaneously twice or three times daily) can prevent venous thrombosis detectable by ^{125}I-fibrinogen scanning in patients at risk (Kakkar *et al.* 1972, Nicolaides *et al.* 1972).

When this had been proven it was then appropriate to conduct a multi-centre study to investigate whether this reduction in calf vein thrombosis was of benefit to patients. Such a trial was organized, from King's College Hospital in London, using low-dose heparin (5000 units of calcium heparin three times daily) for seven days (International Multicentre Trial 1975). The objective of the trial was to determine whether low-dose heparin would prevent fatal pulmonary embolism. The results obtained are shown in Table 42.

Table 42. International Multicentre Trial 1975.

	4121 general surgical patients	
	Heparin	No heparin
	2045	2076
Deaths	80	100

While the difference in deaths did not reach the chosen level of significance, there was some evidence that 16 of the deaths in the control group but only two in the heparin group were due to pulmonary embolism. There were autopsies in 72 per cent of the control deaths and 60 per cent of the 'heparin group' deaths. Inevitably in a multi-centre trial the autopsies were done by many different pathologists. The results of this study are highly suggestive that low-dose heparin is of value, but the final certainty is missing. Sagar, Massey and Sanderson (1975), after their investigation of this issue, supported the conclusions of the International Multicentre Trial; on the other hand, Gruber *et al.* (1977), while agreeing that subcutaneous heparin reduced the incidence of post-operative calf vein thrombi, found no evidence that it reduced the incidence of pulmonary embolism.

2.   LOW-DOSE HEPARIN IN OTHER SURGICAL SETTINGS

(a)   *Fracture of the femoral neck*

In the International Multicentre Trial in general surgical patients, the first dose of heparin was given two hours before the operation, i.e. before any tissue damage had occurred; when low-dose heparin was tested by Morris and Mitchell (1977a) in patients with fractured hips there was no prevention of venous thrombosis. However, Gallus *et al.* (1973) in a similar study reported a definite protective effect. The issue is therefore confused.

(b)   *Total hip replacement*

The evidence here is also conflicting; Hampson *et al.* (1974) found heparin to be ineffective whereas Morris, Henry and Preston (1974) and Sagar *et al.* (1976) reported the reverse. There is agreement that for hip operations the heparin should be started immediately after the hospital admission has occurred and be continued for 14 days post-operatively.

Hip operations are undoubtedly more thrombogenic than most other types of surgery, since there is direct manipulation of the femoral vein, and in the case of fractured neck of femur there is already local tissue damage before the operation has started. It is not unexpected that prevention of thrombus in the femoral vein at the site of operation is difficult. Kakkar *et al.* (1979) combined low-dose heparin with dihydroergotamine (DHE); the concept was that the DHE, a vasoconstrictor, would increase the velocity of venous blood flow. The result of the trial was that heparin with DHE was more effective than heparin alone in preventing both calf vein thrombi and femoral vein thrombi.

Hohl and colleagues (1980) demonstrated that the dose of low-dose heparin could be halved (from 5000 units twice daily to 2500 units twice daily) if dihydroergotamine was given simultaneously; in gynaecological patients, the prophylactic value was the same, as measured by the iodinated fibrinogen test.

3. LOW-DOSE HEPARIN AFTER MYOCARDIAL INFARCTION

Deep vein thrombosis and pulmonary embolism is a recognized complication of myocardial infarction. Conventional anticoagulants make a small contribution in reducing deaths in acute myocardial infarction; it is possible, but unproven, that this benefit was conferred by reducing the small number of fatalities in that disease by preventing pulmonary embolism.

As the management of patients with myocardial infarction is changing constantly, it is difficult to apply studies of the incidence of venous thrombosis performed in the past to patients in 1984. In the early 1970s, using the ^{125}I-fibrinogen technique, the incidence of calf vein thrombosis was about 30 per cent; this could be markedly reduced by low-dose heparin (Gallus *et al.* 1973, Warlow *et al.* 1973). Miller *et al.* in 1976 reported that the incidence was 10 per cent. If the incidence of ^{125}I-fibrinogen-positive calf vein thrombosis is down to 10 per cent then routine low-dose heparin use in coronary care units may no longer be applicable. There have been no trials demonstrating that low-dose heparin usefully prevents pulmonary embolism in patients with myocardial infarction. It is possible that performance of such trials on patients in high-risk groups would prove valuable.

PROPHYLAXIS OF DEEP VENOUS THROMBOSIS IN CEREBROVASCULAR DISEASE

Deep venous thrombosis in the legs occurs in about 50 per cent of patients with stroke, causing hemiplegia or hemiparesis; pulmonary embolism is present in 50 per cent of those that die and is the immediate cause of death in a smaller percentage.

Any form of anti-haemostatic drug is likely to make undetected primary intracerebral haemorrhage worse; understandably, there has been no trial of oral anticoagulants. Low-dose heparin could reasonably be used provided the CT scan has indicated infarction, but so far as we know results from such a study are not available.

C.   Thromboembolism in pregnancy

The suspicion of leg vein thrombosis commonly arises because of the frequency of ankle swelling and discomfort in the legs during pregnancy. Isotopic methods and venography are not permissible as diagnostic methods because of the risk to the fetus. Doppler ultrasound and impedence plethysmography alone or in combination are acceptable but frequently the diagnosis is clinically based. As a result it is not surprising that this is an area in which sound clinical trials have not been concluded and it is doubtful whether they ever will be. Clinicians will wish to use anticoagulants in pregnant patients with deep venous thrombosis without further studies because of the major risk of pulmonary embolism in these young women. The acute episode should be treated with continuous intravenous heparin and for the remainder of the pregnancy low-dose subcutaneous heparin given 12-hourly (Bonnar 1977) should be used. Heparin is preferred to coumarin as the latter crosses the placental barrier and further depresses the immature fetal liver's production of factors II, VII, IX and X. Therefore, while the literature strongly suggests that oral anticoagulants are remarkably effective in reducing maternal mortality after clinically diagnosed deep vein thrombosis or pulmonary embolism, it is not surprising that there is a high perinatal mortality in the off-spring of mothers treated till term, attributable to fetal haemorrhage caused by birth trauma (Villasanta 1965). Oral anticoagulants are also said to be teratogenic when used during the first three months of pregnancy, reported fetal abnormalities including skeletal deformities, mental retardation, deafness and blindness. These have not been recorded when coumarins have been used after the third month (Di Saia 1966, Pettifor and Benson 1975). From this evidence, if oral anticoagulants are to be used they should only be employed after the first trimester; low-dose heparin can be used in the early stages of gestation and substituted for oral anticoagulants again in the last weeks of pregnancy, a manoeuvre which reduces the haemorrhagic risk to the fetus (Hirsch, Cade and O'Sullivan 1970, Ramsay 1975).

Of the causes of maternal death in this country abortion is the commonest and pulmonary embolism is the next most frequent. The period of greatest risk is, however, the puerperium. Here the constraints on the diagnostic methods used are removed by delivery of the child and the clinician can also manage thrombotic events without the limitations imposed by the pregnancy. Uterine bleeding has not been a major problem in the use of heparin or oral anticoagulants in the puerperium.

D.   Other therapeutic agents in deep venous thrombosis

1.   DEXTRAN

The dextrans are a group of polysaccharides with differing molecular weights. Their clinical use began as plasma volume expanders and subsequently their potential antithrombotic role was appreciated. Dextran 70 (molecular weight 70 000) is in common use and Dextran 40 (molecular weight 40 000) probably to a lesser extent. The probabilty is that there is interference with platelet function, as the bleeding time becomes prolonged and measurements of platelet adhesion have shown a reduction (Cronberg *et al.* 1966); there is also disturbance of the polymerization of fibrin.

Dextran 70 is the preparation most commonly used. The usual method of administration in the surgical situation is to give 500 ml intravenously during the operation and a further 500 ml at the end of the operation. Additional infusions each of 500 ml may be given on the two following post-operative days. Use of Dextran 70 is not usually complicated by haemorrhage. However, allergic reactions, circulatory overload and renal failure have been reported with low molecular weight dextrans (Data and Nies 1974, Feest 1976), and their use in patients with cardiac failure should be avoided.

Establishment of the value of these agents is incomplete. A review of the evidence has suggested a four-fold reduction in the incidence of pulmonary embolism by using dextran (Bygdeman, Svensjo and Tollerz 1970). The value of Dextran 40 was compared with that of low-dose heparin in elective major abdominal surgery by Gruber and his colleagues in 1977. ^{125}I-fibrinogen positive calf vein thrombus was prevented more effectively by low-dose heparin than by dextran, but the incidence of pulmonary embolism was the same in these two treatment regimens. Kline *et al.* (1975) reported a randomized double-blind trial, in patients undergoing abdominal surgery, of Dextran 70 against saline. The positive fibrinogen tests were not reduced by Dextran 70, but there was a significant reduction in the incidence of pulmonary embolism. Browse and associates (1976), combined dextran with pneumatic leg compression. As in the previous studies there was no reduction in positive fibrinogen tests but a significant reduction in the incidence of pulmonary embolism detected by lung scanning. The final proof of efficacy is incomplete, but dextran is widely used by surgeons and is worthy of further appraisal.

2.   ASPIRIN, DIPYRIDAMOLE AND OXYPHENBUTAZONE

While the main component of a venous thrombus is fibrin, there is nevertheless a small platelet head, and a reasonable theoretical case for establishing the place, if any, of antiplatelet agents in prevention of venous thrombosis. Available evidence again is confused and contradictory.

Some have reported that aspirin alone or dipyridamole alone or both in combination may be effective (Browse and Hall 1969, Salzman, Harris and De Sanctis 1971, Clagett *et al.* 1975, Dechavanne *et al.* 1975, Renney, O'Sullivan and Burke 1976, Harris *et al.* 1977). Others have not been able to confirm this (O'Brien, Tulevski and Etherington 1971, Medical Research Council 1972, Morris and Mitchell 1977b). Tilberg (1976) claimed that oxyphenbutazone, administered by suppository, and leg bandaging reduced the incidence of venous thrombosis following hip surgery. Detailed reviews of the use of antiplatelet agents in venous thrombosis are available (Kakkar 1981, Turpie 1981).

3. HYDROXYCHLOROQUINE

Hydroxychloroquine has been used as an antiplatelet drug in the prophylaxis of post-operative thromboembolism. Carter and Eban (1974) gave this to patients (over 45 years of age) having elective major surgery. Episodes of venous thrombosis indicated by the labelled fibrinogen test were reduced in the treated group. Chrisman *et al.* (1976) used this agent in fractures of the thigh and pelvis. Fatal and non-fatal pulmonary embolism occurred in the controls but no such events occurred in the treated group.

Like dextran, hydroxychloroquine seems worthy of further study.

4. LOW MOLECULAR WEIGHT HEPARIN

Such heparin is only now becoming available for sizeable clinical trials; at the time of writing the authors do not know of the results. Low molecular weight heparin fosters a powerful antagonistic system to factor Xa, but has a relatively lesser effect on the thrombin–fibrinogen reaction. It may, therefore, be found to be effective as an antithrombotic drug, but to be less haemorrhagic.

E. Ancrod

Ancrod, the purified extract from the Malayan pit viper venom, can be used intravenously and subcutaneously. It reduces plasma fibrinogen and as a result plasma viscosity falls; total defibrination may be produced. It has not found a firm place in the antithrombotic field in routine hospital practice but is again an agent with promise and worthy of further evaluation. Lowe and colleagues (1978) report a well-conducted trial of subcutaneous ancrod in the prevention of deep vein thrombosis after surgery for fractured neck of femur. The ancrod was begun after surgery. Daily injections were given for five days post-operatively and there was no increased incidence of bleeding. Venography, performed 6–16 days after surgery, showed venous thrombi in 73 per cent of the control patients and 45 per cent in the treated group; of possibly greater importance, the venograms showed a reduction of *major* venous thrombi from 65 per cent to 30 per cent. We have ourselves found that initiation of ancrod treatment pre-operatively is associated with significant intra-operative bleeding, even at dosages well short of defibrination.

F.   Therapeutic combinations

Schöndorf and Hey (1976) reported that in hip operations aspirin in combination with low-dose heparin was a more effective prophylaxis than aspirin alone. Loew *et al.* (1977) found that aspirin and low-dose heparin were more effective than either drug alone in elective thoracic or abdominal surgery.

Serious gastrointestinal haemorrhage is sufficiently common with aspirin alone, however, to suggest that the combination might carry high risk of bleeding.

G.   Conclusions on prophylaxis

It is not easy to take from the above a clear set of guidelines. Many of the studies have tested the ability of an antithrombotic regimen to lower the incidence of venous thrombosis as detected by the labelled fibrinogen uptake test. It is, however, the thrombus in the large veins which carries the risk of fatal pulmonary embolism. The limited evidence available suggests that about one quarter of those patients with a positive iodinated fibrinogen scan have dangerous thrombus extending proximally. There is, however, disturbing inconsistency in the literature on the relationship of a positive fibrinogen scan and the occurrence of pulmonary embolism. As, therefore, the clinical implications of a positive finding using this test are imprecisely defined, recommendations based on studies using it as the end-point remain to be validated by those with clinical end-points.

Firstly, modifiable high risk factors, such as obesity or use of oestrogen-containing contraceptive preparations, must be dealt with appropriately if time allows. Then the clinician must be selective. Factors conferring high risk of thromboembolism are well known but methods for more precise identification of high-risk patients will be welcome. A relatively young patient undergoing hysterectomy has a low risk of pulmonary embolism, and graded pressure stockings with early ambulation and leg exercises may be all that is required for the prevention of venous thrombosis. For major abdominal surgery in a patient over the age of 50 years, especially in the presence of malignancy, many surgeons would use low-dose heparin prophylaxis. Low-dose heparin is also commonly given to medical patients at risk—especially those with congestive cardiac failure.

The greatest thrombotic challenge is the high incidence of venous thrombosis and pulmonary embolism in patients following hip fractures and total hip replacement. The balance of evidence is in favour of coumarin prophylaxis introduced, established and carefully controlled prior to the operative procedure.

Management of established disease

Deep venous thrombosis

Once a diagnosis of venous thrombosis is identified as a high probability on clinical grounds it should if possible be confirmed by one or other of the objective methods described above; a small number of patients with the classical signs of pain, erythema and swelling may have cellulitis, ruptured Baker's cysts or haematomas. This done, what action should be taken? Anticoagulation with continuous intravenous heparin with concurrent oral coumarin therapy to rapidly establish appropriate prolongation of the prothrombin time is conventional and widely employed. Heparin has been in use since the late 1930s and coumarins since the late 1940s. The achievements of such regimens have not been subjected to rigorous examination by the type of clinical trial described above and probably never will be. It is the authors' practice to continue oral anticoagulant therapy after deep venous thrombosis for six weeks to three months in the absence of contraindications to their use.

There are two situations in which the policy of using anticoagulant therapy is not universally agreed. The first is the presence of thrombosis clearly shown to be restricted to the calf veins with no more proximally placed thrombus. Some would say that early ambulation and the use of graded pressure stockings are the only measures needed. The authors, however, presently treat patients with calf vein thrombosis with anticoagulant therapy as described above. A second situation in which there may be diversity of opinion on management occurs when venography has shown that the proximal end of the thrombus is free floating and when presumably the risk of embolization is greater. Here thrombolytic therapy or surgical thrombectomy has been advocated (Browse 1977). Thrombolytic therapy may dissolve such thrombi but whether this confers protection against pulmonary embolism here is not established. Surgical thrombectomy and thrombolytic therapy separately or sequentially clearly have a role in the management of major thrombotic occlusion of proximal veins when venous gangrene is a possible complication (thrombolytic therapy is discussed in Chapter 17).

Pulmonary embolism

In hospital wards minor pulmonary emboli probably occur frequently and pass undiagnosed. A much smaller number cause sudden death. Between these two extremes pulmonary embolism with infarction of the lung may masquerade as pleurisy, pneumonia, cardiac failure and myocardial infarction. Even the combination of clinical assessment, electrocardiography, conventional radiology and ventilation/perfusion scanning may leave this diagnosis sometimes in doubt. Pulmonary angiography is the definitive diagnostic method but is only occasionally available or practicable. When the presence of pulmonary embolism is established the basis of management is the use of heparin and oral anticoagulants subjected first to a controlled clinical trial by Barritt and Jordan (1960). This was a prospective, controlled and randomized study which was closed after 35 patients had been admitted. There were then five deaths and five non-fatal occurrences of pulmonary embolism among the 19 patients in the control group whereas among 16 patients treated with anticoagulants only one death had occurred and this was not clearly ascribable to pulmonary embolism. The understandable reaction of these investigators was that, once a patient had received his first injection of heparin, life was almost secure and this area has rarely been subjected to study in larger groups, and it is unlikely that there will be in the future trials containing untreated controls. It is the authors' practice to use full intravenous heparinization by continuous infusion followed by oral anticoagulation for 3–6 months after an established pulmonary embolism.

Thrombolytic therapy (Chapter 17) is a conceptually attractive means of managing major pulmonary emboli. The Urokinase Pulmonary Embolism Trial (1973) did not show a clear benefit in terms of mortality as a result of the routine use of urokinase in patients with pulmonary embolism, but treatment with streptokinase or urokinase should be considered in individual patients with massive pulmonary embolism. Embolectomy is so seldom available as a practical proposition in these patients that it hardly merits mention. If the patient survives the first hour after an episode of embolism the prognosis with the use of thrombolytic agents and conventional anticoagulants is reasonable.

Recurrent pulmonary embolism is managed by reinstitution of anticoagulant therapy or by addition of heparin to warfarin therapy if it is established. Caval interruption can be undertaken by plication or insertion of a device permitting flow but catching emboli; this is seldom practiced in the UK, but is widely used in North America if recurrent pulmonary embolism occurs despite adequate anticoagulant therapy. Such an approach is more acceptable than the older practice of caval ligation, which carries post-operative mortality of about 10 per cent with one-third continuing to have pulmonary embolism (Coupland and Reeve 1975, Morris and Mitchell 1977b).

The excellent short monograph by Pitney (1981) gives a fuller account of venous thromboembolic disease and is recommended additional reading.

ARTERIAL DISEASE

Anticoagulant therapy in coronary artery disease

A.   Short-term in acute myocardial infarction

The vast majority of the trials of oral anticoagulants are not reviewed in detail. A recent reappraisal of them can be found in the paper by Chalmers and associates (1977). The early studies have been much criticized because of their design. In fairness many of the essentials of sound trial design in this field have only been appreciated in the last 15–20 years and one has sympathy with earlier investigators. The early studies will not be considered for another cogent reason; the current management of acute myocardial infarction is so different from that of 15–30 years ago, that evidence obtained from some of the studies in the past is of dubious relevance now.

If the benefit claimed for the use of anticoagulants in the late 1940s and throughout the 1950s and 1960s was real, it may have been due to their prevention of deep venous thrombosis and pulmonary embolism. Early ambulation, shorter hospitalization, the use of newer drugs including the β-blockers and anti-arrhythmic drugs may have altered the situation and changed the need for anticoagulant therapy.

The trials of good design appear in Table 43 (Chalmers *et al.* 1977).

The conclusions which can be drawn from them are as follows:

1   The differences in favour of anticoagulant therapy are small and have therefore usually not reached a chosen level of significance. However, the fact that all six point in the same direction is suggestive of a small benefit. The problem has been that clinicians have been guilty of therapeutic greed (Mitchell 1981a), expecting too much and tending to dismiss small benefits, because expectation was too great.

2   If 'lumped together' as was done by Chalmers *et al.* (1977) the benefit is of the order of reduction of total mortality by about 20 per cent or one-fifth. This is similar to the findings in *long-term* coumarin administration in secondary prevention studies (see below).

3   These data also show the falling mortality rate for patients with acute myocardial infarction reaching hospital alive as being as follows:

	Death rate
1960	30–35
1965	15–20
1970	15–18
1973	10

This highlights the problem of trying to decide on the current role of

Table 43. Anticoagulants in the 'short-term' after acute myocardial infarction.

	Patient numbers			Case fatality rates	
	Total	Controls	Anti-coagulated	Controls	Anti-coagulated
Carleton, Sanders & Burack (1960)	92	47	45	38.3	28.9
Wasserman *et al.* (1966)	147	70	77	21.4	15.6
Medical Research Council (1969)	1427	715	712	18.0	16.2
Drapkin and Merskey (1972)	1136	391	745	21.2	14.9
Handley, Emerson & Fleming (1972)	53	26	27	7.7	7.4
Veterans Administration Co-operative Trial (1973)	999	499	500	11.2	9.6

anticoagulant or any therapy in 1982 in a disorder whose behaviour and mortality rate is changing producing a situation to which the results of earlier studies may not be applicable.

B.   Long-term after myocardial infarction

The evidence on this rests on the analysis of nine controlled trials conducted between 1950 and 1965. Again the evidence on which to base a decision is about 20 years old. The trials are as follows: Bjerkelund 1957, MacMillan, Brown and Watt 1960, Clausen *et al.* 1961, Harvald, Hilden and Lund 1962, Aspenstrom and Korsan-Bengsten 1964, Conrad *et al.* 1964, Medical Research Council 1964, Lovell *et al.* 1967, Veterans Administration Co-operative Study 1969. Under the leadership of the late Professor Donald Reid (International Anticoagulant Review Group 1970) the above trialists co-operated in a pooling of the data. For each patient the investigators completed a record giving in uniform fashion the essential clinical features of the case according to simple agreed diagnostic criteria, his allocation group and his experience up to the time of death or to the end of effective follow-up.

There were 2205 males and 282 females. The mortality experience of 'anticoagulant' and 'comparative' series, which were shown to be alike in relevant clinical characteristics, was significantly lower (by 20 per cent) in males given anticoagulants. The number of females was probably too small to merit conclusions. The benefit in males was amongst those who had angina or had suffered a second infarction since the initial event.

Again then, as in acute myocardial infarction, there was a reduction in deaths of about 20 per cent in survivors in myocardial infarction studied about 20 years ago.

C. The effect of stopping long-term oral anticoagulant therapy in survivors of myocardial infarction

This has been studied in Holland (report of the Sixty-Plus Reinfarction Study Research Group 1980). In Holland there has continued to be widespread use of oral anticoagulants in survivors of myocardial infarction, despite its decline in the rest of the Western world. In a randomized double-blind multi-centre clinical trial the effect of stopping anticoagulants in half of a group of patients over the age of 60 years was examined. These patients had been on anticoagulants for at least six months since their myocardial infarction. All were followed for two years. The desired intensity of anticoagulant therapy was 5–10 per cent thrombotest activity.

The two-year mortality in the patients who stopped anticoagulants was 13.4 per cent in the placebo group and 7.6 per cent in the group continued on anticoagulants. The survival curves showed a steadily widening gap indicating that the efficacy of therapy was present throughout the entire observation period. The lack of a dip shortly after initiation of the placebo treatment suggests that there was no rebound effect on discontinuation of long-term anticoagulant therapy.

This study provides evidence that there is still a role for anticoagulant therapy; in management of myocardial infarction, however, clinicians in this country have, on the whole, paid the report little heed.

Antiplatelet therapy

The three drugs which have now been tested for their role in arterial disease are aspirin, Persantin (dipyridamole) and Anturan (sulphinpyrazone). Aspirin acetylates cyclooxygenase irreversibly for the lifetime of the platelet *in vivo* and this may impair production of thromboxane. Its effect on nucleated endothelial cells is temporary but it may similarly decrease their production of prostacyclins thus modifying any benefits gained by suppression of thromboxane production. The debate on the possibilities of a balance between thromboxane and prostacyclin production as a haemostatic mechanism and a description of the pharmacological actions of aspirin on platelet function and biochemistry appear elsewhere (Chapters 13 and 15). Of clinical importance is the suggestion that high and low doses of aspirin have different effects on the bleeding time, presumably reflecting differential effects on platelet and endothelial function. Some have found that 300–1000 mg of aspirin daily will prolong the bleeding time while 2000–4000 mg daily will shorten it. These observations have not been confirmed by all workers but clearly in the design of therapeutic trials it is desirable that a dose of aspirin is used which produces maximum depression of thromboxane with minimum depression of prostacyclin production in order to impair maximally platelet sequestration at the blood/endothelial interface.

Congenital deficiency of cyclooxygenase, however, results in a mild haemorrhagic, not a thrombotic, disorder. On the basis of this finding, even if aspirin does block both the cyclooxygenase of vessel wall and the platelet the haemostatic balance is against thrombosis, which encourages the belief that trials, concerning aspirin already carried out, have used dosages worth evaluating.

A.   Coronary heart disease

The Boston Collaborative Drug Surveillance Group (1974) made the suggestion that regular aspirin ingestion might reduce the incidence of non-fatal myocardial infarction. They observed that patients discharged from hospital after an episode of myocardial infarction were less likely to be regular aspirin users than were patients with other diagnoses. The group recognized that its data did not represent evidence that aspirin provided primary prevention of myocardial infarction.

Aspirin is currently under test for primary prevention of myocardial infarction and stroke amongst volunteer British doctors, but this study will take several years before completion.

SECONDARY PREVENTION STUDIES

1.   *Aspirin*

There have been six well-conducted trials of aspirin given long-term after myocardial infarction (Tables 44 and 45).

All these studies provided data on the basis of 'intention to treat', all patients randomized, and all deaths/all causes; the percentage reduction in mortality in each is shown in the table. Five trials showed a trend in favour of a protective effect for the regime tested although no one trial result reached the chosen level of significance. The AMIS trial was the exception.

Two biostatisticians have independently reviewed the data provided by these six trials and independently concluded that they can be 'lumped together', using accepted statistical techniques. When this is done, Canner (1980) and Peto (1980, 1982) agree that there is a reduction in total mortality, 'in the vicinity of 10 per cent', and about one-sixth (say 15 per cent), respectively.

Table 44. Six trials of aspirin in secondary prevention.

Reference/Trial	Daily dosage	Reduction in mortality (%)
Elwood *et al.* (1974)	300 mg	23
Coronary Drug Project (1976)	1000 mg	30
Breddin *et al.* (1979)	2000 mg	15
Elwood & Sweetnam (1979)	900 mg	11
AMIS 1980*	1000 mg	(excess of 12)
PARIS 1980 (aspirin plus dipyridamole)†	1000 mg	18

* Aspirin Myocardial Infarction Study Research Group.
† Persantine-Aspirin Re-Infarction Study Research Group.

The overall evidence is, therefore, that aspirin in a dose varying from 300–2000 mg studied in about 12 000 patients resulted in a reduction in mortality of 10–15 per cent. Only one of the trials (Breddin *et al.* 1979) gave more than one gram per day.

Two trials were conducted by Elwood and his colleagues (1974). In the first study male patients following myocardial infarction and after hospital discharge were assigned to 300 mg aspirin per day or placebo. This study was started in Cardiff where favourable results were obtained. When it was extended beyond Cardiff the final results were less favourable to aspirin, but there was still a 23 per cent reduction in mortality at 12 months after admission to the trial. In this study (as in the PARIS study) there was a suggestion that those patients admitted early (less than six weeks after the acute event) obtained the largest benefit.

Elwood and Sweetnam (1979) reported a second MRC trial, including men and women entering the study within seven days of their myocardial infarction; the aspirin dosage was 900 mg per day. In PARIS (1980) 800 patients were given aspirin alone and 400 given placebo. There was an 18 per cent reduction in mortality (see Table 45).

In the Coronary Drug Project (1976), 1 g of aspirin per day was given to 'stable' survivors of coronary thrombosis. The majority had their qualifying myocardial infarction at least five years previously. At the end of follow-up of 10–28 months there was a 30 per cent reduction in mortality.

The exception in trend was the study of aspirin alone in the Aspirin Myocardial Infarction Study (AMIS 1980) in which there was an excess of 26 deaths in the aspirin-treated group in a study containing 4000 patients. There was, however, good evidence when the final analysis was conducted that randomization had not worked well and that there was an excess of poor prognosis risk factors in the aspirin-treated group.

Table 45. Results of six trials of aspirin in secondary prevention

| | Aspirin | | Controls | |
Reference/Trial	Deaths	Patient numbers	Deaths	Patient numbers
Elwood *et al.* (1974)	47	615	61	624
Coronary Drug Project (1976)	44	758	64	771
Breddin *et al.* (1977)	27	317	32	309
Elwood & Sweetnam (1979)	102	832	126	850
AMIS (1980)	245	2267	219	2257
PARIS (1980)	85	810	53	406*

* Control group only half the size of the aspirin group

2.   *Dipyridamole (Persantin) with aspirin*

The case for this antiplatelet regime rests on the results of the Persantin Aspirin Re-infarction Study (PARIS) (1980). This was an international study conducted at 20 centres in the USA and the UK and compared aspirin plus Persantin, aspirin alone and placebo in patients surviving their first myocardial infarction. This was double-blind, randomly allocated, and conducted with objective assessment of events. Predetermined primary end-points, used as the basis of the central conclusions, were as follows:

1   All deaths.

2   Coronary deaths (sudden death within one hour or non-sudden death within 30 days of a definitive or suspected myocardial infarction). Coronary deaths accounted for three-quarters of total mortality.

3   Coronary incidence (this is coronary death plus non-fatal definite myocardial reinfarction; an individual patient only entered this statistic once). The clinical investigators were blind as to the choice of therapy, and so also was the Mortality and Morbidity Committee whose conclusion on events was final. Coronary incidence was therefore not a soft end-point, but was objective.

The statistical level chosen was a Z value equal to or greater than 2.6. In the circumstances of the study a Z value equal to or greater than 2.6 has a *P* value equivalent or better than 1 in 20 but less than 1 in 100. This takes into account multiple looks at the data, three treatment groups and three primary end-points (as defined above).

For all end-points over the first two years of follow-up Persantin plus aspirin did better than aspirin alone, which did better than placebo. For total mortality and coronary mortality the differences from the control group did not reach the statistical level chosen. For coronary incidence the differences in the comparison between Persantin/aspirin and placebo were in favour of patients taking the active therapy; these differences were consistent and significant over the first 24 months. This is the only trial of antithrombotic therapy in secondary prevention after myocardial infarction in which a primary objective and predetermined end-point 'coronary incidence' has been significantly different at the statistical level chosen in favour of therapy.

After 36 months of follow-up the total mortality reduction in the Persantin/aspirin group was 18 per cent as compared with the rate in the placebo group. This difference did not reach the chosen level of significance. The mean time of entry to the trial was 20 months after the qualifying myocardial infarction, i.e. these patients were, in the main, at a stable stage of their disease, when the mortality rate is 3–5 per cent per annum. It is not surprising that with only 2000 patients the favourable trend did not reach significance. The significant reduction in coronary incidence suggests that the differences in total mortality are real. In total mortality Persantin and aspirin showed more favourable trends than aspirin alone during the first two years of the study, but by the end of three years the rates were similar in the two active treatment groups. The window for entry into the trial was six weeks to five years after the qualifying myocardial infarction with a mean entry time of 20 months. The number of patients who had entered the study under six months from qualifying myocardial infarction was only one-eighth of the total number of patients studied—approximately 250 patients. When the trial had been completed, an analysis was made of those patients who had entered the study less than six months from the date of infarction. It was found that nearly all of the benefit was in this group; as this is data-dredging, no conclusion is permissible from this, but this finding has formed the basis of a new study, PARIS II, in which entry is four weeks to four months after the qualifying myocardial infarction.

3. *Sulphinpyrazone*

Only one major study of sulphinpyrazone has been reported (Anturan Reinfarction Trial Research Group 1978, 1980). 1629 patients who had had a myocardial infarction were allocated at random to sulphinpyrazone 200 mg four times daily or to placebo for 12–24 months. Entry to the study was at 25–35 days after the incident of myocardial infarction.

This study was designed on the explicative basis and has been criticized since 43 of the deaths were 'non-analysable' and 71 patients were declared ineligible and excluded after randomization. These patients were excluded, sometimes months after the trial began.

The details of the criticisms of this trial are described by Kolata (1980). Other independent review of the data is being conducted and any final conclusion on this study must await its outcome.

For the present, the most which can be taken from the data is an analysis of the deaths on an 'intention to treat' basis (McNicol 1980) as follows:

	Sulphinpyrazone	Placebo
Patients	813	816
Deaths	74	89

If these are the final figures then this represents a 17 per cent reduction which is not dissimilar to aspirin or oral anticoagulants, but not as good as the recent reports on β-blockers given to survivors of myocardial infarction.

The Food and Drug Administration has decided that at present sulphinpyrazone cannot be labelled and advertised for the prevention of death in the critical months after a heart attack. The quality of scientific evidence required by American law to permit the approval of the drug for use after myocardial infarction is not available.

B. Ingravescent angina ('impending myocardial infarction' or 'acute coronary insufficiency')

This is an ill-defined clinical state between exertional angina and myocardial infarction. These patients present with intensification of angina on effort or the development of angina at rest. The patients may have had a previous identified episode of myocardial infarction and often proceed to a new episode of infarction. Strong claims have been made for the role of anticoagulant therapy (Wood 1961) but this is one of the areas in which the value of any drug needs substantiation by controlled clinical trials.

In 1983 a Veterans Administration Co-operative Study published the results of an important trial of aspirin to prevent acute myocardial infarction and death in men with unstable angina. This was a multi-centre, double-blind, placebo-controlled randomized trial for 12 weeks in 1266 men with unstable angina. Both death and acute myocardial infarction were reduced by half (Lewis *et al.* 1983). The daily dose of aspirin was 324 mg in buffered solution.

C. Prosthetic heart valves

In patients with valve replacement, shortened platelet survival and its correction by antiplatelet agents support the suggestion that continuous platelet deposition on prosthetic valves occurs (Harker and Slichter 1970, Weily and Genton 1970) which would presumably set the scene for embolism.

While there are no unimpeachable trials of the use of anticoagulants to prevent systemic emboli this has become accepted clinical practice in patients with prosthetic valves which should continue despite the lesser risk with more modern valves. The most common clinically apparent site of embolism is the brain where even a small embolus is likely to cause significant symptoms. Other lodgments giving clinical features are in the coronary circulation, retina and limb vessels. Visceral emboli may or may not cause symptoms or signs. Reasonably well-designed studies of anticoagulants in patients with aortic valve prostheses have shown a reduction in incidence of emboli by 75 per cent (Duvoisin, Brandenburg and McGoon 1967, Akbarian *et al.* 1968), and have emphasized the importance of good anticoagulant control in the efficacy of therapy.

Thromboembolism is even more common in patients with mitral valve prostheses. The presence of atrial fibrillation and a large left atrium are additional risk factors. The lesser risk of embolism with improved valve design is accepted (Barnhorst *et al.* 1975, Boncheck and Starr 1975). With porcine valves embolization is probably less common but can still occur from the mitral valve, especially if atrial fibrillation persists and left atrial enlargement is still present. It would appear wise to continue oral anticoagulant for life in patients with any type of prosthetic valve. In the case of porcine valves this is probably not necessary; the incidence of significant embolism from these is low and the place of anticoagulants will be clarified with the passing of time.

There is also a reasonable consensus of opinion that oral anticoagulants are more effective than antiplatelet drugs in preventing embolism although shortened platelet survival may be restored towards normal using dipyridamole, dipyridamole plus aspirin and sulphinpyrazone (Harker and Slichter 1970, Weily and Genton 1970). Sullivan, Harken and Gorlin (1971) suggest that dipyridamole plus oral anticoagulants is more effective than coumarins alone. In practice, the addition of dipyridamole should be considered in those patients who have a new incident of embolism despite a satisfactory anticoagulant effect from coumarins.

D.   Aortocoronary vein bypass surgery

Saphenous vein bypass is now a well-established procedure for angina pectoris; the symptomatic relief can be very dramatic. However, there is a proportion of patients in whom the graft does not remain patent and there is recurrence of symptoms. The maximal occlusion rate occurs in the first three months post-operatively. The state of the distal vascular bed may be the single most important determinant of graft patency, those grafts with a high flow rate and good run off-doing best. In the longer term, intimal proliferation occurs with accelerated atheroma in the graft. It is theoretically possible that the progression of this could be slowed by antithrombotic therapy on the argument that the fewer platelets that adhere to and damage the endothelium or release mitogenic factor the better. Many cardiac surgeons use some form of antithrombotic regimen—anticoagulants, dipyridamole, aspirin, dipyridamole plus aspirin or sulphinpyrazone. The only controlled trial known to the authors is that by Chesebro and colleagues (1982).

A platelet-inhibitor drug trial in coronary artery bypass operations was reported by Chesebro *et al.* (1982); this demonstrated a benefit of peri-operative dipyridamole plus aspirin on early post-operative vein graft patency. Dipyridamole therapy was started two days before the operation and aspirin was added seven hours after the operation. The total patient population was 407; vein graft angiography was performed in 360 patients within six months of the operation (mean time eight days). In the placebo group occlusion of distal anastomosis was three times more common than in the dipyridamole/aspirin-treated group.

E.   Mitral valve disease

While well-designed controlled trials are not to be found there is general acceptance that oral anticoagulants reduce the incidence of emboli arising in patients with mitral valve disease (Cosgriff 1953, McDevitt and associates 1958, Owren 1963). As with prosthetic valves, the commonest site in which emboli lodge is the brain, but coronary, retinal, visceral and limb vessel may also be involved.

Embolism is most common in mitral stenosis, but can also complicate mitral incompetence, even when the lesion is associated with only minor haemodynamic change (Coulshed *et al.* 1970). The risk of embolism in this situation (as in other thrombotic disorders) increases with age; the development of atrial fibrillation also increases the risk; the larger the left atrium the greater the hazard.

The indications for anticoagulants therefore include a tight mitral stenosis, a large left atrium, atrial fibrillation or a previous history of embolism. Apart from these major risk factors, however, it is not possible to identify high- or low-risk patients and most should be anticoagulated. Possible exclusions are those with trivial mitral disease and with with none of the risk factors just described (Pitney 1981).

F.   Cerebrovascular disease

The application of antithrombotic therapy to management of cerebrovascular disease has been a preoccupation of many workers since oral coumarins became available 30–35 years ago. It was realized at an early stage, however, (1960–62) that there was a major danger of intracerebral bleeding as a consequence of these drugs.

1. SHORT-TERM THERAPY IN COMPLETED STROKES

Marshall and Shaw (1960) studied the use of anticoagulant therapy in 'acute strokes' and concluded that the rate and degree of recovery were not improved by anticoagulants as compared with conservative management. In their study patients with suspected cerebral embolism were excluded and thereafter patients were randomly allocated to control and treated groups; the results were measured by survival to six weeks. They found an excess of deaths in the treated group, possibly reflecting the problem of differentiating between infarction and haemorrhage as a cause of stroke.

The above observations were made 20 years before CT scanning became available. In spite of the better distinction of thrombotic from haemorrhagic strokes that this allows, such sophisticated investigative facilities are irrelevant to present practice as CT scanning remains available only in major centres in the UK. More strokes are due to occlusion of cerebral arteries than to intracerebral haemorrhage but the distinction of these is difficult without scanning; it is now known, for instance, that the presence of blood in the cerebrospinal fluid identifies only about half of the episodes due to intracerebral bleeding (Warlow 1981). The use of coumarins in the presence of an undiagnosed intracerebral haemorrhage is likely to be disastrous and even cerebral infarcts due to vascular occlusion may become haemorrhagic if blood flow is re-established into vessels subjected to ischaemic damage. Where CT scanning *is* available, the identification of those strokes due to infarction and those due to haemorrhage will be much more precise and it is possible that studies on newer antithrombotic agents in patients with cerebral infarction thus identified could be undertaken. The very wide variation in the natural history of occlusive cerebrovascular disease and in the prognosis of patients with strokes, the difficulties in assessing end-points other than death or its absence, and the concern that treatment may cause even minor local haemorrhage, suggests that these will not be enthusiastically embarked upon.

2. LONG-TERM THERAPY AFTER CEREBROVASCULAR INCIDENTS

Hill, Marshall and Shaw (1962) reported the results of a long-term trial of anticoagulant therapy in cerebrovascular disease. All the patients included were under 70 years of age and had suffered one or more disturbances of neurological function lasting more than 24 hours and attributed to non-haemorrhagic cerebral carotid or vertebral arterial disease. The authors concluded that, in patients selected on the criteria stipulated, anticoagulant treatment failed to provide protection against recurrent cerebrovascular incidents and added further evidence to substantiate the hazard of cerebral haemorrhage when anticoagulant drugs are used in the context. The majority of other studies of anticoagulant therapy in cerebrovascular disease are not well designed and lack appropriate control groups.

3. TRANSIENT ISCHAEMIC ATTACKS (TIA)

A transient ischaemic attack (TIA) is an episode of focal neurological or retinal dysfunction with symptoms lasting less than 24 hours. Once they commence, the risk of stroke is 5 per cent per annum thereafter and of stroke and/or death is 10 per cent per annum.

In a clinical trial in TIAs there are particular problems. The condition is not very common and has a variable natural history. The analysis of frequency of new attacks is rather a soft end-point; the incidence of stroke and death are harder end-points, but death from myocardial infarction is as common as that from cerebrovascular disease. The problem is similar to that encountered in trials in survivors of myocardial infarction. It is most unlikely that an antithrombotic regimen is capable of abolishing all further events. The most that can be hoped for is a reduction in the event rate; a stroke rate of 5 per cent per annum might be reduced to 3 per cent per annum. Small trials have little hope of identifying such a difference as significant.

Oral anticoagulants

The track record of studies of oral anticoagulants in TIAs is very similar to that in secondary prevention following myocardial infarction. Favourable case studies are: Rose (1950) and Millikan, Siekert and Schick (1955a,b). Larger trials but lacking some of the essentials of sound design are: Millikan, Siekert and Whisnant (1958), Whisnant, Matsumoto and Elveback (1973), Olsson Muller and Berneli (1976), and Whisnant, Cartlidge and Elveback (1978). Randomized trials, but with too few patients are as follows: Veterans Administration (1961), Baker *et al.* (1962), Pearce, Gubbay and Walton (1965), Baker, Schwartz and Rose (1966), and Bradshaw and Brennan (1975).

In total these randomized trials only had about 225 patients. About ten times this number would have been required to show that a reduction in events of 20 per cent was significant. There may well be a benefit from anticoagulants in TIAs but this has not been proven beyond reasonable doubt and it is unlikely that further trials will be conducted.

Aspirin

There have been three randomized trials in TIAs. The numbers of patients studied was as follows:

Canadian Cooperative Study Group (1978) 585
Fields *et al.* (1977, 1978)   303
Reuther and Dorndorf (1978)   58
                                                   ———
                                                   946

While the numbers entered were relatively small, the trial reported by the Canadian Cooperative Study is the best yet conducted in cerebrovascular disease. Thirty-nine per cent of the patients entered had some kind of residual neurological disability 'capable of subsequent observable further deterioration'; these were not, therefore, TIAs as usually understood. The trial was multi-centre and prospective, and was by the so-called 'two by two factorial design'. There were four study groups receiving:

1   Aspirin 325 mg four times a day;
2   Sulphinpyrazone 200 mg four times a day;
3   Aspirin plus sulphinpyrazone;
4   Placebo.

The groups were successfully randomized so that factors influencing prognosis were equally matched. The follow-up was thorough and patients withdrawn were accounted for. The design was 'explicative'. Compliance was good. Since the drug combination showed no synergism nor antagonism it was permissible to analyse all non-aspirin takers against aspirin takers:

	Aspirin	No aspirin
Strokes and/or deaths, sulphinpyrazone takers	20	38
Non-sulphinpyrazone takers	26	30
	——	——
	46	68

Once again, the trial is too small to allow certainty that the protection from stroke or death apparently afforded by aspirin was real. There was an astonishingly large difference in the effect of aspirin in males and females—men receiving it showed a reduction in events of 48 per cent whereas in women 42 per cent more events occurred in those taking the drug.

The second randomized trial of aspirin was in the USA— the 'Fields trial' (Fields *et al.* 1977, 1978). TIAs were reduced in number and there was a non-significant trend in favour of aspirin when stroke, retinal infarction and death were examined. In both the Canadian and the Fields trial many patients were excluded. In the Fields study a large group was excluded to be dealt with surgically and the remainder were randomized for the study. The characteristics of the Fields and the Canadian trials are outlined in Table 46. The German trial by Reuther and Dorndorf (1978) adds little of importance to the previous two.

On this evidence (to the surprise of some of us) the Food and Drug Administration has recommended the use of aspirin for men with TIAs but not women.

Further studies are indicated by the above numerically modest endeavours. The AMIS study confirms a beneficial effect of aspirin in cerebrovascular disease (Klimt 1981). An MRC funded study is in progress in the UK testing two dosage levels of aspirin (600 mg twice daily and 300 mg daily) against placebo in patients following TIAs. It is hoped that patients will be entered into such studies of aspirin in order that its effect on TIAs can be clearly established. Difficulties in the design and interpretation of the studies on TIAs are as follows (Mitchell 1981b):

1   TIAs are unlikely to be a single homogeneous group. The Fields study and the Canadian study differ substantially in construction of criteria for patient entry. Even if the trends they demonstrated were shown to be real, neither allows extrapolation to a more general TIA population.

2   The majority of TIAs and completed stroke patients die of myocardial infarction. The prevention of TIAs by themselves does not necessarily relate to

Table 46. Trials of aspirin in transient ischaemic attacks.

	'Fields' AITIA*	Canadian
Entry requirements ⎱ Nature of episodes ⎰	Monocular blindness Hemisphere TIA	Retinal/cerebral Ischaemic attacks in year 1 Revised to allow single episode thereafter
Timing	Within 3 months	Within 3 months

Duration of 'attacks'	Not specified	Under 24 hours, but
		  patients with residue
		  also recruited

Arteriography	Required Surgically treatable patients not entered	Optional
Number screened	1300	1341
Entered	178	585
Follow-up at time of report	6 months	Average of 26 months

Drug regime tested	Aspirin
	  650 mg twice daily
		Aspirin 325 mg × 4 (A)
		Sulphinpyrazone
		  200 mg × 4 (S)
		A with S in the same dosage

* Aspirin in Transient Ischaemic Attacks.

an effect on mortality. A reduction in death rate may occur because the antithrombotic drug prevents stroke *or* myocardial infarction, possibly by different mechanisms.

3   The most appropriate dose of aspirin remains uncertain.

Is there a difference in the therapeutic role of aspirin in men as compared to women?

On the basis of the evidence in trials of aspirin in patients who have had transient ischaemic attacks, the Food and Drug Administration in the USA has recommended the use of aspirin in men, but not women. There is a similar suggestion in some of the trials of aspirin in venous thrombotic disease. The evidence for a sex difference in response to aspirin is, however, too slender to permit final conclusions.

Other antiplatelet drugs in TIAs

Sulphinpyrazone was tested in the Canadian TIA study and found to be ineffective. Dipyridamole has not been examined sufficiently but is under clinical trial at present in the USA.

4.   CEREBRAL EMBOLISM

Cerebral embolism in patients with mitral valve disease or prosthetic heart valves is discussed on pp. 526–8.

While the evidence is incomplete there is reasonable evidence from the era in which acute myocardial infarction was treated with anticoagulants to suggest that the incidence of mural thrombus embolizing to the brain was reduced.

5.   STROKE IN EVOLUTION (PROGRESSING STROKE)

In the early 1960s this was one of the clinical situations in which the value of oral anticoagulants was studied. The groups, however, must have been so heterogeneous that the patients studied will have included those with a whole range of problems. Most strokes are sudden in onset, or develop during sleep. It is usual for the patient's deficit to be somewhat worse on the second or third day. The physician cannot know whether the deficit has stabilized at the time the patient is first seen, or whether it will worsen or improve. Even if the deficit is worsening over a matter of hours of observation, there may be several causes for such a progression; a thrombus may extend or a part may embolize peripherally. Further haemorrhage may occur into an area, if the primary lesion was haemorrhage, or thrombotic infarcts may develop haemorrhagic areas. The neurological damage at an area of infarction may extend because of the development of cerebral oedema. It is extraordinary, with hindsight, that oral anticoagulants were used at all in the heterogeneous disorders covered by the clinical syndrome of 'stroke' before CT scanning became available. With CT scanning it will become possible to conduct trials of antithrombotic therapy, other than oral anticoagulants, in cerebrovascular disease shown to be thromboembolic in nature if, indeed, the will to do so exists.

G.   Transplantation

Antiplatelet drugs have been used in renal and cardiac transplantation, but again their role has not been established.

Prostacyclin(Epoprosterol-flolan)

This has proved a very powerful antithrombotic in the management of extracorporeal circulations—renal dialysis, cardiopulmonary bypass or charcoal haemoperfusions. The second possible application is in those conditions where acute deficiency of endogenous prostacyclin exists—haemolytic uraemic syndrome and thrombotic thrombocytopenia purpura. Other applications will doubtless be studied in the future; clinical evaluation is on-going.

GUIDELINES

Venous thromboembolic disease

1   Prophylaxis using oral anticoagulants (provided contraindications such as peptic ulcer, recent stroke, etc. are absent).
   (a) Hip fractures proceeding to surgery—provided the will to prevent pulmonary embolism exists and careful control of anticoagulant therapy is possible.
   (b) High-risk medical patients.
   Prophylaxis with low-dose subcutaneous heparin:
   (a) Average-risk surgical and gynaecological patients.
   (b) Average-risk medical patients.

2   Established disease—venous thrombosis; pulmonary embolism. Continuous intravenous infusion of heparin; warfarin started concurrently and continued for 3–6 months. Thrombolytic therapy and/or surgery for special situations.

Arterial disease—secondary prevention after myocardial infarction

Conventional anticoagulants

1   In the acute phase—conventional anticoagulants reduce mortality by approximately 20 per cent. Most will take the view that the trials justifying this are too out of date to merit this as a routine practice.
2   In the long-term, coumarin therapy lowers mortality by about 20 per cent.

Antiplatelet drugs

1   Aspirin (1 g per day) reduces mortality by about 10–15 per cent.
2   Aspirin plus dipyridamole produce the same order of mortality reduction as aspirin alone. Aspirin with dipyridamole produces a significant reduction in coronary incidence (coronary death plus non-fatal but definite myocardial reinfarction); each patient is counted only once in this statistic.

Treatment is likely to be most effective within six months of the qualifying myocardial infarction. Widespread application of this should await the results of PARIS II.

Secondary prevention after the onset of TIAs

Pending the results of the UK TIA trial, 1–2 g of aspirin per day given to men is provisionally justified.

THE FUTURE

The only hope of clarifying the present muddled position is to run further trials. Many authors advocate this, but very few are prepared to put their hands to the helm. Even for the most enthusiastic they are tedious and lacking in glamour. They strain resources and patience and create unwelcome antagonism amongst professional groups. When published, the authors are almost invariably attacked for some imperfection and no single trial is ever accepted as definitive until it has been repeated and the same result obtained. But trials have to be conducted in the real world; however well motivated and designed, compromise on lesser issues may well occur and imperfections are to be expected.

The clinical trial as a tool requires to be sharpened. This might be done in the future in secondary prevention in arterial disease by establishment of better predictors of further events.

The evidence is that the currently available antithrombotic drugs can make a considerable impact on venous thrombosis and embolism but have only a small influence on arterial disease. It is unlikely that new drugs will be immediately available for widespread trial. The next generation of drugs will include thromboxane synthetase inhibitors, prostacyclin analogues and thromboxane antagonists but it is unlikely that these will be available for major clinical trials for a long time. There is still opportunity for further examination of heparin, coumarins, ancrod, aspirin, dipyridamole and sulphinpyrazone.

REFERENCES

Akbarian M., Austen W.G., Yurchak P.M. & Scannel J.G. (1968) Thrombo-embolic complications of prosthetic cardiac valves. *Circulation* **37**, 826–31.

Anturane Reinfarction Trial Research Group (1978) Sulphinpyrazone in the prevention of sudden death after myocardial infarction. *New England Journal of Medicine* **298**, 289–95.

Anturane Reinfarction Trial Research Group (1980) Sulphinpyrazone in the prevention of sudden death after myocardial infarction. *New England Journal of Medicine* **302**, 250–6.

Aspenström G. & Korsan-Bengsten K. (1964) A double blind study of dicoumarol prophylaxis in coronary heart disease. *Acta Medica Scandinavica* **176**, 563–75.

Aspirin Myocardial Infarction Study (AMIS) Research Group (1980) A randomized controlled trial of aspirin in persons recovered from myocardial infarction. *Journal of the American Medical Association* **243**, 661–9.

Baker R.N., Broward J.A., Fang H.C., Fisher C.M., Groch S.N., Heyman A., Karp H.R., McDevitt E., Scheinberg P., Schwartz W. & Toole J.F. (1962) Anticoagulant therapy in cerebral infarction. Report on co-operative study. *Neurology* **12**, 823–35.

Baker R.N., Schwartz W.S. & Rose A.S. (1966) Transient ischaemic strokes. A report of a study of anticoagulant therapy. *Neurology* **16**, 841–7.

Barnhorst D.A., Oxman H.A., Connolly D.C., Pluth J.R., Danielson G.K., Wallace R.B. & McGoon D.C. (1975) Long-term follow-up of isolated replacement of the aortic or mitral valve with the Starr–Edwards prothesis. *American Journal of Cardiology* **35**, 228–33.

Barritt D.W. & Jordan S.C. (1960) Anticoagulant drugs in the treatment of pulmonary embolism. A controlled trial. *Lancet* **I**, 1309–12.

Bjerkelund C.J. (1957) The effect of long term treatment with dicoumarol in myocardial infarction; a controlled clinical study. *Acta Medica Scandinavica*, Suppl. 330, 1–212.

Boncheck L.I. & Starr A. (1975) Ball valve prosthesis, current appraisal of late results. *American Journal of Cardiology* **35**, 843–54.

Bonnar J. (1977) Acute and chronic coagulation problems in pregnancy. In *Recent Advances in Blood Coagulation*. Vol. 2, Chapter 14. Poller L. (ed.). Churchill Livingstone, Edinburgh.

Bonnar J. & Walsh J. (1972) Prevention of thrombosis after pelvic surgery by British Dextran 70. *Lancet* **I**, 614–16.

Borgstrom S., Greitz T., van der Linden W., Molin J. & Rudics J. (1965) Anticoagulant prophylaxis of venous thrombosis in patients with fractured neck of the femur; a controlled clinical trial using phlebography. *Acta Chirurgica Scandinavica* **129**, 500–8.

Boston Collaborative Drug Surveillance Group (1974) Regular aspirin intake and acute myocardial infarction. *British Medical Journal* **I**, 440–3.

Bottomley J.E., Lloyd O. & Chalmers D.G. (1964) Postoperative prophylactic anticoagulants in gynaecology. A ten-year study. *Lancet* **II**, 835–6.

Bradshaw P. & Brennan S. (1975) Trial of long-term anticoagulant therapy in the treatment of small stroke associated with a normal carotid angiogram. *Journal of Neurology, Neurosurgery and Psychiatry* **38**, 642–7.

Breddin K., Loew D., Lechner K., Uberla K. & Walter E. (1979) Secondary prevention of myocardial infarction. Comparison of acetyl salicylic acid, phenprocoumon and placebo. A multicentre two-year prospective study. *Thrombosis and Haemostasis* **41**, 225–36.

Browse N.L. (1977) Personal views on published facts. What should I do about deep vein thrombosis and pulmonary embolism? *Annals of the Royal College of Surgeons of England* **59**, 138–42.

Browse N.L., Clemenson G., Bateman N.T., Gaunt J.I. & Croft D.N. (1976) Effect of intravenous dextran 70 and pneumatic leg compression on incidence of postoperative pulmonary embolism. *British Medical Journal* **II**, 1281–4.

Browse N.L. & Hall J.H. (1969) Effect of dipyridamole on the incidence of clinically detectable deep vein thrombosis. *Lancet* **II**, 718–20.

Bygdeman S., Svensjo E. & Tollerz G. (1970) Prevention of deep venous thrombosis. *Lancet* **II**, 419–20.

Canadian Cooperative Study Group (1978) A randomised trial of aspirin and sulphinpyrazone in threatened stroke. *New England Journal of Medicine* **299**, 53–9.

Canner P.L. (1980) Personal communication. Paper presented at the First Annual Meeting of the Society for Clinical Trials, Philadelphia, Pennsylvania, 8 May, 1980.

Carleton R.A., Sanders C.A. & Burack W.R. (1960) Heparin administration after acute myocardial infarction. *New England Journal of Medicine* **263**, 1002–5.

Carter A.E. & Eban R. (1974) Prevention of postoperative deep vein thrombosis in legs by orally administered hydroxychloroquine sulphate. *British Medical Journal* **III**, 94–5.

Chalmers T.C., Matta R.J., Smith H. & Kunzler A.-M. (1977) Evidence favouring the use of anticoagulants in the hospital phase of acute myocardial infarction. *New England Journal of Medicine* **297**, 1091–6.

Chesebro J.H., Clements I.P., Fuster V., Elveback L.R., Smith H.C., Bardsley W.T., Frye R.L., Holmes D.R., Vlietstra R.E., Pluth J.R., Wallace R.B., Puga F.J., Orszulak T.A., Piehler J.M., Schaff H.V. & Danielson G.K. (1982) A platelet-inhibition-drug trial in coronary-artery bypass operations. *New England Journal of Medicine* **307**, 73–8.

Chrisman O.D., Snook G.A., Wilson T.C. & Short J.Y. (1976) Prevention of venous thromboembolism by administration of hydroxychloroquine. A preliminary report. *Journal of Bone and Joint Surgery* **58A**, 918–20.

Clagett G.P. & Salzman E.W. (1974) Prevention of venous thromboembolism in surgical patients. *New England Journal of Medicine* **290**, 93–6.

Clagett G.P., Schneider P., Rosoff C.B. & Salzman E.W. (1975) Influence of aspirin on post-operative platelet kinetics and venous thrombosis. *Surgery* **77**, 61–74.

Clausen J., Andersen P.E., Anderson P., Grullund S., Harslof E., Andersen U.H., Jorgensen J. & Mose C. (1961) Long-term anticoagulant treatment after acute coronary occlusion. Material with complete comparison with control material. *Ugeskrift for Laegdr* **123**, 987–94.

Clayton J.K., Anderson J.A. & McNicol G.P. (1976) Preoperative prediction of postoperative deep vein thrombosis. *British Medical Journal* **II**, 910–12.

Conrad L.L., Kyriacopoulos J.D., Wiggins C.W. & Honick G.L. (1964) Prevention of recurrences of myocardial infarction, a double-blind study of the effectiveness of long-term oral anticoagulant therapy. *Archives of Internal Medicine* **114**, 348–58.

Coronary Drug Project (1976) Aspirin in coronary heart disease. *Journal of Chronic Diseases* **29**, 625–42.

Cosgriff S.W. (1953) Chronic anticoagulant therapy in recurrent embolism of cardiac origin. *Annals of Internal Medicine* **38**, 278–87.

Coulshed N., Epstein E.J., McKendrick C.S., Galloway R.W. & Walker E. (1970) Systemic embolism in mitral valve disease. *British Heart Journal* **32**, 26–34.

Coupland G.A.E. & Reeve T.S. (1975) The sequelae inferior vena caval interruption. *Australian and New Zealand Journal of Surgery* **45**, 245–51.

Cronberg S., Robertson B., Nilsson I.M. & Nilehn J.E. (1966) Suppressive effect of dextran on platelet adhesiveness. *Thrombosis et Diathesis Haemorrhagica (Stuttgart)* **16**, 384.

Data J.L. & Nies A.S. (1974) Drugs 5 years later: Dextran 40. *Annals of Internal Medicine* **81**, 500–4.

Dechavanne M., Ville D., Viala J.J., Kher A., Faivre J., Pousset M.B. & Dejour H. (1975) Controlled trial of platelet anti-aggregating agents and subcutaneous heparin in prevention of postoperative deep vein thrombosis in high risk patients. *Haemostasis* **4**, 94–100.

Dick W., Matis P. & Mayer W. (1959) Results of alternating anticoagulant prophylaxis in surgery. *Thrombosis et Diathesis Haemorrhagica* **3**, 11–19.

Di Saia P.J. (1966) Pregnancy and delivery of a patient with Starr–Edwards mitral valve prosthesis. *Obstetrics and Gynecology* **28**, 469–72.

Drapkin A. & Merskey C. (1972) Anticoagulant therapy after acute myocardial infarction. Relation of therapeutic benefit to patient's age, sex and severity of infarction. *Journal of the American Medical Association* **222**, 541–8.

Duvoisin G.E., Brandenburg R.O. & McGoon D.C. (1967) Factors affecting thromboembolism associated with prosthetic heart valves. *Circulation* **35** (Suppl. 1), 70–6.

Elwood P.C., Cochrane A.L., Burr M.L., Sweetnam P.M., Williams G., Welsby E., Hughes S.J. & Renton R. (1974) A randomized controlled trial of acetyl salicylic acid in the secondary prevention of mortality from myocardial infarction. *British Medical Journal* **I**, 436–40.

Elwood P.C. & Sweetnam P.M. (1979) Aspirin and secondary mortality after myocardial infarction. *Lancet* **II**, 1313–15.

Eskeland G., Solheim K. & Skjorten F. (1966) Anticoagulant prophylaxis, thromboembolism and mortality in elderly patients with hip fracture. A controlled clinical trial. *Acta Chirurgica Scandinavica* **131**, 16–29.

Feest T.G. (1976) Low molecular weight dextran; a continuing cause of acute renal failure. *British Medical Journal* **II**, 1300.

Fenech A., Hussey J.K., Smith F.W., Dendy P.P., Bennett B. & Douglas A.S. (1981) Diagnosis of deep vein thrombosis using autologous indium-III-labelled platelets. *British Medical Journal* **282**, 1020–2.

Fields W.S., Lemak N.A., Frankowski R.F. & Hardy R.J. (1977) Controlled trial of aspirin in cerebral ischaemia. *Stroke* **8**, 301–15.

Fields W.S., Lemak N.A., Frankowski R.F. & Hardy R.J. (1978) Controlled trial of aspirin in cerebral ischaemia. Part II. *Surgical Group Stroke* **9**, 309–18.

Gallus A.S., Hirsch J., Tutle R.J., Trebilcock R., O'Brien S.E., Carroll J.J., Minden J.H. & Hudecki S.M. (1973) Small subcutaneous doses of heparin in prevention of venous thrombosis. *New England Journal of Medicine* **288**, 545–51.

Gruber U.F., Duckert F., Fridrich R., Torhorst J. & Rem J. (1977) Prevention of postoperative thromboembolism by dextran 40, low doses of heparin and xantinal nicotinate. *Lancet* **I**, 207–10.

Hampson W.G.J., Harris F.C., Lucas H.K., Roberts P.H., McCall I.W., Jackson P.C., Powell N.L. & Staddon G.E. (1974) Failure of low-dose heparin to prevent deep-vein thrombosis after hip replacement arthroplasty. *Lancet* **II**, 795–7.

Hampton J.R. (1981) Presentation and analysis of the results of clinical trials in cardiovascular disease. *British Medical Journal* **282**, 1371–3.

Handley A.J., Emerson P.A. & Fleming P.R. (1972) Heparin in the prevention of deep vein thrombosis after myocardial infarction. *British Medical Journal* **II**, 436–8.

Harker L.A. & Slichter S.F. (1970) Studies of platelet and fibrinogen kinetics in patients with prosthetic heart valves. *New England Journal of Medicine* **283**, 1302–5.

Harris W.H., Salzman E.W., Athanasoulis C.A., Waltmann A.C. & De Sanctis R.W. (1977) Aspirin prophylaxis of venous thromboembolism after total hip replacement. *New England Journal of Medicine* **297**, 1246–9.

Harvald B., Hilden T. & Lund E. (1962) Long-term anticoagulant therapy after myocardial infarction. *Lancet* **II**, 626–30.

Hill A.B., Marshall J. & Shaw D.A. (1962) Cerebrovascular disease: trial of long-term anticoagulant therapy. *British Medical Journal* **II**, 1003–6.

Hirsch J., Cade J.F. & O'Sullivan E.F. (1970) Clinical experience with anticoagulant therapy during pregnancy. *British Medical Journal* **I**, 270–3.

Hohl M.K., Luscher K.P., Annahleim M., Fridrich R. & Gruber U.F. (1980) Dihydroergotamine and heparin or heparin alone for the prevention of postoperative thromboembolism in gynecology. *Archives of Gynecology* **230**, 15–19.

International Anticoagulant Review Group (1970) Collaborative analysis of long-term anticoagulant administration after acute myocardial infarction. *Lancet* **I**, 203–9.

International Multicentre Trial (1975) Prevention of fatal postoperative pulmonary embolism by low doses of heparin. *Lancet* **II**, 45–51.

Kakkar V.V. (1981) Prevention of venous thromboembolism. In *Clinics in Haematology* Vol. 10:2, pp. 543–82. Prentice C.R.M. (ed.). W.B. Saunders London.

Kakkar V.V., Corrigan T., Spindler J., Fossard D.P., Flute P.T., Crellin R.Q., Wessler S. & Yin E.T. (1972) Efficacy of low doses of heparin in the prevention of deep-vein thrombosis after major surgery. A double-blind randomised trial. *Lancet* **II**, 101–6.

Kakkar V.V., Stamatakis J.D., Bentley P.G., Lawrence D., de Haas H.A. & Ward V.P. (1979) Prophylaxis for postoperative deep-vein thrombosis. Synergistic effect of heparin and dihydroergotamine. *Journal of the American Medical Association* **241**, 39–42.

Kistner R.W. & Smith G.V. (1954) A ten year analysis of thromboembolism and dicoumarol prophylaxis. *Surgery, Gynecology and Obstetrics* with *International Abstracts of Surgery* **98**, 437.

Klimt C. (1981) Personal communication on AMIS results in cerebrovascular disease.

Kline A., Hughes L.E., Campbell H., Williams A., Zlosnick J. & Leach K.G. (1975) Dextran 70 in prophylaxis of thromboembolic disease after surgery; a clinically oriented randomized double-blind trial. *British Medical Journal* II, 109–12.

Kolata G.B. (1980) FDA say no to Anturane. *Science* **208**, 1130–2.

Lewis H.D., Davis J.W., Archibald D.G. Steinke W.E., Smitherman T.C., Doherty J.E., Schnaper H.W., Le Winter M.M., Linares E., Pouget J.M., Sabharwal S.C., Chesler E. & De Mots H. (1983) Protective effects of aspirin against acute myocardial infarction and death in men with unstable angina. *New England Journal of Medicine* **309**, 396–403.

Loew D., Brocke P., Simma W., Vinazzer H., Dienstl E. & Boehme K. (1977) Acetylsalicylic acid, low dose heparin, and a combination of both substances in the prevention of postoperative thromboembolism. A double blind study. *Thrombus Research* **11**, 81–6.

Loew D. & Vinazzler H. (1976) Dose dependent influence of acetyl salicylic acid on platelet functions and plasmatic coagulation factors. *Haemostasis* **5**, 239–49.

Lovell R.R.H., Denborough M.A., Nestel P.J. & Goble A.J. (1967) A controlled trial of long-term treatment with anticoagulants after myocardial infarction in 412 male patients. *Medical Journal of Australia* **2**, 97–104.

Lowe G.D.O., Reavey M.M., Johnston R.V., Forbes C.D., Prentice C.R.M. & Cummings S.W. (1978) Subcutaneous ancrod in prevention of deep vein thrombosis after operation for fractured neck of femur. *Lancet* II, 698–700.

McDevitt E., Carter S.A., Gatje B.W., Foley W.T. & Wright I.S. (1958) Use of anticoagulants in cerebral vascular disease; ten-year experience in treatment of thromboembolism. *Journal of the American Medical Association* **166**, 592–7.

McKenna R., Bachmann F., Kaushal S.P. & Galante J.O. (1976) Thrombotic disease in patients undergoing total knee replacement. *Journal of Bone and Joint Surgery* **58A**, 928.

Mackie M. & Douglas A.S. (1984) Drug induced disorders of coagulation. In *Clinical Disorders of Haemostasis*. Ratnoff O.D. (ed.). Grune & Stratton, New York.

MacMillan R.L., Brown K.W.G. & Watt D.L. (1960) Long-term anticoagulant therapy after myocardial infarction. *Canadian Medical Association Journal* **83**, 567–70.

McNicol G.P. (1980) Antiplatelet drugs in the secondary prevention of myocardial infarction. One view of the present position. *Lancet* II, 736–8.

Marshall J. & Shaw D.A. (1960) Anticoagulant therapy in acute cerebrovascular accidents: a controlled trial. *Lancet* I, 995–8.

Matis P. (1961) Results of alternating anticoagulant prophylaxis in surgery. In *Proceedings of the Sijkzigt Conference in the Prevention of Thromboembolism in Surgery, Rotterdam 1961*. Greep J.M., Loeliger E.A. & Roos J. (eds). Excerpta Medica International Congress Series **40**, 22.

Medical Research Council (1964) An assessment of long-term anticoagulant administration after cardiac infarction. *British Medical Journal* II, 837–43.

Medical Research Council (1969) Working Party report on Anticoagulant therapy in Coronary Thrombosis. Assessment of short term anticoagulant administration after cardiac infarction. *British Medical Journal* I, 335–42.

Medical Research Council—Steering Committee (1972) Effect of aspirin on postoperative venous thrombosis. *Lancet* II, 441–5.

Miller R.R., Lies J.E., Carreta R.F., Wampold D.B., DeNardo G.L., Kraus J.F.,

Amersterdam E.A. & Mason D.T. (1976) Prevention of lower extremity venous thrombosis by early mobilization. Confirmation in patients with acute myocardial infarction by I^{125}-fibrinogen uptake and venography. *Annals of Internal Medicine* **84**, 700–3.

Millikan C.H., Siekert R.G. & Shick R.M. (1955a) Studies in cerebrovascular disease III. The use of anticoagulant drugs in the treatment of insufficiency or thrombosis within basilar arterial system. *Staff Meetings of Mayo Clinic* **30**, 116–26.

Millikan C.H., Siekert R.G. & Shick R.M. (1955b) Studies in cerebrovascular disease. The use of anticoagulant drugs in the treatment of intermittent insufficiency of the internal carotid arterial system. *Mayo Clinic Proceedings* **30**, 578–86.

Millikan C.H., Siekert R.G. & Whisnant J.P. (1958) Anticoagulant therapy in cerebral vascular disease—current status. *Journal of the American Medical Association* **166**, 587–92.

Mitchell J.R.A. (1981a) Anticoagulants in coronary heart disease—retrospect and prospect. *Lancet* **I**, 257–62.

Mitchell J.R.A. (1981b) Anticoagulants, aspirin and anturan in transient cerebral ischaemic attacks. In *Advanced Medicine*—Newcastle. Tunbridge W.N.G. (ed.). pp. 276–86. Pitman Medical, London.

Morris G.K., Henry A.P.J. & Preston B.J. (1974) Prevention of deep vein thrombosis by low dose heparin in patients undergoing total hip replacement. *Lancet* **II**, 797–800.

Morris G.K. & Mitchell J.R.A. (1976a) Warfarin sodium in prevention of deep venous thrombosis and pulmonary embolism in patients with fractured neck of femur. *Lancet* **II**, 869–72.

Morris G.K. & Mitchell J.R.A. (1976b) Prevention and diagnosis of venous thrombosis in patients with hip fractures. A survey of current practice. *Lancet* **II**, 867–9.

Morris G.K. & Mitchell J.R.A. (1977a) Preventing venous thromboembolism in elderly patients with hip fractures: studies of low-dose heparin, dipyridamole, aspirin and flurbiprofen. *British Medical Journal* **I**, 535–7.

Morris G.K. & Mitchell J.R.A. (1977b) The aetiology of acute pulmonary embolism and the identification of high risk groups. *British Journal of Hospital Medicine* **18**, 6–12.

Morris G.K. & Mitchell J.R.A. (1978) Clinical management of venous thrombo-embolism. *British Medical Bulletin* **34**, 169–75.

Neu L.T., Waterfield J.R. & Ash C.J. (1965) Prophylactic anticoagulant therapy in the orthopaedic patients. *Annals of Internal Medicine* **62**, 463–7.

Nicolaides A.N., Dupont P.A., Desai S., Lewis J.D., Douglas J.N., Dodsworth H., Fourides G., Luck R.J. & Jamieson C.W. (1972) Small doses of subcutaneous sodium heparin in preventing deep venous thrombosis after major surgery. *Lancet* **II**, 890–3.

O'Brien J.R., Tulevski V. & Etherington M. (1971) Two *in-vivo* studies comparing high and low aspirin dosage. *Lancet* (Letter) **I**, 399–400.

Olsson J.E., Muller R. & Berneli S. (1976) Long-term anticoagulant therapy for transient ischaemic attacks and minor strokes with minimum residuum. *Stroke* **7**, 444–51.

Owren P.A. (1963) The results of anticoagulant therapy in Norway. *Archives of Internal Medicine* **111**, 240–7.

Pearce J.M.S., Gubbay S.S. & Walton J.N. (1965) Long-term anticoagulant therapy in transient cerebral ischaemic attacks. *Lancet* **I**, 6–9.

Persantine Aspirin Reinfarction Study Research Group (PARIS) (1980) Persantin and aspirin in coronary heart disease. *Circulation* **62**, 449–61.

Peto R. (1980, 1982) Personal communications.

Pettifor J.M. & Benson R. (1975) Congenital malformations associated with the administration of oral anticoagulants during pregnancy. *Journal of Pediatrics* **86**, 459–62.

Pitney W.R. (1981) *Venous and Arterial Thrombosis.* Churchill Livingstone, Edinburgh.

Poole J.C.F. (1959) A study of artificial thrombi produced by a modification of Chandler's method. *Quarterly Journal of Experimental Physiology and Cognate Medical Sciences* **64**, 378.

Poole J.C.F. (1960) Microscopical appearances of artificial thrombi. In *Pathogenesis and Treatment of Occlusive Vascular Arterial Disease.* Proceedings of a Conference at the Royal College of Physicians, London, 1959. McDonald L. (ed.) p. 231. Pitman Medical Publishing Co., London.

Ramsay D.M. (1975) Thromboembolism in pregnancy. *Obstetrics and Gynecology* **45**, 129–32.

Renney J.T.G., O'Sullivan E.F. & Burke P.F. (1976) Prevention of post-operative deep vein thrombosis with dipyridamole and aspirin. *British Medical Journal* **I**, 992–4.

Reuther R. & Dorndorf W. (1978) Aspirin in patients with cerebral ischaemia and normal angiograms or non-surgical lesions. The results of a double blind trial. In *Acetylsalicylic Acid in Cerebral Ischaemia and Coronary Heart Disease.* Breddin K., Dorndorf W., Loew D. & Marx R. (eds). pp. 97–106. F.K. Schuttauer Verlag, Stuttgart.

Rose W. McI. (1950) Anticoagulants in the management of cerebral infarction: A record of the poor result obtained. *Medical Journal of Australia* **1**, 503–4.

Sackett D.L. & Gent M. (1979) Controversy in counting and attributing events in clinical trials. *New England Journal of Medicine* **301**, 1410–12.

Sagar S., Massey J. & Sanderson J.M. (1975) Low-dose heparin prophylaxis against fatal pulmonary embolism. *British Medical Journal* **IV**, 257–9.

Sagar S., Nairn D., Stamatakis J.D., Maffei F.H., Higgins A.F., Thomas D.P. & Kakkar V.V. (1976) Efficacy of low-dose heparin in prevention of extensive deep vein thrombosis in patients undergoing total-hip replacement. *Lancet* **I**, 1151–4.

Salzman E.W., Harris W.H. & De Sanctis R.W. (1966) Anticoagulation or prevention of thromboembolism following fractures of the hip. *New England Journal of Medicine* **275**, 122–30.

Salzman E.W., Harris W.H. & De Sanctis R.W. (1971) Reduction in venous thromboembolism by agents affecting platelet function. *New England Journal of Medicine* **284**, 1287–92.

Schöndorf T.H. & Hey D. (1976) Combined administration of low dose heparin and aspirin as prophylaxis of deep vein thrombosis after hip joint surgery. *Haemostasis* **5**, 250–7.

Sevitt S. & Gallagher N.G. (1959) Prevention of venous thrombosis and pulmonary embolism in injured patients. A trial of anticoagulant prophylaxis with phenindione in middle-aged and elderly patients with fractured necks of femur. *Lancet* **II**, 981–9.

Sevitt S. & Gallagher N.G. (1961) Venous thrombosis and pulmonary embolism. A clinico-pathological study in injured and burned patients. *British Journal of Surgery* **48**, 475–89.

Simon T.L. & Stengle J.M. (1974) Antithrombotic practice in orthopedic surgery. Results of a survey. *Clinical Orthopaedics and Related Research* **102**, 181–7.

Sixty-Plus Reinfarction Study Research Group (1980) A double-blind trial to assess long term oral anticoagulant therapy in elderly patients after myocardial infarction. *Lancet* II, 989–94.

Storm O. (1958) Anticoagulant protection in surgery. *Thrombosis et Diathesis Haemorrhagica* 2, 482.

Sullivan J.M., Harken D.E. & Gorlin R. (1971) Pharmacologic control of thromboembolic complications of cardiac-valve replacement. *New England Journal of Medicine* 284, 1391–4.

Tilberg B. (1976) Prevention of postoperative deep vein thrombosis by leg bandaging and oxyphenbutazone. *British Medical Journal* I, 1256–7.

Turnbull A.C. (1960) Prophylaxis by anticoagulants after gynaecological operations. In *Thrombosis and Anticoagulant Therapy*. Walker W. (ed.). Churchill Livingstone, Edinburgh.

Turpie A.G.G. (1981) Antiplatelet therapy. In *Clinics in Haematology*. Vol. 10:2. pp. 497–520. Prentice C.R.M. (ed.). W.B. Saunders, London.

Urokinase Pulmonary Embolism Trial (1973) A national co-operative study. *Circulation* 47, (II) 1–108.

Veterans Administration (1961) An evaluation of anticoagulant therapy in the treatment of cerebrovascular disease. *Neurology* 11, 132–8.

Veterans Administration Co-operative Study (1969) Long-term anti-coagulant therapy after myocardial infarction. *Journal of the American Medical Association* 207, 2263–7.

Veterans Administration Co-operative Trial (1973) Anticoagulants in acute myocardial infarction: results of a co-operative clinical trial. *Journal of the American Medical Association* 225, 724–9.

Villasanta U. (1965) Thromboembolic disease in pregnancy. *American Journal of Obstetrics and Gynecology* 93, 142–60.

Warlow C.P. (1981) Cerebrovascular disease. In *Clinics in Haematology*. Vol. 10:2. pp. 631–51. Prentice C.R.M. (ed.). W.B. Saunders, London.

Warlow C., Beattie A.G., Terry G., Ogston D., Kenmure A.C.F. & Douglas A.S. (1973) A double-blind trial of low doses of subcutaneous heparin in the prevention of deep vein thrombosis after myocardial infarction. *Lancet* II, 934–6.

Wasserman A.J., Gutterman L.A., Toe K.B., Kemp V.E. & Richardson D.W. (1966) Anticoagulants in acute myocardial infarction; the failure of anticoagulants to alter mortality in randomised series. *American Heart Journal* 71, 43–9.

Weily H.S. & Genton E. (1970) Altered platelet function in patients with prosthetic mitral valves. Effects of sulphinpyrazone therapy. *Circulation* 42, 967–72.

Whisnant J.P., Cartlidge N.E.F. & Elveback L.R. (1978) Carotid and vertebral-basilar transient ischaemic attacks: effect of anticoagulants, hypertension and cardiac disorders on survival and stroke occurrence. A population study. *Annals of Neurology* 3, 107–15.

Whisnant J.P., Matsumoto N. & Elveback L.R. (1973) The effect of anticoagulant therapy on the prognosis of patients with transient cerebral ischaemic attacks in a community. Rochester Minnesota 1955 through 1969. *Mayo Clinic Proceedings* 48, 844–8.

Winter J.H. & Douglas A.S. (1981) Oral anticoagulants. In *Clinics in Haematology*. Vol. 10:2. pp. 459–80. Prentice C.R.M. (ed.). W.B. Saunders, London.

Wood P. (1961) *Acute Coronary Insufficiency*. Symposium on anticoagulant therapy, London, 1960. Harvey-Blythe, London.

Chapter 19
Statistics of Bioassay of
Blood Coagulation Factors

T. B. L. KIRKWOOD *and* T. J. SNAPE

Measurement of individual components of the blood coagulation system plays a central role in the diagnosis and treatment of haemorrhagic disorders and in the understanding of normal haemostasis. These measurements are complicated by the fact that each factor is but a part of an intricate network of interrelated enzyme–substrate–inhibitor interactions, many factors becoming activated only after the system is triggered. Although many of the activated components of the coagulation system are enzymes, the sequential nature of the reaction, and the frequent requirement for one or more cofactors to accelerate the process, renders the application of classical enzyme kinetics both complex and inexact (Hemker, Hemker and Loeliger 1965, Hemker *et al.* 1967). Furthermore, in the majority of *in vitro* assays, the component to be measured is often several steps removed from the end point, the formation of a fibrin clot.

These difficulties have led to recognition of the fact that, although most coagulation factor assays are carried out under semi-artificial test-tube conditions, they are best regarded as *bioassays*. A bioassay may be defined as the measurement of a substance in terms of its biological activity (see Finney 1978). In the case of a coagulation factor, the biological response is the time taken for formation of a fibrin clot, in a reaction system where the concentration of the factor is made rate-limiting.

The central element of a bioassay is the establishment of an empirical dose-response relationship. For varying concentrations of the factor to be assayed, a progressive change in the biological response must be observed. This provides the means of converting *responses* measured for preparations of unknown concentration to *potencies*, on a scale of activity defined by a reference preparation.

Principles of bioassay

Standard curves and their limitations

In the simplest form of bioassay, a dose-response relationship for a reference preparation (which commonly may be pooled normal plasma), is constructed by testing it over an extensive series of dilutions. A graphical plot of response (clotting time) against concentration then defines a *standard curve* (Fig. 54).

To use the standard curve subsequently, a sample plasma is tested at a given dilution, $1/d$, and the resultant clotting time, say t, is noted. This clotting time is equated, by means of the standard curve, to a concentration, say z, of the standard material. The concentration of the clotting factor in the sample plasma is then determined as $x = z \times d$. Provided the standard curve is strictly monotonic, that is it goes only up or down and does not show a peak, trough or plateau, the estimated value of x is determined uniquely, whatever the shape of the curve. It is necessary, of course, that the clotting time t is within the range over which the standard curve has been measured. Values outside this range may sometimes be estimated by extrapolation, but such a procedure rests heavily on assumptions about the form of the standard curve and is not to be recommended.

The attraction of the standard curve method is its simplicity, but its drawbacks are several. Perhaps the most serious of these is the unpredictable lability of various components of the assay systems normally used, which means that the standard preparation cannot be relied upon to give the same dose-response relationship from one occasion of testing to the next, let alone from day to day, or from week to week. Thus, tests of plasma samples which are referred to a predetermined standard curve can give potencies which are in

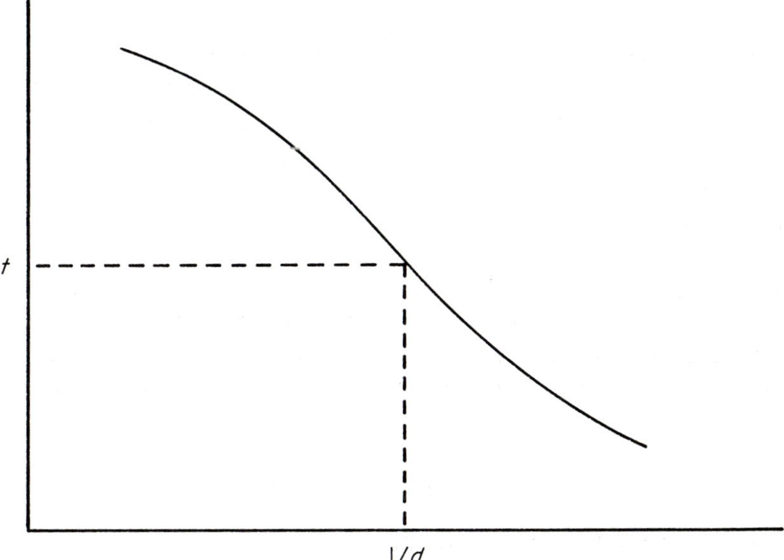

Fig. 54. Typical standard curve obtained by plotting clotting time against concentration ($=$ 1/dilution).

error by a significant amount. A second drawback is that if a plasma sample behaves on dilution in a way qualitatively different from the standard material, perhaps because it is abnormal in some respect, the potency estimate will depend on the dilution at which it happens to be tested. This means that the potency estimate is likely not to be valid (although this will not be noticed if only a single point is read off the standard curve). To overcome these drawbacks, it is necessary to set up the measurement of blood coagulation factors in the form of comparative bioassays, where a fresh sample of the reference preparation is included within each test.

Comparative bioassay

The basic idea of a comparative bioassay is that if two preparations are truly comparable, and they are tested together on the same occasion, their dose-response relationships should be identical apart from an adjustment to take account of any difference in potency between them. In other words, the weaker preparation should behave exactly as if it were a simple dilution of the stronger. When this is the case, the activity of one preparation can be described in terms of the other as a *potency ratio*. Should one of the preparations be a standard for which the potency is known (or arbitrarily defined), say P units ml^{-1}, then if R is the potency ratio of the other preparation in terms of the standard, its potency can be determined as $R \times P$ units ml^{-1}. In this way, through the use of a common system of standards (see Chapter 20), all potency measurements can be made on the same scale.

To put the principle of the comparative bioassay into practice, two alternative methods are used, both of which involve the graphical plotting of the dose-response relationships for the two preparations. For convenience, we shall refer to these preparations as the standard, S, and the unknown, U. Often there will be several unknowns (U_1, U_2, ... U_n) to be compared with a single standard in the same assay, but we restrict our attention to the simplest case since the analysis of a multiple assay is essentially the same. In the first method the response (clotting time, t) is plotted directly against the concentration c ($= 1/d$, where d is the dilution factor). This will result in two diverging curves the shapes of which are, in fact, the same, apart from a scaling factor in the horizontal dimension (Fig. 55a). In the second method the response is plotted against the logarithm of the concentration c. This has the special, and very useful, property that on the logarithmic scale the horizontal scaling factor is converted into a simple horizontal displacement through a distance equal to log R (Fig. 55b). This convenient mathematical device makes it much easier to tell at a glance if the dose-response relationships for the standard and unknown are of the same shape. Either graphical method can be used for the

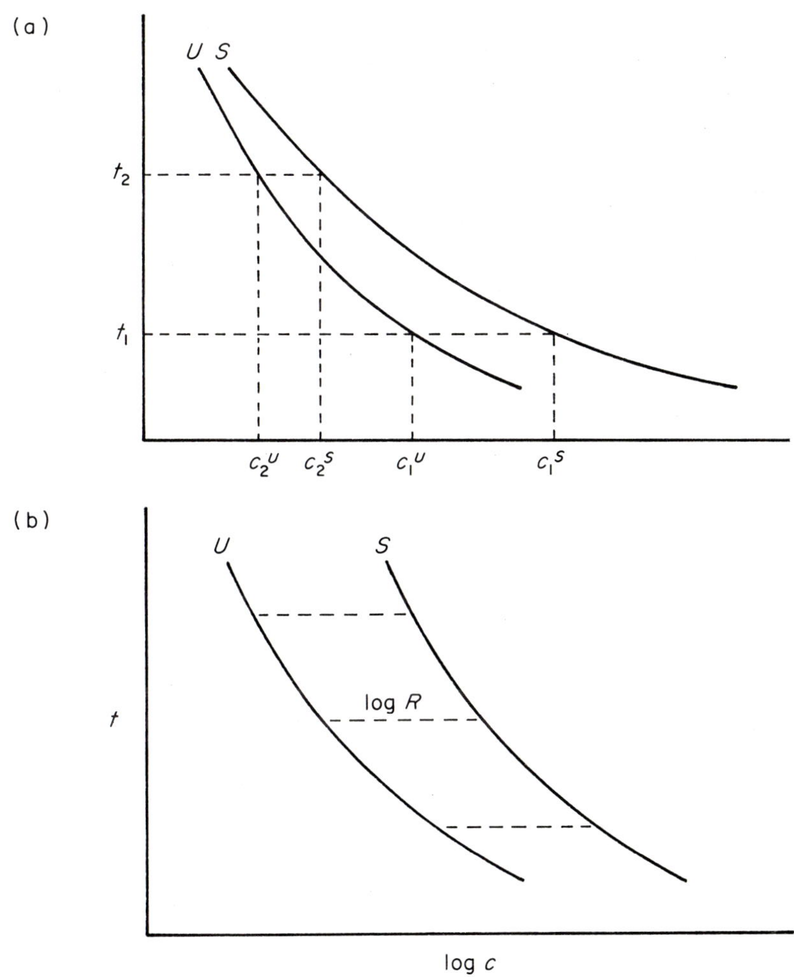

Fig. 55. Dose-response relationships for a standard and unknown preparation which differ only in potency. (a) Clotting time is plotted against concentration; for any value of t, the ratio c^S to c^U is the same, so the curves diverge; the potency ratio for the unknown in terms of the standard is $R = c_1{}^S/c_1{}^U = c_2{}^S/c_2{}^U$. (b) Clotting time is plotted against log concentration; the curves are parallel with a constant horizontal distance between them equal to log R.

purposes of comparative bioassay, but this last property represents a considerable advantage for the log concentration plot.

Whichever method is used it is more convenient from several points of view if the dose-response relationships are straight lines, at least over the concentration range in which tests are usually carried out. If the relationship is not already straight, this can often be arranged by the simple operation of changing the vertical scale on which response (clotting time) is plotted, for example to a logarithmic scale. This is, of course, just a mathematical ploy, but it is not in any way a dishonest one as it has no fundamental effect on the potency ratio, which is determined only by *horizontal* comparisons and is therefore unaffected by anything that is done to the vertical axis. The operation of changing the vertical scale is known as 'transformation' of the response variable, and much the most common transformation in coagulation factor assays is the logarithmic one. Others, such as taking the square root, or a transformation called the logit, may occasionally be required.

Assuming the dose-response relationships are linear, or have been made so by transformation, the graphical plots will show either two lines of differing slope intersecting the vertical axis ($c = 0$) at a common point (Fig. 56a), or two parallel lines (Fig. 56b). In the former representation, the potency ratio of the unknown in terms of the standard is equal to the ratio of the slopes of the corresponding lines. This is known, therefore, as a *slope ratio* assay. In the latter representation, the potency ratio is the antilogarithm of the horizontal distance measured from the line of the unknown to the line of the standard, distances in a left to right direction being counted as positive and in the reverse direction as negative. This is known as a *parallel line* assay. The derivation of these methods of calculating the potency ratio follows naturally if one writes down the equations of the lines in either of the two cases (see Finney 1978).

It should be clear that since the slope ratio and parallel line assay methods differ really only in the way the data are plotted, there is no reason why a given assay should not be analysed according to either model. The only exception is when the 'blank' clotting time (i.e. the clotting time at zero concentration) has been measured and is to be included in the analysis. In such instances the logarithm of zero is at minus infinity on the log concentration scale, so the parallel line method cannot be used unless the blank clotting times are omitted. In the absence of this complication the choice of method is likely to depend on the following:

1   Established precedent.
2   The relative ease of linearization.
3   The availability of data analysis programs.
4   The particular preference of the user.

The greater ease of comparison of the shapes of dose-response relationships in the parallel line method has tended to make this the method of choice in the great majority of coagulation assays.

Statistical analysis

Although it is increasingly common for the data of coagulation factor assays to be subjected to statistical analysis, it should perhaps be stated clearly that an

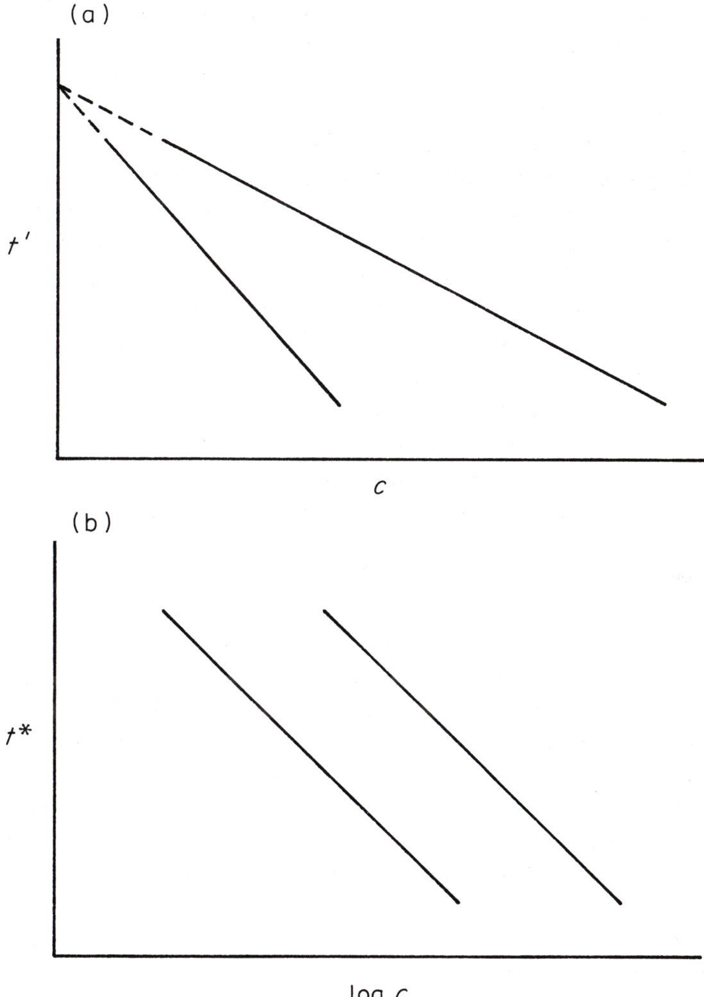

Fig. 56. Dose-response relationships as in Fig. 55 except that the vertical scales have been transformed to give linearity. t' and t^* are transformed values of the clotting times, the transformations in general being different. In some instances the dose-response relationships are linear without the need for transformation.

estimate of the potency ratio can, in fact, be obtained quite simply from a hand-drawn graph. The reasons why a statistical analysis is to be preferred, however, are as follows. Firstly, a numerical analysis is more objective. Secondly, statistical analysis permits more detailed tests to be made of the validity of the assay than can be made by eye. Thirdly, statistical analysis provides an estimate of the precision of the potency ratio.

Assay validity

If the individual clotting times in an assay were determined without error, it would be an easy matter to decide if the data fitted the assumed slope ratio or parallel line model. In practice, this is not the case, and each clotting time is in error by an amount which is an aggregate of the small technical imprecisions of dilution, pipetting and clot detection. The result is that at the end of, say, a parallel line assay, the assayist is confronted with a set of data which do not show straight parallel lines. An example of typical data from a two-stage assay of factor VIII:C is shown in Table 47 and is illustrated in Fig. 57. The question is whether the deviations from the parallel line model are just the result of purely random error, or whether they suggest that the model is fundamentally incorrect. (The possibility of fundamental invalidity has to be constantly borne in mind when trying to measure a single activity present in two different preparations one of which might, for example, contain an abnormal molecule or an inhibitor.) On the other hand, it may simply be the case that a gross technical error, such as an incorrect dilution, has occurred unnoticed.

To check the validity of the assay the statistical technique of analysis of variance can be used (Finney 1978, Kirkwood and Snape 1980). In this technique, the total variation among all of the individual clotting times is split up into a set of components, each of which corresponds to a relevant factor, such as non-parallelism. These components are then compared with the

Table 47. Data from a typical two-stage factor VIII assay.

Preparation	Dilution	Clotting time (s)		
		Duplicate 1	Duplicate 2	Average
Standard, *S*	1:64	16.8	17.0	16.9
	1:128	20.2	20.2	20.2
	1:256	26.2	26.4	26.3
Unknown, *U*	1:64	17.8	18.4	18.1
	1:128	21.0	21.6	21.3
	1:256	27.2	27.8	27.5
Unknown, *U**	1:64	16.6	17.6	17.1
	1:128	20.8	22.0	21.4
	1:256	26.0	27.0	26.5
Standard, *S**	1:64	16.2	16.0	16.1
	1:128	19.8	20.2	20.0
	1:256	27.0	25.0	26.0

* Independent replicate dilutions.

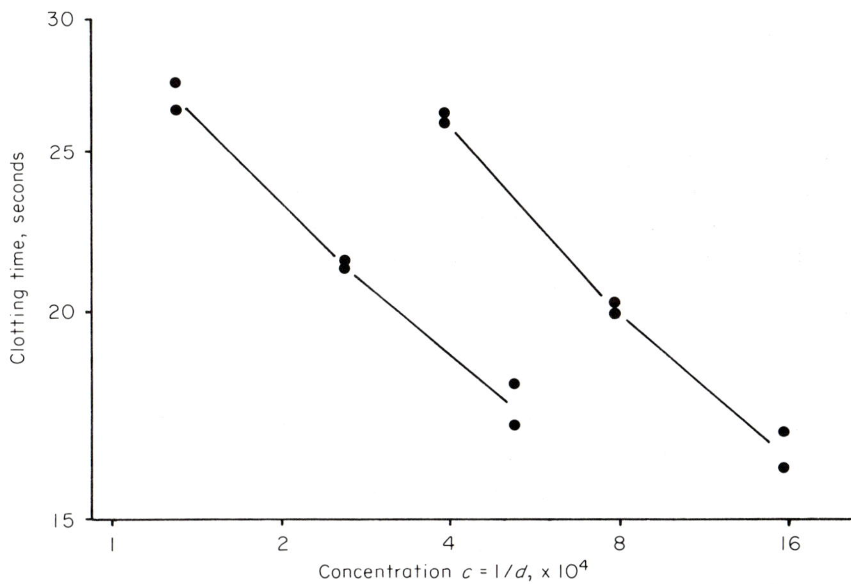

Fig. 57. Graphical representation of the data in Table 47 from a two-stage assay of factor VIII:C.

'residual' or background error of the clotting times to see if they are larger than could be due to chance.

The analysis of variance for the assay data in Table 47 is shown in Table 48. The total variation, given as the total 'sum of squares' has been split into five parts. The first part is due to differences in the average lengths of clotting times recorded for the two preparations. The second is due to the change in clotting time with changing concentrations, on the assumption that the dose-response relationships are straight and parallel. The third is due to

Table 48. Analysis of variance table for the data in Table 47.

Source	df	Sum sqs.	Mean sq.	F	Sig. level
Preparations	1	0.00154	0.00154	13.6	—
Regression	1	0.07452	0.07452	657.9	$P<0.001$
Non-parallelism	1	0.00010	0.00010	0.88	$P>0.05$
Curvature	2	0.00038	0.00019	1.66	$P>0.05$
Residual error	6	0.00068	0.00011	—	—
Total	11	0.07722	—	—	—

differences in the slopes of the dose-response relationships of the two preparations. The fourth is due to deviations from linearity of the dose-response relationships; this is an aggregate for both preparations, but a further subdivision into a separate curvature component for each preparation could be made. The fifth and last part is the residual error, which measures the variation among the replicate pairs of clotting times. The corresponding fragments of the total sum of squares are listed in the column headed 'Sum sqs' and they add up to the total which is shown at the bottom.

Associated with each component of variation is a number of 'degrees of freedom,' and what really matters is the amount of variation per degree of freedom, or 'mean square' variation. The figures in the 'Mean sq.' column are obtained by dividing the sums of squares by the corresponding degrees of freedom. Finally, to compare the mean square variation for each component with the mean square residual error, the entries in the 'Mean sq.' column are divided by the mean square residual error and these values, known as variance ratios, are entered in the column headed 'F'. It is on the F values that the assessment of assay validity is based.

A value of F around 1 means that the mean square variation was about the same as would be expected by chance if there was no underlying difference due to that particular component. A value of F much greater than 1 suggests, however, that the source of variation was real. To determine the precise statistical significance of a value of F, reference should be made to statistical tables of the F-distribution. These give figures above which the calculated value of F should be regarded as evidence of real variation, at the chosen level of significance. For example, the F value for non-parallelism in Table 48 was 0.88. The tabled F figure for significance at the 5 per cent level of a variance ratio, whose numerator has 1 degree of freedom, and whose denominator has 6 degrees of freedom, is 5.99. Since 0.88 is less than 5.99 the conclusion would be that there was no significant evidence ($P > 0.05$) for non-parallelism in this assay.

The important determinants of validity in a parallel line assay are the F values for non-parallelism, curvature and regression. Neither of the first two should be significant, but the third should be highly significant as otherwise there is no evidence that response changes with dose, and obviously such an assay would be valueless. The F value for 'preparations' is of much less importance, although preferably this should be small since this indicates that the standard and unknown have been compared over closely similar ranges of response. The level of statistical significance for the preparations F value does not matter.

In the example in Table 48 there is no indication that the assay may have been invalid and the conclusion is easily reached that it was sound. This will not always be the case, however, and properly used, the analysis of variance is an invaluable diagnostic guide to assay invalidity, which, with practice, may be appraised at a glance. For a parallel line assay the most serious evidence of invalidity, assuming a satisfactorily significant regression slope, is a significant F value for non-parallelism. This suggests that the standard and unknown have different forms of dose-response relationship, and in such cases it is meaningless to try to estimate a potency ratio. An assay showing this type of validity must usually be discarded. A second, less serious form of invalidity is where only the curvature F value is significant. When this happens, it may be possible to remove the curvature by appropriate transformation of the responses, and the assay may be re-analysed. In marginal cases it may be helpful to draw the data as a graph as well, to aid in making a decision.

For routine assay analyses, it is helpful to decide on rejection/acceptance criteria which may be applied consistently, and which can be easily taught to new staff. In selecting these criteria, it must be recognized that there is no sure way to reject all invalid assays and accept all valid ones. Increasing the stringency of the validity tests, by rejecting assays at lower levels of statistical significance for non-parallelism and curvature, decreases the risk of inadvertently accepting unsound assays but raises the likelihood of rejecting good ones. An example of a criterion which would reject only fractionally more than 1 in 20 sound assays, and which gives greater protection against non-parallelism than against the less serious risk of curvature, would be to discard an assay as invalid if either the non-parallelism F value is significant at the 5 per cent level, or the curvature F value is significant at the 1 per cent level.

For slope ratio assays an analysis of variance comparable to that of Table 48, but with different validity tests, can be carried out (see Finney 1978).

Potency ratio estimation and precision

Having established that an assay is valid, it is straightforward to calculate the potency ratio of the unknown in terms of the standard. This is done in a parallel line assay by fitting the best pair of straight parallel lines to the data, and determining the horizontal distance between them (or, in a slope ratio assay, by fitting the best straight lines which intersect at zero concentration, and calculating the ratio of their slopes). In either case, the best lines are determined by the statistical technique of least squares, and the calculation can be done at the same time as the analysis of variance.

The precision of the potency ratio estimate is worked out from the random error of the clotting times, which is given by the residual error mean square of the analysis of variance. This results in a figure for the precision of the potency ratio estimate, which is based on error arising from sources entirely within the assay, and from this a 95 per cent confidence interval for the potency ratio estimate can be calculated (see Fig. 58). It is important to be aware, however,

```
****************** PARALLEL-LINE ASSAY PROGRAM, VERSION 2A/7 ****************

ASSAY TITLE:FACTOR VIII                                     SEQ NO: 0
OPERATOR:MEH                                                DATE:010383

***** DATA INPUT *****

   Dose level:        1st        2nd        3rd
Preparation 1
   Dose (/ 10 )        4          2          1
   Resp            16.9/16.1  20.2/20.0  26.3/26.0
Preparation 2
   Dose (/ 30 )        4          2          1
   Resp            18.1/17.1  21.3/21.4  27.5/26.5

***** TRANSFORMED DATA *****              Response transform:    LOG

   Dose level:        1st        2nd        3rd        Overall
Preparation  1
   Mean LOG dose   0.602060   0.301030   0.000000   0.301030
   Mean LOG resp   1.217356   1.303191   1.417465   1.312671
   Variance        0.000222   0.000009   0.000012   0.000244
Preparation  2
   Mean LOG dose   0.602060   0.301030   0.000000   0.301030
   Mean LOG resp   1.245337   1.329397   1.431289   1.335341
   Variance        0.000305   0.000002   0.000129   0.000436

***** ANALYSIS OF VARIANCE *****

SOURCE              SSq          DF       MSq          F-ratio     SIG.LEVEL
Preparations        0.001542      1      0.001542       13.61
Regression          0.074521      1      0.074521      657.93
Parallelism         0.000100      1      0.000100        0.88     OK; P>.05
Curvature           0.000376      2      0.000188        1.66     OK; P>.05
Residual            0.000680      6      0.000113
Total               0.077219     11

Preparation         Curv SSq              Slope
   1                0.000270             -0.332373
   2                0.000106             -0.308859
   Common           -                    -0.320616

***** RESULTS *****

PREPARATION              LOG POTENCY     WEIGHT     POTENCY     95% CONFID. INT.
1:81/537DIL                                           3.50
2:8P1769/5DIL            0.950480        2667.44     8.92        8.00 TO   9.95
```

Fig. 58. A typical computer print-out for the analysis of data from a factor VIII assay.

that there may be additional sources of error which arise only between one assay and another (e.g. errors in making initial dilutions), and which therefore are not represented in the within-assay error. These additional, or between-assay, errors, may be quite as large as the within-assay error, and a proper assessment of the true precision of the potency ratio may require due consideration of both (see the section 'Combination of Potencies' below).

Method of calculation

Although not impossibly lengthy, the calculations required for the statistical analysis of a bioassay are tedious to do on a hand calculator, and there is the likelihood of an arithmetical error. This calculation is ideally suited, however, to a microcomputer which may be stationed in or near to the coagulation laboratory. Alternatively, a programmable calculator or, of course, a mainframe or minicomputer could be used.

The attraction of a programmed calculation is that once the program is set up, the user need only know how to enter the data and how to interpret the results. With a suitable printer, the computer can also be programmed to produce a convenient form, providing a complete record of the assay and its analysis. An example of such a print out is contained in Fig. 58. The data can also be drawn graphically on a visual display screen or graph plotter, if desired.

Computer programs in Fortran for the analysis of clotting factor assays have been described (Williams, Davidson and Ingram 1975, Counts and Hays 1979), and detailed instructions on constructing a flexible data analysis routine in this, or any other programming language, were given by Kirkwood and Snape (1980).

Assay design

No assay can be properly interpreted which has not been properly designed. The two main priorities in the design are as follows:

1 to ensure a reliable estimate of random error;
2 to prevent systematic error, or bias.

In addition, it is necessary to select an adequate number and range of dilutions.

Assessment of random error

The estimate of random error plays a central role in the assay analysis, firstly as the residual error mean square in the analysis of variance, and secondly in calculating the precision of the potency ratio. Because the residual error mean square is the yardstick against which the other components of variation are measured for statistical significance, it is important that it should be neither over-, nor under-estimated. Over-estimation diminishes the chance of the analysis picking up genuine invalidity; under-estimation increases the probability that a sound assay is falsely rejected.

The size of the random error is determined by comparing replicate clotting times, that is, clotting times which have been independently re-tested within the assay. It is therefore necessary to repeat tests for at least some of the concentrations of at least one of the preparations. The greater the number of repeats, the more dependable is the estimate of random error likely to be, because it is then less prone to chance fluctuations. As a general principle, a total of six repeats (replicates) should be regarded as a minimum.

For the estimated random error to be an accurate measure of the true within-assay variability it is necesary that in repeating the clotting times *all* potentially error-contributing steps are replicated. In particular, the duplicate testing of subsamples from a single set of dilutions is not adequate as replication—the dilutions themselves must also be repeated. Unless this is done, the residual error mean square will tend usually to be smaller than the sum of squares for the deviations from parallelism and linearity, and the likelihood of a sound assay being rejected will be significantly increased.

In one important instance, however, the differences between duplicates may be larger than the true error. This occurs in two-stage assays when one of the duplicate subsamples falls on the response 'plateau', and the other falls off it. In this case the problem is that the two duplicates are not measuring exactly the same thing. The essential point, therefore, is that whatever the difference between duplicates does represent, it *does not* represent an indication of residual error.

There is no reason why duplicate subsamples should not be tested, since this may be a useful safeguard against gross technical error or, as in the case of the two-stage assays for factors VIII and IX, agreement between duplicates is an indication of the proper operation of the assay mechanism. The duplicate clotting times so obtained should first be averaged to give a single value, and should not be entered into the analysis as if they were independent data points (replicates).

Control of bias

Any factor which causes a progressive change in the clotting time from the start of the assay to its finish may cause bias in the resulting potency ratio, and should be eliminated, or taken into account in the assay design. For example, if there is a tendency for clotting times to become more prolonged as the assay proceeds, and if the standard is always tested before the unknown, the potency of the unknown will be estimated on average to be too low. Also, this kind of temporal drift may cause spurious invalidity by introducing a change in the slope of the dose-response relationship from start to end of the assay, or it may mask genuine invalidity by inflating the difference between replicates, and hence the error mean square. Other kinds of bias may arise where differences in the nature of the preparations being tested necessitate minor differences in their handling (perhaps an absorption step required to remove an interfering agent present in one preparation and not the other). This is especially a problem when concentrate preparations have to be assayed against plasmas

(Kirkwood *et al.* 1977, Barrowcliffe, Tydeman and Kirkwood 1979, Barrow-cliffe and Kirkwood 1980).

The existence of systematic bias, due to differences between reagent systems and between assay methods, comes to light for the most part during multi-centre collaborative studies and is of particular concern to the standardization authorities (see Chapter 20). However, it is important that the individual laboratory should be aware of this, especially since a step change in the assay results may occur when a batch of reagent is replaced. This is discussed further in a later section.

The control of bias within the individual assay is best secured, firstly, by trying to prevent it from occurring and, secondly, by designing the assay so it may be detected should prevention fail. The prevention of temporal drift depends, for the most part, on selecting only reagents of proven stability, and on keeping each assay as short as possible. The detection of drift is most easily arranged by performing repeat tests in balanced reverse order, for example *SUUS* or *USSU* (see Table 47). With this scheme, pronounced temporal drift is readily detected by comparing the first set of replicate clotting times with the last. The design also has the advantage that minor drift, although inflating the residual error mean square and thus weakening the validity tests, is averaged out across the preparations and should have little or no effect on the potency ratio. Should temporal drift continue to be a problem despite these measures, the approach of Williams, Davidson and Ingram (1975), in which the effect of temporal drift is separated in the analysis of variance as 'regression on order', might be considered appropriate. In general, however, the approach should be to eliminate, rather than to accommodate, drift.

Choice of dilutions

The number and range of dilutions has an important bearing, both on the tests of validity, and on the precision of the potency ratio. In general, the precision of the potency ratio is greatest when the number and range of dilutions is largest (though beyond three dilutions a situation of diminishing returns applies (Finney 1978)), and when these dilutions are selected to lie on the steepest part of the dose-response relationship.

For the tests of validity, a minimum of two dilutions for each preparation is required if a test for non-parallelism is to be made, and a minimum of three dilutions is needed to test for curvature. In addition, the dilutions for each preparation should be selected to overlap in their clotting times as much as possible, so that the comparison between the preparations can be made with the minimum need for extrapolation.

The exact design of the assay will depend to a great extent on the precise application, and on the number of unknowns it is required to test. At one extreme, it may be required to screen a large number of plasma samples rapidly when a high level of precision is not especially important. In this case the standard should be tested over many (perhaps up to six) dilutions, covering the linear part of the dose-response relationship as widely as possible, particularly to allow many unknowns of varying potency to be accommodated. The tests of the standard should be replicated at the beginning and end of the assay, and possibly in between, both to provide an estimate of the residual error mean square and as a precaution against drift. The unknown samples can be tested at fewer dilutions, possibly only one, although two are preferable to check on parallelism and to guard against one or other dilution being out of range. The order of testing should be either balanced, if replication is possible for the unknowns, or should follow the order in which the unknowns were collected.

At the opposite extreme, it may be required to determine the potency of a single preparation with great care and precision, as for example when calibrating one standard against another. When this is the case, detailed tests of statistical validity are essential, and each material should be tested over at least three dilutions, carefully chosen to give comparable clotting times for each preparation. A balanced order of testing should be used. An example of such a study was described by Barrowcliffe and Kirkwood (1978) for the calibration of the 2nd International Standard for factor VIII.

For everyday purposes, the basic balanced assay design, *SUUS*, as in Table 47, with three dilutions of each preparation is recommended. This can be extended easily to include more than one unknown, e.g. $SU_1U_2U_2U_1S$.

Combination of potencies

In cases where several assays have been made of the same unknown against the same standard, a combined estimate of the potency ratio will usually be required. The natural thing would seem to be simply to average the individual potency ratios, but there are two reasons why this may not be an appropriate procedure.

In the first place, estimates of potency ratio tend to follow a skew distribution called the log-normal distribution (Fig. 59). This is true whether the assays are of the parallel line or slope ratio variety. A property of this form of distribution is that the average, or arithmetic mean, which is calculated as $\Sigma R_i/n$ (R_i being the ith individual potency ratio and n the number of potency ratios), is usually an *over-estimate* of the true value. A better way to estimate the true value is to calculate what is called the geometric mean. The geometric mean is the antilogarithm of the mean of the log potency ratios, or in a formula, antilog $[\Sigma \log Ri/n]$. It is thus standard practice in combining potency ratios to calculate a geometric mean.

The second point to consider in combining a set of potencies is that the

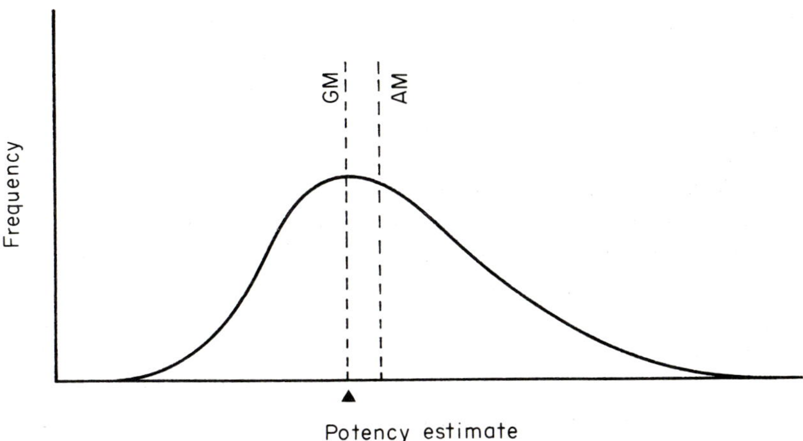

Fig. 59. Log-normal distribution of repeated potency estimates of a single preparation. The distribution is skewed towards high values, and the arithmetic mean (AM) is an over-estimate of the true value, marked by ▲. The geometric mean (GM) coincides with the true value, although, in reality, there will be some deviation due to random error.

individual values may have different degrees of precision. If one figure is known to be very precise and another to be very imprecise, it is desirable that the combined value should be slanted towards the more precise one. The precision of an individual potency ratio is commonly described in terms of its statistical 'weight', which is the reciprocal of the variance (i.e. the square of the standard error) of the log potency ratio. The more precise the estimate, i.e. the smaller its standard error, the greater is its weight.

The value of the weight which is calculated by analysing each assay singly is a measure of within-assay variation. When multiple assays are considered, however, it may be necessary to take account of between-assay variation as well. A statistical test, called a homogeneity test, can be used to determine whether there is a significant amount of between-assay variation (Table 49).

To carry out this test, a statistic X^2 is calculated by the formula:

$$X^2 = \Sigma W_i (M_i - \bar{M}_w)^2$$

where $M_i = \log R_i$

W_i = the weight based on within-assay error for the ith assay

$\bar{M}_w = \Sigma W_i M_i / \Sigma W_i$

If the value of X^2 is greater than the tabled value of a χ^2 distribution with $n-1$ degrees of freedom at the chosen level of statistical significance, the potencies are regarded as heterogeneous. Otherwise, they are accepted as homogeneous.

Table 49. Examples of combination of homogeneous and heterogeneous potency estimates.

Homogeneous

Potency, R	Log potency, M	Weight, W	df*
10.4	1.017	2143	6
11.1	1.045	3060	6
10.8	1.033	1992	6

$\bar{M}_w = 1.032$

$$X^2 = 2143 \times (1.017 - 1.032)^2$$
$$+ 3060 \times (1.045 - 1.032)^2$$
$$+ 1992 \times (1.033 - 1.032)^2 = 1.01$$

The 5% significance level for χ^2 with $(n-1)$ df $= 5.99$, so X^2 is not significant ($P > 0.05$).

Combined potency $= $ antilog $(\bar{M}_w) = 10.8$

95% confidence interval $=$ antilog $(\bar{M}_w - t/\sqrt{\Sigma W_i})$

to antilog $(\bar{M}_w + t/\sqrt{\Sigma W_i})$

(where t has $6 + 6 + 6 = 10$ df)

$= 10.2 - 11.4$

Heterogeneous

Potency, R	Log potency, M	Weight, W	df
2.8	0.4472	1482	6
3.4	0.5315	3621	6
3.1	0.4914	2497	6

$X^2 = 7.88$ (calculated as above)

which is greater than 5.99 so X^2 is significant ($P < 0.05$).

$\bar{M}_u = \Sigma M_i / n$ $\quad = 0.490$

s $\quad = 0.042$

Combined potency $= $ antilog $(\bar{M}_u) = 3.09$

95% confidence interval $=$ antilog $(\bar{M}_u - ts/\sqrt{n})$

to antilog $(\bar{M}_u + ts/\sqrt{n})$

(where t has $n - 1 = 2$ df)

$= 2.25 - 4.24$

---

* Associated with residual error mean square of assay.

Homogeneous potency estimates do not show evidence of significant additional between-assay variation. Thus, the weights W_i are an adequate description of assay precision. The combined potency estimate is usually calculated as the *weighted geometric mean*, antilog $\bar{M}_w$. The weight for this combined potency is ΣW_i, and the number of degrees of freedom, d, associated with this weight is the sum of the degrees of freedom associated with the residual error mean squares of the individual assays. A 95 per cent confidence interval for the combined potency may be calculated as the range:

$$\text{antilog } (\bar{M}_w - t/\sqrt{\Sigma W_i}) \text{ to antilog } (\bar{M}_w + t/\sqrt{\Sigma W_i})$$

where t is the 5 per cent percentage point of a t-distribution with d degrees of freedom.

When the potency estimates are heterogeneous, the single assay weights, W_i, are an insufficient description of assay-to-assay variation, and the weighted geometric mean is not appropriate. In this case, common practice is to use simply the unweighted geometric mean,

$$\text{antilog } \bar{M}_u, \text{ (where } \bar{M}_u = \Sigma M_i/n),$$

although a compromise procedure called 'semi-weighting' may sometimes be used instead (Bliss 1952). If the unweighted geometric mean is used for the combined potency estimate, its own weight is calculated as n/s^2 where s is the standard deviation of the individual log potencies, M_i. The associated number of degrees of freedom is $n-1$, and a 95 per cent confidence interval is calculated as the range:

$$\text{antilog } (\bar{M}_u - ts/\sqrt{n}) \text{ to antilog } (\bar{M}_u + ts/\sqrt{n})$$

where t is the 5 per cent percentage point of a t-distribution with $n-1$ degrees of freedom.

In practice there is seldom any major difference between the combined potencies calculated as weighted and unweighted geometric means, provided the weights of the individual potencies do not vary greatly. There may, however, be considerable differences in the widths of the confidence intervals to these combined potencies. The confidence interval for the unweighted geometric mean is generally much wider than the confidence interval for the weighted geometric mean. This is due to two effects. Firstly, by taking account of the extra between-assay variation for heterogeneous potencies, the weight for the unweighted geometric mean is usually much smaller. Secondly, the number of degrees of freedom $(n-1)$ associated with the weight for the unweighted geometric mean is usually much less than the number of degrees of freedom (d) for the weighted geometric mean. This results in a larger value of t in the formula for calculating the confidence interval. The latter is an especially serious problem when the number of assays is small, say five or less.

One way round this difficulty, in a laboratory where assays are performed routinely in a uniform manner, is to substitute for s in the formula above a standard deviation, σ, derived from previous experience. If the number of degrees of freedom on which σ is based is large, say 60 or more, a value of 2 can be substituted for t, giving a 95 per cent confidence interval ranging from antilog $(\bar{M}_u - 2\sigma/\sqrt{n})$ to antilog $(\bar{M}_u + 2\sigma/\sqrt{n})$. The advantage is that this confidence interval will usually be narrower than one based on s, although there is a slight risk that occasionally a set of assays will be genuinely less precise than usual, and this may pass unrecognized.

Statistical trouble-shooting

Routine statistical analysis of clotting factor assays is a straightforward and inexpensive way to enhance the reliability and amount of information which can be extracted from the data. It also offers the means to monitor the quality of the assay system over a period of time, and to detect, at an early stage, changes which may require action.

The three things to be watched are as follows:

1 The frequency with which assays are rejected as invalid.

2 The assay slope.

3 The residual error mean square.

The frequency of assay rejections is an indication of the quality of the assay design in accurately determining the within-assay error, and thus in providing a check on fundamental validity. If all assays were truly valid the long-term frequency of rejections should be $F = 1 - (1 - P_1) \times (1 - P_2)$, where P_1 is the significance level of non-parallelism beyond which an assay is rejected, and P_2 is similarly the significance level for curvature. For example, if $P_1 = 0.05$ and $P_2 = 0.01$ then $F = 0.0595$, so one would expect approximately 6 per cent of assays to be failed on the validity tests. A rejection rate much lower than this would indicate that the residual error mean square was over-estimated, thereby increasing the risk of failing to detect genuinely invalid assays. A higher rejection rate would be due in part to the fact that some assays are genuinely invalid, but it is unlikely that this could account for more than, say, another 5–10 per cent. Thus, a rejection rate higher than 15 per cent should be regarded as suggestive of under-estimation of the residual error mean square.

The assay slope is important because, other things being equal, an assay is more precise if its slope is steeper. If the assay slope begins to show signs of consistent change, usually a flattening, this is a likely sign that a batch of reagent has deteriorated and needs to be replaced.

The residual error mean square indicates the level of within-assay variation, and any change (progressive or sudden) deserves close study. It may be that a reagent is no longer reliable, or that an automated coagulometer is developing a fault or requires service. In the case of manual assays it is not uncommon that different assayists obtain different residual error mean squares and so each should monitor his results separately. It should perhaps be noted in passing that the residual error mean square does not provide a sound basis for smug comparisons, as by itself it is but a part measure of assay quality!

Finally, as a check that the assay result itself is consistent over time it is good practice to assay an 'in-house control sample' at regular intervals—perhaps a sample of a lyophilized or deep-frozen preparation. A drift in the potency estimate may reveal deterioration in some aspect of the assay system, provided it can be established that the standard or the control sample has not itself suffered degradation.

Any of these monitoring systems is likely to be facilitated by use of quality control charts, such as a cusum chart (Murdoch 1979).

Conclusions

Experience over many years, and in many different centres, has established that the statistical techniques of bioassay are well suited to the analysis of blood coagulation factor assays. The establishment of a dose-response relationship using the biological response of fibrin clot formation permits one preparation to be compared quantitatively with another. The techniques may also be used where the substrate of the reaction is an artificial chromogenic peptide (see, for example, Gaffney *et al.* 1977), or where the assay is one based on immunological recognition (see Kirkwood and Barrowcliffe 1980).

Statistical analysis of the assay data permits the maximum amount of useful information to be extracted. Firstly, through checks on the statistical validity of the assay, the assumption that the preparations can be properly compared may be tested. Secondly, the precision of the resulting potency ratio estimate can be calculated. With the wide-scale availability of low-cost portable computing equipment it is now an easy matter to set up a system for routine and flexible assay analysis directly within the coagulation laboratory. From the assay analyses it is, furthermore, possible to extract indices such as assay slope, and residual error mean square, which can be used to monitor the stability of the assay system over time.

In order that the assay should be amenable to analysis, and that its result should be free from systematic bias, it should be carefully designed. For optimal reliability and precision the following points should be considered:

1   To estimate within-assay error, and to test assay validity, at least some of the responses must be properly replicated.

2   A minimum of two dilutions of each preparation is required to estimate a slope and to test for non-parallelism.

3   A minimum of three dilutions is required to test for curvature.

4   The dilutions should be chosen so that the ranges of responses of the different preparations overlap as extensively as possible.

5 For greatest precision, the dilutions should cover as much of the linear part of the dose-response relationship as possible.

6 Temporal drift should be guarded against by use of a balanced design, and the total duration of testing kept as short as possible.

The application of statistical analysis to an assay conforming to these design principles is unreservedly recommended.

REFERENCES

Barrowcliffe T.W. & Kirkwood T.B.L. (1978) An international collaborative assay of factor VIII clotting activity. *Thrombosis and Haemostasis* **40**, 260–71.

Barrowcliffe T.W. & Kirkwood T.B.L. (1980) Standardization of Factor VIII. I. Calibration of British Standards for factor VIII clotting activity. *British Journal of Haematology* **46**, 471–81.

Barrowcliffe T.W., Tydeman M.S. & Kirkwood T.B.L. (1979) Major effect of pre-diluent in factor IX clotting assay. *Lancet* **II**, 192.

Bliss C.I. (1952) *The Statistics of Bioassay.* Academic Press, New York.

Counts R.B. & Hays J.E. (1979) A computer program for analysis of clotting factor assays and other parallel-line bioassays. *American Journal of Clinical Pathology* **71**, 167.

Finney D.J. (1978) *Statistical Method in Biological Assay.* Academic Press, New York.

Gaffney P.J., Lord K., Brasher M. & Kirkwood T.B.L. (1977) Problems in the assay of thrombin using synthetic peptides as substrates. *Thrombosis Research* **10**, 549–56.

Hemker H.C., Hemker P.W. & Loeliger E.A. (1965) Kinetic aspects of the interaction of blood-clotting enzymes. *Thrombosis et Diathesis Haemorrhagica* **13**, 155–75.

Hemker H.C., Siepal T.V., Altman R. & Loeliger E.A. (1967) Kinetic aspects of the interaction of blood-clotting enzymes. II. The relation between clotting time and plasma concentration in prothrombin-time estimations. *Thrombosis et Diathesis Haemorrhagica* **17**, 349–57.

Kirkwood T.B.L. & Barrowcliffe T.W. (1980) Standardization of Factor VIII. II. A British Standard for factor VIII related antigen. *British Journal of Haematology* **46**, 483–90.

Kirkwood T.B.L. & Snape T.J. (1980) Biometric principles in clotting and clot lysis assays. *Clinical and Laboratory Haematology* **2**, 155–67.

Kirkwood T.B.L., Rizza C.R., Snape T.J., Rhymes I. & Austen D.E.G. (1977) Identification of sources of inter-laboratory variation in factor VIII assay. *British Journal of Haematology* **37**, 559–68.

Murdoch J. (1979) *Control Charts.* The Macmillan Press Ltd, London.

Williams K.N., Davidson J.M.F. & Ingram G.I.C. (1975) A computer program for the analysis of parallel-line bioassays of clotting factors. *British Journal of Haematology* **31**, 13–23.

Chapter 20
Standards and Controls in Assays of Blood Coagulation Factors

TREVOR W. BARROWCLIFFE

In virtually all studies of the blood coagulation process, whether for clinical purposes or for research, measurements of individual clotting factors, or of sections of the clotting process, have to be made. The overall purpose of standardization is to ensure that these measurements have the same meaning, regardless of the time and place of origin, and the methodology used. It is important to recognize that this is a long-term process which goes hand in hand with the development of improved assay techniques and with our fundamental knowledge of the substance being measured. One view of standardization is that it involves rigid specification of methodology, and should not be attempted until knowledge of the system being studied is at an advanced stage. In fact, the reverse is the case: the less our knowledge, the greater the need for some sort of standardization at an early stage, so that results with different methods and in different laboratories can be related to one another. Indeed, the process of standardization starts right at the beginning once a substance has been discovered, with an agreed terminology. Fortunately, the blood coagulation field has been well served in this respect by the activities of an international committee on nomenclature, which established the Roman numeral system for clotting factors, originally introduced by Owren in 1947. Recent developments, particularly in our understanding of the contact system (Griffin 1981) and of factor VIII-related activities (Zimmermann and Meyer 1981), have emphasized the importance of agreement on terminology as a first step in standardization and, in the case of factor VIII, an international subcommittee was convened to make recommendations on nomenclature.

In this chapter, the process of standardization of measurement of blood coagulation factors will be viewed from three different levels. The first level concerns the practical provision and use of laboratory standards and control samples, as a means of internal quality control. Secondly, systems of relating results from one laboratory to those in others, at regional or national level, will be described. The third and most difficult level which will be discussed is the extent to which international agreement has been reached in measurements of the most important clotting factors. Finally, some problems of standardization of individual components of the coagulation system will be considered in detail, to show how the process of standardization can contribute towards our understanding of the measurement of these substances.

Units of biological activity

Once nomenclature has been established, the next most important step in standardization is to achieve agreement on the definition of a unit of biological activity. Three different methods of definition of units have been used to standardize measurements of clotting factors.

'Absolute' units

Here the unit is defined as the activity obtained under a certain set of precisely delineated reaction conditions. This has been mostly used for the enzymes thrombin and plasmin; the National Institute of Health (NIH) unit of thrombin was originally defined as the amount of thrombin which will clot a standardized solution of fibrinogen in 15 seconds. Recently a similar type of unit, the inhibitor unit, has been proposed for antithrombin III. Although such units may appear to be 'absolute', in the sense that they do not involve comparison with a reference standard, they are of course related to the materials with which the active substance interacts, and thus the problem of standardization is effectively transferred from one substance to another. In the case of the enzymes of the coagulation system, the introduction of synthetic peptide substrates has simplified this problem, and led to the possibility of expression of activities in classical enzyme terminology, e.g. katals (for a recent review of synthetic substrates in coagulation, the reader is referred to Blombäck 1981). However, the main disadvantage of this system is that the measurements depend critically on precise fulfilment of a specified set of reaction conditions. While this may be relatively easy within one laboratory, it is difficult to achieve on an inter-laboratory basis, especially in complex assays involving labile components.

This basic drawback, which exists for many other biological systems in addition to coagulation, has led to the recognition that adequate standardization can only be achieved by comparison of the activity of the unknown sample against that of a standard of defined activity, assayed under the same conditions. Variations in the test system from assay to assay, and from one laboratory to another, affect the standard and test sample in the same way, so that the final measurement should be mostly independent of such variations.

Normal plasma units

Because assays for most coagulation factors were developed before they had been purified, the first standard to be established consisted simply of normal plasma, the unit of activity being defined as that amount in 1 ml of 'average normal plasma'. One advantage of this system of units is that the severity of a clotting factor deficiency in a patient can be easily related to normal on a percentage scale. Another important advantage is that the denaturation which tends to occur on purification is avoided and, since most assays of clotting factors are carried out on plasma, normal plasma is an appropriate standard on the basis of a general preference for assaying 'like against like' in bioassays.

The main disadvantage of normal plasma as a reference is the very wide range in levels of clotting factors in the normal population, due to differences associated with age, sex, race and blood group, as well as intrinsic biological variability and the influence of drugs such as oral contraceptives. The combined effects of these differences can result in appreciable variations in the clotting factor content of multi-donor pools: it is not uncommon in many laboratories to find differences of 20 per cent in the factor VIII content of successive pools of plasma from 20 donors, and pools from different laboratories may differ even more widely. A further problem is that successive pools can only be assayed against the previous pool and, because of the poor stability of some clotting factors, especially V and VIII, this can result in a 'drift' of the value of the unit over a period of time. It is being increasingly recognized that the only satisfactory solution to these problems is the provision of stable reference standards against which successive batches of working standard can be compared.

Reference standards

In most areas of biological measurement, greatest uniformity has been achieved through the establishment of stable reference standards. The general principle of defining a unit of biological activity as the activity in a specified amount of a single reference substance was first established for insulin in 1925 by Sir Henry Dale; it has since been applied to many other biological substances, and only lately to clotting factors. In setting up reference standards for coagulation, use has been made of the general principles of biological standardization which have been developed over many years for other substances. The basic processes in establishing such a reference standard are as follows:

1 *Ampouling* of one or more candidate reference preparations. An important feature of any standard is that all ampoules should be identical in content. An accuracy of filling of less than 1 per cent is considered desirable for international and national standards, and the steps taken to achieve this have been described in detail by Campbell (1974).

2 *Preliminary testing* of proposed standards against the current standard, and

comparison with test substances likely to be assayed against the proposed standards. This is normally done in the laboratory responsible for preparing the standard and is a basic check on whether the proposed reference substance has adequate activity and gives valid assays against the materials with which it is going to be compared.

3 *Testing stability of proposed standards.* Another important feature of a standard is its stability. To act as a long-term reference preparation, the proposed standard should display no significant losses in potency when stored under its normal conditions (usually $-20°C$) for up to 10 years, and should also be able to withstand short periods at higher temperatures, so that it can be mailed at ambient temperatures without losses of activity. The general principle used in producing stable biological standards is that of removal, as far as possible, of the main agents of chemical change, i.e. water, oxygen, heat and light. Thus most standards are freeze-dried and the drying process has been developed both to ensure minimum losses of biological activity and to reduce moisture levels as low as possible, i.e. less than 1 per cent (Campbell 1974). Oxygen is eliminated by preparing all materials under nitrogen before sealing in glass ampoules. Rubber-stoppered vials are unsatisfactory because significant accumulation of atmospheric oxygen can occur inside the vial. Finally all standards are stored at $-20°C$ in the dark. Stability testing is normally done using the accelerated degradation method. Ampoules are stored at a range of temperatures, including some at higher temperatures to accelerate the degradation process and obtain measurable losses of activity. The usual range of temperatures is: $-20°C$ (reference), $+4°C$, $+20°C$, $+37°C$ and, occasionally, $+45°C$. From the losses in potency measured at the higher temperatures, it is possible to predict the degradation rates at $-20°C$, using a modified Arrhenius equation (Kirkwood 1977). Preliminary testing of a number of candidate preparations is normally done in the standards laboratory, and may lead to selection of one or more suitable preparations for collaborative study. This aspect is particularly important when setting up a standard for the first time; even when previous stability data exist, it can be misleading if samples have not been prepared under the conditions used for biological standards.

4 *Collaborative study.* Once suitable candidate preparations have been identified from the preliminary investigations, they are then subjected to an international collaborative study. This is the major part of establishment of a standard, and the general principles of such studies have been outlined by WHO (World Health Organisation 1978). The following represents a brief summary of the guidelines adopted at the National Institute for Biological Standard and Control (NIBSC), though it should be emphasized that many of these have been decided on pragmatic grounds.

(a) *Materials.* The two main types of material usually included are samples of plasma and one or more purified preparations; these should represent the degree of purity of the test samples against which the standard will be compared. For establishment of a new standard it is preferable to include more than one purified preparation, prepared by different methods. For studies carried out to replace existing standards, information gained from the first study may be used to limit the choice of materials.

(b) *Methods.* In virtually all studies, each laboratory is asked to use its own assay methods. However, some degree of control is applied in the form of instructions for reconstitution of ampoules, number of dilutions and order of testing. Good assay design is an important part of any collaborative study, and the statistical principles of assay design are described in the previous chapter. Also described in Chapter 19 are the methods of analysis used to calculate potencies from the raw data, and to test for validity of the assays.

(c) *Comparison with existing unit.* When any new standard is established, comparison is always made with the previously accepted unit, which in the case of most clotting factors is 'average normal plasma'. Thus participants are asked to collect normal plasma locally for comparison against the proposed standard, and samples of local standards, consisting of frozen or freeze-dried plasma pools, are included. Such comparisons, as well as being the basis of the unitage for the new standard, also serve to illustrate the divergences usually found between different laboratories' concepts of 'normal plasma'.

(d) *Assignation of potency.* From the raw data submitted, a mean potency estimate is calculated for each laboratory and the individual laboratory estimates are then combined into an overall weighted mean (see Chapter 19 for further details). It is customary to include all assays except those which are statistically invalid, even when it is clear that assays by different methods give different results. The problems arising from these methodological differences are discussed later in this chapter. For a new standard, the unitage is assigned by comparison with the existing unit, as already mentioned. A replacement standard is usually calibrated against the previous standard, but it may be desirable to compare also against normal plasma, as a check for possible 'drift' in the unit over many years (see section on factor VIII). The final assignation of potency, and establishment of the standard, is done by WHO for International Standards, and NIBSC for British Standards.

Practical use of laboratory standards and controls

The hierarchy of standardization

Where International Standards and Reference Preparations have been established as described in the previous sections, these can then be used to standardize measurements of clotting factors in any test sample. The 'hierarchy' of quantitation is illustrated in Fig. 60, and involves the concept of calibration of local 'working' standards against the International Standard (IS). In the case of frequently assayed factors such as factor VIII, there may be a need for an additional level of standardization, at the national or regional level, to be inserted between the international and local standards, in order to conserve supplies of the IS. This additional step can sometimes cause problems, because of the errors of the calibration process (see section on factor VIII) and, where this is the case, as in the manufacture of clotting factor concentrates, a direct link between the international and local standards may be preferable.

International standards and reference preparations have now been established for a number of clotting factors and related substances, and Table 50 gives a summary of the reference materials currently available. Measurement of all these substances can now be made in international units by calibration of local standards against the appropriate primary reference standard.

Calibration of local and national standards

As in the case of international collaborative studies, few formal rules exist for the calibration process, but some general guidelines can be given. The most important principle is that of repetition, to minimize the errors of the calibration process at each stage. For local standards, it is essential to carry out at least four independent assays, preferably six. By 'independent assay' is meant a completely fresh set of standard and test solutions; for concentrate preparations a new initial dilution should be made and, for freeze-dried standards, a fresh ampoule reconstituted. Since the supply of international standards is often limited to a few ampoules for each laboratory, a useful

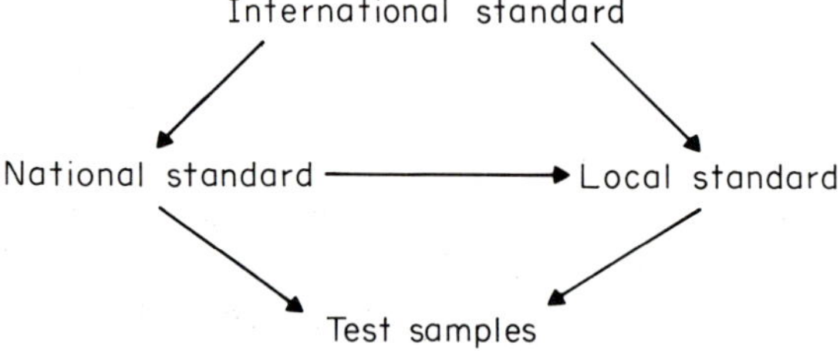

Fig. 60. The hierarchy of standardization. The International Standard provides a fixed reference point for all other preparations and defines the unitage. National standards are calibrated against International Standards. Local, or 'house' standards (including manufacturers' standards) are calibrated against the national standards or, where these do not exist, directly against the International Standard. Samples to be assayed are compared against either local standards or national standards.

Table 50. International standards and reference materials in haemostasis and thrombosis.

Substance	Current standard	Date established	Code No.
Human factor VIII (concentrate)	3rd IS	1982	80/556
Human factor VIII (plasma)	1st IRP	1982	80/511
Human factor IX (concentrate)	1st IS	1976	72/32
Thromboplastin (human plain)	2nd IRP	1983	BCT/253
Thromboplastin (rabbit, plain)	2nd IRP	1982	RBT/79
Thromboplastin (bovine, combined)	2nd IRP	1983	OBT/79
Thrombin (human)	1st IS	1975	70/157
Plasmin (human)	2nd IRP	1982	77/588
Streptokinase	1st IS	1964	62/7
Urokinase	1st IRP	1966	66/46
Ancrod	1st IRP	1976	74/581
Heparin (porcine mucosal)	4th IS	1983	82/502
Human antithrombin III (plasma)	1st IRP	1978	72/1

IS   International Standard; IRP International Reference Preparation. An IRP designation has been used in the past to indicate that the preparation may require further characterization. However, for all the above materials, IRP and IS are equivalent in status.

All the above preparations are available from: NIBSC, Holly Hill, Hampstead, London NW3 6RB, UK, except thromboplastins, which are obtained from: Centraal Laboratorium voor de Bloedtransfusiedienst, PO Box 9190, 1006 AD Amsterdam, The Netherlands.

compromise to obtain the required number of assays is to perform two or more assays from the same ampoule, provided that this can be done within the period of stability of the reconstituted standard (usually 1–2 hours). Repetition of testing of both materials should also be carried out within each assay, using two separate sets of dilutions of each. Ideally, a fresh set of reagents, even if from the same batches, should be used for each assay. In practice, this is not always possible, but some attempt should be made to spread the work over more than one day, to allow for possible day-to-day variation in reagents and environmental conditions. The calibration process is often a good opportunity to involve more than one operator, and indeed to compare accuracy and precision between operators. For the latter purpose it is important that the potency and precision of each assay, and of the combined assays, be assessed by standard statistical methods (see Chapter 19).

For calibration of national standards, essentially the same principles apply as for local standards, except that several laboratories are involved instead of just one, and so the calibration exercise needs to be coordinated and the results analysed by a central laboratory. It is in this situation that discrepancies in results between laboratories, and between assay methods, often arise. However, except in very rare cases, the results from all laboratories and methods are always combined into a single potency figure for the national standard.

Use of local standards in assays

Once a local standard has been reliably calibrated, it is then a simple matter to use it to assay test samples. However, a number of points about the design of clotting assays needs to be considered. The concept of 'design' arises from the need to compare standard and test preparations *under the same conditions* for the potency estimate to be valid. The main problem is the biological nature and instability of the reagents and test samples, so that in many assays the clotting times obtained with the same sample dilutions and the same reagents may change considerably during the course of a working day. The practice of comparing a large number of test samples against a standard curve prepared at the beginning of the day is not only statistically unsound, but gives unreliable potency estimates because of the likelihood of temporal drift. It becomes necessary, therefore, to set a particular time period during which it can be safely assumed that the test system has remained stable. This time may vary considerably with different assay methods but, for most clotting assays, it is preferable to aim to complete the assay within one hour, after which a new standard curve, with fresh reagents, should be prepared. Within this period there is considerable scope for variation in numbers of samples tested, number of dilutions, order of testing, etc., and it is not possible to give a single 'best design' to cover all situations. Some general principles are given as follows:

1   *Standard curve.* Whenever possible, two separate sets of dilutions of the standard should be prepared and tested at the beginning and end of each assay.

2   *Dilution range.* The range of dilutions tested should cover the linear part of the dilution curve as widely as possible.

3   *Number of dilutions.* At least three dilutions are required to define the standard curve. At least two, and preferably three, dilutions of each test sample should be tested. Estimates of potency from a single dilution should never be relied upon except as a rough screening procedure.

4   *Clotting times.* Dilutions of test samples should be chosen so that the clotting times fall within the range of those obtained for the standard. The standard curve should not be extrapolated beyond this range.

5   *Duplicates and replicates.* Duplicate clotting times are obtained from the same dilution of sample and often by subsampling from the same incubation mixture. A replicate is a true repeat, involving a fresh dilution of sample and

addition of reagents to form a separate incubation mixture. Ideally, both should be used, but if it is only possible to measure two clotting times, these should be replicates rather than duplicates; the use of duplicates alone gives a false impression of the precision of the assay. Further details of assay design and analysis are given in Chapter 19.

Use of controls

The use of 'control' samples, i.e. samples of known potency, is less widespread in assays of clotting factors than in the 'screening' tests such as the prothrombin time (PT) and activated partial thromboplastin time (APTT). Because the test samples are assessed by comparison with a standard, there is no need for a control sample in each assay. The use of control samples as a 'check' on the correctness of test assay results can be misleading. For instance, if standard and control samples are both freeze-dried, the same error of reconstitution may be made for both, giving a 'spot-on' result for the control sample in the presence of a large error in measurement of the test sample of fresh plasma. In general, there is no easy way of ensuring that the result of a clotting assay is the 'right' result. Each assay has its own intrinsic error which can only be determined by statistical assessment of repeated measurements (see Chapter 19).

However, control samples can be useful in a number of situations as an aid to internal quality control, and these are summarized as follows:

1 *Comparison of operators.* For comparison of accuracy and precision of operators, it is clearly useful to have the same test sample which can be assayed repeatedly against the standard.

2 *Comparison of assay methods.* When an existing assay method is modified or a new one developed there is often a need to compare results with the old method on the same sample. Similarly, even when batches of reagents are changed, it is useful to check results on a control sample.

3 *Checking stability of standard.* When frozen plasma is used as a local standard, stability of some factors, notably factor VIII, may be a problem and, if the standard is used for more than a few months, its potency will need to be monitored. Comparison against control samples can be used for this purpose, provided of course that the control samples themselves have guaranteed stability. For standards which are intended for more long-term use, e.g. over one year, it is preferable to carry out recalibration exercises against the original reference standard.

For some of these purposes control samples can be prepared in the laboratory, e.g. by admixture of normal and deficient plasmas. Control samples of defined potency can also be obtained commercially but these are usually determined only with the manufacturer's assay method and laboratories using different methods may not always get the same results.

Proficiency assessment schemes

Although the provision of reference standards is a major aspect of standardization of clotting factors, it does not of course guarantee that results will be the same in all laboratories. Some information on the extent of agreement (or disagreement) between laboratories can be obtained from collaborative studies, which are carried out to establish standards. However, this is not the primary aim of these studies and, since they involve only a small number of laboratories selected for their expertise, such results may give a false impression of the overall variation between laboratories.

Proficiency assessment schemes normally involve all laboratories and, by assessing their performance in assaying the same samples, give a more complete picture of the 'state of the art'. Such schemes have been run successfully for the prothrombin time in the UK (Poller, Thomson and Yee 1979) and in the USA (Koepke *et al.* 1977). Samples for assays of clotting factors, however, have been only recently included in these schemes and as yet only preliminary data are available. More details are given later in this chapter under the appropriate headings for individual clotting factors.

Standardization of specific clotting factors

Factor VIII

Factor VIII is one of the most frequently assayed of the clotting factors; in a recent survey (Haemophilia Centre Directors 1981), it was estimated that at least 25 000 assays are carried out annually in the UK. The bulk of these assays are carried out in connection with control of haemophilia therapy. In the early days of treatment with plasma and cryoprecipitate, local standardization was probably adequate and a pool of normal plasma was invariably used as the standard. The problems of normal plasma as a standard have already been mentioned, and are particularly acute for factor VIII, because of a very wide normal range (50–200 per cent of average normal) and its instability in plasma. With the advent of freeze-dried concentrates of factor VIII, distributed widely around the world from a few manufacturers, it became clear that local standardization was inadequate and that some kind of stable reference standard was needed. In 1967, the World Health Organisation launched a large international collaborative study with the aim of establishing an international standard for factor VIII and, at the same time, comparing assay methods in different laboratories. The results of this study were reported in detail by Bangham *et al.* (1971). Briefly, it was found that wide divergences existed in different laboratories' concepts of 'average normal plasma', thus emphasizing the need for a standard. In comparisons of assay methods, the two-stage assay methods were generally more precise than the one-stage. With both methods, greatest precision was achieved in assays of 'like vs. like' (e.g. plasma vs. plasma) than 'like vs. unlike' (plasma vs. concentrate) samples. The instability of factor VIII in plasma was confirmed, but the freeze-dried factor VIII concentrate used in the study was found to be much more stable. On grounds of stability and its similarity to the freeze-dried concentrates being used for therapy, the concentrate was chosen as the First International Standard for factor VIII, and established as such by WHO in 1971 (World Health Organisation 1971). The unitage of the standard was assigned by comparison with fresh normal plasma in the 20 participating laboratories; the average figure, against a total of 167 donors, was 2.6 'normal plasma units' per ampoule, which became 2.6 international units.

Assays of concentrates

With the establishment of a stable reference standard, it became possible for all countries using or manufacturing factor VIII concentrates to adopt the same unitage, the international unit (iu). This is inevitably a gradual process, but it is now true to say that all major manufacturers of factor VIII concentrates assay their products in international units, i.e. directly or indirectly against the IS. As with all such standards, the IS for factor VIII is intended as the primary reference preparation, and intermediate standards, national or local, must be used for assays of batches of concentrate, as indicated in Fig. 60. Because calibration of one standard against another is subject to error, it is best if the path between the IS and the samples for assay be made as short as possible. In the UK, this has been achieved by the adoption of a common standard, the British Working Standard for Factor VIII Concentrate, by the production laboratories and by the NIBSC. This concentrate standard is carefully calibrated against the IS by all laboratories using it, and is then used directly as a working standard in the assay of production batches. As with imported factor VIII, batches of UK-produced concentrate are checked at NIBSC and the agreement on potency has been remarkably good. In the USA, each manufacturer has his own 'house standard' and, until recently, these have been calibrated against the USA standard, issued by the Bureau of Biologics (BoB), of the Food and Drug Administration (FDA), which is in turn calibrated against the IS. This 'double calibration' has led to discrepancies, with potencies of most manufacturers' products being 15–25 per cent higher against the BoB standard than when assayed directly against the IS. The causes of these discrepancies have been difficult to establish, but are probably related to the fact that the BoB standard was a plasma, whereas the IS and the therapeutic materials are concentrates. As already mentioned, comparison of dissimilar materials gives less precise assays and is more likely to lead to discrepancies. It has recently been agreed that the USA manufacturers of concentrates will calibrate their working standards directly against the IS, instead of indirectly via the BoB standard, and this should eliminate the discrepancies previously mentioned.

It is preferable for manufacturers of concentrates to use samples of their own product as a working standard; in both the calibration process and the assay of production batches, 'like' is then being assayed against 'like'. Calibration of such working standards should be carried out carefully, with a minimum of six assays against the IS to obtain adequate precision. Although factor VIII appears to be very stable in concentrates, the potency of working standards should be checked annually against the IS if they are going to be used for much longer than one year.

It should be recognized that, with the widespread adoption of international units, there is less need for the clinician to assay the dose sample on a routine basis. This is particularly so in the UK, since each batch is checked at NIBSC and the labelled potency adjusted if necessary before release. Although additional checks are always useful, these should be carried out properly by performing several assays, using a standard calibrated in international units. A single assay on a dose sample may give a misleading result, because of the large coefficient of variation on a single assay, and the discrepancies which arise when concentrates are assayed against the plasma standards used in clinical assays (see next section).

The first IS for factor VIII was replaced in 1977 by the second IS, a similar intermediate purity concentrate. The new concentrate was compared with the first IS and also with samples of fresh normal plasma, in an international collaborative study (Barrowcliffe and Kirkwood 1978). The relationship between the international unit and average normal plasma was found to have remained reasonably constant and the new standard was established by WHO with a potency of 1.1 iu per ampoule (World Health Organisation 1977). One of the main findings of this study was that when samples of a common freeze-dried plasma were assayed against the IS (concentrate), the two-stage assays gave significantly lower potencies than the one-stage assays. This finding, which was later shown to be a general phenomenon (Kirkwood and Barrowcliffe 1978), has far-reaching implications for the standardization of factor VIII, particularly in the calibration of plasma standards and in the assessment of recovery.

More recently, the second IS has been replaced by the third IS, also an intermediate purity concentrate (Barrowcliffe *et al.* 1983). The new standard was assayed against both the old standard and against the plasma reference standard for factor VIII (see next section), which had previously been calibrated against fresh normal plasma. As in the previous collaborative study, there was close agreement between the international unit, as defined by the concentrate standard, and average fresh normal plasma.

Plasma standards

The standardization of factor VIII assays in plasma has been more problemati-cal than standardization of concentrates. Clearly, for assay of patients' plasmas, a pooled plasma standard is most appropriate, but the difficulties of ensuring 'normality' in a pool have already been stressed. Standardization of local pools can only be achieved by comparison with an external reference standard and, in principle, each local standard could be assayed against the IS. However, because of the large number of laboratories involved, this is wasteful of resources, and some sort of regional or national scheme is preferable. In the UK, the system established by Bangham and Brozović (1974) was for national plasma standards to be issued from NIBSC, after calibration against the IS by several laboratories. However, as recently described (Barrowcliffe and Kirkwood 1980), a major problem with this system has been the occurrence of wide discrepancies, up to two-fold, between different laboratories' potency estimates. These discrepancies are of two kinds: first, there is an overall discrepancy between one-stage and two-stage assays, the one-stage methods giving higher potencies for the plasma standards by an average of 20 per cent (Kirkwood and Barrowcliffe 1978). Additionally, within each method there are differences between laboratories due to variations in reagents and techniques. Both these types of discrepancy arise from the dissimilar nature of the materials (plasma and concentrate) and are not seen when one plasma standard is compared against another. Although some progress has been made in finding the causes of the discrepancies (see next section), it is clear that calibration of plasma standards against the IS (concentrate) is unsatisfactory in the long term. It has therefore been decided to establish an international reference plasma for factor VIII, to coexist alongside the concentrate standard. Improvements in methods of collection and freeze-drying have led to increased stability of factor VIII in plasma, and current stability data indicate that such a standard should have a lifespan of at least five years (Barrowcliffe and Kirkwood 1980). The 1st International Reference Preparation for Factor VIII Related Activities in Plasma has now been established (World Health Organisation 1983) and has been calibrated by comparison with a large number of normal plasma samples in an international collaborative study (Barrowcliffe *et al.* 1983). Values for the other factor VIII-related activities have been determined in the standard, in addition to its factor VIII clotting activity. The British plasma standard for factor VIII will continue to be issued, but in future will be calibrated against the international plasma standard instead of the international concentrate standard. This should minimize the discrepancies between laboratories and avoid the need to assign an unsatisfactory compromise figure for the potency.

Although the British plasma standard is intended for use as a working standard in everyday assays, limitations of supply mean that some larger laboratories have to use their own local standard, calibrated by reference to the British standard. Although this is less preferable, it still ensures reasonable homogeneity of measurement of factor VIII among all laboratories using the British standard. Some UK laboratories prefer to use commercial plasma standards. These are calibrated against either a local pool or the international standard (concentrate), but usually by the manufacturer's methods alone and not in a collaborative study. Although each manufacturer is careful to ensure batch-to-batch consistency, there is no coordination between different manufacturers to ensure that each brand is based on the same unitage. This is a particular problem in the USA, where several brands of commercial plasma standard are widely used and no national working standard is available. It is hoped that the establishment of the international plasma standard for factor VIII will lead to greater uniformity, through manufacturers being persuaded to use it for calibration of their plasma standards.

Standardization of reagents and techniques

Since factor VIII in a test sample is always measured in comparison with a standard, the influence of reagents and technical factors is less crucial than in the case of screening tests, such as the PT and APTT. Nonetheless, the importance of reagents as a cause of inter-laboratory discrepancy is illustrated by the results of a workshop set up to investigate the causes of the discrepancies already mentioned in assays of plasma against concentrate (Kirkwood *et al.* 1977). In this study, it was found that the differences between laboratories using variations of the same method (one-stage or two-stage) were eliminated when all used the same reagents, although a difference between one-stage and two-stage methods remained. Clearly it would be impossible for all laboratories to use the same reagents for routine assays. However, standardized agents have been tried in the collaborative studies to calibrate British plasma standards (Barrowcliffe and Kirkwood 1980). In these studies, there was considerable improvement in inter-laboratory agreement when the same reagents were used for the two-stage assays. This was particularly so when a combined freeze-dried reagent (prepared by mixing large batches of activated serum, phospholipid and factor V, and freeze-drying the mixture) was used. Such combined reagents have been used in our laboratory for several years and have proved helpful in internal quality control, avoiding day-to-day differences in serum activation and the need for frequent changes of batches. On average, batches have been changed every six months, although it appears that the reagents are stable for at least a year. In the one-stage assays, standardization of either the phospholipid or haemophilic plasma separately did not substantially improve inter-laboratory agreement (Barrowcliffe and

Kirkwood 1980), suggesting that other influences, such as activation method, may also be important. As with the two-stage assays, it is preferable for internal quality control to avoid frequent changes of reagents, and the factor VIII-deficient substrate plasma should be collected in reasonable quantity from several haemophiliacs, all with less than one per cent detectable factor VIII.

The causes of the one-stage/two-stage discrepancy have been less easy to identify. A collaborative study was set up to investigate one possible cause, the aluminium hydroxide $(Al(OH)_3)$ adsorption step, used in the two-stage method but not in the one-stage (Barrowcliffe, Kirkwood and Rizza 1980). It was found that omission of the adsorption step from the two-stage method reduced the discrepancy to less than 10 per cent. However, for technical reasons, the two-stage assay without adsorption is not entirely satisfactory for clinical samples, and further studies are in progress on other modifications of the adsorption technique. At present, it is not possible to say which method, if either, is 'correct'. In a study of *in vivo* recovery (Nilsson, Kirkwood and Barrowcliffe 1979), the one-stage assays gave recoveries of approximately 100 per cent, whereas the two-stage method gave about 80 per cent recovery. Many clinicians prefer the one-stage method because of the 100 per cent recovery figure, but it should be recognized that many proteins give less than 100 per cent recovery and the true figure for factor VIII is unknown. The different figures for *in vivo* recovery should be borne in mind if a change of method is contemplated.

Proficiency assessment

Samples for factor VIII assay have only recently been included in proficiency assessment trials. The first survey in the USA reported results from around 530 laboratories on two plasma samples sent by the College of American Pathologists (Harris, Triplett and Koepke 1978). There was considerable variability of results, with coefficients of variation ranging from 55.5–76.5 per cent on the mild haemophilic plasma sample (around 10 per cent factor VIII) and somewhat less for the other sample, of normal plasma. About two-thirds of the laboratories used a variety of commercial standards; the remainder used local plasma pools. It is considered by the authors of the report that the different standards used are the main source of variability. In the UK, samples for factor VIII assay have recently been included in the proficiency assessment scheme run by the Department of Health and Social Security, and it will be interesting to see whether the availability of a common standard has influenced the overall precision as compared with the USA results: as yet, only preliminary data are available.

Factor IX and other clotting factors

Many of the problems of standardization of factor VIII apply also to factor IX. A stable reference standard is needed for assay of the therapeutic concentrates used for treatment of factor IX deficiency, and an international collaborative study was carried out in which freeze-dried concentrate and plasma samples were compared with samples of fresh normal plasma (Brozović, Robertson and Kirkwood 1976). Factor IX is more stable than factor VIII, and the plasma sample in this study was only slightly less stable than the concentrate. However, the concentrate was chosen because of its similarity to the therapeutic concentrates, and established by WHO as the First International Standard for Factor IX with a unitage of 5.6 iu per ampoule (WHO 1977b). As with factor VIII, 'like against like' gives greatest precision, and concentrate working standards are preferable for assay of therapeutic materials. In the UK, a British working standard for factor IX concentrate is calibrated against the IS, and used by the production laboratories and by NIBSC. In the UK, plasma standards have also been calibrated against the IS for factor IX; for the last few batches the practice has been to use the same plasma standard for both factor VIII and factor IX. These plasma versus concentrate assays have come up against the same sort of discrepancies as for factor VIII. In a workshop study, it was found that the predilution method used for the concentrate was an important source of variability; using factor IX-deficient plasma instead of buffer as a prediluent for the IS altered the potency of the plasma by as much as 50 per cent (Barrowcliffe, Tydeman and Kirkwood 1979). With factor IX-deficient plasma as a prediluent, the potencies of the plasma standards are somewhat lower (around 0.6 iu/ampoule) than would be obtained by assay against normal pooled plasmas. However, this method has been adopted, as it gives a value which is more consistent with the post-infusion samples obtained after injection of concentrate into factor IX-deficient patients.

Congenital deficiencies of the other clotting factors are extremely rare and the need for therapeutic materials correspondingly very small. Factor IX concentrates are used to a certain extent to treat acquired deficiencies of factors II, VII and X, but as yet no international standards have been established for these clotting factors. For assay of clotting factors other than VIII or IX in plasma, reliance must be placed on commercial standards or local pools. Since the other factors have narrower normal ranges than factor VIII and, with the exception of factor V, are more stable, a well-collected normal pool provides adequate standardization. Subjects taking drugs known to affect clotting factors, e.g. anticoagulants, oral contraceptives, should be excluded but, apart from this, no other exclusion should be made. The number of donors should be at least 20 and the age-range not too narrow. Plasma should be centrifuged immediately after collection, snap frozen and stored at as low a temperature as possible, preferably − 70°C or below.

Fibrinogen

Fibrinogen is the only clotting factor which can in principle be determined without recourse to a standard, because of its unique clottability. A variety of different methods has evolved, depending on measurement of the opacity or weight of the clot, turbidity, tyrosine content or measurement of the thrombin time. The method of Ratnoff and Menzie (1951), involving measurement of the tyrosine content of a carefully collected and washed clot, is widely regarded as a reference method. The thrombin clotting time is best performed as a comparative assay against a fibrinogen standard, using several dilutions and calculating the results graphically as described for other clotting factors. Plasmas of known fibrinogen content are available commercially. Samples for fibrinogen assay have been included in the UK proficiency assessment scheme since 1976. The most popular methods are the fibrinogen titre and the Clauss thrombin time method. All techniques performed reasonably well with fibrinogen levels in the normal range but, for low fibrinogen levels, the thrombin time method tended to differ from the others. The turbidity technique, fibrinogen titre and heat precipitation methods were also relatively unreliable.

Similar variability in type of method and results was reported in the USA from the initial proficiency assessment studies of the College of American Pathologists, with coefficients of variation for all methods ranging from 21–90 per cent in 1967 and 1971. However, since 1971, a new thrombin time method introduced by Dade has become very popular, and is now preferred by more than 80 per cent of laboratories in the USA. The new method, based on comparison against a standard, has given much improved accuracy and precision, with overall coefficients of variation in the region of 5–10 per cent in the 1978 survey (Koepke 1978).

Thrombin

Although assays of thrombin are rarely carried out for clinical purposes, thrombin is widely used as a reagent, and it is important that its unitage be standardized. For this purpose, an International Standard for Human Thrombin is available and all manufacturers of diagnostic reagents are encouraged to calibrate their thrombin against it, using the comparative bioassay method already described. In the international collaborative study (Robertson, Gaffney and Bangham 1975), there were no consistent differences in precision and potency estimates when plasma or fibrinogen, from either bovine or human sources, was used as substrate.

Antithrombin III

The recognition that a deficiency of antithrombin III (AT III), whether congenital or acquired, can be a major predisposing factor in the development of thrombosis, has led to increased interest in the measurement of this inhibitor (Barrowcliffe and Thomas 1981). This interest has also been stimulated by the introduction of synthetic peptide substrates for measurement of thrombin and other enzymes, which has simplified the technique and improved the precision of AT III assays. However, the fact that residual enzyme is measured by a chemical reaction should not obscure the biological nature of the interaction between AT III in plasma and the thrombin added in the assay, and it is important to apply the basic principles of bioassay already discussed. Two types of situation are commonly encountered in which these principles are not followed. The first is in the expression of results as 'inhibitor units', as described by the manufacturer of one commercial kit, instead of the more usual percentage activity in comparison with a normal plasma standard. These inhibitor units are defined in terms of the amount of thrombin inhibited under certain specified reaction conditions. The difficulty of reproducing the conditions exactly and the basic biological variability of the system make this an unreliable method of standardization and it is essential if using this method to compare the inhibitor units given by the test sample with a standard curve prepared with the same reagents. The second common practice is to assay test samples at a single dilution only, usually in duplicate. Although this is an understandable economy in view of the cost of the synthetic substrates, such single point estimates have a high intrinsic error, and economic savings should be weighed against the very real possibility of an incorrect clinical judgment resulting from a false single point estimate. Ideally, three dilutions of test samples should be assayed but, if only two measurements are to be made, it is better that these be two independent dilutions in different parts of the standard curve, rather than duplicates from the same single dilution. Although the precision will probably be less than with duplicates, the value obtained will be a truer assessment of the AT III level. In recognition of the importance of AT III assays, an international collaborative study was carried out with the aim of establishing a stable reference standard (Kirkwood, Barrowcliffe and Thomas 1980). Samples of highly purified AT III and freeze-dried plasma were compared with local pooled plasma in 11 laboratories. Considerable discrepancies were found between the different assay methods when the purified AT III samples were assayed against the common freeze-dried plasma; this can now be seen as a general pattern in comparing purified materials and plasma (cf. factors VIII and IX). In contrast, comparison of the freeze-dried plasma with local pools gave remarkably good agreement between different methods. The plasma was also more stable than the purified materials and, in view of these findings, and the fact that most AT III assays are performed on plasma samples, the freeze-dried plasma was chosen as the 1st International Reference Preparation for AT III. It is intended for calibration of both local and commercial standards though, as with factor VIII, some sort of regional or national standardization scheme is preferable. In the UK, batches of British plasma standard for factor VIII have also been calibrated for AT III, so that laboratories can use it as a working standard for both substances.

REFERENCES

Bangham D.R., Biggs R., Brozović M., Denson K.W.E. & Skegg J.L. (1971) A biological standard for measurement of blood coagulation factor VIII activity. *Bulletin of the World Health Organisation* **45**, 337–51.

Bangham D.R. & Brozović M. (1974) International Units and reference materials. *Thrombosis et Diathesis Haemorrhagica* **31**, 3–11.

Barrowcliffe T.W., Curtis A.D. & Thomas D.P. (1983) Standardisation of Factor VIII. IV: Calibration of the 3rd International Standard for Factor VIII (concentrate). *Thrombosis and Haemostasis* **50**, 697–702.

Barrowcliffe T.W. & Kirkwood T.B.L. (1978) An international collaborative assay of Factor VIII clotting activity. *Thrombosis and Haemostasis* **40**, 260–71.

Barrowcliffe T.W., Kirkwood T.B.L. & Rizza C.R. (1980) Aluminium hydroxide adsorption and Factor VIII clotting assays. *Lancet* **I**, 820.

Barrowcliffe T.W. & Kirkwood T.B.L. (1980) Standardisation of Factor VIII. I: Calibration of British standards for Factor VIII clotting activity. *British Journal of Haematology* **46**, 471–81.

Barrowcliffe T.W. & Thomas D.P. (1981) Antithrombin III and heparin. In *Haemostasis and Thrombosis*. Bloom A.L. & Thomas D.P. (eds). pp. 712–24. Churchill Livingstone, Edinburgh.

Barrowcliffe T.W., Tydeman M.S. & Kirkwood T.B.L. (1979) Major effect of prediluent in Factor IX clotting assay. *Lancet* **II**, 192.

Barrowcliffe T.W., Tydeman M.S., Kirkwood T.B.L. & Thomas D.P. (1983) Standardisation of Factor VIII. III: A plasma reference standard for Factor VIII-related activities. *Thrombosis and Haemostasis* **50**, 690–6.

Blömback M. (1981) Chromogenic substrates in the laboratory diagnosis of clotting disorders. In *Haemostasis and Thrombosis*. Bloom A.L. & Thomas D.P. (eds). pp. 809–23. Churchill Livingstone, Edinburgh.

Brozović M., Robertson I. & Kirkwood T.B.L. (1976) Study of a proposed international standard for blood coagulation factor IX. *Thrombosis and Haemostasis* **35**, 222–36.

Campbell P.J. (1974) International biological standards and reference preparations. II: Procedures used for the production of biological standards and reference preparations. *Journal of Biological Standardisation* **2**, 259–67.

Griffin J.H. (1981) The contact phase of blood coagulation. In *Haemostasis and Thrombosis*. Bloom A.L. & Thomas D.P. (eds). pp. 84–97. Churchill Livingstone, Edinburgh.

Haemophilia Centre Directors' Working Party on Standardization of Factor VIII Assay

(1981) A survey of VIII:C assay in the United Kingdom. *Clinical and Laboratory Haematology* **3**, 186–9.

Harms C.S., Triplett D.A. & Koepke J.A. (1978) Factor VIII (antihemophilic factor) assay results in the 1976 College of American Pathologists survey program *American Journal of Clinical Pathology* **70**, 560–2.

Kirkwood T.B.L. (1977) Predicting the stability of biological standards and products. *Biometrics* **33**, 736–42.

Kirkwood T.B.L. & Barrowcliffe T.W. (1978) Discrepancy between one-stage and two-stage assay of Factor VIII:C. *British Journal of Haematology* **40**, 333–8.

Kirkwood T.B.L., Barrowcliffe T.W. & Thomas D.P. (1980) An international collaborative study establishing a reference preparation for antithrombin III. *Thrombosis and Haemostasis* **43**, 10–15.

Kirkwood T.B.L., Rizza C.R., Snape T.J., Rhymes I.L. & Austen D.E.G. (1977) Identification of sources of inter-laboratory variation in Factor VIII assay. *British Journal of Haematology* **37**, 559–68.

Koepke J.A. (1978) An innovative method for the determination of normal values in hematology using peer group laboratories. *American Journal of Clinical Pathology* **70**, 577–9.

Koepke J.A., Gilmer P.R. Jr, Triplett D.A. & O'Sullivan M.B. (1977) The prediction of prothrombin time performance using secondary standards. *American Journal of Clinical Pathology* **68**, 191–4.

Nilsson I.M., Kirkwood T.B.L. & Barrowcliffe T.W. (1979) *In vivo* recovery of Factor VIII: a comparison of one-stage and two-stage assay methods. *Thrombosis and Haemostasis* **42**, 1230–9.

Poller L., Thomson J.M. & Yee K.F. (1979) Quality control trials of the prothrombin time: an assessment of the performance in serial studies. *Journal of Clinical Pathology* **32**, 251–3.

Ratnoff O.D. & Menzie A.B. (1951) A new method for the determination of plasma fibrinogen in small samples of plasma. *Journal of Laboratory and Clinical Medicine* **37**, 316–20.

Robertson I., Gaffney P.J. & Bangham D.R. (1975) Standard for human thrombin. *Thrombosis et Diathesis Haemorrhagica* **34**, 3–19.

World Health Organisation (1971) *Technical Reports Series* **463**, 14.

World Health Organisation (1977a) *Technical Report Series* **610**, 12–13.

World Health Organisation (1977b) *Technical Report Series* **610**, 13.

World Health Organisation (1978) *Technical Report Series* **626**, 101–39.

World Health Organisation (1983) *Technical Report Series* **687**, 23–4.

Zimmerman T.S. & Meyer D. (1981) Structure and function of factor VIII (von Willebrand factor). In *Haemostasis and Thrombosis*. Bloom A.L. & Thomas D.P. (eds). pp. 111–23. Churchill Livingstone, Edinburgh.

Index

Factor VIIIR (*cont*)
  haemostasis physiological role 68–9
  immunological properties 65–6
  molecular weight 64–5
  plasma concentration 65
  ristocetin cofactor ratio 66–7
  synthesis 69
Factor VIIIR:Ag 206–7
  assay 183–4
  deficiency, von Willebrand's disease
    108
  von Willebrand variants,
    electrophoresis 183
Factor IX
  acquired deficiency 154–5
  activation, gel electrophoresis
    14–15
  antibody assay 193
  assays 179–81
  bioassay standards 578–9
  concentrates
    haemophilia B 292
    VIII:C antibody therapy 236
  conversion to factor IXab 13
  deficiency *see* Haemophilia B
  factor VIII interaction 13–19
  gene polymorphism 111, 137
  levels, haemostasis 292
  one-stage assay 180
  variants 180–1
Factor X
  activation, kinetics 49
  amino acid chains, molecular weights
    48
  assay, Russell's viper venom 179
  congenital deficiency,
    management 257, 299
  conversion requirements 17
  deficiency 100–1, 149–50, 257,
    299
    acquired 154
    prevalence 97
  human, differences from bovine 48
  peptide cleavage 48
  tissue factor and factor VII
    interactions 49–50
  transfused, half-life 1448
Factor Xa
  ATIII effects 84
  generation test (XaGT) 255–6
  prothrombin cleavage 41–2
Factor XI 11–13, 20–1, 48–9

congenital deficiency, management
    299–300
  contact activation 3
  deficiency 12, 112, 149, 259–60
    prevalence 97
  HMWK complexes 12
  platelet-derived activator 4
  structure 12
Factor XIa 3
  factor IX conversion 13
Factor XII 5–7
  binding, activation effects 6
  contact activation 3
  deficiency 112, 149
    congenital, management 301–2
    plasminogen activator 420
  kaolin-bound, activation 6
  platelet aggregation cofactor 332
Factor XIIa 3
α-factor XIIa 5
β-factor XIIa 5
Factor XIII
  assay 187
  concentrate, placental 301
  deficiency 100, 144–5
    acquired 301
    prevalence 97, 144
    replacement therapy 260
  prophylactic 301
  transfusion half-life 187
Families, psychological problems,
    haemophilia 133
FEIBA 289–90
Femur, fractured neck
  low-heparin 509
  oral anticoagulants 507–8
Fibrin
  breakdown products 428–30
  formation 28–30
  plasmin generation 427
  plasminogen activator
    binding 426–7
  polymerization defect 153
  polymerization sites, peptide masking
    29–30
  role in fibrinolysis 426–7
  solubility 30
  stabilization 30
Fibrin/fibrinogen-related antigens 430
Fibrin stabilizing factor
  assay 187
  deficiency 97, 100, 144–5